QUANTITATIVE CLINICAL PATHOLOGY

EDITED BY

Peter W. Hamilton
BSc, PhD
Lecturer in Quantitative Pathology
Institute of Pathology
The Queen's University of Belfast
Belfast, UK

AND

Derek C. Allen
MD, MRCPath
Honorary Lecturer and Consultant
in Histopathology and Cytopathology
Histopathology Laboratory
Belfast City Hospital
The Queen's University of Belfast
Belfast, UK

b

Blackwell
Science

Editorial Offices:
Osney Mead, Oxford OX2 0EL
25 John Street, London WC1N 2BL
23 Ainslie Place, Edinburgh EH3 6AJ
238 Main Street, Cambridge
Massachusetts 02142, USA
54 University Street, Carlton
Victoria 3053, Australia

Other Editorial Offices:
Arnette Blackwell SA
1, rue de Lille, 75007 Paris
France

Blackwell Wissenschafts-Verlag GmbH
Kurfürstendamm 57
10707 Berlin, Germany

Feldgasse 13, A-1238 Wien
Austria

First published 1995

Set by Setrite Typesetters Ltd, Hong Kong
Printed and bound in Great Britain
at the University Press, Cambridge

DISTRIBUTORS

Marston Book Services Ltd
PO Box 87
Oxford OX2 0DT
(*Orders*: Tel: 01865 791155
Fax: 01865 791927
Telex: 837515)

North America
Blackwell Science, Inc.
238 Main Street
Cambridge, MA 02142
(*Orders*: Tel: 800 215-1000
617 876-7000
Fax: 617 492-5263)

Australia
Blackwell Science Pty Ltd
54 University Street
Carlton, Victoria 3053
(*Orders*: Tel: 03 347-0300
Fax: 03 349-3016)

A catalogue record for this title is available from the British Library

ISBN 0 632 03286 3

Library of Congress
Cataloging in Publication Data

Quantitative clinical pathology/
edited by Peter W. Hamilton and Derek C. Allen.
p. cm.
Includes bibliographical references and index.
ISBN 0-632-03286-3
1. Cytodiagnosis.
2. Cells—Measurement.
3. Histology, Pathological.
I. Hamilton, Peter W., Ph. D.
II. Allen, Derek C.
[DNLM: 1. Cytological Techniques.
2. Pathology, Clinical—methods.
QY 95 Q112 1995]
RB43.Q354 1995
616.07′582—dc20 94-9864
CIP

This book is dedicated to the memory of Dr Patrick C.H. Watt (1953–1989)

Patrick Watt qualified in medicine in 1977 after a distinguished undergraduate career at The Queen's University of Belfast. He quickly attained his FRCS (with gold medal) and during the course of his surgical research fellowship year became increasingly interested in pathology. He completed his MD thesis with honours, investigating dysplasia in the post-operative stomach. He then made a brave career move into pathology where he worked in the University Department of Pathology, Royal Victoria Hospital, Belfast and obtained the MRCPath. He developed a comprehensive knowledge of and skill for diagnostic histopathology and fine-needle aspiration cytology. His consultant appointment was with special responsibility for co-ordinating breast-screening pathology in Northern Ireland. He initiated, established and encouraged others in new diagnostic and research techniques and had a particular interest in quantitative pathology. He published many papers, co-authored the very successful textbook *Pathology for Surgeons* and formulated the outline of this book. He was without doubt one of the most talented pathologists of his generation and achieved much in his short career which was tragically cut short by acute leukaemia. His generosity of spirit, friendliness and example are fondly remembered by his family, friends and colleagues.

P.W.H, D.C.A

I often say that when you can measure
what you are speaking about, and express it in numbers,
you know something about it;
but when you cannot measure it,
when you cannot express it in numbers,
your knowledge is of a meagre
and unsatisfactory kind

William Thompson [Lord Kelvin] 1883

CONTENTS

CONTRIBUTORS

D. C. ALLEN MD, MRCPath, *Honorary Lecturer and Consultant in Histopathology and Cytopathology, Histopathology Laboratory, Belfast City Hospital, The Queen's University of Belfast, Belfast, UK*

P. H. BARTELS PhD, *Professor, Optical Sciences and Pathology, Optical Sciences Center and Department of Pathology, The University of Arizona, Tucson, Arizona, USA*

G. BRUGAL PhD, *Professor of Cell Biology, Laboratoire de Microscopie Quantitative, CERMO, Université Joseph Fourier, Grenoble Cedex, France*

R. S. CAMPLEJOHN MSc, PhD, *Senior Lecturer, Richard Dimbleby Department of Cancer Research, UMDS, St Thomas's Hospital, London, UK*

J. S. A. COLLINS MD, FRCP (Lond), FRCP (Ed), *Consultant Gastroenterologist, Royal Victoria Hospital, Belfast, UK*

M. J. COOKSON BSc, MSc, MPhil, FIMA, CMath, MBSC, *Head, Hill Centre, The London Hospital Medical College, University of London, London, UK*

A. D. CROCKARD BSc, PhD, MRCPath, *Consultant Clinical Scientist, Regional Immunology Laboratory, Royal Victoria Hospital, Belfast, UK*

S. S. CROSS BSc, MB, BS, MRCPath, *Senior Lecturer, Department of Pathology, University of Sheffield Medical School, Sheffield, UK*

F. GIROUD PhD, *Assistant Professor of Cell Biology, Laboratoire de Microscopie Quantitative, CERMO, Université Joseph Fourier, Grenoble, France*

P. W. HAMILTON BSc, PhD, *Lecturer in Quantitative Pathology, Institute of Pathology, The Queen's University of Belfast, Belfast, UK*

R. W. LYNESS MD, FRCPath, *Consultant Histopathologist, Belfast City Hospital, Belfast, UK*

J. C. MACARTNEY BSc, MD, FRCPath, *Consultant Histopathologist, Alexandra Hospital, Redditch, UK*

J. McCLURE BSc, MD, FRCPath, *Proctor Professor of Pathology, University of Manchester, Manchester, UK*

R. MONTIRONI MD, *Associate Professor of Pathology, Institute of Morbid Anatomy and Histopathology, Nuovo Ospedale Regionale, The University of Ancona, School of Medicine, Ancona, Italy*

C. C. PATTERSON BSc, MSc, PhD, FSS, *Senior Lecturer in Medical Statistics, Department of Epidemiology and Public Health, The Queen's University of Belfast, Belfast, UK*

J. S. PLOEM PhD, *Emeritus Professor of Cellbiology, Laboratory of Cytochemistry and Cytometry, Leiden University, Leiden, The Netherlands*

E. K. W. SCHULTE, *Anatomisches Institut, Fachbereich Medizin, Johannes Gutenberg Universitat, Mainz, Germany*

C. S. SCOTT MSc, PhD, MRCPath, *Head of Leukaemia Diagnostic Unit, Department of Haematology, Regional Radiotherapy Centre, Cookridge Hospital, Leeds, UK*

D. SEIGNEURIN MD, PhD, *Cytopathologist, Service de Cytogenetique et Cytologie, Centre Hospitalo-Universitaire A, Michallon, Grenoble, France*

D. THOMPSON MSc, *Principal Systems Programmer, Optical Sciences Center, The University of Arizona, Tucson, Arizona, USA*

J. E. WEBER PhD, *Professor of Statistics, Department of Statistics, The University of Arizona, Tucson, Arizona, USA*

W. F. WHIMSTER MD, FRCP, FRCPath, *Head, Department of Morbid Anatomy, King's College School of Medicine, London, UK*

K. E. WILLIAMSON FIMLS, PhD, *Department of Surgery, The Queen's University of Belfast, Belfast, UK*

G. D. WILSON BSc, PhD, *Senior Research Scientist, GRC Gray Laboratory, Mount Vernon Hospital, Middlesex, UK*

PREFACE

Measurement in pathology is important not only in the scientific investigation of pathogenesis but as a means of improving routine diagnostic and prognostic decisions. As an investigative tool, the advantage of measurement is not questioned. However, the role of measurement in routine diagnostic practice has found only a few well-established applications. Lack of standardization, education, clear statistical guidelines, large conclusive studies and perhaps a fear of numbers are detracting factors. Nevertheless, the demand for reproducibility and consistency in diagnosis will require us further to investigate and employ measurement as a diagnostic aid. Hopefully its adoption, under strict standardized protocols, in those areas where conventional diagnosis is difficult, will provide the objectivity we need.

In this book we have attempted to include those subjects currently relevant to the field of quantitative pathology. It has been written with the practising clinical pathologist in mind and an attempt has been made to explain the subject matter clearly and keep it on a practical level. We hope this book will provide valuable guidelines for those who are wanting to use quantitative methods as part of their research or who wish to develop and apply measurement in their routine diagnostic practice. It should also provide a wide-ranging reference manual for the specialist in the field.

The book has been divided into four parts, each containing several chapters. In a multiauthor work such as this, it is inevitable that overlap will exist and where possible, repetition has been minimized. Where it occurs, we hope it will serve to emphasize rather than distract. The editors have attempted to cross-reference relevant topics.

The first part deals with measurement in microscopic pathology and includes chapters on stereology (Chapter 1), computer-aided morphometry (Chapter 2), photocytometry (Chapter 6) and automated cytometry (Chapter 7). This should give the casual reader a greater insight into these techniques used to obtain quantitative data from microscopic images. For the expert we hope it will provide material useful for teaching and reference. Chapter 4 provides a detailed review of the literature regarding the application of morphometry in diagnostic pathology. For ease of consultation in this chapter the references for each subject are given at the end of each subsection. Chapter 6 examines the measurement of nuclear DNA content using light microscopy and this is followed by a chapter on the automated analysis of microscopic features, including nuclear DNA content. These chapters independently review these important areas of application in pathology. Other subjects covered in this part include mitotic counts (Chapter 3) and the quantitation of AgNORs (Chapter 5). Both of these topics continue to be important in pathological investigation, mitotic counts being a long-standing quantitative tool in diagnostic histopathology, while AgNORs represent a more recent development.

The second part of the book deals with the technique and applications of flow cytometry. This has been a rapidly growing discipline and it would be impossible in a general book such as this to review all applications and avenues of research. Three principal areas were considered to be central to pathological investigation – DNA content (Chapter 10), cell cycle analysis (Chapter 11) and immunology (Chapter 12). Technical details concerning the principle of flow cytometry (Chapter 8) and the preparation of tissue (Chapter 9) are also provided.

Part 3 is entitled 'Current Developments'. The topics included in this part are largely technique-oriented and are still undergoing rapid development. The concept of computerized expert systems (Chapter 13) and their role in decision-making is not new but it is only relatively recently that they have begun to find their feet as a tool in pathological diagnosis and image understanding. Similarly, three-dimensional reconstruction (Chapter 14) has been used by anatomists for many years but again only recently, with the availability of the digital computer, has it been reconsidered as a practically feasible tool for the investigation of disease. Finally, the fractal dimension (Chapter 15) introduces the pathologist to a new way of looking at (and quantifying) biological shape – a method which has emerged from the world of theoretical physics, applied mathematics and chaos theory. The nature of these subjects is such that the material therein will rapidly become out of date but we hope the text serves to familiarize and enlighten the reader, and perhaps encourage involvement, in these growing areas of pathological research.

The last part is important as it deals with study design and statistical considerations (Chapters 16 and 17). The content should be sufficient to guide the reader in using statistics in quantitative pathology from the design of the study to the analysis of the data.

We are very grateful to those who contributed to the compilation of this book – the various expert authors of international reputation who wrote chapters and the staff at Blackwell Science. Our own team of helpers included Mrs Priscilla Clarke, Ms Moira Cunningham and Mr Graham Kennedy, who enabled the collation of numerous references. Mrs Bridie Kelly typed part of the manuscript and Mr Roy Creighton and Mr Michael Sinclair prepared a number of the photographs.

We trust you will enjoy reading this book and find it helpful and informative.

Peter W. Hamilton
Derek C. Allen
Belfast

PART 1
MEASUREMENT IN MICROSCOPIC PATHOLOGY

1

STEREOLOGY

P. W. HAMILTON

In order to view the internal components of an opaque tissue a thin section is necessary. A tissue section provides us with an (almost) two-dimensional (2D) translucent slice and reduces the dimensionality of features which exist in the three-dimensional (3D) conglomerate (Table 1.1). Viewing tissue and cellular components in this way yields information regarding tissue organization, cellular function and disease processes, upon which histopathological diagnosis is largely based. It is vital to remember, however, that tissue constitutes a 3D structure and that disease is a 3D process.

Reconstruction of serial sections can be a useful method to observe the appearance of tissue structures in the third dimension and this is discussed in Chapter 14. However, there are more basic methods which allow us to obtain 3D quantitative information such as volume, surface area and feature number from the 2D information seen in tissue sections. These methods are collectively termed stereology. They are based on the assumption that a quantitative relationship exists between the dimensions of a randomly sectioned structure on profile and the dimensions of that structure in 3D space. The proof of this relationship is found in the realms of geometric statistical probability, as are the methods used to derive stereological measurements. It is this close association between stereology and mathematical formulation that has perhaps discouraged many pathologists from using it as an analytical tool. However, while the derivation of these formulae may indeed be complex, the practical application of stereological techniques and their associated formulae is easy. Proof of this comes from the fact that all the calculations described in this chapter can be made using a pocket calculator. As such they form a cheap and reliable means of retrieving quantitative information from tissue sections. The power and accuracy of stereology over methods such as interactive image analysis are often vastly under-rated. Gundersen *et al.* [1] have shown that worthwhile measurements can often be obtained more rapidly than interactive image analysis, yet give comparable results. Indeed, stereology can provide accurate estimates of 2D as well as 3D features, as shall be illustrated later. Additionally, the conception that stereology is excessively time-consuming is unfounded (see Section 1.9).

Many stereological variables are derived from ratios of two or more related measurements and so do not give absolute values. Indeed, quoting stereological ratios alone is discouraged, particularly for number and surface area measurements [2]. To obtain absolute values, a reference space is needed which has been measured in real units. Often this

Table 1.1 The reductions of dimensions when a tissue section is examined

3D tissue block	2D tissue section*
Volumes (3D)	Profiles (2D)
Surfaces (2D)	Boundaries (1D)
Filaments (1D)	Points (0D)

* A tissue section is not strictly 2D as it does have a depth, but for the purposes of stereological analysis we must treat it as such.
D, Dimensional.

is only usefully represented by the whole organ that is being assessed. So, by calculating the absolute volume of the organ and treating component measurements as a fraction of the whole, the actual value of the fraction can be determined. While this can be a time-consuming exercise, it does provide valuable data.

The tool of the stereologist is the geometric probe which is used to sample the structures being investigated. Probes can be in the form of points which are zero-dimensional (0D), lines (1D), frames (2D) and volumes (3D). These probes hit features in 3D space with different probabilities and so they can be used to measure features of various dimensions which exist in the 3D space (Table 1.2). This shall become clear later.

Recent developments in stereology have provided new tools which may be novel to some readers. These include the disector, the fractionator, the selector, point-sampled intercepts and the nucleator. They are design-based methods and differ from previous methods in that they make no assumptions about the features to be measured. They do, however, rely on careful study design which must fulfil certain criteria. This being considered, they are relatively easy to apply. A full review of these design-based methods has been given previously by Gundersen *et al.* [3,4].

It is the aim of this section to consider some of the available stereological methods which can be used to obtain quantitative data from histopathological tissue sections. This will be done with minimal statistical derivation and with simple histological examples. Those wishing to read further into the statistical background of stereology are referred to several leading texts on the subject [3–7]. Some of the techniques mentioned allow only the measurement of 2D features and so would not be called stereology by the purist. Whilst they are biased by their nature, they do however illustrate how geometric probes (the tools of a stereologist) can be used to estimate 2D measurements.

Table 1.2 Geometric probes, their dimensions and the features which they can be used to measure

Geometric probe	Feature
Point (0D)	Volume (3D)
Line (1D)	Surface (2D)
Surface (2D)	Length (1D)
Volume (3D)	Number (0D)

D, Dimensional.

1.1 NUMBER OF PROFILES PER UNIT AREA OR LENGTH

One of the simplest measurements that histopathologists often want to make is to count the number of objects (e.g., nuclei, mitoses, neurons, glomeruli, etc.) in a microscopic field. This can be done simply by counting the number of events within a frame of known area and expressing this as number per square millimetre or square micrometre. The confusion lies in deciding whether we should count those objects straddling the edge of the frame. It has been demonstrated that in order to obtain an unbiased estimate of number, a measuring frame, illustrated in Fig. 1.1, should be used [8]. The measuring frame should be smaller than the field of vision and all objects outside the frame or touching the left and lower bold margins of the frame and their extensions should be excluded from the count [8]. In Fig. 1.1 the area of the frame is 0.120 mm² and using the exclusion lines, a total of 42 alveolar profiles can be counted. The number of profiles per unit area is termed Q_a and is calculated as follows:

$$Q_a = \frac{\text{number of objects}}{\text{are of frame}} = \frac{42}{0.120\,\text{mm}^2}$$

In Fig. 1.1, therefore, $Q_a = 350$ alveoli per mm².

In certain circumstances this method may pose problems. For example, when counting plasma cells in the lamina propria of small intestinal biopsies, often the lamina propria will not occupy the whole frame [6]. In such instances, the area of lamina propria within the frame needs to be measured; then the plasma cell count can be related to this. If the frame possesses a grid of points, area can be assessed using point-counting technique, as detailed in Sections 1.2.1 and 1.2.2.

In other studies, counting the number of objects per unit length (e.g., muscularis mucosae, epithelium) may be more appropriate. This is facilitated if the length can be measured with a straight

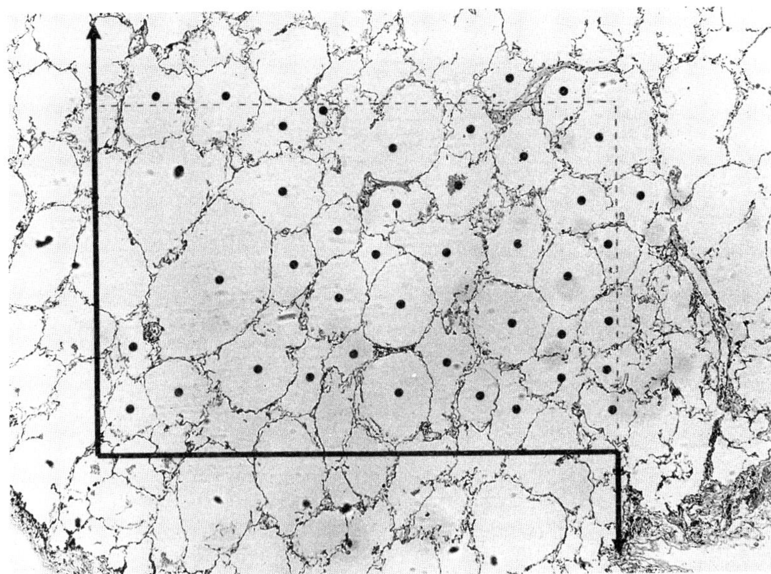

Fig. 1.1 An unbiased measurement of alveolar number (Q_a) from a section of human lung tissue. A counting frame is superimposed over the image, with exclusion lines shown in bold. The area of the frame is $0.120\,mm^2$. Alveolar profiles included in the count are identified by a dot.

rule or graticule. If the length is curved, as is more likely to be the case, then the boundary length must be estimated. This can be done simply by counting intercepts with lines of known length [9] or by more sophisticated surface density measuring techniques (Section 1.5).

It should be remembered that counting objects from a single section is inherently biased. A tissue section will cut objects in 3D space in relation to their height perpendicular to the plane of section: longer or larger objects will have a greater probability of being included in the section than shorter or smaller objects. In order to remove bias, numbers need to be assessed in 3D space (see Section 1.7).

1.2 AREA AND VOLUME MEASUREMENTS

1.2.1 Area fractions

Simple methods can be used to measure the *fraction* of area (A_a) occupied by a particular tissue component. For example, we can estimate the area fraction of a lung section occupied by alveoli (Fig. 1.2). By superimposing a grid of points over the lung section, the total number of points hitting the section (= 54) and the number falling within the alveolar spaces (= 40) can easily be counted. We can therefore estimate that 40/54 = 0.77, i.e., 77% of that field was occupied by alveolar air space. In stereological notation this is represented by the formula:

$$A_a = \frac{P_p}{P_t}$$

where: A_a = area fraction; P_p = number of points hitting component of interest (i.e., alveoli); and P_t = total number of points hitting section.

It is important to think of the points as *probes* which, when randomly positioned on a tissue section, will hit objects proportional to their cross-sectional area. If, however, the tissue section is randomly obtained from a 3D composite, then in reality the points are probing 3D space and will hit objects proportional to their volume. This conveys one of the fundamental principles of stereology – that the ratio of areas (A_a) on sectioned profile is directly related to the ratio of volumes (V_v) in the 3D equivalent.

$$A_a = V_v$$

This is true providing that the sections examined are at random, the point grid is randomly positioned on the tissue section, and samples are sufficient in

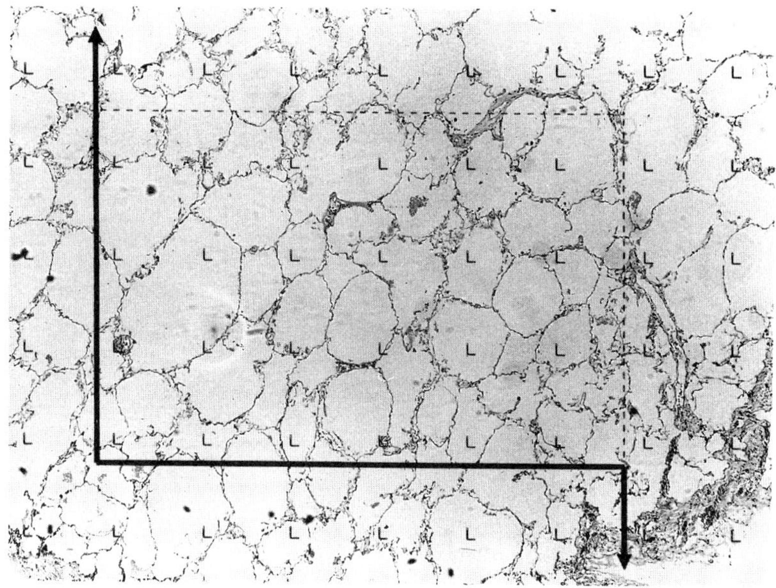

Fig. 1.2 A measurement of alveolar area (volume) fraction from the same section as shown in Fig. 1.1. The fraction of points (corners of L-shaped probes) falling within the alveolar spaces are counted irrespective of the frame boundary. The small box indicates the area represented by each point and is termed $a(p)$.

number to be representative of the tissue. Therefore, if 77% of the tissue area is occupied by alveoli, it is assumed that they also constitute 77% of lung volume.

This only gives us a *ratio* of component volume to the containing reference space. Absolute values of component volume can only be calculated if the actual volume of the reference space is known. If the reference space constitutes an organ (lung in the above example), then various methods can be used to measure its volume (e.g., water displacement; see Aherne and Dunnill [6] for review) and the absolute volume of alveoli can then be calculated.

An alternative method which allows the mean volume of objects to be measured is the *point-sampled intercept* technique. This is discussed in Section 1.6.

1.2.2 Absolute area measurements

Whilst point counting in the above example only allows a volume fraction to be calculated, we can estimate absolute values for 2D parameters (e.g., profile area) on sectioned tissue. By knowing the area of the frame and the percentage of that frame occupied by alveoli (Fig. 1.2), we can calculate the absolute area of alveoli $a(prof)$, i.e., 77% of $0.120\,\text{mm}^2 = 0.77 \times 0.120 = 0.0924\,\text{mm}^2$. Dividing this by the number of profiles in the field (= 42) gives us the mean profile area $\bar{a}(prof)$, i.e., $0.0924/42 = 0.0022\,\text{mm}^2$ or $2200\,\mu\text{m}^2$. Alternatively, and perhaps more simply, $\bar{a}(prof)$ can be calculated by dividing the profile area fraction (A_a) by the relative number of profiles (Q_a). These absolute values are only measures of cross-sectional profile area and cannot be extrapolated to the third dimension.

1.2.3 Cavalieri volume

A method of obtaining *absolute* volume measurements of whole structures is called the Cavalieri estimate and is described by Gundersen *et al.* [3]. As this requires complete serial sectioning of the total structure to be examined, this method has been mainly used for estimating the volume of macroscopic structures [10] and can be used to estimate total organ volume. The example here is taken from a study by Braendgaard *et al.* [11] which measured the cortex volume in human brain. The brain was serially sectioned into slices of approximately equal thickness (t). A point grid was superimposed on each section and the sum of points (P_p) hitting the cortex counted. The area that each point on the grid represents, $a(p)$, must be known (see Fig. 1.2 for explanation). We can then solve for the cortex volume by:

$$V(struct) = t \times a(p) \times P_p$$

For example, if the thickness of each brain slice is 10 mm, $a(p)$ is 20 mm^2, and the number of points hitting the cortex over all brain sections is 21, then:

$$V(cortex) = 10 \times 20 \times 21 = 4200\,\text{mm}^3$$

This is a very simple procedure and gives an unbiased estimate of true volume. As for the number of sections and points to sample, Gundersen *et al.* [3] claim that for the measurement of human brain cortex volume, 10–15 uniform and random consecutive sections with a total of 200 points counted on each will provide an accurate result. However, this would need to be confirmed for other applications using the methods described in Section 1.9.

1.3 PROFILE BOUNDARY MEASUREMENTS

Another feature which may be of histological interest is the length of structure boundaries as seen in sectioned profile. Again, as this is purely based on 2D information, it is biased by orientation. The method requires the use of a grid of lines of known length superimposed over the tissue and we shall use nuclear profiles to demonstrate this (Fig. 1.3). The ends of the lines represent the points used to calculate volume estimates. The total summed length of these lines (L) is 420 µm. Next, the number of times that the lines intersect with the boundaries (I) must be counted. Boundary length per unit area (B_a) of section is then calculated as follows:

$$B_a = \frac{\pi}{2.L} \,.\, I\,\mu\text{m}$$

where L = total length of test lines and I = total number of intersects of lines with profile boundaries.

In the example, $L = 420\,\mu$m, $I = 30$ and so $B_a = 0.112\,\mu$m. This is only the relative profile boundary length. To obtain an absolute value of total boundary length, $b(prof)$, we must multiply B_a by the area of the field (i.e., $b(prof) = 0.112\,\mu\text{m} \times 4872\,\mu\text{m}^2 = 546\,\mu\text{m}$). The mean boundary length, $\bar{b}(prof)$, may then be easily calculated as before by dividing $b(prof)$ by Q_a.

This must be repeated over a number of fields and sections to obtain a more reliable estimate, but generally counting as few as 200 intersections is sufficient.

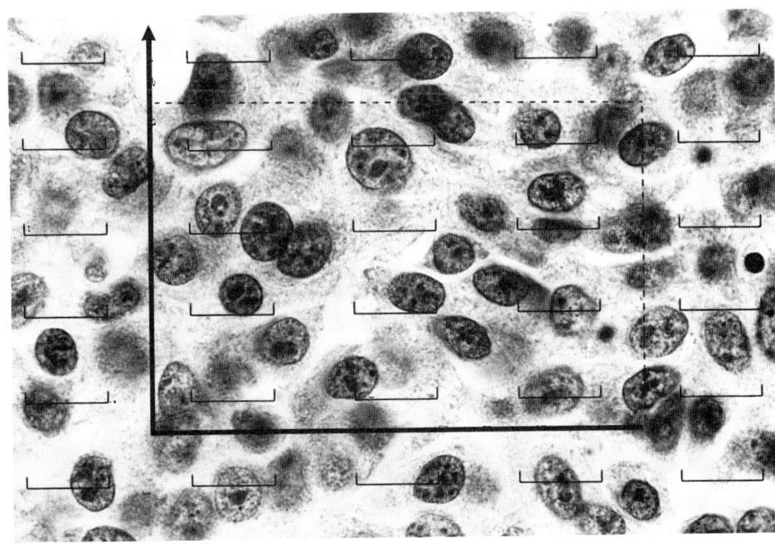

Fig. 1.3 A measurement of relative nuclear boundary length. A grid of 30 lines (each 14 µm in length) is superimposed over the section. The area of the frame is 4872 µm^2. By counting the number of intersections of lines with nuclear boundaries, boundary length measurements can be made. This grid style can also be used for area measurements by using the ends of the lines as point probes.

1.4 ISOTROPY, ANISOTROPY AND VERTICAL SECTIONS

When measuring the area or volume fraction or the number of profiles, the sections must have a random position in 3D space to be statistically representative of the tissue. For stereological estimations of surface density (Section 1.5) or volume using point-sampled intercepts (Section 1.6), additional criteria must be observed — either the features which are being measured need to be *isotropic*, i.e., have uniform random properties in all directions, or else random isotropic line probes need to be applied.

Many tissues when sectioned for histological consideration show some form of morphological order or direction and are therefore *anisotropic*. If these tissues are sectioned randomly in three dimensions then isotropy of tissue features may be obtained. A method for producing true isotropic sections, called the *orientator*, has been reviewed by Gundersen *et al.* [3]. However, random sectioning of layered tissue (e.g., skin) results in the loss of the preferred direction of section (i.e., through the layers) and the morphological information that is associated with that direction. Additionally, the feature which is to be measured (e.g., the surface) may be absent in randomly taken sections. The solution to these problems is found in *vertical sections* [12]. Vertical sections retain the preferred direction of section yet, in combination with an appropriate random sampling regime, ensure the unbiased measurement of anisotropic components.

A vertical section is by definition a section perpendicular to a defined horizontal plane [3]. The horizontal plane can be a characteristic of the tissue itself. For example, colorectal mucosa has a natural horizontal plane, parallel to the muscularis mucosae, in that a section vertical to this plane will reveal the various layers of the mucosa. Alternatively, where a natural horizontal plane does not exist, it can be arbitrarily defined by the observer. Using the colon as an example, vertical sections may be made, as shown in Fig. 1.4. Random positioning of the vertical sections only takes place in the last step of Fig. 1.4. The preferred morphology of the tissue will be retained and the direction of the vertical axis will be identifiable on tissue section. Each vertical section used should be in a different and

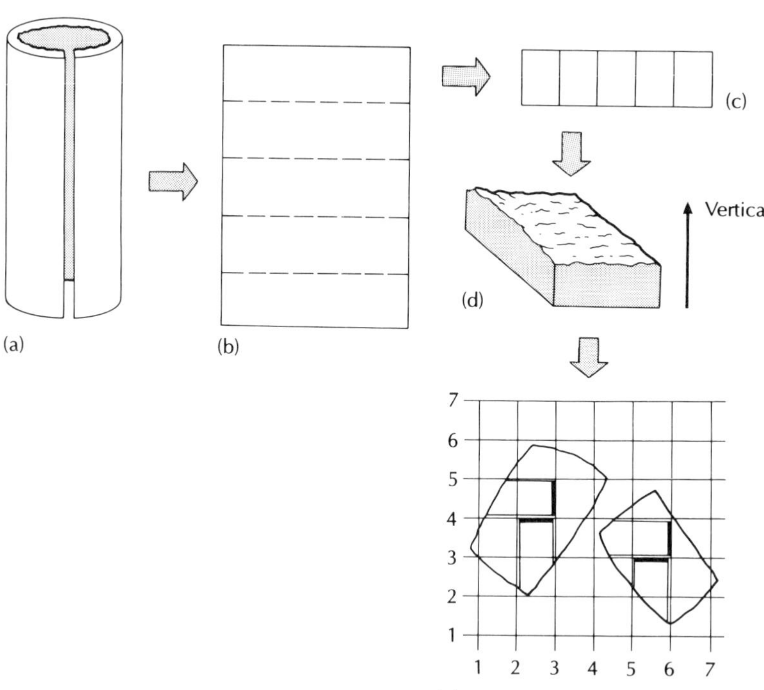

Fig. 1.4 Vertical sections of colonic mucosa. (a) The bowel is opened and layed out as a flat block of tissue (b), which is then sliced into long strips of bowel (c) and further sliced into blocks of tissue (d). These blocks, which are oriented mucosa side upwards, are then spun randomly around their vertical axis and placed randomly on a grid (e). Finding the highest co-ordinate that the tissue covers defines the point where final blocks are taken in the *x* and *y* direction. Vertical sections are taken from the end of the block, labelled with a bold line.

random plane. If tissue biopsies are to be examined, it is sufficient to orient them, with the horizontal plane flat on the table-top, spin them around an imaginary axis, and take a vertical section parallel to the edge of the table or other suitable marker.

As vertical sections are not isotropic, the line probes must be designed to be isotropic, uniform and random in 3D space. This will be illustrated in the following section with the use of the cycloid arc to measure surface area. One stipulation is that the test system of probes is aligned with the known vertical axis of the section. Various microscopic stages are available to facilitate this [3]. In this way unbiased measurements can be made regardless of tissue anisotropy.

1.5 SURFACE AREA MEASUREMENTS

Surface to volume ratio (S_V) or surface density is an important measurement of significance at the tissue and cellular level. As with boundary measurements (Section 1.3), this requires counting intersections with a line grid. A typical application for this in histopathology might be the measurement of epithelial surface density in small intestinal biopsies from individuals with coeliac disease [13]. Unlike lung tissue, which is fairly isotropic, small-intestinal mucosa shows component orientation with a regular or recurring glandular pattern. The use of line grids which are strongly oriented in one direction (as used in Fig. 1.3) will give falsely high or low transection counts depending on the direction of the tissue in relation to the graticule lines. An attempt to overcome this problem led to the development of grids with lines of random orientation [6]. Such lines, however, are only random in 2D space and so still give a biased estimate of surface area.

A new and much more efficient method for estimating surface density has been developed [12] using *vertical sections* described previously, and specific test line systems, which are isotropic and random in 3D space. It has been shown that for test lines to be effectively isotropic and random in 3D space, their angle relative to the vertical axis must be sine-weighted (for more detail see Baddeley *et al.* [12]). A more practical approach, however, is to use test curves whose length is proportional to sine θ. Such curves are termed *cycloid arcs* and a typical test system is shown in Fig. 1.5. The vertical axis of the test system must be aligned with the vertical axis of the section (which must be known).

To measure the surface area of the epithelium in a small-intestinal biopsy (Fig. 1.5), the number of times the cycloid lines intercept the boundary of

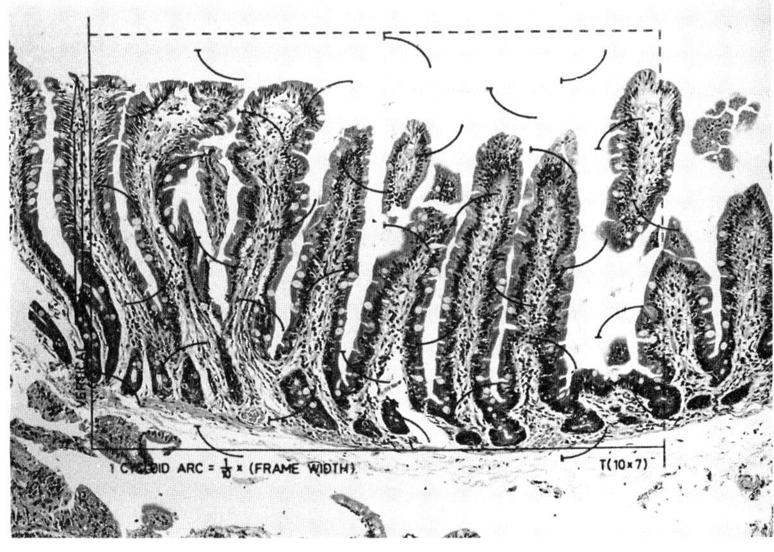

Fig. 1.5 The measurement of epithelial surface area of small-intestinal mucosa using the cycloid test system (grid reproduced from Gundersen *et al.* [3]). The cycloid is proportional to the sine of the angle to vertical axis. The left edge of the frame indicates the vertical axis of the test system, which must be aligned with the vertical axis of the section. Surface to volume ratio (S_V) is estimated by counting the number of intersections of cycloid lines with surface of epithelium (see text). Volume fraction of underlying tissue can be estimated by counting the ends of cycloid lines as point probes.

the epithelial surface is counted (I). Underlying tissue volume can be assessed by counting the total number of points falling within the epithelium and lamina propria. The S_V ratio of epithelium can then be calculated using the following formula:

$$S_V = 2 \cdot \frac{I}{L}$$

where L = total length of test lines and I = intersections with test lines. In the example shown in Fig. 1.5, $L = 5.25$ mm, $I = 33$ and therefore $S_V = 12.57\ \text{mm}^2/\text{mm}^3$. Total surface area ($S$) can be calculated if we know the absolute volume of the reference space $V(ref)$ (e.g., whole small intestine or a length of small intestine) by multiplying S_V by $V(ref)$.

Changes in magnification significantly alter surface to volume measurements. Magnification should, therefore, be kept constant to allow comparison of results.

1.6 VOLUME ESTIMATES USING POINT-SAMPLED INTERCEPTS

A simple method exists which allows the unbiased measurement of object volume by point sampling. The measurement of nuclear volume provides an ideal example. The test system shown in Fig. 1.6 is superimposed over the population of nuclei. For each point that hits a nucleus, the distance of the nuclear intercept (I) through that point in a random direction is measured and raised to the third power (I^3). This is done for a number of nuclear profiles and averaged. The mean volume of nuclei (V_V) is then given by:

$$\bar{V}_V = \frac{\pi}{3} \cdot \bar{I}^3$$

In Fig. 1.6, the mean I^3 is 785.36 and so the mean volume of nuclei, $V_V = 822.43\ \mu\text{m}^3$.

This volume estimate is weighted. That is, larger nuclei will have a greater chance of being hit by a point and of being measured. This has been shown to be of benefit in several histological studies on malignancy [14–16] where the larger nuclei tend to be of greater diagnostic or prognostic importance [4].

Of course, for the intercept length (I) to be unbiased, the lines must have a random orientation. In isotropic, uniform, random sections (in which the nuclei have a random position and shape in 3D space), random positioning of a grid of parallel lines is sufficient [15,16]. If IUR sections cannot be readily obtained, then the tissue needs to be sampled using *vertical sections* (Section 1.4). As tissue anisotrophy may exist in vertical sections, the test system must be oriented with the vertical axis of the section and the lines need to be given a random

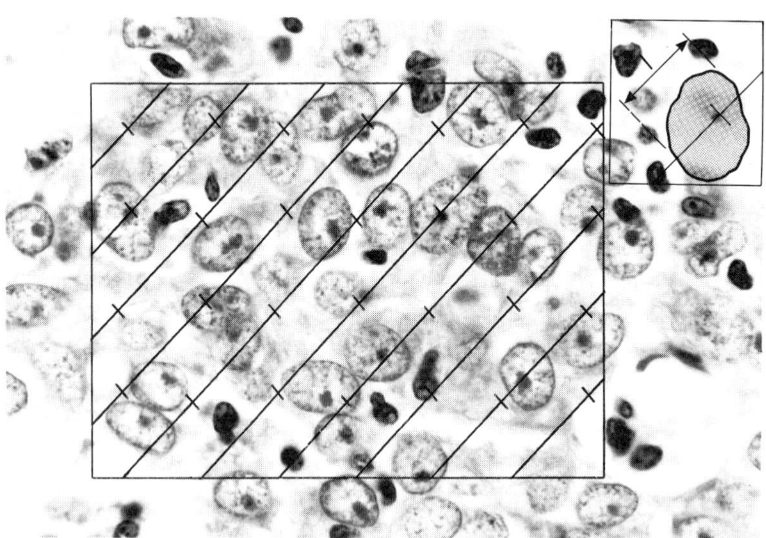

Fig. 1.6 Illustration of the measurement of nuclear volume by point-sampled intercept analysis. The length of the line transecting each of the nuclei hit by a point (cross-line) is measured. If vertical sections are used, the vertical axis of the section needs to be aligned with the vertical axis of the grid and the direction of the lines needs to be random.

direction for each field measured. This can be done using a frame which has directional markers on its border. The choice of a random starting number, with constant increments from this, will provide random directions for the point-intercept sampling procedure [4,17]. Nuclear volume can then be calculated with the described formula, regardless of anisotropy.

In order to speed up the process of point-sampled intercept stereology, Moss *et al.* [18] have described a computer-enhanced method for measuring intercept lengths from digitally stored images. This is now available in a number of commercially available instruments including the Finestra Image Analysis System (Confocal Technology, Liverpool) and PRODIT (Buro Medische Automatisering, The Netherlands). This represents a necessary step fowards in the integration of computerized image analysis and stereology.

1.7 NUMBER OF OBJECTS IN A VOLUME

Estimating the number of objects per unit volume (N_V) of tissue using stereology has until recently been a complex and statistically unsatisfactory task. The accuracy of these methods strongly relied on model-based assumptions about the size and shape of the objects that were being counted, which could never be fulfilled in biological microscopy. A new method which is unbiased and based upon design, called the disector, has been proposed.

1.7.1 The disector

In previous sections, we have made use of points, lines and frames as probes to retrieve information from tissue sections (see Table 1.2). In order to measure the number of objects in a 3D volume, we require a 3D probe.

The disector is the name given to a unique 3D probe which simply comprises a pair of parallel sections, a known height apart (Fig. 1.7). One of these sections is termed the *sampling* plane and the other the *reference* plane. A measuring frame of known area is applied to the sampling plane. The volume of the disector can then be calculated by multiplying the area of the measuring frame by the height (h) between the two sections. To get an unbiased estimate of number per volume of the disector, one must attempt to match the profiles seen on the two sections, i.e., the sampling and reference plane. Profiles are only counted if they: (i) appear in focus on the sampling plane; (ii) comply with the exclusion rules of the measuring frame; and (iii) *do not* appear in the reference plane (see Fig. 1.7). The number of profiles counted in this way is termed Q^- and the reference space is the volume of the disector, $v(dis)$. Further parallel sections can be used to add to the disector, the next section using the previous one as the reference plane and so on. As each section is examined, the volume of the disector increases.

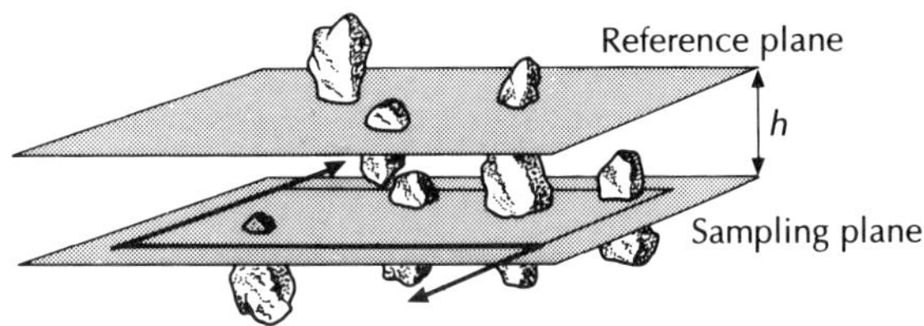

Fig. 1.7 The principle of the disector. Two parallel sections are taken through a number of objects in space. The distance between the sections is h. The lower section is the sampling plane upon which a counting frame (see Section 1.1) is superimposed. Objects are counted if they are sectioned by the sampling plane only, and do not appear on the reference plane. In this example only three objects are included in the count.

If Q^- is measured over several fields, the number per volume (numerical density) is given by:

$$N_V = \frac{Q^-}{v(dis)}$$

Either the total Q^- and $v(dis)$ or the means can be used in the formula. When the height of the disector is variable, as in tissue sections, the mean may be the best way to express $v(dis)$ with the mean number of cell counts as the numerator.

So how can the disector be applied in practice? Parallel sections can be obtained in two ways:

1 Physical sections can be used for the disector, although section thickness should be less than one-quarter to one-third the height of the objects that are being counted [3,4]. The major problem with this approach is that the images from the section pairs need to be compared. This can be done using two projection microscopes which project the images side by side for comparison [10,19] or by finding corresponding areas on the section by section mapping [20]. Photographing the sampling and reference plane is another option but would be expensive and time-consuming. The use of digitized images may also provide a useful means of aligning and comparing the reference and sampling planes of the disector.

2 Optical sections of the tissue can be made on thick sections by moving the microscopic plane of focus up and down (Fig. 1.8). A special instrument called a microcator is required for this; it is sensitive

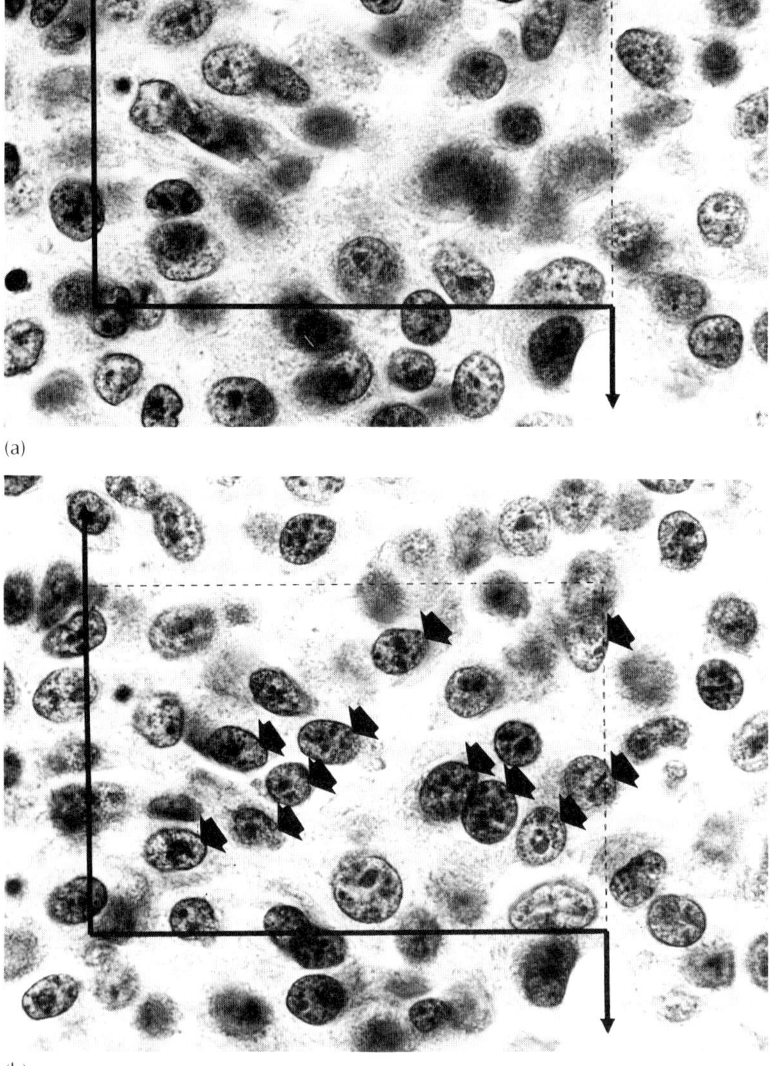

Fig. 1.8 The optical disector using two planes of focus a known distance apart (4 μm). (a) The reference plane. (b) The sampling plane. Eleven nuclei are present on the sampling plane (arrows) but not seen in the reference plane, therefore $Q^- = 11$. Note that only clearly focused nuclei are recorded in both the reference and sampling plane.

to movement of the microscopic stage in the z direction and so can measure the distances between focal planes (i.e., the height of the disector). The optics of the microscope should be adjusted to give the smallest depth of field possible and only oil immersion lenses used [3,4]. The high-resolution optical sections obtained by Confocal Laser Scanning Microscopy (CLSM) provide ideal images for use with the disector [21], although its use is limited to fluorescent or reflected light images. The obvious advantage of optical sections is that they are already aligned and this greatly facilitates measurement of numerical density using the optical disector.

To calculate the total number of objects (N) in a volume of reference tissue, $V(ref)$, for example in an organ, then:

$$N = N_V \cdot V(ref)$$

Of course the volume of the reference tissue would need to be calculated. This might be done using the Cavalieri estimator of volume (Section 1.2.3) or by determining water displacement by the organ (for review of such methods, see Aherne and Dunnill [6]). However, it is important to determine if any tissue shrinkage occurs due to fixation, embedding and sectioning which is not present in the whole organ, as this will influence the estimation of N_V and ultimately N.

An alternative way to determine the total number of objects in a reference volume is by using the fractionator principle.

1.7.2 Fractionator

This is a simple principle based on the random sampling of a fraction of the original tissue reference space which is then assessed for object density (Q^-) using the disector. The total number of objects is given by multiplying Q^- by the sampling probability of the fraction of tissue measured. This is well-illustrated in a study by Ogbuihi and Cruz-Orive [20] who were attempting to estimate the total number of lymphatic valves in lungs of children who died from sudden infant death syndrome. The lung was fixed and cut into sagittal slices each 8–10 mm thick; each slice was then further sectioned into strips 8–10 mm wide. From this set of strips, every fourth (f_1) strip (the interval number is immaterial) was selected and entered into the next stage of the sampling programme. The selected strips were then cut into blocks, of which every sixth (f_2) block was selected. All selected blocks of tissue were then embedded in paraffin and exhaustively sectioned at 5 μm. Every 400th (f_3) section and its neighbour were then selected as disectors for measurement of Q^-. To estimate the total number (N) of valves in that lung then:

$$\begin{aligned} N(valves) &= f_1 \cdot f_2 \cdot f_3 \cdot Q^- \\ &= 4 \cdot 6 \cdot 400 \cdot Q^- \end{aligned}$$

The fractionator tool is extremely resilient, as it is not affected by magnification, section thickness or tissue shrinkage [4].

1.8 OTHER STEREOLOGICAL METHODS

Several other stereological tools are available but all are based on the methods or combinations of the methods already described. For example, the *nucleator* is another method of measuring mean nuclear or cell volume, similar to that discussed in Section 1.6, but measures the intercept distance through a *fixed* point in the object. Nucleoli have been used as fixed points in several studies. A tool termed the *selector* which is a combination of the disector and point-sampled intercept methods allows a measure of object size and number to be estimated. These additional tools are fully discussed by Gundersen *et al.* [4].

Understanding the principles and methods laid out in this chapter will readily promote the application of these other tools. New advances in stereological methodology are being made frequently and these are generally reported in the *Journal of Microscopy*. It is important that those involved in applying quantitative methods in pathology should keep abreast of the advances in this increasingly important field.

1.9 SAMPLING IN STEREOLOGICAL STUDIES

Efficiency in stereology, as in any quantitative study, is measured by the degree of variation that exists in the measuring system and the cost that is required to reach this. Variation is present at the different levels of sampling, e.g., between patients, biopsies, sections and fields. It has been the practice of stereological studies in the past to measure each individual field as precisely as possible, thus requiring large numbers of points/lines on the grid. However, as variation is generally greater between fields, measuring each field precisely is less important than measuring a larger number of fields roughly [22,23]. For volume estimation, therefore, it is better to use grids which have a small number of points and use these to count a larger number of fields. Similarly, as variation may be greater between different tissue samples, it is more appropriate to assess a greater number of tissue samples with less precision than a small number with great precision. Hence the stereologist's motto: 'Do more less well!' [23]. In general terms, a total of 100–200 points and/or intersections per subject is sufficient to give precise results [23]. It is also important to consider the cost, principally with regards to time, that is required to reach a desired accuracy (see Chapter 15). *Sampling design* is therefore of vital importance in stereological studies as it is in all quantitative analyses. Methods to determine optimal sample numbers in quantitative analyses are given in Chapter 16 and a simple step-by-step approach for determining sampling design is given by Gundersen *et al.* [22].

1.10 THE USE OF LINE/POINT GRIDS

Various methods can be used to superimpose counting grids over a histological image. The conventional approach in light microscopy has been to use eyepiece graticules which can be inserted into the optical path of a microscope. Counting can then be done directly from the histological section. Alternatively, transparencies of the tissue can be projected on to a screen on which a suitable grid has been drawn. If photomicrographs are being used, the negative can be printed using a grid mask inserted in the light path, so leaving a permanent grid on each photographic print. Other simple methods include the use of grid transparencies which can be overlaid in photomicrographs of the tissue. These can be made easily by photocopying drawn grids on to acetate sheets, although any distortion in photocopied material should be checked [24]. The use of digital overlay boards on most image analysis systems allows various computer-stored grids to be superimposed over a video image of the section. This approach is currently being advanced with the use of computer-controlled head-up displays in the visual column of the microscope [25].

1.11 CONCLUSION

It is a common misconception that stereology is a dying practice being replaced solely by computerized measuring systems. This is not the case! Stereology remains a growing science with new techniques continually being developed. Its importance in quantitative pathology has been expressed in many recent papers [14,16,25–27]. It is perhaps disappointing that the developments in stereology and image analysis have occurred largely independently of each other [28]. We should, therefore, seek to see a closer marriage of these two powerful tools. Image analysis systems should be designed to aid the stereological analysis of biological images and enhance the collection, handling and analysis of stereological data. This would promote the use of these important techniques in pathological research and practice.

Acknowledgement

I would like to thank Dr Vyvyan Howard for his useful comments on this chapter.

References

1 Gundersen HJG, Boysen M, Reith A. Comparison of semi-automatic digitizer-tablet and simple point counting performance in morphometry. *Virchows Arch [Cell Pathol]* 1981; 37: 317–325.

2 Gundersen HJG. Stereology and sampling of biological surfaces. In: Echlin P. (ed.) *Analysis of Organic and Biological Surfaces*. New York: John Wiley, 1984: 477–506.

3 Gundersen HJG, Bendtsen TF, Korbo L *et al.* Some new, simple and efficient stereological methods and their use in pathological research and diagnosis. *Acta Pathol Microbiol Immuno Scand* 1988; 96: 379–394.

4 Gundersen HJG, Bagger P, Bendtsen TF *et al.* The new

stereological tools: disector, fractionator, nucleator and point sampled intercepts and their use in pathological research and diagnosis. *Acta Pathol Microbiol Immuno Scand* 1988; 96: 857–881.

5 Weibel ER. *Stereological Methods*, vol. I. *Practical Methods for Biological Morphometry*. London: Academic Press, 1979.

6 Aherne WA, Dunnill MS. *Morphometry*. London: Edward Arnold, 1982.

7 Gundersen HJG. Stereology of arbitrary particles. A review of unbiased number and size estimators and the presentation of some new ones. *J Microsc* 1986; 143: 3–5.

8 Gundersen HJG. Notes on the estimation of the numerical density of arbitrary profiles: the edge effect. *J Microsc* 1977; 111: 219–223.

9 Skinner JM, Whitehead R. Morphological methods in the study of the gut immune system in man. *J Clin Pathol* 1976; 29: 564–567.

10 Pakkenberg B, Gundersen HJ. New stereological method for obtaining unbiased and efficient estimates of total nerve cell number in human brain areas. Exemplified by the mediodorsal thalamic nucleus in schizophrenias. *Acta Pathol Microbiol Immuno Scand* 1989; 97: 677–681.

11 Braendgaard H, Evans SM, Howard CV, Gundersen HJ. The total number of neurons in the human neocortex unbiasedly estimated using optical disectors. *J Microsc* 1990; 157: 285–304.

12 Baddeley AJ, Gundersen HJG, Cruz-Orive LM. Estimation of surface area from vertical sections. *J Microsc* 1986; 142: 259–276.

13 Dunnill MS, Whitehead R. A method for the quantitation of small intestinal biopsy specimens. *J Clin Pathol* 1972; 25: 243–246.

14 Nielsen K, Colstrup H, Nilsson T, Gundersen HJ. Stereological estimates of nuclear volume correlated with histopathological grading and prognosis of bladder tumour. *Virchows Arch A [Cell Biol]* 1986; 52: 41–54.

15 Nielsen K. Stereological estimates of nuclear volume in normal mucosa and carcinoma *in situ* of the human urinary bladder. *Virchows Arch B [Cell Pathol]* 1988; 55: 233–236.

16 Aru A, Nielsen K. Stereological estimates of nuclear volume in primary lung cancer. *Pathol Res Pract* 1989; 185: 735–739.

17 Braendgaard H, Gundersen HJG. The impact of recent stereological advances on quantitative studies of the nervous system. *J Neurosci Methods* 1986; 18: 39–78.

18 Moss MC, Browne MA, Howard CV, Joyner DJ. An interactive image analysis system for mean particle volume estimation using stereological principles. *J Microsc* 1989; 156: 79–90.

19 Moller A, Strange P, Gundersen HJ. Efficient estimation of cell volume and number using the nucleator and the disector. *J Microsc* 1990; 159: 61–71.

20 Ogbuihi S, Cruz-Orive LM. Estimating the total number of lymphatic valves in infant lung with the fractionator. *J Microsc* 1990; 158: 19–30.

21 Howard V, Reid S, Baddeley A, Boyde A. Unbiased estimation of particle density in the tandem scanning reflected light microscope. *J Microsc* 1985; 138: 203–212.

22 Gundersen HJG, Gotzsche O, Osterby R. Sampling efficiency in morphometry simplified. *Metab Bone Dis Relat Res* 1980; 2: 443–448.

23 Gundersen HJG, Osterby R. Optimising sampling efficiency of stereological studies in biology: or 'Do more less well!'. *J Microsc* 1981; 121: 65–73.

24 Steer MW. *Understanding Cell Structure*. Cambridge: Cambridge University Press, 1981.

25 Oberholzer M, Bianchi L, Dalquen P, Landmann L, Heitz PU. Stereology in the extraction of information from images. *Anal Quant Cytol Histol* 1985; 7: 197–204.

26 Tosi P, Luzi P, Baak JPA *et al.* Gastric dysplasia: a stereological and morphometrical assessment. *J Pathol* 1987; 152: 83–94.

27 Baak JPA, Nauta JJ, Wisse-Brekelmans EC, Bezemer PD. Architectural and nuclear morphometrical features together are more important prognosticators in endometrial hyperplasia than nuclear morphometrical features alone. *J Pathol* 1988; 154: 335–341.

28 Weibel ER. Measuring through the microscope: development and evolution of stereological methods. *J Microsc* 1989; 155: 393–403.

2

INTERACTIVE COMPUTER-AIDED MORPHOMETRY

P. W. HAMILTON

The digital computer has been of great benefit in the storage, handling, statistical analysis and display of numerical data. In addition, the ability of the computer to display complex graphics and digitally stored images has greatly enhanced the analysis of visual data. These benefits have been exploited in the collection and analysis of quantitative histological information. *Computerized image analysis* has been used to describe that area of work which utilizes computers in the morphometric measurement of histological or cytological features.

Two approaches to measurement using computers can be defined.

1 *Interactive image analysis* systems rely on the operator physically to define the structure of interest using a specialized drawing device. Co-ordinate data from the drawing device are read by the computer and from these, various geometric dimensions are calculated relating to the drawn object.

2 *Automatic image analysis* uses a more complex approach which requires histological images from a video camera to be stored digitally in computer memory. Once stored in this way, images can be processed and features automatically detected by the computer and measured. The ultimate objective behind such an approach is to remove the need for an operator and increase the rate at which morphometric measurements can be made. Unfortunately, the complexity of most histological images makes the application of fully automated procedures difficult, although not impossible (see Chapter 13).

The distinction between these two methods is by no means strict. Interactive methods can benefit from the image storage, retrieval and processing functions commonly used for automated image analysis. As total automation in the identification and measurement of important histological features is rarely straightforward, interaction can be used to check and correct mistakes made by the computer. For example, a commonly quoted problem in automation is that overlapping nuclei are often identified and measured as a single object. Interaction by the user will allow the erroneously defined object to be removed from the analysis or alternatively, a separating line can be drawn between the two nuclei, allowing the computer to measure the nuclei independently. Automatic image analysis is discussed in Chapter 7.

As has already been mentioned, interactive computer systems rely on an operator to interact with the computer by providing it with geometric data on the object to be measured. This is done by tracing the individual objects (e.g., cells, nuclei, etc.) or distances (e.g., crypt length) using specialized drawing devices. Data on the tracing are entered into the computer in the form of co-ordinates, which the software reads and from which various morphometric variables can be calculated. Such systems have also been called semiautomatic or optomanual image analysers.

The rapid drop in the cost of computer hardware and memory has resulted in a marked decrease in the cost of image analysis equipment. Commercially available interactive image analysers are relatively cheap and basic systems can be purchased for less than the cost of a research microscope. Cost increases with features such as digital overlay (Section 2.1), computer processing speed, software requirements, e.g., statistical analysis and digital boards capable of image capture or for communications with other devices. At the top end of the market spectrum would be systems capable of image storage, processing and automated analysis, yet most retain the ability for interactive measurement. With the widespread popularity and availability of IBM PC clones and Apple Macs, most can now be upgraded at low cost to perform simple and also more complex image measurement functions.

2.1 INTERACTIVE DRAWING DEVICES

Several drawing devices are available for the collection of co-ordinate data. The digitizing tablet and cursor (Fig. 2.1) are probably the most widely used tracing devices. The digitizing tablet essentially consists of a mesh of fine wires strung in x and y directions under the surface. In most systems, the cursor generates an electromagnetic field which is detected by the tablet, the position of the cursor being entered into the computer in the form of x and y co-ordinates. Movement of the stylus on the tablet is, therefore, continually registered by the computer. By pressing a button on the cursor, the co-ordinates of a tracing action can be stored in the memory and from this various geometric variables can be derived. In this way histological features can be traced and morphometric measurements made.

Histological images can be presented to the digitizing tablet for measurement in a number of ways. Photomicrographs can be placed on the tablet (Fig. 2.2) and features of interest outlined. Similarly, 2 × 2 transparencies can be projected on to the tablet surface and special tablets can be purchased which allow back-projection. Projection allows enlargement of histological features with high resolution, permitting the measurement of microscopically small objects. As the production of numerous photomicrographs or transparencies is expensive, images can be projected on to the tablet directly from the microscope using a prism which deflects the microscopic image away from the eyepieces on to the graphic tablet. One of the most effective means of making measurements directly from the microscope is by sending a video image of the tissue to a television monitor on to which is superimposed a computer-generated cross-hair (Fig. 2.3) which represents the position of the cursor on the tablet.

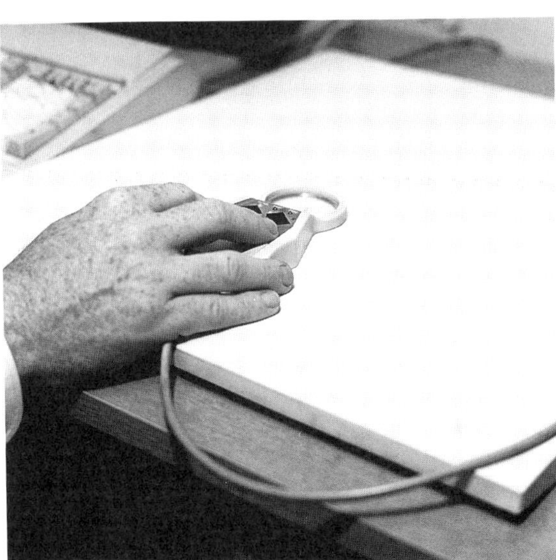

Fig. 2.1 Digitizing tablet and hand-controlled drawing device (cursor).

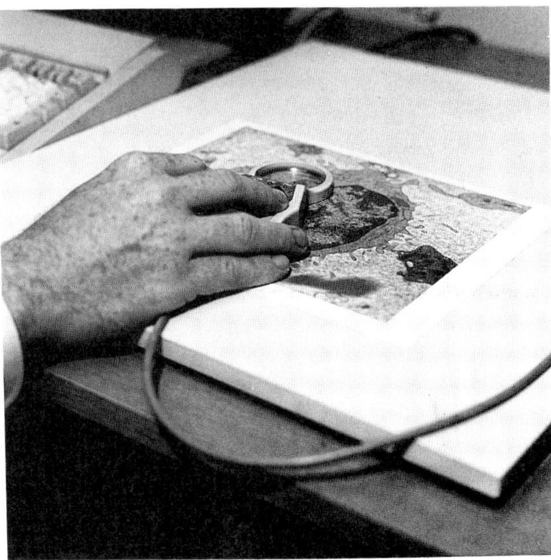

Fig. 2.2 Graphic tablet with photomicrograph. Features can be measured by pressing a button on the drawing device, tracing the feature of interest (e.g., nucleus) and releasing the button. The computer automatically calculates the morphometric parameters relating to the traced object.

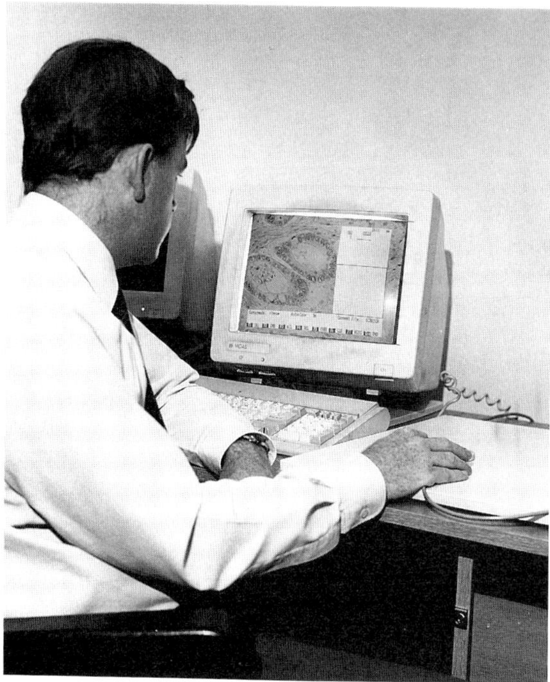

(a)

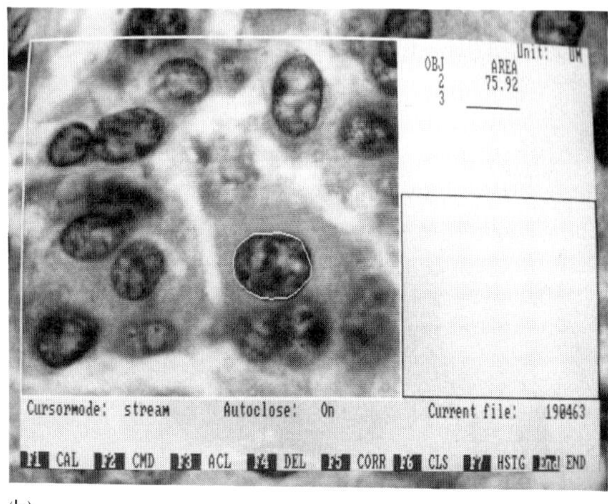

(b)

Fig. 2.3 (a) Features can be traced from an on-line video image. A digital cursor is generated overlying the image and manoeuvred using the drawing device. (b) Tracing objects is carried out as before and morphometric parameters derived.

This is called *digital overlay* and requires specialist hardware and software which can 'mix' the analog video image with digital graphics. In this way, the position of the cross-hair on-screen can be controlled by moving the drawing device over the tablet. Various features can then be traced on the screen and measured as before.

A *mouse* can be used to guide a cursor on-screen to trace features for measurement. The mouse does not require a position-sensitive tablet. Movement of a roller-ball on the underside of the mouse as it moves over a normal table surface directs the cursor on-screen and allows features to be traced. It is perhaps not as sensitive as a dedicated digitizing table for measurement.

Light pens are sensitive to light intensities provided by the monitor and in this way are used to generate co-ordinates of image structures by tracing them directly on the monitor screen. In a similar way, *touch-sensitive screens* can be used to trace and measure image features. Both these methods, however, are limited by their low resolution and are now seldom implemented in commercial systems.

2.2 INTERACTIVE MEASUREMENTS

In most commercially available instruments, a wide range of measurement capabilities are available which can be freely selected by the user. Enclosed structures (e.g., nuclei) can be traced and numerous measurements relating to size and shape calculated simultaneously for each profile (Table 2.1a). Various factors which describe object shape are listed in Table 2.2. Simple measurements of area alone (Table 2.1b) can provide information on the quantity of tissue components or act as a reference space for the assessment of object number and simple object counts alone can be facilitated (Table 2.1c). Additionally, by defining two end-points or by tracing a continuous line, linear distance or length can be measured respectively (Table 2.1d). A similar range of variables may be determined using automatic image analysis but the advantage of interactive systems is that the user's visual acumen is retained in the definition of histological features. Examples of measurements using interactive analysis can be found throughout the literature on histological morphometry. These include ovary [1],

Table 2.1 Examples of measurements and features which can be obtained using interactive methods

(a) *Area*
Perimeter
Maximum diameter
Minimum diameter
e.g., nuclei, cells, etc.

(b) *Area*
e.g., stroma, epithelium, duct, islet, etc.

(c) *Number*
e.g., lymphocytes, mitoses, Ki-67-positive cells, nuclei, mast cells, etc.

(d) *Length*
e.g., epithelial length, mucosal height, depth of invasion, glomerular width, fibre width, etc.

Table 2.2 Examples of shape descriptors that can be computed from traced profiles

Form factor $(AR) = 1/4 \times \pi \times$ (longest axis) $\times$ (shortest axis)
Form factor $(PE) = (4\pi$ area$)/$perimeter$^2)$
Roundness factor = perimeter$/(2\sqrt{\pi \text{ area}})$
Contour index = perimeter$/\sqrt{\text{area}}$

endometrium [2,3], breast [4], lymph node [5], prostate [6], stomach [7,8], jejunum [9] and colorectum [10–12]. The wealth of studies illustrates the ease and versatility with which interactive systems can be used to provide useful histometric data and highlights the increasing availability of such instruments in pathological circles.

2.3 CAVEATS IN INTERACTIVE IMAGE ANALYSIS

Several factors need to be considered when using interactive image analysis and these are outlined below.

2.3.1 User variation

Whilst one of the main advantages of interactive systems is that they allow the user to define the features to be measured, this may also introduce additional variation to the study. First, the manual tracing of morphological features can be relatively slow and tedious, can result in operator fatigue and give rise to measurement error [13]. Second, as the operator must decide on what is to be measured, biased results can be obtained even without a conscious effort on the part of the operator [13]. This emphasizes the need for the proper design of, and strict adherence to, an appropriate random sampling regime. Variation introduced by the user includes differing interpretation of the histological image influencing the choice of fields or objects for measurement and varying ability to delineate features using the interactive drawing devices. The first of these is related to histological experience and is difficult to reduce if selective methods of sampling are being used, save a more closely defined protocol for field or object selection. The second relates to experience in the use of the drawing device. Gamel *et al.* [14] demonstrated that a person with 16 months' experience in tracing nuclear images was able to retain higher levels of reproducibility than a novice with experience of 1 week. Further work in this area has also shown that tracings made with a pen on a graphic tablet show greater variation than those made with a flat cursor in the same way [15].

2.3.2 Image size

Experiments using graphic tablet measuring systems have shown that the size of the measured object has a dramatic effect on the variation of results [15]. Images larger than 15 mm on the graphic tablet are reported to be more suitable, showing lower coefficients of variation [15] and better reproducibility [16].

In most systems the tablet can be appropriately scaled to the magnification of the images being examined. This allows image dimensions to be expressed in real units rather than arbitrary values. Scaling can be carried out by entering two positions on the tablet using the stylus and informing the system what the distance between the two points is, at image magnification. This is achieved with a microscopic slide graticule, if measurements are to be made directly from the microscope, or from a generated scale bar if photographs are used (e.g., in electron microscopy). If a scale bar is not employed, care must be taken to ensure consistent enlargement of micrographs from negatives and accurate calculation of the final magnification. If the magnification is known, a magnification factor can be entered, which results in automatic scaling of the graphic tablet.

2.3.3 Hardware/software

The optimal functioning of the computer, drawing device and the controlling software is crucial if accurate measurements are to be made. Most currently available systems can be purchased 'ready to measure' and it is all too easy to assume that measurements made by the instrument are accurate. A software miscalculation or hardware problem may lead to erroneous measurement data. For example, early versions of the Kontron MOP Videoplan software were shown to overestimate linear measurements such as length [17], although this has now been corrected [15]. This highlights the importance of testing any commercial instrument for accuracy and reliability before embarking on the collection of morphometric data. Measurement accuracy can be checked by measuring profiles of known dimensions. These are sometimes provided by the manufacturers of image analysis equipment.

2.3.4 Tracing speed

Fleedge *et al.* [15] showed that the speed at which features are traced is an important contributor to measurement variation. The higher the tracing speed, the higher the variation. This would be expected, as the faster one traces around a feature, the less care can be paid to its accurate delineation. In addition, it is unclear what part the processing speed of the computer plays in this phenomenon [18].

2.4 THE HOME PROJECT

An important recent development in interactive morphometry has been the HOME (Highly Optimized Microscope Environment) project. This is a European multilaboratory endeavour [18] to interface the microscope and the computer in such a way that measurement in routine pathology is made practical (Fig. 2.4). The principal advantage of the system is that computer and microscopic images can be simultaneously viewed through the eyepieces of a conventional but modified microscope. This is made possible by using a video display unit, built into the microscope head, allowing digital images (graphics, text, etc.) to be overlayed on to the microscope image (Fig. 2.4b). By moving a hand-controlled mouse, a digital cursor can be manoeuvred over the microscopic image and various measurements made, as previously described. This means that the operator can look at a microscopic slide and make measurements without raising his/her head from the field of view – a major advantage.

In addition, the HOME system has an integrated encoding scanning stage. This permits microscopic features to be marked, stored in computer memory and relocated on the slide at a future date [19]. This has been shown to be of particular benefit in diagnostic cytology [20].

Much effort has gone into providing a friendly computer interface. It is menu-driven and slide identification, object marking, relocation and choice of measurement are easily controlled. It is evident that this system has been designed by pathologists for pathologists and several applications for use in routine diagnosis are currently being integrated into the software. Whether a system of this type will eventually find itself on the desk of every practising histo- and cytopathologist remains to be seen, but there is no doubt that it represents a vital step forward in promoting measurement in a routinely acceptable fashion.

2.5 CONCLUSION

The ability to interact with computerized measuring instruments will remain the cornerstone of diagnostic morphometry, as this combines the visual skill and knowledge of the pathologist with the precision of the computer. The successful application of morphometry as a routine diagnostic tool for the pathologist will depend on the adoption of cheap and simple interactive computer systems and their integration with the standard microscope.

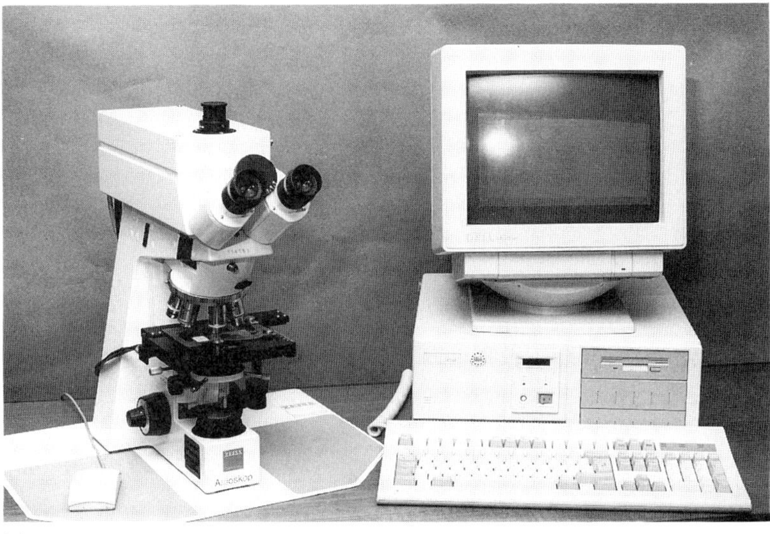

(a)

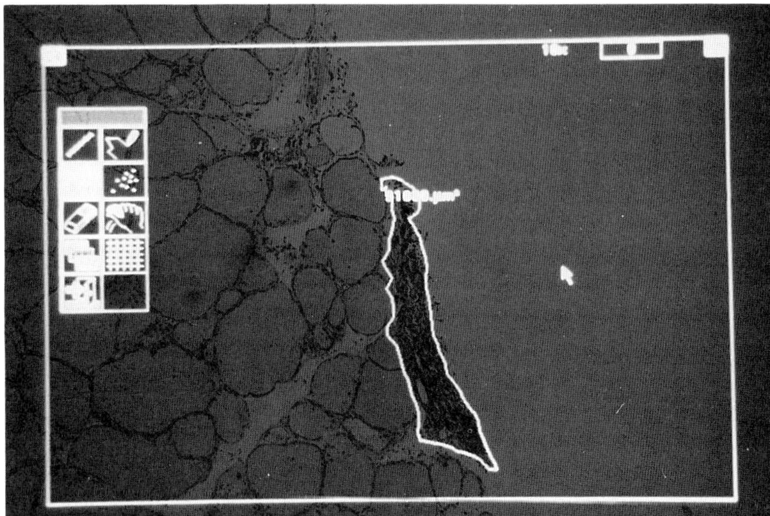

(b)

Fig. 2.4 (a) The Highly Optimized Microscope Environment (HOME) prototype: a standard microscope but with a head-up display attachment behind the eyepieces. Software is run on a standard computer, digital graphics overlay the microscope image and measurements made using the mouse. (b) A display down the eyepiece of the HOME system, showing how histological features can be traced and measured. Courtesy of Dr James Tucker.

References

1 Baak JPA, Agrafojo Blanco A, Kurver PHJ *et al.* Quantitation of borderline and malignant mucinous ovarian tumours. *Histopathology* 1981; 5: 353–360.

2 Baak JPA, Kurver PHJ, Diegenbach PC *et al.* Discrimination of hyperplasia and carcinoma of the endometrium by quantitative microscopy – a feasibility study. *Histopathology* 1981; 5: 61–68.

3 Skaarland E. Morphometric analysis of nuclei in epithelial structures from normal and neoplastic endometrium: a study using the Isaacs cell sampler and Endoscann instruments. *J Clin Pathol* 1985; 38: 496–501.

4 Baak JP, Kurver PH, De Snoo-Niewlaat AJ, De Graef S, Makkink B, Boon ME. Prognostic indicators in breast cancer – morphometric methods. *Histopathology* 1982; 6: 327–339.

5 Crocker J, Jones EL, Curran RC. Study of nuclear diameters in non-Hodgkin's lymphomas. *J Clin Pathol* 1982; 35: 954–958.

6 Bocking A, Auffermann W, Schwartz H, Bammert J, Dorrjer G, Vucicuja S. Cytology of prostatic carcinoma. Quantification and validation of diagnostic criteria. *Anal Quant Cytol Histol* 1984; 6: 74–88.

7 Jarvis LR, Whitehead R. Morphometric analysis of gastric dysplasia. *J Pathol* 1985; 47: 133–138.
8 Tosi P, Luzi P, Baak JPA *et al.* Gastric dysplasia: a stereological and morphometrical assessment. *J Pathol* 1987; 152: 83–94.
9 Slavin G, Sowter C, Robertson K, McDermott S, Paton K. Measurement in jejunal biopsies by computer-aided microscopy. *J Clin Pathol* 1980; 33: 254–261.
10 Brown LJR, Smeeton NC, Dixon MF. Assessment of dysplasia in colorectal adenomas: an observer variation and morphometric study. *J Clin Pathol* 1985; 38: 174–179.
11 Hamilton PW, Allen DC, Watt PCH, Patterson CC, Biggart JD. Classification of normal colorectal mucosa and adenocarcinoma by morphometry. *Histopathology* 1987; 9: 901–911.
12 Allen DC, Hamilton PW, Watt PCH, Biggart JD. Morphometrical analysis in ulcerative colitis with dysplasia. *Histopathology* 1987; 9: 913–926.
13 Henderson G. Automation. In: Aherne WA, Dunnill MS (eds) *Morphometry*. London: Edward Arnold, 1982: 191–197.
14 Gamel JW, Gleason J, Williams H, Greenberg R. Reproducibility of nucleolar measurements of human intraocular melanoma cells from standard histologic microslides. *Anal Quant Cytol Histol* 1985; 7: 174–177.
15 Fleege JC, Baak JPA, Smeulders AWM. Analysis of measuring system parameters that influence reproducibility of morphometric assessments with a graphic tablet. *Hum Pathol* 1988; 19: 513–517.
16 Dardick I, Caldwell D. Reproducibility of morphometric image analysis (letter). *Hum Pathol* 1985; 16: 1178.
17 Cornelisse JTWA, van den Berg TJTP. Profile boundary length can be overestimated by as much as 41% when using a digitiser tablet. *J Microsc* 1984; 136: 341–344.
18 Fleedge JC, van Diest PJ, Baak JPA. Reliability of quantitative pathological assessments, standards, and quality control. In: Baak JPA (ed.) *Manual of Quantitative Pathology in Cancer Diagnosis and Prognosis*. Berlin: Springer Verlag, 1991: 151–181.
19 Brugal G, Dye R, Krief B, Chassery J-M, Tanke H, Tucker JH. HOME: Highly Optimised Microscope Environment. *Cytometry* 1992; 13: 109–116.
20 Morens A, Krief B, Brugal G. The HOME microscope workstation. A new tool for cervical cancer screening. *Anal Quant Cytol Histol* 1992; 14: 289–294.

3

MITOTIC COUNTS

P. W. HAMILTON AND D. C. ALLEN

Assessment of mitotic activity is an important aspect of tumour grading and mitotic counts are probably one of the measurements most used by histopathologists. The thesis behind this is that mitotic numbers reflect the proliferative activity of the tumour and the growth rate of the tissue. Whether the enumeration of mitoses is truly indicative of the proliferative status of a tumour is difficult to prove, although the clinical relevance of assessing mitoses for diagnosis and prognosis has been shown. Mitotic counts are a significant criterion in the diagnosis of malignant smooth-muscle tumours but have also been shown to be valuable in assessing several other tumours, including breast and ovarian carcinoma as well as sarcomas. Several methods have been proposed for counting mitoses.

3.1 MITOSES PER 10 HIGH-POWER FIELDS (HPFs)

It is customary in most centres to express mitoses as the number per 10 HPFs. While this method has been shown to be reproducible when using a standardized approach [1], it can be subject to several sources of error. The main criticism is the lack of a well-defined reference space against which to relate the count. These problems are detailed below.

1 While a 40× objective magnification is commonly used, a review of a range of microscopes [2] has shown that high-powered field areas can vary from 0.071 to 0.414 mm^2. This degree of disparity would result in a sixfold difference in mitotic counts. While it is now becoming accepted practice to quote the optical details and microscopic field size in studies involving mitotic counts, it makes it difficult to compare results from different centres.

2 Even if the size of microscopic fields could be standardized, mitotic counts will vary depending on the amount of tissue present or the cellularity within different fields. For example, the centre of a scirrhous breast carcinoma may be paucicellular while its peripheral rim is abundantly cellular. This can be overcome by calculating mitotic counts as a ratio of either the area of tissue or the total number of cells present (see later).

3 The criteria involved in defining what actually constitutes a mitotic figure are subjective. This is discussed in more detail later.

4 Finally, one must question whether 10 fields is a sufficient sample to obtain a representative value [3]. This has rarely been tested in studies quoting mitotic counts and is certain to vary in different tissues depending on intratumoural heterogeneity.

Despite its practical convenience, these limitations must make practising histopathologists question the credibility of assessing mitotic counts per 10 HPFs [4], particularly when the reproducibility of the technique is questionable [5]. The following methods provide a more objective and statistically acceptable means for assessing mitotic activity in histological tissue.

3.2 MITOSES PER SQUARE MILLIMETRE

Counting mitotic figures within a reference space of known area allows results to be expressed as mitoses per square millimetre. This can be achieved using appropriate eyepiece graticules and overcomes the problems of differing microscopic field sizes. The accurate method for doing this is detailed in Section 1.1. However, if the area of known size is a square (as it often is), then it is likely that on some occasions the tissue from which the mitoses are being sampled will not occupy the whole field. This can be overcome using interactive image analysis to measure the area of tissue from which counts are to be made or, perhaps more conveniently, by point-counting methods to estimate the area fraction of the field covered by tissue.

3.3 VOLUME-CORRECTED MITOTIC INDEX

This method was proposed by Haapasalo *et al.* [6] as a suitable solution to the above problems. It relies on measuring within a microscopic field of known radius the fraction of area occupied by tumour tissue and then counting the number of mitoses within the tissue. This is carried out on several fields to obtain a representative sample. The area fraction is taken to estimate the volume fraction (V_V) of tissue (see Section 1.2.1) and the mitotic index is then calculated from the following formula:

$$M/V_{\text{index}} = \frac{k(M)}{V_V}$$

where $k = 100/\pi r^2$, in which r = the radius of the microscopic field in millimetres; M = the number of mitotic figures in the neoplastic tissue; and V_V = the volume fraction of neoplastic tissue as a percentage of the whole microscopic field.

This method is reported to show better reproducibility [7] and to act as a powerful prognostic indicator in ovarian [8], bladder [9] and pancreatic [10] carcinoma.

While this method does take into account the amount of tissue present, the volume of tissue is not always an accurate indicator of the number of interphase cells. If the cells are densely packed then the number of mitoses per square millimetre will be higher than if the cells are loosely packed. Cell density varies between fields, sections, samples and tumours. This is caused not only by intratumoural heterogeneity in growth pattern but also by factors such as necrosis or myxoid degeneration. In addition, variation in nuclear size will determine the number of nuclei per square millimetre and so comparison of tumours showing widely varying nuclear sizes may give spurious results [4].

3.4 THE MITOTIC INDEX

The problems discussed above indicate that the only true measure of mitotic state is one which calculates the number of mitoses present as a fraction of the total number of cells. The denominator can be calculated by directly counting the total numbers of cells on which the fraction is to be based. Alternatively, the total number of cells in a field can be estimated using geometric probes (see Chapter 1). For example [11], total cells within a microscopic field can be estimated by counting the number of cells (n) that intersect a single line bisecting the field (using a suitable eyepiece graticule) and feeding this into the formula: $\pi(n/2)^2$. The mitotic events are counted as normal and the mitotic index is expressed as mitoses/$\pi(n/2)^2$.

It is peculiar that the true mitotic index has been used in so few studies, especially since this is the common means used to quantify the labelling indices of other proliferative cell markers. This may be because it is more time-consuming and close consideration needs to be given towards the size of sample to obtain a representative index. Nevertheless, a desire for meaningful data on the proliferative status of neoplasms and its role in diagnosis and prognosis should encourage histopathologists to adopt the most accurate techniques [3].

3.5 OTHER CONSIDERATIONS

Regardless of the method used, accurate identification of mitotic figures is vital and experience seems to play an important role [12]. Distinction of mitoses from karyorrhectic or pyknotic nuclei is important and adherence to strict morphological criteria is essential. Baak *et al.* [13] give such guidelines in the grading of breast carcinoma (Table 3.1) Staining of the section must be optimal. While the May–Gruenwald–Giemsa stain is particularly use-

Table 3.1 Criteria for selection of mitotic figures. Summarized from Baak *et al.* [13]

Absent nuclear membrane
Clear hairy extensions of nuclear material (condensed chromosomes):
clotted – metaphase
in a plane – metaphase/anaphase
separate clots – telophase
Cell cytoplasm often purple/blue/larger

ful, the development of special stains which highlight mitotic figures [14] will also go a long way to enhance identification and improve the reproducibility of counts.

Delay in fixation is known to result in a decreased mitotic count by as much as 50% [15,16]. This may be due to cell cycle continuation and completion of mitosis after tissue removal in the absence of oxygen [17,18] or simply diminished preservation and a reduced ability to be able to identify mitoses histologically. Regardless of the reasons, it is vital that tissue is fixed promptly after removal to provide optimal conditions for mitotic counting [15].

The number of mitoses present in a defined field will also be related to the thickness of the section [2]. It is desirable, therefore, to have uniform section thickness before comparisons of counts between samples are made. If a single unadjusted focal plane is used and only mitotic figures in that plane are counted then section thickness is less important [6]. However, in practice, focusing 'up and down' is a useful way to confirm the identification of suspected mitotic figures.

Appropriate and sufficient sampling of tissue is important to provide statistically valid results. Intratumoural heterogeneity of mitotic counts needs to be assessed so that adequate samples are taken at the various levels (fields, sections, blocks, tumours). This can be done using the methods outlined in Chapter 16.

The method of sampling is also important. Some authors feel that mitotic counts should be made on the 'worst areas of the tumour' or 'in the area of highest cellularity'. Selection of such areas, however, is a subjective process and will vary between different observers, thus undermining the objectivity of the measurement. Unless these areas are also defined by means of quantitative measurement [4] then the statistical accuracy of such selective sampling is in doubt. However, it is important to appreciate that random sampling from a tumour with localized areas of high mitotic activity may dilute the final result.

Some tissues require careful consideration before examination and quantitation of mitoses. Gastrointestinal epithelium is a prime example as cellular proliferation is spatially distributed along the length of the gland (i.e., in the normal colon the proliferating compartment occupies the lower third of the crypt). For this reason, complete glands need to defined where the base, middle and mouth of the gland are in the same plane of section [19]. This is difficult and rarely possibly in neoplasia. Alternative methods for counting mitoses in gastrointestinal tissue with respect to their spatial distribution within the gland have been proposed [20,21].

3.6 CONCLUSION

Counting of mitoses is and will remain an important tool for the bench pathologist in establishing diagnoses and giving prognostic information. It is vital that a standardized protocol for the staining, identification, counting and numerical expression of mitotic figures be established by a multinational panel of recognized experts. This should permit the comparison of results from different centres, allowing a more definitive examination of the association between mitotic counts and cell proliferation, and the histopathological significance of mitoses in diseased tissue.

References

1 Van Diest P, Baak JPA, Matze-Cok P *et al.* Reproducibility of mitosis counting in 2469 breast cancer specimens: results from the Multicentre Morphometric Mammary carcinoma project. *Hum Pathol* 1992; 23: 603–607.

2 Ellis PSJ, Whitehead R. Mitosis counting – a need for reappraisal. *Hum Pathol* 1981; 12: 3–4.

3 Quinn CM, Wright NA. Letter. *J Pathol* 1991; 163: 362–364.

4 Quinn CM, Wright NA. The clinical assessment of proliferation and growth in human tumours: evaluation of methods and applications as prognostic variables. *J Pathol* 1990; 160: 93–102.

5 Silverberg SG. Reproducibility of the mitosis count in the histological diagnosis of smooth muscle tumours of the uterus. *Hum Pathol* 1976; 7: 451.

6 Haapasalo H, Pesonen E, Collan Y. Volume corrected mitotic index (M/V-index). The standard of mitotic activity in neoplasms. *Pathol Res Pract* 1989; 185: 551–554.

7 Haapasalo H, Collan Y, Seppa A, Gidlund A-L, Atkin NB, Personen E. Prognostic value of ovarian carcinoma grading methods – a method comparison study. *Histopathology* 1990; 16: 1–7.

8 Haapasalo H, Collan Y, Atkin NB, Personen E, Seppa A. Prognosis of ovarian carcinomas: prediction by histoquantitative methods. *Histopathology* 1989; 15: 167–168.

9 Lipponen PK, Collan Y, Eskelinen MJ, Pesonen E, Sotarauta M. Volume corrected mitotic index (M/V index) in human bladder cancer; relation to histological grade (WHO) clinical stage (UICC) and prognosis. *Scand J Nephrol* 1990; 24: 39–45.

10 Lipponen P, Eskelinen M, Collan Y, Marin S, Alhava E. Volume corrected mitotic index (M/V index) in pancreatic cancer: relation to histological grade, clinical stage and prognosis. *Scand J Gastroenterol* 1990; 25: 548–554.

11 Simpson JF, Dutt PL, Page DL. Expression of mitoses per thousand cells and cell density in breast carcinomas: a proposal. *Hum Pathol* 1992; 23: 608–611.

12 Donhuifensen K. Mitosis counts: reproducibility and significance in grading of malignancy. *Hum Pathol* 1986; 17: 1112–1125.

13 Baak JPA, Van Diest PJ, Ariens A Th *et al.* The multicentre morphometric mammary carcinoma project (MMMCP). A nationwide prospective study on reproducibility and prognostic power of quantitative assessments in The Netherlands. *Pathol Res Pract* 1989; 185: 664–670.

14 Busch C, Vasko J. Differential staining of mitosis in tissue sections and cultured cells by a modified nethenamine-silver method. *Lab Invest* 1988; 59: 876–878.

15 Cross SS, Start RD, Smith JHF. Does delay in fixation affect the number of mitotic figures in processed tissue? *J Clin Pathol* 1990; 43: 597–599.

16 Donhuijsen K, Schmidt U, Hirche H, Van Beuningen D, Budach V. Changes in mitotic rate and cell cycle fractions caused by delayed fixation. *Hum Pathol* 1990; 21: 709–714.

17 Bullough WS. Mitotic activity in the tissues of dead mice, and in tissues kept in physiological salt solutions. *Exp Cell Res* 1950; 1: 410.

18 Graem N, Helweg-Larsen K. Mitotic activity and delay in fixation of tumour tissue. *Acta Pathol Microbiol Immunol Scand (A)* 1979; 87: 375.

19 Wright N, Alison M. *The Biology of Epithelial Cell Populations*, vol. 2. Oxford: Clarendon Press, 1984.

20 Goodlad RA, Levi S, Lee CY, Mandir N, Hodgson H, Wright N. Morphometry and cell proliferation in endoscopic biopsies: evaluation of a technique. *Gastroenterology* 1991; 101: 1235–1241.

21 Hamilton PW, Grimes J, Arthur K, Wilson RH. Three-dimensional analysis of proliferation patterns in gastrointestinal epithelium – a new technique. *J Pathol* 1993; 169(suppl): 173.

4

GENERAL APPLICATIONS OF MORPHOMETRY

D. C. ALLEN
With contributions by J. S. A. Collins, J. McClure and R. W. Lyness

4.1 GASTROINTESTINAL DISEASE

4.1.1 Mouth

Using a semiautomatic image analysis system (IBAS-1), Shabana *et al.* [1] studied a series of 100 oral mucosal white lesions. In particular they noted the size and shape of the basal layer epithelial cells. The nuclear features (area, perimeter, maximum diameter) showed a progressive increase from normal controls through traumatic keratoses, lichen planus, leucoplakia and a 'risk' group, to squamous-cell carcinoma. A mean nuclear area cut-off value of $>40\,\mu m^2$ incorporated 10, 82 and 94% of the leucoplakic, high-risk and carcinomatous lesions, respectively. They advocated that basal cell nuclear size is of diagnostic value in assessing the risk of malignant transformation. Stereology can accurately characterize differentiation in squamous carcinomas of the mouth [2] and head and neck [3]. In the latter a combination of subjective criteria (differentiation, necrosis, inflammatory component) and quantitative parameters (prominence of nucleoli, surface area to volume ratio) were found to predict tumour DNA ploidy accurately and patient response to chemotherapy and survival.

4.1.2 Oesophagus

Barrett [4] originally envisaged his description of columnar epithelium-lined oesophagus as a failure of embryonic maturation. Subsequently it has been recognized as a consequence of distal mucosal metaplasia due to chronic reflux oesophagitis. It has an association with the development of oesophagogastric junctional adenocarcinoma [5]; this correlates with an increased tritiated thymidine labelling index and expanded proliferative zone found in a minority of cases [6]. In a study of epithelial abnormalities present adjacent to oesophageal squamous carcinomas, Lindholm *et al.* [7] obtained 100% discrimination between normal squamous epithelium and dysplasia/carcinoma *in situ*. The morphometric analysis effected this by dividing the epithelium into three equal zones and identifying the following significant variables: (i) nuclear area in the superficial zone; (ii) nuclear perpendicularity in the intermediate zone; (iii) nuclear density in the total epithelial thickness; and (iv) the interzonal variation of these parameters. In established squamous-cell carcinoma a tumour cell mean nuclear area $>70\,\mu m^2$ has been found to be significantly associated with transmural oesophageal penetration and diminished patient survival [8]. The micro TICAS system used also allowed DNA ploidy estimates on the Feulgen-stained sections but only the automated karyometric measurements were of value. Morphometry has also shown that there is no difference in the proportion of tumour to stroma before and after chemotherapy in oesophageal adenocarcinoma, whereas squamous-cell carcinoma shows a marked reduction [9]. Cell counts indicate that p53 oncogene product expression correlates with the proliferation indices Ki-67 and proliferating cell nuclear antigen (PCNA) in oesophageal squamous carcinoma and adjacent dysplasia [10].

4.1.3 Stomach

Intestinal metaplasia

Gastric intestinal metaplasia is characterized by mucin-producing goblet cells with or without absorptive columnar cells, Paneth cells and pseudovillous structures [11]. Its significance as a lesion antedating gastric adenocarcinoma remains the subject of much debate, as it is associated with not only neoplasms but also benign gastric pathology. The concept of the possible progression of chronic atrophic gastritis through intestinal metaplasia, dysplasia and finally to the intestinal form of carcinoma [12] is supported by the prevalence of the latter with the sulphomucin-secreting incomplete variant (type III) of metaplasia. Non-sulphomucin-secreting metaplasia (types I and II) is usually found in situations where the cancer risk is low [13,14]. However, the high iron diamine alcian blue technique employed to demonstrate the mucin secretion can be capricious and its assessment has been visual and somewhat arbitrary. In a series of papers Rubio *et al.* [15–17] have quantified more objectively the presence of alcian blue-positive goblet cells and Paneth cells as a methodological prequel to mapping the occurrence of metaplasia in gastric dysplasia and adenocarcinoma. Tosi *et al.* [18] have directed their attention to the stereological and morphometric differences between the various subtypes of intestinal metaplasia. Type III intestinal metaplasia had significantly greater nuclear pleomorphism, higher nuclear cytoplasmic ratios, and smaller and less numerous goblet cell vacuoles in the upper and lower parts of the crypts. This suggests impaired maturation and aberrant differentiation in keeping with the previous histochemical and qualitative studies. It is only with such standardization of approach that the true biological role of gastric intestinal metaplasia will emerge.

Gastric dysplasia and carcinoma

Gastric dysplasia is a precancerous lesion and its appearances have been well-characterized in both flat [19] and polypoidal mucosa [20]. Follow-up studies show that it may regress, remain static or progress to carcinoma [21]. This tendency is also much stronger with dysplasia occurring in the context of an adenoma [20], where up to 75% may be associated with infiltrating malignancy [22]. This highlights the importance of making its accurate and reproducible diagnosis. Difficulties arise in separating regenerative hyperplasia from dysplasia due to the subjective criteria used to distinguish them. Quantitative studies have attempted to address these issues.

Jarvis and Whitehead [23] used computer-aided morphometry to study a large number of gastric epithelial segments graded as regenerative, mild, moderate or severe dysplasia or cancer. Each segment was quantified by defining nuclear area and its variability, nuclear crowding, nuclear elongation, nuclear cytoplasmic ratio and epithelial thickness. Discriminant analysis reduced the original variables to a function which described over 90% of the dataset variance. It was mainly contributed to by nuclear area and its variation, i.e., factors descriptively termed as nuclear size. Further analysis produced classification coefficients which were used to calculate a probability score for membership of a particular case to the defined histological groups. There was only a 46.9% agreement between the histological and computer-predicted groups, with most errors occurring in the regenerative category. Despite this, the study is useful in showing the relative weight of the various cytological criteria used in diagnostic assessment. Judging the classification rule performance against original groups which were predefined subjectively is another potential source of error.

The effect of this and also architectural features were examined by Tosi *et al.* [24]. The data were obtained by a combination of semiautomatic image analysis and stereological techniques. The importance of architectural features was shown by discriminant analysis, indicating that the volume density of glands (a measure of gland crowding and quantity of epithelium) and the nuclear distance (a measure of stratification from the centre of the nucleus to the basement membrane) were the features of greatest importance. Statistically they also used cluster analysis, a technique in which predefined subjective groups are not necessary. Eight stereological and morphometric parameters produced three statistically separate clusters and resulted in a total 35.2% disagreement with the histological categories of mild, moderate and severe dysplasia. In a subsequent parallel study [25] the same authors used a similar classification rule to separate reliably (> 96%) and reproducibly (maximum intra- and interobserver coefficients of variation: 5 and 8%) ulcer-associated regenerative hyperplasia and cancer-associated severe dysplasia. The rule performed equally well in both training and test sets. They also stated that quantitation advocated two groups of dysplasia: low-grade and high-grade, the latter with a significant risk of cancer development. The virtue of combining stereological and morphometric data in assessing gastric dysplasia has also been stressed elsewhere [26].

In a densitometric analysis of Feulgen-stained sections of gastric hyperplastic and adenomatous polyps, nuclear area was measured in the lesion and its adjacent normal mucosa [27]. Higher values occurred in the adenomas than the hyperplastic polyps. There were also significantly greater differences found between the adenomas with severe dysplasia and those associated with invasive growth and their adjacent mucosae.

Danno [28] used morphometry to interpret gastric cytological smears and emphasized the importance of nuclear cytoplasmic ratio in separating benign and malignant epithelium. Subsequently Boon *et al.* [29] measured nuclear perimeter and area, cell perimeter and area, nuclear cytoplasmic ratio and their standard deviations. A discriminant function using mean nuclear cytoplasmic ratio and the standard deviation of nuclear area gave 100% correct classification of 33 test cases of known histology. In a test set of 39 cytologically difficult cases there were no false positives and only two false negatives. They suggested that morphometry could therefore be constructively applied in diagnoses where 25 cells or more are available for study. A further report [30] separating benign and malignant gastric epithelium adopted a more sophisticated densitometric analytical approach. It generated a three-dimensional cell image in which morphometric shape factors were represented by the *x*- and *y*-axes while the cell light absorbance (a quantitative measurement of features related to nuclear texture, e.g., hyperchromasia, irregularity of chromatin pattern) constituted the *z*-axis. There was perfect distinction of benign and malignant cases, with nuclear staining intensity and parameters corresponding to cell size being of most importance.

The morphometric characteristics of gastric carcinoma show that quantitative differences exist between the categories of the World Health Organization (WHO) classification and intestinal and diffuse carcinomas (Lauren's classification) [31]. Schmitz-Moormann *et al.* [32] measured tumour size and volume, inflammatory cell counts, and also quantified stromal infiltration and peritumoural fibrosis using stereology. Nodal staging and Lauren's classification were important prognostic indicators but none of the other measured parameters was related to patient survival. In a detailed study of gastric carcinoma Hamilton *et al.* [33] combined semiautomatic image analysis with flow cytometry. Morphometric analysis of nuclear and cellular features was found to be objective and reproducible but of little help in predicting patient survival. Nuclear size was however greater in intestinal than diffuse carcinomas and in tumours that showed a more advanced degree of local infiltrative and lymphatic spread. It was not directly associated with the DNA proliferative index and could not identify those tumours which were DNA aneuploid in nature.

Sections of gastric carcinoma have been stained with a monoclonal antibody to PCNA as a means of assessing tumour proliferation status [34]. The PCNA index (percentage of positive cells per 1000 tumour cells) and a semiquantitative PCNA grading system (< or > 50% positive cells in tissue sections) were compared. Neither correlated with histological variables, tumour stage, lymph node involvement or flow cytometry S-phase fraction. However, patients with a high PCNA index had a worse prognosis and those with a low PCNA grade had better survival. PCNA grade emerged more strongly from the analysis, perhaps because it allowed for intratumoural variation better than absolute cell counts.

4.1.4 Large intestine

Diverticular disease and neuromuscular abnormalities

In diverticulosis the widths of both muscle layers are greatly increased and in the taeniae coli this is due to an increase in the number and circumferential pericellular distribution of elastin fibrils [35]. This leads to diminished colonic wall compliance, shortening and compensatory thickening of the circular coat. The lumen diameter decreases and there are short segments of high intraluminal pressure between opposed circular muscle folds, resulting in the formation of diverticular pouches. Mucosal herniation and measurable thickening of the muscularis layers are also noted in chronic inflammatory bowel disease [36].

Simple morphometric techniques based on ganglion and nerve fibre counts have contributed to the understanding and diagnosis of the neuromuscular disorder Hirschsprung's disease and its related variants, such as aganglionosis and neuronal colonic dysplasia [37–39].

Chronic inflammatory bowel disease

Insights into the pathogenesis of ulcerative colitis and Crohn's disease have arisen from quantifying cell populations and their functions [40]. Enumerating immunoglobulin-containing cells in mucosal biopsies is a relatively simple and reproducible procedure [41]. It shows immunocyte numbers in diseased bowel to be increased by a factor of four, mainly due to a 30-fold increase in immunoglobulin G (IgG)-containing cells [42]. Others [43] have obtained similar results and also confirmed elevated plasma cell counts to varying extents in the different immunoglobulin classes [44]. The total mucosal counts correlate with the level of disease activity [45] and are predominantly IgG B cells [46]. It is postulated that antigen exposure leads to a local immune response and that these antibodies in turn may cocontribute to disease pathogenesis by immune cross-reactivity or complex formation [40]. There is variation in the reporting of the distribution of immunoglobulin classes in Crohn's disease and ulcerative colitis and as to whether these profiles aid in their discrimination [41,47,48].

Both automated [49] and semiautomatic [50] morphometric procedures allow the quantitation of tissue components and cell populations in colonic biopsies. The number and type of immunoglobulin-containing cells [51], total mucosal cellularity and the distribution of inflammatory cells within the lamina propria [50] help to differentiate between normal mucosa, acute infectious colitis and chronic inflammatory bowel disease. Bacterial colitis shows a preferential increase in IgA-producing plasma cells [45,51]. Crohn's disease and ulcerative colitis have increased cellularity with disproportionately heavy mononuclear inflammation in the deepest one-third of the mucosa [50], consisting of IgG and IgA immunocytes [51]. Lamina propria mononuclear inflammatory cell densities are greater in distal proctocolitis than in extensive or left-sided colitis [52]. This has led to the suggestion that distal proctocolitis results from a more intense immune response, which leads to localization of the disease in that part of the bowel. Eosinophil numbers have been postulated as an index of activity [53] and prognosis in proctocolitis [54]. A Quantimet study of goblet cell mucin content has confirmed that it is diminished more in ulcerative colitis than in Crohn's disease [55].

Using graticule measurements clinical improvement in colitis correlates with normalization of architectural variables such as mucous membrane thickness, crypt depth and epithelial height [56]. Normal mucosa, ulcerative colitis in remission and chronic active disease score differently on assessment of features such as glandular lumen diameter, gland density and the linear space of lamina propria between consecutive glands [57,58]. Inflamed mucosa has enlarged, sparse glands set in abundant lamina propria [59]. Image analysis has shown the ratios of surface to mucosal lengths and surface to crypt epithelial heights, in combination with lamina propria cellularity, to be highly predictive for chronic inflammatory bowel disease [50]. An interesting extension of this has been the monitoring of some of these parameters in active disease and ulcerative colitis in remission as a means of comparing the response to and efficacy of oral 5-amino-salicylic acid and rectal prednisolone treatment [60]. Surface villus regeneration, which is one of the most reproducible biopsy criteria for assessing ulcerative colitis [61,62] has been confirmed with an increase in mucosal height [63] due predominantly to inflammatory expansion of the lamina propria [64] and also in the surface to mucosal length ratio [50]. Surface ulceration and crypt regeneration are emphasized by decreased surface and increased crypt epithelial heights [63]. This study also reflected the difficulty in separating quantitatively ulcerative colitis and Crohn's disease.

Collagenous and lymphocytic colitis

Collagenous colitis denotes a clinical syndrome of chronic watery diarrhoea associated with thickening of the mucosal subepithelial collagen table [65]. The normal collagen layer is elaborated by the pericryptal fibroblast sheath and measures up to 7 μm [66]. In collagenous colitis this thickness can increase up to 50 μm and it appears as an eosinophilic subepithelial hyaline band [67]. A suggested pathogenetic mechanism is that it causes a barrier to water absorption [65], but its exact relationship to the aetiology of chronic diarrhoea remains uncertain [68].

There is a further group of patients with chronic diarrhoea who have normal endoscopic findings but mucosal inflammatory changes on biopsy. The term microscopic or lymphocytic colitis has been coined and its features recently quantified [69]. Its possible relationship to collagenous colitis and coeliac-associated colonic lymphocytosis [70] is further discussed by Yardley *et al.* [71].

Transitional mucosa

Transitional mucosa consists of elongated, branched glandular crypts with dilated goblet cells containing alcian blue-staining sialomucins instead of the usual high iron diamine-positive sulphomucins [72]. Its significance is controversial [73] with two main lines of interpretation. It is regarded as an early premalignant change due to its frequent occurrence in the mucosa adjacent to colorectal carcinoma [74]. A corollary to this has been recommendation of its detection in biopsy surveillance of patients with chronic ulcerative colitis [75]. Alternatively it may be secondary to mucosal inflammation, ischaemia or prolapse, and present in conjunction with dysplastic or malignant tissues as a consequence of maturation from them [76]. Quantitation shows an increased mucosal height in transitional mucosa: range 0.8–2 mm [77], normal range 0.5–0.8 mm [78]. Densitometry confirms goblet cell *O*-acyl sialomucin levels intermediate between those of normal mucosa and carcinoma [79]. Analysis of multiple nuclear and cellular variables failed to show any differences from control mucosa or the trend encountered in other premalignant colonic conditions (see below) and could therefore not support transitional mucosa as an early neoplastic change [77]. Other workers have shown quantitative differences at both architectural [80] and cytological levels [81], but no increase in either the Ki-67 proliferative or enzyme markers that might suggest a higher than expected risk for malignant change [80].

Epithelial dysplasia

This precancerous mucosal lesion has a variable potential for progression to adenocarcinoma. It is commonly encountered in sporadic adenomas, familial adenomatous polyposis and in a small proportion of patients with chronic ulcerative colitis. Its recognition and grade assessment are subject to wide inter- and intraobserver variation [82,83]. Morphometry has been studied as a means to reducing this.

Adenomas

Adenoma formation is postulated as glandular growth due to the infolding of proliferating surface epithelium between normal, pre-existing glands. The proliferative region in normal mucosa is confined to the lower one-third of the crypt. In patients with colonic polyps incorporation of the thymidine analogue bromodeoxyuridine shows a higher labelling index in the polyps and also an expansion of the proliferative compartment of the intervening mucosa [84]. This has also been confirmed by assessing the proliferation antigen Ki-67 [85]. In villous adenomas there is also a similar shift with extension of both epithelial and mesenchymal proliferation to the crypt neck, resulting in upwards papillary projections [86]. Stereological [87] and scanning electron microscopic studies of adenoma [88] confirm this, showing an increased epithelial surface area thrown into villi consisting of branched folia and intervening crypts. Low-resolution image analysis can separate normal mucosa, adenomas and adenocarcinoma using the following variables: the minimum diameter of glands, minimum distance between and the number of neighbouring glands, and area and circumference of glands [89]. This can also be achieved by ultrastructural analysis of nuclear size [90]. Morphometric features shown to exhibit a trend between the varying grades of dysplasia in adenomas are nuclear cytoplasmic ratio, nuclear size variation and stratification [82,91].

The dysplasia–carcinoma sequence [92] is highlighted by the greater likelihood of malignant change where adenomas are multiple [93], >2 cm in diameter (50% malignancy rate) and show a villous architecture and severe dysplasia [92]. These features are also more likely to be associated with DNA aneuploidy [94], which in turn is more frequently encountered with increasing lesional nuclear size [95]. Therefore, quantitation of adenomas can lead to more consistent grading and identification of those most likely to contain carcinoma. This is highlighted by Rubio and Porwit-McDonald [96], who found that the mean nuclear area increased significantly along the following spectrum: hyperplastic polyps, hamartomatous polyps, tubular/villous adenomas with low-grade dysplasia and tubular/villous adenomas with high-grade dysplasia. The nuclear area in villous adenomas with invasive growth was significantly higher than in all other adenomas without invasive growth ($P < 0.001$). Discriminating nuclear differences in various grades of adenoma have also been described using syntactic structure analysis [97].

Studies of the mucosa and polyps in familial adenomatous polyposis have mostly related to work on cell proliferation using tritiated thymidine [98] or flow cytometry [99].

Ulcerative colitis with dysplasia and carcinoma

Tritiated thymidine [100], stathmokinetic [101] and Ki-67 [102] studies have shown ulcerative colitis to be a hyperproliferative epithelial condition. Patients with long-standing disease have an increased risk of mucosal dysplasia and carcinoma [103,104]. The designation of this dysplasia is subject to observer variation, with distinction from regenerative hyperplasia sometimes being difficult, although this is important in patient follow-up and treatment [83] (Fig. 4.1). Image analysis of multiple nuclear and cellular geometric variables gives an insight into the morphologic differences between histological groups and allows the construction of classification rules in an attempt to achieve more accurate and reproducible categorization of individual lesions. Analysis of normal mucosa, regenerative hyperplasia, dysplasia and carcinoma in ulcerative colitis identified variables such as nuclear size, stratification, shape, polarity and nuclear cytoplasmic ratio as those subjective features that are useful in making the histological diagnosis [105]. Discriminant analysis reduced the variables and used them to construct an allocation rule or scoring system. In this way normal colorectal mucosa and adenocarcinoma were perfectly separated [106] (Fig. 4.2a). The system was verified against a test set and then applied to colitic mucosa [105]. This grouped high-grade dysplasia with adenocarcinoma and led to the intermediate placement of regeneration and low-grade dysplasia. The close association between high-grade dysplasia and adenocarcinoma (Fig. 4.2b) suggests a possible role for quantitation in confirming such a diagnosis as it is an indication for colectomy. The overlap between regeneration and low-grade dysplasia emphasizes the continuous morphological spectrum that exists and the necessity of also taking into account inflammatory and architectural changes. The latter component was quantified in a parallel low-power image analysis study [64]. The classification rule based on epithelial height and lamina propria area completely separated normal mucosa, regeneration and high-grade dysplasia (Fig. 4.3a). Subsequently the same authors [107] incorporated stereological parameters into a combined architectural and cytological assessment. Variables describing nuclear size and

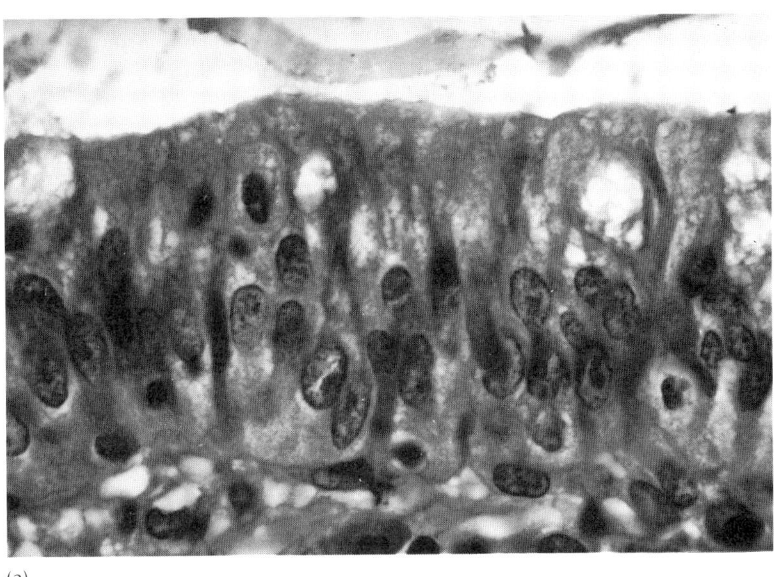

(a)

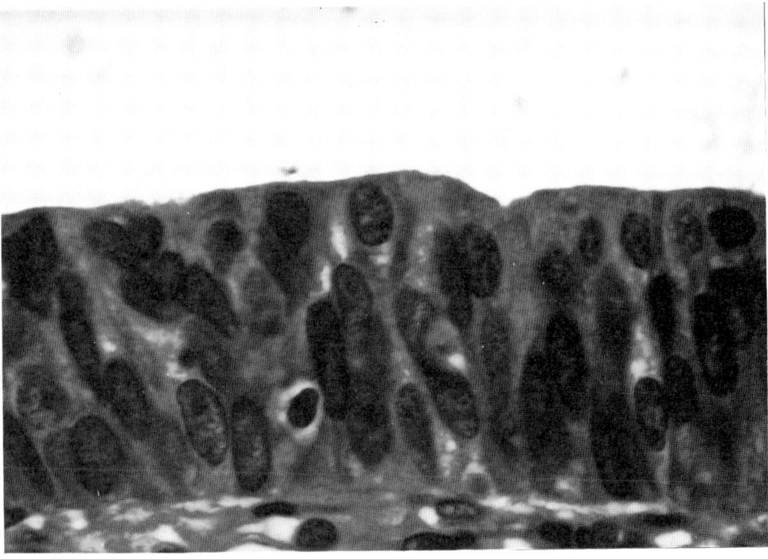

(b)

Fig. 4.1 (a) Ulcerative colitis: mucosa negative for dysplasia. There is nuclear enlargement, crowding and stratification with an open chromatin pattern and prominent nucleoli. (b) Ulcerative colitis: mucosa positive for dysplasia, high grade. There is nuclear enlargement, crowding and stratification of the full epithelial width. Nuclear chromatin is coarsened. From Allen *et al.* [105].

stratification, epithelial height and crypt crowding were emphasized to varying extents. Bayesian decision boundary lines were also superimposed on the bivariate scatter plots of the discriminant scores (Fig. 4.3b) and probability densities calculated to estimate the likelihood of histological group membership. This refinement on the previous work improved the separation of low- and high-grade dysplasia, although some overlap was still evident. The system needs further validation before it can be employed as a quantitative index in the classification of biopsy material.

Adenocarcinoma

Light and electron microscopic quantitation is capable of separating normal colorectal mucosa and adenocarcinoma. Significant discriminating

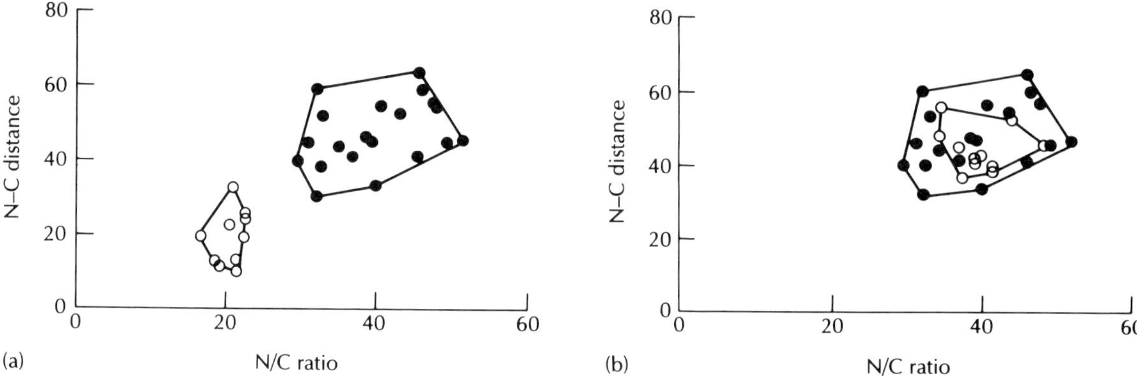

Fig. 4.2 Scatter plots of the discriminating variables mean nuclear cytoplasmic ratio (N/C ratio) against coefficient of variation of nucleus to cell apex distance (N–C distance) in ulcerative colitis for: (a) normal colorectal mucosa (○) and adenocarcinoma (●); and (b) high-grade dysplasia (○) and adenocarcinoma (●). (a) From Hamilton *et al.* [106] and (b) from Allen *et al.* [105].

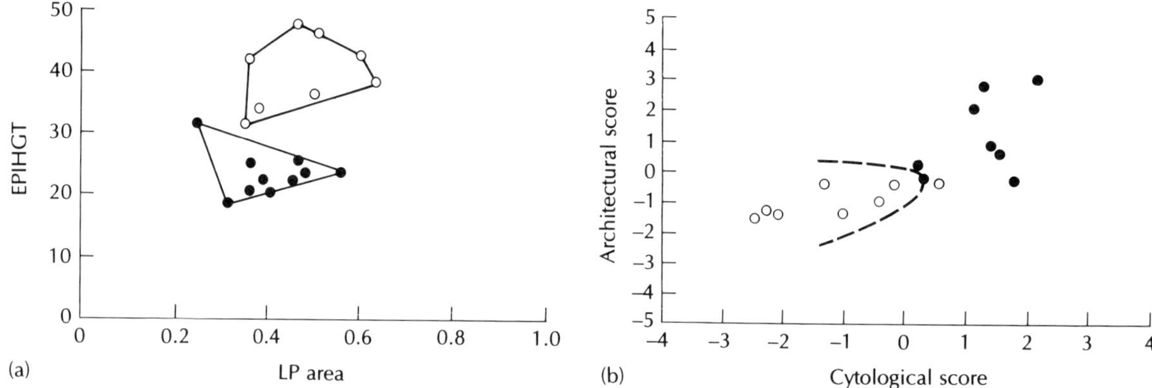

Fig. 4.3 (a) Scatter plot of the discriminating variables lamina propria area per unit length of muscularis mucosae (LP area) against epithelial height (EPIHGT) in ulcerative colitis for regenerative changes (●) and high-grade dysplasia (○). (b) Scatter plot of low-grade dysplasia (○) and high-grade dysplasia (●) scores showing separation of cases. The position of the Bayesian decision boundary is shown. (a) From Allen *et al.* [64] and (b) from Hamilton *et al.* [107].

variables are nuclear volume and nuclear cytoplasmic ratio [108] and a combination of the latter with measures of nuclear stratification [106]. In this study discrimination was achieved with high reproducibility by an observer with minimal histological knowledge who was unaware of the diagnosis. Sato *et al.* [90] have shown a trend of nuclear and nucleolar enlargement correlating with malignant transformation from normal mucosa through dysplasia to carcinoma. They postulated a possible role for the quantitative diagnosis of epithelial lesions by measuring the area of 50 nuclei and their nucleoli.

Bufo *et al.* [109] used an automatic video shape analytical morphometry (SAM) system to compare adenomas with severe dysplasia, normal mucosa and carcinoma. They found statistically significant differences between the diagnostic groups in relation to nuclear quantitative and shape-descriptor parameters. In another study using similar material and techniques [110] there was further morphometric (nuclear size), densitometric (DNA content) and textural (chromatin pattern) confirmation of the dysplasia–carcinoma sequence. This group are evaluating use of their preliminary data to categorize prospectively endoscopic cytology smears as an aid to preoperative diagnosis.

In established colorectal adenocarcinoma, Lowe *et al.* [111] noted a DNA aneuploidy rate of 51% in a group of Dukes' stage B carcinomas. Morphometric differences from the DNA diploid tumours were in the mean nuclear profile area (62.9 vs 48.2 μm^2; $P < 0.001$) and the percentage of large nuclei in a given carcinoma (6.2 vs 1%; $P < 0.001$). Their findings allowed the construction of a simple algorithm to determine nuclear size by a single linear graticule measurement taken over six fields. This gave a 74% accurate prediction of DNA ploidy status and it was recommended for use in routine histological assessment. Morphometry has been studied as a prognostic indicator in 'curative' resection for colorectal adenocarcinoma using ocular micrometers [112] and semiautomatic image analysis [113,114]. Ambros *et al.* [112] found that patient outcome correlated with serosal involvement, the number of diseased lymph nodes, and the tumour cell mean nuclear area. The most important predictor of patient survival was the number of involved nodes but this also showed significant colinearity with nuclear area. Deans *et al.* [113] studied a series of 312 patients with a minimum follow-up of 5 years. Multivariate survival analysis showed that no morphometric parameter significantly added to a prognostic model consisting of patient age, Dukes' stage and tumour differentiation. Nuclear shape varied with tumour differentiation but did not relate to survival.

Carter *et al.* [114] showed a strong correlation between the variation in tumour cell nuclear size and both the character of the invasive margin and extent of local spread (Dukes' stage). Morphometry was only able to distinguish between groups 1 and 2 of a four-tier prognostic system which scores depth of local spread, the number of involved nodes, character of the invasive margin and the presence of peritumoural lymphocytic infiltration [115]. It appears to give broadly similar prognostic information to the traditional Dukes' staging [116]. Interestingly, one of the components of Jass's index is the degree of peritumoural lymphocyte infiltration. Several other authors have also noted beneficial prognostic significance of increased tumoural densities of eosinophils, plasma cells and mast cells – presumably a manifestation of local immune response [117,118]. Morphometry of cytological scrapings has shown that the nuclear cytoplasmic ratio is better than nuclear area in distinguishing adenomas, locally irradiated bowel and recurrences in the postoperative follow-up of rectal carcinoma [119]. The PCNA proliferation index is significantly elevated in cancers and their adjacent mucosa in patients who died compared with survivors [120].

Stromal tumours

Irrespective of their site within the gastrointestinal tract, suggested predictors of behaviour are tumour size ($>$ 7.5 cm), mitotic count ($>$ three per 10 high-power fields; HPFs) and DNA aneuploidy [121]. Morphometric measurements do not refine this any further [122].

4.1.5 Conclusion

Quantitation of cell populations and geometric features in gastrointestinal disease has increased our understanding of the pathogenesis and morphology of idiopathic inflammatory bowel disease, infective proctocolitis, collagenous colitis, gastric dysplasia and premalignant colorectal adenomas. Its main applications have been in grading of dysplasia and the search for prognostic factors in established disease. In the former it has confirmed the dysplasia–cancer sequence and shown the difficulty in subdividing what is a morphologic spectrum. However, it has given important insights into the relative weight given to the various subjective features used in histological diagnosis. This should result in a more analytical, standardized and hopefully reproducible assessment combining cytological and architectural components. In gastrointestinal adenocarcinoma the most important factor affecting prognosis remains depth of local spread and nodal status. It appears to relate to tumour cell nuclear size and it remains to be seen if more detailed morphometric and proliferation studies will result in a multiparameter prognostic index that will more truly reflect the biology of gut cancer.

References

1 Shabana AHM, El-Labban NG, Lee KW. Morphometric analysis of basal cell layer in oral premalignant white lesions and squamous cell carcinoma. *J Clin Pathol* 1987; 40: 454–458.

2 Barry JD, Sharkey FE. Morphometric grading of squamous cell carcinoma. *Histopathology* 1986; 10: 1143–1152.

3 Helliwell TR, Atkinson MW, Cooke TG, Cooke LD, Stell PM. Morphometric analysis, ploidy and response to chemotherapy in squamous carcinomas of the head and neck. *Pathol Res Pract* 1989; 185: 755–759.

4 Barrett NR. The lower oesophagus lined by columnar epithelium. *Surgery* 1957; 41: 881–894.

5 Haggitt RC, Tryzelaar J, Ellis FH, Colcher H. Adenocarcinoma complicating columnar epithelium-lined (Barrett's) esophagus. *Am J Clin Pathol* 1978; 70: 1–5.

6 Pellish LJ, Hermos JA, Eastwood GL. Cell proliferation in three types of Barrett's epithelium. *Gut* 1980; 21: 26–31.

7 Lindholm J, Rubio CA, Kato Y, Hata J. A morphometric method to discriminate normal from dysplastic/carcinoma *in situ* squamous epithelium in the human esophagus. *Pathol Res Pract* 1989; 184: 297–305.

8 Stephens JK, Bibbo M, Dytch M, Maiorana A, Ruol A, Little AG. Correlation between automated karyometric measurements of squamous cell carcinoma of the esophagus and histopathologic and clinical features. *Cancer* 1989; 64: 83–87.

9 Darnton SJ, Allen SM, Edwards CN, Matthews HR. Histological findings in oesophageal carcinoma with and without preoperative chemotherapy. *J Clin Pathol* 1993; 46: 51–55.

10 Sasano H, Miyazaki S, Gooukon Y, Nishihira T, Sawai T, Nagura H. Expression of p53 in human esophageal carcinoma: an immunohistochemical study with correlation to proliferating cell nuclear antigen expression. *Hum Pathol* 1992; 23: 1238–1243.

11 Ming SC, Goldman H, Freiman DG. Intestinal metaplasia and histogenesis of carcinoma in human stomach. Light and electron microscopic study. *Cancer* 1967; 20: 1418–1429.

12 Correa P. A human model of gastric carcinogenesis. *Cancer Res* 1988; 48: 3554–3560.

13 Jass JR, Filipe MI. Sulphomucins and precancerous lesions of the human stomach. *Histopathology* 1980; 4: 271–279.

14 Filipe MI, Edwards MR, Ehsanullah M. A prospective study of dysplasia and carcinoma in the rectal biopsies and rectal stump of eight patients following ileorectal anastomosis in ulcerative colitis. *Histopathology* 1985; 9: 1139–1153.

15 Rubio CA, Lindholm J, Rodensjo M. Mapping intestinal metaplasia by histochemistry and morphometry. *Pathol Res Pract* 1989; 184: 525–528.

16 Rubio CA, Porwit-McDonald A, Rodensjo M, Duvander A. A method of quantitating Paneth cell metaplasia of the stomach by image analysis. *Anal Quant Cytol Histol* 1989; 11: 115–118.

17 Rubio CA, Saraga EP, Lindholm J. Improved method for mapping gastric intestinal metaplasia using selective histochemical morphometry. *Anal Quant Cytol Histol* 1990; 12: 122–126.

18 Tosi P, Filipe MI, Baak JP *et al.* Morphometric definition and grading of gastric intestinal metaplasia. *J Pathol* 1990; 161: 201–208.

19 Morson BC, Sobin LH, Grundmann E, Johansen A, Nagayo T, Serck-Hanssen A. Precancerous conditions and epithelial dysplasia in the stomach. *J Clin Pathol* 1980; 33: 711–721.

20 Nakamura T, Nakano GI. Histopathological classification and malignant change in gastric polyps. *J Clin Pathol* 1985; 38: 754–764.

21 Oehlert W, Keller P, Henke M, Strauch M. Gastric mucosal dysplasia: what is its clinical significance? *Front Gastrointest Res* 1979; 4: 173–182.

22 Rubio CA, Kato Y, Sugano H. The intramucosal cysts of the stomach in Japanese subjects having focal (elevated) dysplasia. *Gan* 1983; 7: 391–397.

23 Jarvis LR, Whitehead R. Morphometric analysis of gastric dysplasia. *J Pathol* 1985; 47: 133–138.

24 Tosi P, Luzi P, Baak JPA *et al.* Gastric dysplasia: a stereological and morphometrical assessment. *J Pathol* 1987; 152: 83–94.

25 Tosi P, Baak JPA, Luzi P, Miracco C, Lio R, Barbini P. Morphometric distinction of low- and high-grade dysplasias in gastric biopsies. *Hum Pathol* 1989; 20: 839–844.

26 Yan RF, Zhang YC, Wu YQ. Morphometric indexes and computerized diagnosis of gastric dysplasia. *Proc Chin Acad Med Sci Peking* 1989; 4: 43–47.

27 Rubio CA, May I. A method for quantitating the nuclear area of gastric polyps using image analysis. *Anal Quant Cytol Histol* 1990; 12: 117–121.

28 Danno M. Statistical criteria for the cytology of gastric cancer. A proposal of distance index. *Acta Cytol* 1975; 20: 466–468.

29 Boon ME, Kurver PHJ, Baak JPA, Thompson HT. The application of morphometry in gastric cytological diagnosis. *Virchows Arch Pathol Anat* 1981; 393: 159–164.

30 Weinreb M, Zajicek G, Levij IS. Discrimination between normal and malignant gastric epithelial cells by computer image analysis. *Anal Quant Cytol* 1984; 6: 206–210.

31 Wolf B, Muller E, Schwinde A. An ultrastructural morphometric analysis on ultrathin epon and ultrathin cryosections of normal human gastric tissue and human gastric cancer. *Virchows Arch Pathol Anat* 1985; 407: 209–219.

32 Schmitz-Moormann P, Pohl C, Huttich C, Himmelmann GW. Prediction of prognosis in patients with gastric cancer by quantitative morphology and multivariate analysis. *Scand J Gastroenterol* 1987; 22(suppl 133): 58–62.
33 Hamilton PW, Wyatt JI, Quirke P *et al.* Morphometry of gastric carcinoma: its association with patient survival, tumour stage and DNA ploidy. *J Pathol* 1992; 168: 201–208.
34 Jain S, Filipe MI, Hall PA, Waseem N, Lane DP, Levison DA. Prognostic value of proliferating cell nuclear antigen in gastric carcinoma. *J Clin Pathol* 1991; 44: 655–659.
35 Whiteway J, Morson BC. Elastosis in diverticular disease of the sigmoid colon. *Gut* 1985; 26: 258–266.
36 Allen DC, Biggart JD. Misplaced epithelium in ulcerative colitis and Crohn's disease of the colon and its relationship to malignant mucosal changes. *Histopathology* 1986; 10: 37–52.
37 Meier-Ruge W. Hirschsprung's disease: its aetiology, pathogenesis and differential diagnosis. In: Grundmann E, Kirstein WH (eds) *Current Topics in Pathology*, vol. 59. Berlin: Springer, 1974: 131–179.
38 Risdon RA, Malone M. Paediatric gastrointestinal disease. In: Anthony PP, MacSween RNM (eds) *Recent Advances in Histopathology*, vol. 14. Edinburgh: Churchill Livingstone, 1989: 223–249.
39 Heitz PU, Komminoth P. Biopsy diagnosis of Hirschsprung's disease and related disorders. In: Williams GT (ed.) *Current Topics in Pathology*, vol. 81. Berlin: Springer, 1990: 257–276.
40 MacDermott RP. Symposium on cell mediated immunity in human disease. Part II. Cell mediated immunity in gastrointestinal disease. *Hum Pathol* 1986; 17: 219–233.
41 Seldenrijk CA, Hendriks J, Smeulders AWM *et al.* Reproducibility of counting immunoglobulin-containing cells in colonic mucosal biopsies. *Anal Quant Cytol Histol* 1988; 10: 94–100.
42 Brandtzaeg P, Baklien KI, Fausa O, Hoel PS. Immunohistochemical characterisation of local immunoglobulin formation in ulcerative colitis. *Gastroenterology* 1974; 66: 1123–1136.
43 Keren DF, Appelman HD, Dobbins WO *et al.* Correlation of histopathologic evidence of disease activity with the presence of immunoglobulin-containing cells in the colons of patients with inflammatory bowel disease. *Hum Pathol* 1984; 15: 757–763.
44 Rosekrans PCM, Meijer CJLM, van der Wal AM, Cornelisse CJ, Lindeman J. Immunoglobulin containing cells in inflammatory bowel disease of the colon: a morphometric and immunohistochemical study. *Gut* 1980; 21: 941–947.
45 Scott BB, Goodall A, Stephenson P, Jenkins D. Rectal mucosal plasma cells in inflammatory bowel disease. *Gut* 1983; 24: 519–524.
46 Strickland RG, Husby G, Black WC, Williams RC Jr. Peripheral blood and intestinal lymphocyte subpopulations in Crohn's disease. *Gut* 1975; 16: 847–853.
47 Seldenrijk CA, Meuwissen SGM, Schipper NW, Morson BC, Lindeman J, Meijer CJLM. Value of counting colonic mucosal Ig-containing cells in the differential diagnosis of chronic inflammatory bowel disease. *J Clin Pathol* 1992; 45: 241–247.
48 van Spreeuwel JP, Meijer CJLM, Rosekrans PCM, Lindeman J. Immunoglobulin containing cells in gastrointestinal pathology — diagnostic applications. *Pathol Ann* 1986; 21: 295–310.
49 Salzmann JL, Peltier-Koch F, Bloch F, Petite JP, Camilleri JP. Morphometric study of colonic biopsies: a new method of estimating inflammatory disease. *Lab Invest* 1989; 60: 847–851.
50 Jenkins D, Goodall A, Drew K, Scott BB. What is colitis? Statistical approach to distinguishing clinically important inflammatory change in rectal biopsy specimens. *J Clin Pathol* 1988; 41: 72–79.
51 van Spreeuwel JP, Lindeman J, Meijer CJLM. A quantitative study of immunoglobulin containing cells in the differential diagnosis of acute colitis. *J Clin Pathol* 1985; 38: 774–777.
52 Jenkins D, Goodall AI, Scott BB. Ulcerative colitis: one disease or two? (Quantitative histological differences between distal and extensive disease.) *Gut* 1990; 31: 426–430.
53 Sarin SK, Malhotra VS, Gupta S, Karol A, Gaur SK, Anand BS. Significance of eosinophil and mast cell counts in rectal mucosa in ulcerative colitis. A prospective controlled study. *Dig Dis Sci* 32: 363–367.
54 Heatley RV, James PD. Eosinophils in the rectal mucosa. A simple method of predicting the outcome of ulcerative proctocolitis? *Gut* 1979; 20: 787–791.
55 McCormick DA, Horton LWL, Mee AS. Mucin depletion in inflammatory bowel disease. *J Clin Pathol* 1990; 43: 143–146.
56 Nogaller AM, Nikonenko TH, Averina TK. Clinicomorphological and morphometric characteristics of chronic colitis. *Klin Med (Mosk)* 1983; 61: 82–88.
57 Rubio CA, Johansson C, Kock Y. A quantitative method of estimating inflammation in the rectal mucosa. II. Normal limits in symptomatic patients. *Scand J Gastroenterol* 1982; 17: 1077–1081.
58 Rubio CA, Johansson C, Uribe A, Kock Y. A quantitative method of estimating inflammation in the rectal mucosa. IV. Ulcerative colitis in remission. *Scand J Gastroenterol* 1984; 19: 525–530.
59 Rubio CA, Johannson C, Kock Y. A quantitative method of estimating inflammation in the rectal mucosa. III. Chronic ulcerative colitis. *Scand J Gastroenterol* 1982; 17: 1083–1087.
60 Zaitoun AM, Cobden I, Al Mardini H, Record CO. Morphometric studies in rectal biopsy specimens from patients with ulcerative colitis: effect of oral 5 amino salicylic acid and rectal prednisolone treatment. *Gut* 1991; 32: 183–187.
61 Surawicz CM, Belic L. Rectal biopsy helps to

distinguish acute self-limited colitis from idiopathic inflammatory bowel disease. *Gastroenterology* 1984; 86: 104–113.
62 Dundas SAC, Kay R, Beck S *et al.* Can histopathologists reliably assess dysplasia in inflammatory bowel disease? *J Clin Pathol* 1987; 40: 1282–1286.
63 Thompson EM, Price AB, Altman DG, Sowter C, Slavin G. Quantitation in inflammatory bowel disease using computerised interactive image analysis. *J Clin Pathol* 1985; 38: 631–638.
64 Allen DC, Hamilton PW, Watt PCH, Biggart JD. Architectural morphometry in ulcerative colitis with dysplasia. *Histopathology* 1988; 12: 611–621.
65 Lindstrom CG. 'Collagenous colitis' with watery diarrhoea: a new entity? *Pathol Eur* 1976; 11: 87–89.
66 Gardiner GW, Goldborg R, Currie D, Murray D. Colonic carcinoma associated with an abnormal collagen table. *Cancer* 1984; 54: 2973–2977.
67 Nielsen VT, Vetner M, Harslof E. Collagenous colitis. *Histopathology* 1980; 4: 83–86.
68 Williams GT, Rhodes J. Collagenous colitis: disease or diversion? *Br Med J* 1987; 294: 855–856.
69 Lazenby AJ, Yardley JH, Giardiello FM, Jessurun J, Bayless TM. Lymphocytic ('microscopic') colitis: a comparative histopathologic study with particular reference to collagenous colitis. *Hum Pathol* 1989; 20: 18–28.
70 Wolber R, Owen D, Freeman H. Colonic lymphocytosis in patients with celiac sprue. *Hum Pathol* 1990; 21: 1092–1096.
71 Yardley JH, Lazenby AJ, Giardiello FM, Bayless TM. Collagenous, 'microscopic', lymphocytic, and other gentler and more subtle forms of colitis. *Hum Pathol* 1990; 11: 1089–1091.
72 Filipe MI. Value of histochemical reactions for mucosubstances in the diagnosis of certain pathological conditions of the colon and rectum. *Gut* 1969; 10: 577–586.
73 Williams GT. Commentary. Transitional mucosa of the large intestine. *Histopathology* 1985; 9: 1237–1243.
74 Filipe MI. Mucins of normal, premalignant and malignant colonic mucosa. In: Wolman SR, Mastromarina AJ (eds) *Progress in Cancer Research and Therapy*, vol. 29. New York: Raven, 1984: 237–251.
75 Filipe MI, Potet F, Bogolometz WV *et al.* Incomplete sulphomucin-secreting intestinal metaplasia for gastric cancer. Preliminary data from a perspective study from three centres. *Gut* 1985; 26: 1319–1326.
76 Allen DC, Connolly NS, Biggart JD. High iron diamine–alcian blue mucin profiles in benign, premalignant and malignant colorectal disease. *Histopathology* 1988; 13: 399–412.
77 Hamilton PW, Watt PCH, Allen DC. A morphometrical assessment of transitional mucosa in the colon. *Histopathology* 1988; 13: 519–530.
78 Saffos RO, Rhatigan RM. Benign (non-polypoid) mucosal changes adjacent to carcinoma of the colon. *Hum Pathol* 1977; 8: 441–449.
79 Dawson PA, Patel J, Filipe MI. Variation in sialomucins in the mucosa of the large intestine in malignancy: a quantimet and statistical analysis. *Histochem J* 1978; 10: 559–572.
80 Lawson MJ, White LM, Coyle P, Butler RN, Roberts-Thomson IC, Conyers RA. An assessment of proliferative and enzyme activity in transitional mucosa adjacent to colonic cancer. *Cancer* 1989; 64: 1061–1066.
81 Bibbo M, Michelassi F, Bartels PH *et al.* Karyometric marker features in normal-appearing glands adjacent to human colonic adenocarcinoma. *Cancer Res* 1990; 50: 147–151.
82 Brown LJR, Smeeton NC, Dixon MF. Assessment of dysplasia in colorectal adenomas: an observer variation and morphometric study. *J Clin Pathol* 1985; 38: 174–179.
83 Riddell RH, Goldman H, Ransohoff DF *et al.* Dysplasia in inflammatory bowel disease: standardized classification with provisional clinical applications. *Hum Pathol* 1983; 14: 931–968.
84 Wilson RG, Smith AN, Bird CC. Immunohistochemical detection of abnormal cell proliferation in colonic mucosa of subjects with polyps. *J Clin Pathol* 1990; 43: 744–747.
85 Johnston PG, O'Brien MJ, Dervan PA, Carney DN. Immunohistochemical analysis of cell kinetic parameters in colonic adenocarcinomas, adenomas, and normal mucosa. *Hum Pathol* 1989; 20: 696–700.
86 Maskens AP. Histogenesis of adenomatous polyps in the human large intestine. *Gastroenterology* 1979; 77: 1245–1251.
87 Elias H, Hyde DM, Mullens RS, Lambert FC. Colonic adenomas: stereology and growth mechanisms. *Dis Colon Rectum* 1981; 24: 331–342.
88 Phelps PC, Toker C, Trump BF. Surface ultrastructure of normal, adenomatous and malignant epithelium from human colon. *Scan Electron Microsc* 1979; 3: 169–176.
89 Kayser KK, Modlinger F, Postl K. Quantitative low-resolution analysis of colon mucosa. *Anal Quant Cytol Histol* 1985; 7: 205–212.
90 Sato E, Goto M, Nakamura T. Nuclear ultrastructure in carcinoma, adenoma, Peutz–Jeghers polyp and dysplasia of the large bowel: a morphometric analysis. *Gan* 1981; 72: 245–253.
91 Sassi I, Faravelli A, Freschi M, Ferrari AM, Cantaboni A. Planimetric grading of dysplasia in colorectal adenomas: a step forward? In: *Fourth International Symposium on Morphometry in Morphological Diagnosis*. London: Royal Society of Medicine, 1986: 78.
92 Konishi F, Morson BC. Pathology of colorectal adenomas: a colonoscopic survey. *J Clin Pathol* 1982; 35: 830–841.
93 Bussey HJR. Multiple adenomas and carcinomas. In: Bennington JL (ed.) *Major Problems in Pathology*, vol. 10. *The Pathogenesis of Colorectal Cancer*.

Philadelphia: WB Saunders, 1978: 72–80.

94 Quirke P, Fozard JBJ, Dixon MF, Dyson JED, Giles GR, Bird CC. DNA aneuploidy in colorectal adenomas. *Br J Cancer* 1986; 53: 477–481.

95 Jarvis LR, Graff PS, Whitehead R. Correlation of nuclear ploidy with histology in adenomatous polyps of colon. *J Clin Pathol* 1987; 40: 26–33.

96 Rubio CA, Porwit-McDonald A. A method to quantitate the relative nuclear area of colorectal polyps by image analysis. *Anal Quant Cytol Histol* 1991; 13: 155–158.

97 Meijer GA, van Diest PJ, Fleege JC, Baak JPA. Syntactic structure analysis of the arrangement of nuclei in dysplastic epithelium of colorectal adenomatous polyps. *Acta Cytol* 1993; 37: 106A.

98 Lipkin M, Blattner WA, Gardner EJ *et al.* Classification and risk assessment of individuals with familial polyposis; Gardner's syndrome and familial non-polyposis colon cancer from [^{3}H] thymidine labelling patterns in colonic epithelial cells. *Cancer Res* 1984; 44: 4201–4207.

99 Quirke P, Dixon MF, Day DW, Fozard JBJ, Talbot IC, Bird CC. DNA aneuploidy and cell proliferation in familial adenomatous polyposis. *Gut* 1988; 29: 603–607.

100 Bleiberg H, Mainguet P, Galand P, Chretien J, Dupont-Mairesse N. Cell renewal in the human rectum: *in vitro* autoradiographic study on active ulcerative colitis. *Gastroenterology* 1970; 58: 851–855.

101 Allan A, Bristol JB, Williamson RCN. Crypt cell production rate in ulcerative proctocolitis: differential increments in remission and relapse. *Gut* 1985; 26: 999–1003.

102 Franklin WA, McDonald GB, Stein HO *et al.* Immunohistologic demonstration of abnormal colonic crypt cell kinetics in ulcerative colitis. *Hum Pathol* 1986; 1129–1132.

103 Riddell RH. The precarcinomatous phase of ulcerative colitis. In: Morson BC (ed.) *Current Topics in Pathology. Pathology of the Gastrointestinal Tract.* Berlin: Springer, 1976: 179–219.

104 Lennard Jones JE, Morson BC, Ritchie JK, Williams CB. Cancer surveillance in ulcerative colitis. Experience over 15 years. *Lancet* 1983; 11: 149–152.

105 Allen DC, Hamilton PW, Watt PCH, Biggart JD. Morphometrical analysis in ulcerative colitis with dysplasia and carcinoma. *Histopathology* 1987; 11: 913–926.

106 Hamilton PW, Allen DC, Watt PCH, Patterson CC, Biggart JD. Classification of normal colorectal mucosa and adenocarcinoma by morphometry. *Histopathology* 1987; 11: 901–911.

107 Hamilton PW, Allen DC, Watt PCH. A combination of cytological and architectural morphometry in assessing regenerative hyperplasia and dysplasia in ulcerative colitis. *Histopathology* 1990; 17: 59–68.

108 Nakamura T, Nakaya T, Sato E, Sasano N. Ultramorphometry of the nucleus of human rectal cancer compared with normal mucosal gland. *Tohokn J Exp Med* 1974; 112: 177–188.

109 Bufo P, Ricco R, Potente F, Troia M, Serio G, Pesce-Delfino V. Using analytical morphometry to distinguish severe dysplasia and large bowel carcinoma. *Boll Soc Ital Biol Sper* 1990; 66: 143–150.

110 Verhest A, Kiss R, d'Olne D *et al.* Characterization of human colorectal mucosa, polyps, and cancers by means of computerized morphonuclear image analysis. *Cancer* 1990; 65: 2047–2054.

111 Lowe J, Kent J, Armitage NC, Ballantyne KC, Hardcastle JD. Nuclear morphometry and nuclear DNA content in rectal carcinoma. In: *Fourth International Symposium on Morphometry in Morphological Diagnosis.* London: Royal Society of Medicine, 1986: 19.

112 Ambros RA, Pawel BR, Meshcheryakov I, Kotrotsios J, Lambert WC, Trost RC. Nuclear morphometry as a prognostic indicator in colorectal carcinoma resected for cure. *Anal Quant Cytol Histol* 1990; 12: 172–176.

113 Deans GT, Hamilton PW, Watt PCH *et al.* Morphometric analysis in colorectal cancer. *Dis Colon Rect* 1993; 36: 450–456.

114 Carter CD, Weeks SC, Jarvis LR, Whitehead R. Morphometric analysis of nuclear features, ploidy status, and staging in rectal carcinoma. *J Pathol* 1989; 159: 113–120.

115 Jass JR, Love SB, Northover JMA. A new prognostic classification of rectal cancer. *Lancet* 1987; 1: 1303–1306.

116 Dukes LE. The classification of cancer in the rectum. *J Pathol Bact* 1932; 35: 323–332.

117 Fisher ER, Paik SM, Rockette H, Jones J, Caplan R, Fisher B. Prognostic significance of eosinophils and mast cells in rectal cancer: findings from the National Surgical Adjuvant Breast and Bowel Project (protocol R-01). *Hum Pathol* 1989; 20: 159–163.

118 McGinnis MC, Bradley EL Jr, Pretlow TP *et al.* Correlation of stromal cells by morphometric analysis with metastatic behaviour of human colonic carcinoma. *Cancer Res* 1989; 49. 5989 5993.

119 Gerard F, Guerret S, Gerard JP, Grimaud JA. Usefulness of morphometry in the cytologic assessment of rectal tumors. *Anal Quant Cytol Histol* 1990; 12: 181.

120 Al-Sheneber IF, Shibata HR, Sampalis J, Jothy S. Prognostic significance of proliferating cell nuclear antigen expression in colorectal cancer. *Cancer* 1993; 71: 1954–1959.

121 Cooper PN, Quirke P, Hardy GJ, Dixon MF. A flow cytometric, clinical, and histological study of stromal neoplasms of the gastrointestinal tract. *Am J Surg Pathol* 1992; 16: 163–170.

122 Cunningham RE, Federspiel BH, McCarthy WF, Sobin LH, O'Leary TJ. Predicting prognosis of gastrointestinal smooth muscle tumours. Role of clinical and histologic evaluation, flow cytometry, and image cytometry. *Am J Surg Pathol* 1993; 17: 588–594.

4.1.6 Inflammatory disorders of the upper gastrointestinal tract

J. S. A. COLLINS

Oesophagitis

Reflux oesophagitis has been studied using quantitative histological methods by several authors over the past decade. In the clinical setting, lower oesophageal biopsies may be obtained using endoscopically guided forceps or by the Quinton tube which employs a suction technique. The latter method yields larger and better oriented samples than endoscopic pinch biopsies [1]. Histological changes in the basal and papillary layer of the oesophageal mucosa were not adequately described in relation to reflux oesophagitis until criteria were suggested related to basal-cell hyperplasia and papillary elongation [2]. These workers obtained suction biopsies from 33 subjects with, and 21 without, subjective and objective evidence of oesophageal reflux. They found that the mean basal zone thickness in 'normal' specimens was 10% of mucosal thickness (range 5–14%) while abnormal specimens showed a mean basal zone thickness of 30% mucosal thickness (range 16–80%). From their series, abnormal basal zone thickness was defined as > 15% and papillary length as > 66% of epithelial thickness in specimens taken 2 cm above the lower oesophageal sphincter. Subsequently, other workers defined different values of basal and papillary height as upper values of normal [3–5]. Reported differences in criteria may be explained by sex make-up of study groups, biopsy sites or alcohol intake. Both Johnson and colleagues' [5] and Seefeld and colleagues' [4] studies were more rigorous in their definition of well-oriented papillae within sections, while the usefulness of the 'Ismail-Beigi criteria' was later called into question when a high incidence of biopsies fulfilling these criteria was found in asymptomatic subjects [6].

These studies were similar in their utilization of a simple form of quantitative histology to define a disease state associated, in this case, with gastro-oesophageal reflux. The morphometric measurement of individual nuclear and nucleolar characteristics in oesophageal biopsies was first described in a study of endoscopic pinch biopsies from six patients with endoscopically documented oesophagitis [7]. These authors defined base and intermediate zones of epithelium independent of tissue section orientation. Within each zone, nuclear number and their respective areas were measured using an interactive computer system. The rationale behind this technique was that increased base layer division in oesophageal reflux results in an increased number of nuclei per unit length of base zone epithelium and a reduction in nuclear area. In the intermediate zone, it was postulated that increased cell turnover results in an increased number of nuclei per unit area of the section and a smaller average nuclear size. Nucleolar size and number would be expected to rise in the presence of increased cell turnover. The conclusion of this study was that certain nuclear parameters could provide a useful measure of cell turnover and possibly enhance diagnostic methods by employing quantitative techniques.

The validity of quantitation in poorly oriented endoscopic pinch biopsies from the lower oesophagus and the correlation between acid reflux, assessed by prolonged ambulatory pH monitoring, and nuclear changes were assessed in a subsequent study [8]. Morphometric measurements of nuclear area, concentration and nucleolar dimensions in the tissue zones defined by Jarvis *et al.* [7] were measured in oriented suction biopsies from eight asymptomatic subjects, 17 with reflux symptoms but normal endoscopic findings and 15 patients with severe symptoms and endoscopic appearances of reflux. No significant differences were shown for any parameter between the groups. In a separate group of 16 patients, identical morphometric measurements were made in non-oriented endoscopic pinch biopsies and correlated with prolonged ambulatory pH data – the gold standard for reflux severity. No significant correlation could be shown between the nuclear parameters and degree of acid reflux. The authors suggested that morphometric measurements could not be recommended as a diagnostic technique in the diagnosis of oesophagitis, although it may be appropriate in the assessment of individual patient response in therapeutic trials.

Gastritis

Until recently, most studies on the histopathological changes encountered in gastritis have graded inflammation using subjective or descriptive criteria. While excellent criteria for acute and chronic gastritis have been developed [9], such methods may create problems of reproducibility. Despite the advantages of a method to quantify gastritic change, only recently have workers attempted to use morphometric and counting techniques to this purpose.

Initial studies on gastric biopsy specimens used grid-counting techniques to quantify the effect of chronic alcohol ingestion [10]. These workers counted both lymphocytes and plasma cells in square microscopic fields, and concluded that alcoholic patients had a higher incidence of antral gastritis than non-alcoholics. Using similar grid-counting techniques, other workers have compared differential inflammatory cell counts in gastric biopsy specimens between groups of patients with non-ulcer dyspepsia and asymptomatic subjects [11]. Immunoglobulin-producing cells in the gastric mucosa have been quantified in patients with various gastrointestinal disorders using a cell-counting technique based on photographic slides [12].

The description and subsequent reclassification of chronic gastritis following the reports on *Helicobacter pylori* colonization of the gastric mucosa led to radical reappraisal of aetiological factors pertaining to gastritis and duodenal ulcer disease [13]. Comparative studies of the antral gastritis often described with duodenal ulcer disease and its close association with *H. pylori* infection were associated with varying techniques to grade gastritis.

The quantitative assessment of gastric mucosal inflammation and its relationship to *H. pylori* infection in gastric antral and body biopsies from patients with dyspepsia and controls were subsequently described utilizing an interactive, computer-linked image analyser [14,15]. Measurements were carried out using the MOP Videoplan (Kontron) on all biopsies with the investigators 'blind' to the endoscopic diagnosis. One section from each endoscopic biopsy was chosen for study. Three contiguous fields of the lamina propria were assessed for polymorph concentration and mononuclear cell concentration per square millimetre and three contiguous lengths of surface epithelium were assessed for inflammatory cell number per millimetre.

Analysis of variance was used to calculate the effect on standard error (SE) for each measured parameter of increasing fields analysed and biopsies analysed. The authors concluded that increasing field number had less effect on SE than increasing total number of biopsies analysed. These two studies were able to show statistically significant differences between diagnostic groups using non-parametric statistics. In particular, *H. pylori* positivity was associated with significantly greater antral and body inflammation.

More recently, the same authors have compared the cell-counting technique described above with a different gastritis-grading method based on the use of photographs taken to represent increasing grades or scores of acute and chronic inflammation [16]. Agreement statistics showed that mean score differences (cell-counting minus photographic score) were negative, indicating that the photographic method yields higher mean patient scores. Scatter plots of score difference versus mean score obtained using the two different methods showed that only 3.6% of scores fell outside ± 2 standard deviations (SD) of the mean difference. The authors concluded that the use of graded photographs provided quantitative results comparable to those obtained by direct enumeration of inflammatory cells.

Duodenitis and small-bowel disease

The first study to propose a definitive classification of duodenitis using quantitative histology was based on the conventional histological examination of 747 endoscopic duodenal biopsies [17]. Its validity was tested for increasing grades of inflammation using a cell-counting technique and estimation of section surface/volume ratio. The least severe form of duodenitis was designated mild duodenitis, with increased cellularity of the lamina propria but no change in villous height. Moderate duodenitis was defined by increased cellularity with deformed and shortened villous architecture, while severe duodenitis was characterized by the highest degree of cellularity and frank epithelial erosion.

In a subsequent study, these criteria were used

in the comparison of endoscopic and histological findings in duodenal biopsies from 17 patients with duodenal ulcer and 20 with an endoscopically normal duodenal mucosa [18]. In the ulcer group, biopsies were taken from mucosal areas considered to be inflamed and at least 3 mm from the ulcer crater margin. In normal subjects, random biopsies were taken from the duodenal bulb. The authors concluded that an ulcerated duodenal bulb is invariably associated with duodenitis of varying severity.

The degree of abnormality in duodenal mucosal architecture has been quantitatively assessed using a microdissection technique [19]. Biopsies from patients with duodenal ulcer-associated and non-specific duodenitis were compared with controls. Significant reduction in villous height and increase in mitotic figure count per crypt were found in the duodenitis biopsies compared to control mucosa. No significant differences were noted between ulcer-associated and non-specific duodenitis. The same authors noted a significant decrease in epithelial cell count per villus in the presence of duodenitis compared to controls – an abnormality which was reversed following duodenal mucosal healing [20]. In a later study, the nature of the inflammatory infiltrate in duodenitis was studied using an eye-piece graticule on semithin sections from endoscopic biopsies [21]. Although epithelial polymorphs were frequently seen in controls, substantial numbers were present in the duodenitis groups where infiltration was noted in both lamina propria and superficial epithelium. Chronic inflammatory cells, which were mostly lymphocytes and plasma cells, were significantly more frequent in biopsies from patients with duodenitis.

Several studies have attempted to quantify histological parameters in biopsy sections from the inflamed duodenal bulb. Villous cellularity, length and width were measured in biopsies from 88 normal and 20 inflamed bulbs [22]. These authors concluded that the density of inflammatory cellular infiltration in the lamina propria is a decisive factor in the histological diagnosis of duodenitis. In a later study, the same authors studied 48 patients with duodenitis using quantitative techniques [23]. They showed that villous epithelial height decreases with advancing age and, using multivariate discriminant analysis, concluded that histological examination of the duodenal mucosa should be compared with endoscopically normal mucosa from the third part of the duodenum in order to grade adequately the severity of inflammation.

The effect of alcohol on the duodenal mucosa was studied in 47 alcoholics and 21 controls using a cell-counting technique to quantify mononuclear cells, goblet cells and gastric metaplasia [24]. Mononuclear cells were higher in patients with concomitant gastritis and showed a slight increase with age in controls. Plasma cell populations in duodenal biopsies have been quantified using immunoperoxidase-staining techniques [25]. IgA plasma cells were significantly higher in patients with Whitehead grade 1 and 2 duodenitis compared to controls, suggesting that these cells reflect a local immune response to mucosal damage. In a later study, this group studied plasma cell, polymorph and eosinophil counts in patients with endoscopically normal duodenal bulbs, duodenitis or duodenal ulcer [26]. Using cluster and discriminant analysis, they defined duodenitis of mild grade as characterized by increased plasma cells, mucosal oedema and crypt polymorphs, whereas severe grade showed significant villous atrophy, heavy polymorph infiltrate and decreased plasma cells.

Using computer-linked image analysis, inflammatory cell counts were compared between biopsy sections from duodenal ulcer crater margins, endoscopic areas of duodenitis and control mucosa in groups of patients with active duodenal ulcer, duodenitis only and non-ulcer dyspepsia [27]. Variables measured included polymorph and mononuclear cells per millimetre of superficial epithelium and per square millimetre of lamina propria. Ulcer margin and duodenitis biopsies had significantly higher inflammatory cell counts than endoscopically normal mucosa from patients with non-ulcer dyspepsia and controls. Despite endoscopic appearances, biopsies from non-ulcer patients had significantly higher inflammatory cell counts than control specimens.

Coeliac disease

Quantitative histological methods applied to small-bowel sections have measured villous height, crypt/height ratio and mitotic activity within the crypts

[28,29]. The latter authors have emphasized the importance of obtaining well-oriented suction biopsies cut at right angles to the mucosal surface. These methods have provided the basis for a histological diagnosis of coeliac disease, and the value of reduced villous height/crypt depth ratio has been confirmed in adults, provided that allowance is made for geographical variations [30,31].

A simple stereological method using a template devised by Weibel [32] was first described in an effort to assess accurately surface/volume ratio [30]. Interactive computer-aided image analysis has also been used to measure parameters such as mucosal height/crypt depth ratio [31]. This study confirmed a significant reduction in this variable in sections from patients with untreated coeliac disease. The interactive computerized method requires expensive equipment but has the supposed advantage that histological measurements are made directly within defined fields and derived stereological estimates are not made. However, it has been suggested, in a comparative study between the two methods, that the semiautomatic method is not necessarily superior [33] (see Section 1.1). Similar techniques have measured morphological changes in giardiasis [34] and food allergy [35].

Individual cell types within the small-bowel mucosa have been quantified. Initial reports that intraepithelial lymphocytes (IELs) were increased in relation to the number of villous epithelial cells in untreated coeliac disease [36] were later challenged by other workers [37]. Ferguson and Murray [36] proposed that the number of IELs reverted to normal after the patients were treated with a gluten-free diet. However, Marsh [38] later pointed out that IELs per unit length of muscularis mucosae, which is not changed in coeliac disease, are unchanged after dietary manipulation. Increased activation of lymphocytes and their increased loss into the gut lumen associated with desquamation of enterocytes was described by Marsh [38]. Quantitation of mitotic figures among IELs has been recommended as a reliable diagnostic feature in gluten-sensitive enteropathy and may distinguish true disease from other features of small-bowel biopsy sections distorted by poor orientation [39]. Despite criticism of the techniques involved in the counting of IEL mitoses, the value of the study has been defended [40,41].

IELs in the jejunal mucosa have been identified as suppressor/cytotoxic T cells [42]. The identification of Leu-1 and T_2 antigens has been reported in an increased proportion of the cells, providing evidence that there is increased migration and stimulation of these cells in coeliac disease [43]. An alteration of immune tolerance to dietary gluten in coeliac disease has been suggested by the finding of more stimulated T-helper cells in coeliac mucosa [44].

4.1.7 Conclusion

Quantitative histological techniques applied to oesophageal mucosal biopsies have provided simple criteria for the histological diagnosis of reflux oesophagitis on endoscopic biopsy sections. However, orientation and a variety of definitions of normal make interpretation of most cases difficult. Attempts at more detailed quantitation have been shown to be time-consuming and not practical for routine diagnostic use.

Quantitation of gastric mucosal inflammatory cells probably provides the 'gold standard' for assessment of acute and chronic gastritis, but recent studies suggest that photographic comparison techniques correlate well with quantitative data obtained by semiautomatic image analysis.

Measurement of duodenal and small-bowel sections for a wide variety of parameters has provided valuable data pertaining to the pathogenesis of duodenal ulcer disease and the immunohistological change in coeliac disease.

References

1 Komorowski HA, Lemicke JA. Comparison of fiberoptic endoscope and Quinton tube oesophageal biopsies in esophagitis. *Gastrointest Endosc* 1978; 24: 154–155.
2 Ismail-Beigi F, Horton PF, Pope CE. Histological consequences of gastroesophageal reflux in man. *Gastroenterology* 1970; 58: 163–174.
3 Behar J, Sheahan DG. Histologic abnormalities in reflux oesophagitis. *Arch Pathol* 1975; 99: 387–391.
4 Seefeld U, Krejs GJ, Siebenmann RE, Blum AL. Esophageal histology in gastroesophageal reflux. Morphometric findings in suction biopsies. *Am J Dig Dis* 1977; 22: 956–964.
5 Johnson LF, Demeester TR, Haggitt RC. Esophageal

epithelial response to gastroesophageal reflux. A quantitative study. *Am J Dig Dis* 1978; 23: 498–509.
6 Weinstein WM, Bogosh ER, Bowes KL. The normal human esophageal mucosa: a histological reappraisal. *Gastroenterology* 1975; 68: 40–44.
7 Jarvis LR, Dent J, Whitehead R. Morphometric assessment of reflux oesophagitis in fibreoptic biopsy specimens. *J Clin Pathol* 1985; 38: 44–48.
8 Collins JSA, Watt PCR, Hamilton PW *et al.* Assessment of oesophagitis by histology and morphometry. *Histopathology* 1989; 14: 381–389.
9 Whitehead R, Truelove SC, Gear MW. The histological diagnosis of chronic gastritis in fibreoptic gastroscope biopsy specimens. *J Clin Pathol* 1972; 25: 1–11.
10 Parl FF, Lev R, Thomas E, Pitchumoni CS. Histologic and morphometric study of chronic gastritis in alcoholic patients. *Hum Pathol* 1979; 10: 45–56.
11 Toukan AU, Kamal MF, Amr SS, Arnaout MA, Abu-Romyeh AS. Gastroduodenal inflammation in patients with non-ulcer dysphagia. A controlled endoscopic and morphometric study. *Dig Dis Sci* 1985; 30: 313–320.
12 Valnes K, Brandtzaeg P, Elgjo K, Stave R. Quantitative distribution of immunoglobulin-producing cells in gastric mucosa: relation to chronic gastritis and glandular atrophy. *Gut* 1986; 27: 505–514.
13 Marshall EJ, Warren JR. Unidentified curved bacilli in the stomach of patients with gastritis and peptic ulceration. *Lancet* 1984; i: 1311–1315.
14 Collins JSA, Hamilton PW, Watt PCH, Sloan JM, Love AHG. Superficial gastritis and *Campylobacter pylori* in dyspeptic patients – a quantitative study using computer-linked image analysis. *J Pathol* 1989; 158: 303–310.
15 Collins JSA, Sloan JM, Hamilton PW, Watt PCH, Love AHG. Investigation of the relationship between gastric antral inflammation and *Campylobacter pylori* using graphic tablet planimetry. *J Pathol* 1989; 159: 281–285.
16 Collins JSA, Watt PCH, Hamilton PW, Sloan JM, Love AHG. Grading of superficial antral gastritis: comparison of cell-counting and photographic-based methods. *J Pathol* 1991; 163: 251–256.
17 Whitehead R, Roca M, Meikle DD, Skinner J, Truelove SC. The histological classification of duodenitis in fibreoptic biopsy specimens. *Digestion* 1975; 13: 129–136.
18 Stephen JG, Lesna M, Venables CW. Endoscopic appearance and histological changes in ulcer-associated duodenitis. *Br J Surg* 1978; 65: 438–441.
19 Hasan M, Sircus W, Ferguson A. Duodenal mucosal architecture in non-specific and ulcer-associated duodenitis. *Gut* 1981; 22: 637–641.
20 Hasan M, Ferguson A. Measurements of intestinal villi in non-specific and ulcer-associated duodenitis – correlation between area of microdissected villus and villus epithelial cell count. *J Clin Pathol* 1981; 34: 1181–1186.
21 Hasan M, Hay F, Sircus W, Ferguson A. Nature of the inflammatory cell infiltrate in duodenitis. *J Clin Pathol* 1983; 36: 280–288.
22 Schmitz-Moorman P, Schmidt-Slordahl R, Peter JH, Massarrat S. Morphometric studies of normal and inflamed duodenal mucosa. *Pathol Res Pract* 1980; 167: 313–321.
23 Schmitz-Moorman P, Pittner PM, Reichmann L, Massarrat S. Quantitative histological study of duodenitis in biopsies. *Pathol Res Pract* 1984; 178: 499–507.
24 Lev R, Thomas E, Parl FF, Pitchumoni CS. Pathological and histomorphometric study of the effects of alcohol on the human duodenum. *Digestion* 1980; 20: 207–213.
25 Scott BB, Goodall A, Stephenson P, Jenkins D. Duodenal bulb plasma cells in duodenitis and duodenal ulceration. *Gut* 1985; 26: 1032–1037.
26 Jenkins D, Goodall A, Gillet FR, Scott BB. Defining duodenitis: quantitative histological study of mucosal responses and their correlations. *J Clin Pathol* 1985; 38: 1119–1126.
27 Collins JSA, Hamilton PW, Watt PCH, Sloan JM, Love AHG. Quantitative histological study of mucosal inflammatory cell densities in endoscopic duodenal biopsy specimens from dyspeptic patients using computer-linked image analysis. *Gut* 1990; 31: 858–861.
28 Shiner M, Doniach I. Histopathologic studies in steatorrhoea. *Gastroenterology* 1960; 38: 419–440.
29 Thurlbeck WM, Benson JA, Dudley HR. The histopathological changes of sprue and their significance. *Am J Clin Pathol* 1960; 34: 108–117.
30 Dunnill MS, Whitehead R. A method for the quantitation of small intestinal biopsy specimens. *J Clin Pathol* 1972; 25: 243–246.
31 Slavin G, Sowter C, Robertson K, McDermott S, Paton K. Measurement in jejunal biopsies by computer-aided microscopy. *J Clin Pathol* 1980; 33: 254–261.
32 Weibel ER. Principles and methods for morphometric study of the lung and other organs. *Lab Invest* 1963; 12: 131–155.
33 Corrazza GR, Frazzoni M, Dixon MF, Gasbarrini G. Quantitative assessment of the mucosal architecture of jejunal biopsy specimens: a comparison between linear measurements, stereology and computer-aided microscopy. *J Clin Pathol* 1985; 38: 765–770.
34 Rosekrans PCM, Meijer CJLM, Polanco I, Mearin ML, van der Wal AM, Linderman J. Long term morphological and immunohistochemical observations on biopsy specimens of small intestine from children with gluten sensitive enteropathy. *J Clin Pathol* 1981; 34: 138–144.
35 Rosekrans PCM, Meijer CJLM, Cornelisse CJ, van der Wal AM, Linderman J. Use of morphometry and immunohistochemistry of small intestinal biopsy specimens in the diagnosis of food allergy. *J Clin Pathol* 1980; 33: 125–130.
36 Ferguson A, Murray D. Quantitation of intraepithelial

lymphocytes in human jejunum. *Gut* 1971; 12: 989–994.
37 Guix M, Skinner JM, Whitehead RW. Measuring intraepithelial lymphocytes, surface area and volume of lamina propria in the jejunal mucosa of coeliac patients. *Gut* 1979; 20: 275–278.
38 Marsh MN. Studies of intestinal lymphoid tissue III. Quantitative analysis of intraepithelial lymphocytes in the small intestine of human control subjects and of patients with coeliac sprue. *Gastroenterology* 1980; 79: 481–492.
39 Marsh MN. Functional and structural aspects of the epithelial lymphocyte with implications for coeliac disease and tropical sprue. *Scand J Gastroenterol* 1985; 114(suppl): 55–75.
40 Ferguson A, Ziegler K. Intraepithelial lymphocyte mitoses in a jejunal biopsy correlates with intraepithelial lymphocyte count irrespective of diagnosis. *Gut* 1986; 27: 675–679.
41 Marsh MN. Measurement of intra-epithelial lymphocytes. *Gut* 1986; 27: 1516–1517.
42 Selby WS, Janossy G, Jewell DP. Immunohistological characterisation of intraepithelial lymphocytes of the human gastrointestinal tract. *Gut* 1981; 22: 169–176.
43 Selby WS, Janossy G, Bofill M, Jewell DP. Lymphocyte subpopulations in the human small intestine. The findings in normal mucosa and in the mucosa of patients with adult coeliac disease. *Clin Exp Immunol* 1983; 52: 219–228.
44 Malizia G, Trejdosiewicz LK, Ward GM, Howdle PD, Janossy G, Losowsky MS. The microenvironment of coeliac disease: T cell phenotypes and expression of the T_2 'T blast' antigen by small bowel lymphocytes. *Clin Exp Immunol* 1985; 60: 437–446.

4.2 PANCREAS

Rudimentary quantitation has been used to study lipomatosis of the pancreas, which is partial replacement of the acinar parenchyma by fat, with no evidence of preceding inflammation or scarring. The islet and ductal tissue is usually uninvolved and in severe forms there remain only scattered lobules of exocrine tissue [1]. It is a phenomenon which has been confirmed to correlate statistically with increasing age and obesity, yet is also to an extent reversible, diminishing in terminal illness [2]. It is rarely accompanied by pancreatic insufficiency despite the varying degree to which the parenchymal tissue is disturbed [3].

Microscopical quantitation has mostly been directed at the islet-cell population and the physiology of this will be briefly summarized before a review of its application in pancreatic pathology.

4.2.1 Islet-cell tissue

Enumeration of islet numbers and diameters has been combined with other planimetric and stereological techniques to provide quantitative data such as the relative and absolute values for islet-cell areas and weights. Individual cell identification has been facilitated by the advent of immunohistochemistry but all of this must be viewed against a number of factors limiting precision, such as interindividual differences in cell constitution and distribution, and artefacts such as partial autolysis [4].

In the neonate the islet volume constitutes approximately 10% of the pancreas with about 250 000 islets weighing in total 0.3 g and with diameters ranging from 85 to 210 μm [5]. In the infant of 4–8 months the islet mass forms 5% of the tissue [5] and by the age of 3 years the islet number has increased to its adult population of approximately 1 million [6] and a weight of 1.5 g [5]. An islet-cell diameter above 400 μm is considered enlarged. This marked growth in islet-cell tissue is attributed to a disproportionate increase in B-cell numbers [5]. The pancreatic head is predominated by islets of small volume with the body and tail of the gland containing islets of larger size [7] and greater number [8]. The dimensions and frequency of individual cell cytoplasmic granules are related to pathophysiological demands [4]. A, D and polypeptide (PP) cells have a constant nuclear size [4] while B cells are recognized occasionally to have large nuclei; this is found in normal adults as an expression of polyploidy [9]. Mitoses in the pancreatic islets are rare but may be encountered in replication-stimulated hyperglycaemia [10] and regeneration and hypertrophy in diseases such as cirrhosis or diabetes [11].

4.2.2 Diabetes

The size and weight of the pancreas in long-standing insulin-dependent diabetes mellitus (IDDM) is usually reduced by approximately 50% [12]. In both acute and chronic IDDM the number and size of islets are reduced [13,14]. Saito *et al.* [15] showed a marked negative correlation between the islet volume and the maximum blood sugar level during glucose tolerance testing in both diabetics and controls and advocated such measurements in assessing the pathophysiology of diabetes. Using immunohistochemistry, Kloppel *et al.* [16] found the islet volume in patients with diabetes to be half that of normal controls. Chronic IDDM is characterized by a decreased volume [17] or absence of B cells and, although there is a relative hyperplasia of non-B cells [18], their absolute numbers are actually decreased [16].

In non-insulin-dependent diabetes mellitus (NIDDM) the findings differ from non-diabetics, with the size of islets apparently unchanged [19] but islet numbers [12] and their relative volume dramatically decreased [20]. In the latter study, once allowance was made for amyloid infiltration (hyalinosis), the area occupied by the islets was identified as approximately 25–50% of controls. As in IDDM there is a marked reduction in B cells [16,19].

The newborn of diabetic mothers have islets which have increased volume and size, and elevated numbers of B cells (for review, see Hultquist and Olding [21]). Persistent hyperinsulinaemic hypoglycaemia in infants of non-diabetic mothers also shows nesidioblastosis characterized by a fivefold microadenomatous increase in endocrine tissue [22].

4.2.3 Cystic fibrosis

The lesions of cystic fibrosis are somewhat imperceptible in the newborn and are more amenable to quantitation. Imrie *et al.* [23] used stereology to show that there is a reversal in the normal linear increase in the ratio of acinar/connective tissue volume seen in the first 52 weeks postconception. Thus infants with cystic fibrosis above 42 weeks postconception could be discriminated from controls using a combination of volume percentage lumen and the ratio of acinar to connective tissue. In a group of 16 patients ranging up to 20 years of age who came to autopsy, Kopito *et al.* [24] found a reduction in acinar tissue from 33% of normal values in infants to 5% in severely affec'ed older patients. This was accompanied by a marked increase in fatty connective tissue and ductal elements. Water and soluble mineral content were decreased by over 50% and levels of zinc, calcium, copper, magnesium, potassium and sodium were all significantly ($P < 0.01$) reduced.

A degree of nesidioblastosis has also been demonstrated and this may help to deter the development of diabetes mellitus but may contribute to the pathogenesis of peptic ulcer disease in cystic fibrosis [25]. Islet-cell volume is increased and the ratios of the peptide producing A, B and D cells altered [26].

4.2.4 Pancreatitis

Quantitation in this area has assessed mainly the endocrine tissue component. In severe primary pancreatitis and also that secondary to carcinomatous duct obstruction there is an approximately 50% reduction in the numbers of B cells. This was thought to be due to scarring of the exocrine pancreas affecting islet composition by impairment of the local circulation and of glucose diffusion, leading to a reduction in the number and sensitivity of the B cells [27]. There was also a compensatory hyperplasia of glucagon-producing A and PP cells. The latter have also been found in some cases of pancreatic carcinoma [28].

4.2.5 Pancreatic tumours

The prognosis of pancreatic exocrine carcinoma is related to the usual classical indicators such as site, size, histological type and differentiation, and the presence of nodal and vascular involvement. A combination of morphometric (nuclear area), densitometric (nuclear DNA content) and textural parameters into a malignancy index can separate and reflect histological classification of normal tissue, pancreatitis and grades I, II and III adenocarcinoma [29]. Lipponen *et al.* [30] have shown that the histological grade, clinical stage and volume-corrected mitotic index (M/V index) all correlate with survival. In a series of 59 patients they found that the M/V index related to histology and the presence of metastases but was superior at separating patients into two prognostically different groups. They suggested this as a means of patient selection for different therapeutic modalities. In carcinoma of the ampulla of Vater, stereological estimates of nuclear volume have shown that a volume-weighted mean nuclear volume (nuclear V_v) $> 150\,\mu m^3$ is associated with a lower survival rate [31]. Periampullary carcinoma has a better outlook than pancreatic ductal cancer and prognostic information can be improved by measuring nuclear irregularity, a factor describing nuclear shape corrected for roundness [32].

Pancreatic islet-cell tumours are classified according to their microscopic growth pattern [33] but this does not give an indication of their future biological behaviour. Accepted histological criteria of malignancy are unreliable as features such as nuclear pleomorphism, prominent nucleoli, local infiltration and vascular invasion have all been reported in tumours which did not metastasize. Tumour size has been thought to relate to malignancy [34], but this is not always so [35]. Functionality is associated with malignancy, with 85% of insulinomas being benign and most gastrinomas (approximately 70%) malignant [35]. Using semiautomatic image analysis, Kenny *et al.* [36] examined a series of 31 pancreatic endocrine tumours with a mean follow-up period of 5 years. Discriminant analysis chose tumour-cell nuclear cytoplasmic ratio and the number of nuclei per square millimetre as significant variables to derive a classification rule. It was capable of correctly classifying 92% of the localized and metastatic tumours into their correct categories (Fig. 4.4). The rule was successfully verified on a new set of five test cases. The study also confirmed the lack of information imparted by the increased nuclear size, pleomorphism and mitoses in these tumours. Morphometry was advocated as a means of improving histological assessment and prognostication.

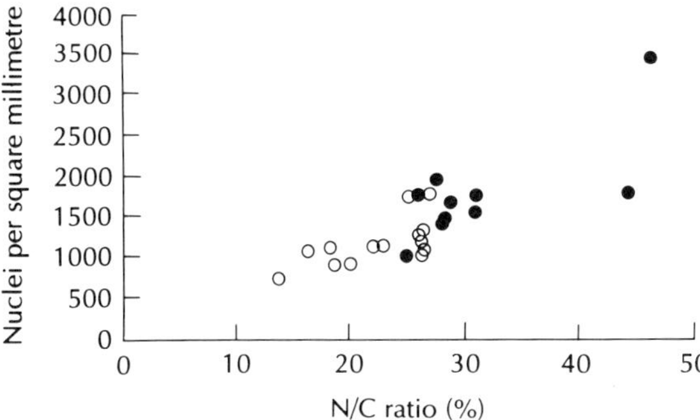

Fig. 4.4 Bivariate scatter plot using nuclei per square millimetre and nuclear/cytoplasmic ratio, showing good separation of localized (○) and metastatic (•) pancreatic endocrine tumours. From Kenny *et al.* [36].

4.2.6 Conclusion

Quantitation in the pancreas has given insight into the pathogenesis and morphology of diseases such as diabetes and cystic fibrosis. It has not been of use in pancreatitis. Potential practical applications are the role of mitotic activity in exocrine carcinomas and, nuclear density and nuclear cytoplasmic ratio in endocrine tumours as a gauge of biological behaviour and prognosis.

References

1 Seifert S. Lipomatous atrophy and other forms. In: Kloppel G, Heitz PU (eds) *Pancreatic Pathology*. Edinburgh: Churchill Livingstone, 1984: 27–31.

2 Olsen TS. Lipomatosis of the pancreas in autopsy material and its relation to age and overweight. *Acta Pathol Microbiol Scand* 1978; 86 (Section A): 367–373.

3 Schmitz-Moormann P, Pittner PM, Heinze W. Lipomatosis of the pancreas — a morphometrical investigation. *Pathol Res Pract* 1981; 173: 45–53.

4 Kloppel G, Lenzen S. Anatomy and physiology of the endocrine pancreas. In: Kloppel G, Heitz PU (eds) *Pancreatic Pathology*. Edinburgh: Churchill Livingstone, 1984: 133–153.

5 Rahier J, Wallon J, Henquin JC. Cell populations in the endocrine pancreas of human neonates and infants. *Diabetologia* 1981; 20: 540–546.

6 Ogilvie RF. Quantitative estimation of pancreatic islet tissue. *Q J Med* 1937; 6: 287–300.

7 Saito K, Iwama N, Takahashi T. Morphometrical analysis on topographical difference in size distribution, number and volume of islets in the human pancreas. *Tokoho J Exp Med* 1978; 124: 177–186.

8 Wittingen J, Frey CF. Islet concentration in the head, body, tail and uncinate process of the pancreas. *Ann Surg* 1974; 179: 412–414.

9 Ehrie MG, Swartz FF. Diploid, tetraploid and octoploid beta cells in the islets of Langerhans of the normal human pancreas. *Diabetes* 1974; 23: 583–588.

10 Logothetopoulos J. Islet cell regeneration and neogenesis. In: Freinkel N, Steiner DF (eds) *Handbook of Physiology*, Section 7, Endocrinology, vol. 1. Baltimore: Williams & Wilkins, 1972: 67–76.

11 Cecil RL. On hypertrophy and regeneration of the islands of Langerhans. *J Exp Med* 1911; 14: 500–519.

12 Doniach I. Postmortem histology of the islets of Langerhans in juvenile diabetes mellitus. *Postgrad Med J* 1974; 50(suppl 3): 544–545.

13 Gepts W. Pathologic anatomy of the pancreas in juvenile diabetes mellitus. *Diabetes* 1965; 14: 619–633.
14 Doniach I, Morgan AG. Islets of Langerhans in juvenile diabetes mellitus. *Clin Endocrinol* 1973; 2: 233–248.
15 Saito K, Takahashi T, Yaginuma N, Iwama N. Islet morphometry in the diabetic pancreas of man. *Tokoho J Exp Med* 1978; 125: 185–197.
16 Kloppel G, Drenck CR, Carstensen A, Morohoshi T, Oberholzer M, Heitz PU. Ultrastructure and immunocytochemistry of the endocrine pancreas in diabetes. *Medicine* 1982; 2: 299–308.
17 Saito K, Yaginuma N, Takahashi T. Differential volumetry of A, B and D cells in the pancreatic islets of diabetic and non-diabetic subjects. *Tokoho J Exp Med* 1979; 129: 273–283.
18 Kloppel G. Islet histopathology in diabetes mellitus. In: Kloppel G, Heitz PU (eds) *Pancreatic Pathology*. Edinburgh: Churchill Livingstone, 1984: 154–192.
19 Maclean N, Ogilvie RF. Quantitative estimation of the pancreatic islet tissue in diabetic subjects. *Diabetes* 1955; 4: 367–376.
20 Westermark P, Wilander E. The influence of amyloid deposits on the islet volume in maturity onset diabetes mellitus. *Diabetologia* 1978; 15: 417–421.
21 Hultquist GT, Olding LB. Endocrine pathology of infants of diabetic mothers. *Acta Endocrinol* 1981; 241(suppl): 1–202.
22 Heitz PU, Kloppel G, Hacki WH, Polak JM, Pearse AGE. Nesidioblastosis: the pathologic basis of persistent hyperinsulinemic hypoglycemia in infants. Morphologic and quantitative analysis of seven cases based on specific immunostanding and electron microscopy. *Diabetes* 1977; 26: 632–642.
23 Imrie JR, Fagan DG, Sturgess JM. Quantitative evaluation of the development of the exocrine pancreas in cystic fibrosis and control infants. *Am J Pathol* 1979; 95: 697–707.
24 Kopito LE, Shwachman H, Vawter TF, Edlow J. The pancreas in cystic fibrosis. Chemical composition and comparative morphology. *Pediatr Res* 1976; 10: 742–749.
25 Brown RE, Madge GE. Cystic fibrosis and nesidioblastosis. *Arch Pathol* 1971; 92: 53–57.
26 Soejima K, Landing BH. Pancreatic islets in older patients with cystic fibrosis with and without diabetes mellitus: morphometric and immunocytologic studies. *Pediatr Pathol* 1986; 6: 25–46.
27 Kloppel G, Bommer G, Commandeur G, Heitz P. The endocrine pancreas in chronic pancreatitis. Immunocytochemical and ultrastructural studies. *Virchows Arch A Pathol Anat Histol* 1978; 377: 157–174.
28 Bommer G, Friedl U, Heitz PU, Kloppel G. Pancreatic PP cell distribution and hyperplasia: immunocytochemical morphology in the normal pancreas, chronic pancreatitis and pancreatic carcinoma. *Virchows Arch A Pathol Anat Histol* 1980; 387: 319–331.
29 Rickaert F, Gelin M, Van Gansbeke D *et al.* Computerized morphonuclear characteristics and DNA content of adenocarcinoma of the pancreas, chronic pancreatitis, and normal tissues: relationship with histopathologic grading. *Hum Pathol* 1992; 23: 1210–1215.
30 Lipponen PK, Eskelinen MJ, Collan Y, Marin S, Alhava E. Volume-corrected mitotic index in human pancreatic cancer. Relation to histologic grade, clinical stage, and prognosis. *Scand J Gastroenterol* 1990; 25: 548–554.
31 Artacho-Perula E, Roldan-Villalobos R, Lopez-Rubio F, Vaamonde-Lemos R. Stereological estimates of nuclear volume in carcinoma of the ampulla of Vater. *Histopathology* 1992; 21: 241–248.
32 Weger AR, Lindholm J, Glaser K, Mairinger T, Mikuz G. Morphometry and prognosis in cancer of the pancreatic head. *Pathol Res Pract* 1992; 188: 764–769.
33 Soga J, Tazawa K. Pathologic analysis of carcinoids. Histologic re-evaluation of 62 cases. *Cancer* 1971; 28: 990–998.
34 Cubilla AL, Hajdu SI. Islet cell carcinoma of the pancreas. *Arch Pathol* 1975; 99: 204–207.
35 Heitz PU, Kasper M, Polak JM, Kloppel G. Pancreatic endocrine tumours: immunocytochemical analysis of 125 tumours. *Hum Pathol* 1982; 13: 263–271.
36 Kenny BD, Sloan JM, Hamilton PW, Watt PCH, Johnston CF, Buchanan KD. The role of morphometry in predicting prognosis in pancreatic islet cell tumors. *Cancer* 1989; 64: 460–465.

4.3 LIVER

4.3.1 Cirrhosis and alcoholic liver disease

The assessment of cirrhosis and alcoholic liver disease are common problems in western society. Quantitation has provided some interesting insights into the morphology of these conditions. A morphometric finding particularly relevant to needle biopsy is that there is close correlation and equivalence of capsule thickness, subcapsular and intralobar non-parenchyma volume fractions in normal and diseased liver [1]. This helps to obviate doubts about how representative needle biopsy is in diffusely fibrotic conditions. The determination of fibrous tissue content is facilitated by connective tissue stains and these colorimetric methods closely parallel their equivalent morphometric measurements [2]. Stereology has shown that there is a bimodal growth pattern of both fibrous septal thickening and elongation in the evolution of cirrhosis [3]. Sinusoidal radius is also increased, while volume fraction and length remain unchanged, suggesting that changes in the sinusoids do not contribute to the resultant portal hypertension [4].

In alcoholic steatosis there is close correlation between visual assessment and image analysis of the mean density (percentage) of steatosis, whereas there are conflicting results for the size distribution of droplets [5]. Pathologists consistently overestimated the proportion of macro- to micro-droplets. The risk of development of cirrhosis can be gauged by the degree of perivascular and perisinusoidal centrilobular fibrosis seen in alcoholic hepatitis [6]. In established cirrhosis the process of fibrosis is associated with a marked shift and diminution in the number and fat content of adipocytes [7].

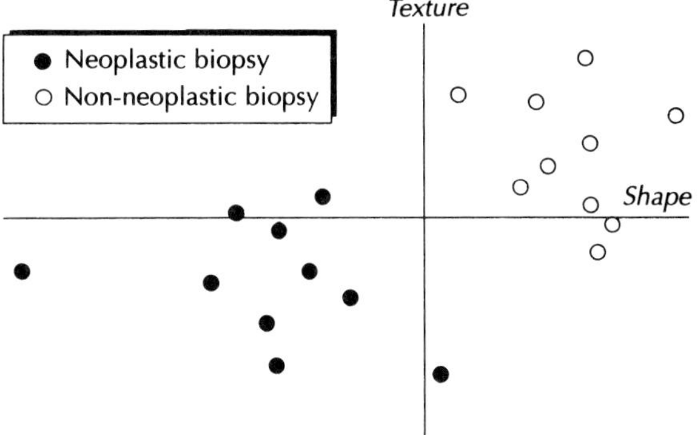

Fig. 4.5 Separation of benign (○) and malignant (●) hepatocellular lesions using a linear discriminant based on nuclear shape and texture. From Jagoe *et al.* [9].

4.3.2 Hepatocellular carcinoma

Morphometry of fine-needle aspirates (200 nuclei per case) in six patients with well-differentiated hepatocarcinoma and six with cirrhosis and atypia showed significant differences between the two diagnostic groups. This was based on larger nuclear size and greater anisonucleosis in carcinoma [8]. Image analysis of needle biopsies in hepatomas identified the range of nuclear sizes within a sample as having only a minor discriminatory effect between benign and malignant tissue. However, this was outweighed by the influence of the variation of nuclear shape measurements within a lesion, such as boundary curvature factor and the distances between the nuclear boundary and its centre of gravity [9]. Discriminant analysis used a combination of the SD of the latter variable with a measurement of the variation in chromatin density to effect complete separation (Fig. 4.5). Other workers have emphasized the importance of a reduction in cell size and an increase in nuclear cytoplasmic ratio (interpreted histologically as nuclear crowding) in diagnosing well-differentiated hepatocarcinoma [10].

The liver has a considerable reserve and regenerative capacity and cellular changes such as polyploidy are encountered in a variety of inflammatory, fibrotic and malignant conditions. The existence of hepatocellular dysplasia as a premalignant condition in cirrhosis has to some extent been elaborated by morphometry, although it has led to differing schools of thought. Visual assessment and measurements define two populations in cirrhotic nodules referred to by various authors as small and large dysplastic cells. The morphometric features of small dysplastic cells are close to those of their corresponding adjacent hepatocellular carcinoma and are considered by some to be the true preneoplastic component [11,12]. There is controversy as to the significance of large dysplastic cells, as their nuclear areas and nuclear cytoplasmic ratios are similar to benign tissue and this is interpreted as a reactive change [11,12]. This has been disputed by Roncalli *et al.* [13], who found the nuclear/cytoplasmic, nucleolar/cytoplasmic, and nucleolar/nuclear ratios of large- and small-cell dysplasia to be significantly higher than a range of benign liver diseases. This suggests confirmation of Anthony and colleagues' original concept [14] of large-cell dysplasia as a premalignant condition.

4.3.3 Miscellaneous conditions

Quantitation has also been applied to a variety of other liver diseases. Cellular and nuclear size increase along the spectrum of convalescent active hepatitis, chronic inactive/active hepatitis and cirrhosis, while nuclear cytoplasmic ratio remains constant [15]. The number of IgM-containing cells is higher and IgG immunocytes lower in primary biliary cirrhosis than chronic hepatitis and there is a close correlation with serum IgM levels [16]. Morphometry has shown possible contributory vascular aetiologies for the conditions nodular regenerative hyperplasia, partial nodular transformation and focal nodular hyperplasia [17]. It has also been used to study infantile syndromes characterized by paucity of bile ducts [18], as well as increased mitochondrial size and reduced numbers in Reye's syndrome [19].

4.3.4 Conclusion

Morphometry has confirmed the usefulness of needle biopsy in diffuse fibrotic liver disease. It also has a potential use in the discrimination of hepatocellular carcinoma from cirrhosis and benign focal hepatic lesions.

References

1 Ryoo JW, Buschmann RJ. Comparison of intralobar non-parenchyma, subcapsular non-parenchyma, and liver capsule thickness. *J Clin Pathol* 1989; 42: 740–744.
2 Jimenez W, Pares A, Caballeria J *et al.* Measurement of fibrosis in needle liver biopsies: evaluation of a colorimetric method. *Hepatology* 1985; 5: 815–818.
3 Pesce CM, Carli FS. Growth patterns of the fibrous septa of cirrhosis. A morphometric and allometric study. *Pathol Res Pract* 1989; 184: 486–488.
4 Pesce C, Colacino R. The sinusoids in cirrhosis. A morphometric study. *Virchows Arch A Pathol Anat Histol* 1986; 40: 217–219.
5 Auger J, Schoevaert D, Martin ED. Comparative study of automated morphometric and semiquantitative estimations of alcoholic liver steatosis. *Anal Quant Cytol Histol* 1986; 8: 56–62.
6 Caulet S, Fabre M, Schoevaert D, Lesty C, Meduri G, Martin E. Quantitative study of centrolobular hepatic fibrosis in alcoholic disease before cirrhosis. *Virchows Arch A Pathol Anat Histol* 1989; 416: 11–17.
7 Mak KM, Lieber CS. Lipocytes and transitional cells in alcoholic liver disease: a morphometric study. *Hepatology* 1988; 8: 1027–1033.
8 Zeppa P, Zabatta A, Fulciniti F *et al.* The role of morphometry in the cytology of well differentiated hepatocarcinoma and cirrhosis with atypia. *Anal Quant Cytol* 1988; 10: 343–348.
9 Jagoe R, Sowter C, Slavin G. Shape and texture analysis of liver cell nuclei in hepatomas by computer aided microscopy. *J Clin Pathol* 1984; 37: 755–762.
10 Kondo F, Wada K, Kondo Y. Morphometric analysis of hepatocellular carcinoma. *Virchows Arch A Pathol Anat Histol* 1988; 413: 425–430.
11 Matturi L, Bauer D. Morphometric characteristics of hepatocellular dysplasia. *Anal Quant Cytol Histol* 1988; 10: 339–342.
12 Giannini A, Zampi G, Bartoloni F, Omer S. Morphological precursors of hepatocellular carcinoma: a morphometrical analysis. *Hepatogastroenterology* 1987; 34: 95–97.
13 Roncalli M, Borziol M, Tombesi MV, Ferrari A, Servida E. A morphometric study of liver cell dysplasia. *Hum Pathol* 1988; 19: 471–474.
14 Anthony PP, Vogel CL, Barker LF. Liver cell dysplasia: a premalignant condition. *J Clin Pathol* 1973; 26: 217–223.
15 Shimazu H, Shinzawa T, Togahi H *et al.* Computerized morphometry of liver cells in diffuse hepatic diseases. *Gastroenterol Jpn* 1988; 23: 124–128.
16 van Spreeuwel JP, van Gorp LH, Nadorp JH, Janssens AR, Lindeman J, Meijer CJ. Immunoglobulin-containing cells in liver biopsies of patients with chronic hepatitis and primary biliary cirrhosis. *Histopathology* 1984; 8: 559–566.
17 Wanless R. The use of morphometry in the study of nodular and vascular lesions of the liver. *Anal Quant Cytol Histol* 1987; 9: 39–41.
18 Hashida Y, Yunis EJ. Syndromatic paucity of interlobular bile ducts: hepatic histopathology of the early and endstage liver. *Pediatr Pathol* 1988; 8: 1–15.
19 Daugherty CC, Gartside PS, Heubi JE, Saalfeld K, Snyder J. A morphometric study of Reye's syndrome. Correlation of reduced mitochondrial numbers and increased mitochondrial size with clinical manifestations. *Am J Pathol* 1987; 129: 313–326.

4.4 BREAST

There have been few quantitative studies on benign breast tissue but Hutson *et al.* [1] used subgross sections, stereology and planimetric techniques to assess the distribution of parenchymal and connective-tissue elements in age-related changes in normal breasts. They found that the relative amounts of these components vary with age and that involution is a pre- rather than a postmenopausal phenomenon. Epithelial elements were unevenly distributed throughout the gland, with the lower quadrants containing more than the upper quadrants. However, the upper outer quandrant had the largest proportion of lobular units and this may relate to the higher incidence of lobular carcinoma that is found there. Stereology has shown that benign fibroadenomas have an active proliferation of epithelium independent of their histological subtype and that it is the stromal component that dictates on which part of the intracanalicular or pericanalicular spectrum they fall [2]. Morphometry of fine-needle aspirates in lactating adenoma has highlighted the nuclear pleomorphism that can occur in this condition and its quantitative similarities to invasive lobular and well-differentiated breast carcinoma [3]. This obviously emphasizes the necessity for a good history and close clinical examination. Phyllodes tumours form a spectrum of lesions, the biological behaviour of which cannot be reliably predicted from their histology. Potential indicators of aggressive behaviour are stromal cellularity, poorly circumscribed margins and mitotic activity [4]. At an ultrastructural level stereology has emphasized the differences that exist between normal breast and its benign and malignant lesions [5]. There can be few diseases to match breast carcinoma for its potential combination of variable subtypes, treatment modalities and outlook. In mammographic screening of impalpable lesions the emphasis is to detect smaller, earlier lesions with a view to improving morbidity and mortality figures. Consequently the range of lesions being encountered by clinical pathology laboratories is changing in line with this. Image analysis is also used to analyse clustered calcifications on mammograms [6]. The purpose of this section is to overview the plethora of literature generated by quantitative studies on breast tissue. They have been carried out to gain fresh insight into the standardization of nomenclature, grading and prognosis of both early and established disease.

4.4.1 Fine-needle aspiration cytology

Quantitative studies on cytological aspirates depend crucially on the method of fixation and staining and this should be ascertained before direct comparisons between studies are made [7]. Duane *et al.* [8] used semiquantitative and interactive analytical approaches to distinguish colloid carcinoma from pregnancy adenoma, fibroadenoma and other forms of breast carcinoma. This is particularly relevant as colloid carcinoma can assume a relatively benign-appearing cytomorphology. The nuclear axis product (a size factor) and ratio (a shape factor) were the most useful parameters. A high degree of correct classification (15/18) has also been achieved by densitometric contextural analysis of benign and malignant breast aspirates [9]. In a comparative study of nuclear area, perimeter and maximum diameter there was good correlation between eyepiece micrometer and semiautomatic image analysis measurements [10]. There were statistically significant differences in these parameters between 14 benign lesions and 49 invasive ductal carcinomas. The latter were split into three groups according to whether 0, 1–3 or >4 lymph nodes were involved. These groups were also successfully identified by the variable mean nuclear perimeter, whereas mean nuclear area and diameter could not discriminate between patients with or without nodal disease. This contrasts with the findings of Cornelisse *et al.* [11] where carcinomas with small nuclei were more frequent in patients with negative lymph nodes.

Mouriquand *et al.* [12] constructed a semiquantitative scoring system based on the visual assessment of cell cluster size, cell size, nuclear regularity and staining, nucleolar size and mitoses. Grade I tumours had a 95% chance of a disease-free interval of 7 years, grade II 70% and grade III 45%. The risk of recurrence was also related to the size of the tumour, the presence of nodal metastases and steroid receptors. Ocular micrometry of tumour-cell nuclear diameter split a series of 249 breast cancers into two groups predominated either by large (LN) or small nuclei (SN), with a demarcation value of 12 μm [13]. Disease-free survival at 5 years was significantly better in the SN group (90%) than in the LN patients (58%). SN cases also had greater intervals between completion of treatment, the appearance of metastases and death. Kuenen-Boumeester *et al.* [14] formulated a prognostic score after multivariate analysis extracted nuclear area and the presence of axillary metastases as valuable factors. The score classified four patient groups with decreasing metastasis-free periods and survival (group I — no cancer deaths; group IV — 81% cancer deaths). As in the previous study [13], they also noted a degree of overlap in nuclear size between benign lesions and small-cell varieties of breast carcinoma, e.g., infiltrating lobular carcinoma. Other studies have found the following variables to be of use in distinguishing between benign and malignant breast aspirates: nuclear overlap and disarray [15], nuclear area [11], SD in nuclear area [16] and nuclear cytoplasmic ratio [17]. A further morphometric analysis of fine-needle aspirates found that mean nuclear area and its SD gave a predictive value for benignity or malignancy in over 85% of cases [18]. This claim was made having excluded lesions such as fibroadenomas, apocrine metaplasia and inflammation prior to the analysis. Densitometric (DNA ploidy content), morphometric (nuclear area) and chromatin texture significantly and positively evolve in parallel with the histopathological grade of invasive ductal breast carcinomas [19]. The same trend is encountered (despite differences in morphonuclear features) irrespective of whether the samples measured are fine-needle aspirates or touch imprints from their corresponding resection specimens. In both aspirates and histology sections, stereology and image analysis have shown clear differences between benign and malignant breast disease for estimates of nuclear volume [20].

The rest of the discussion will mainly deal with the use of quantitation in breast tissue sections. Processing of the latter causes significant shrinkage and therefore direct comparison with results from aspirate material cannot be made and a corrective factor of approximately 1.55× should be used [21].

4.4.2 Intraductal hyperplasia and carcinoma

The distinction between epitheliosis (hyperplasia of the usual type), atypical hyperplasia and intraduct carcinoma is difficult. It is important as the latter two categories have significantly increased relative risks (4×, 10× respectively) of developing invasive carcinoma. The problem is well-illustrated and discussed in standard textbooks [22]. Using a simple eyepiece graticule, Bhattacharjee *et al.* [23] found that, with a cut-off value of 20 μm^2, representing the difference between the mean nuclear area in a diseased duct and its adjacent normal counterpart, they could correctly classify 86% of 16 cases of epitheliosis and 20 cases of intraduct carcinoma. They measured 50 nuclei per case, the procedure taking 1 h and resulting in a standard error (SE) of less than 2%. In a subsequent semiautomated technique Norris *et al.* [24] distinguished intraduct carcinoma with atypia from ductal hyperplasia, atypical hyperplasia and intraduct carcinoma without atypia. However, based on DNA content and nuclear perimeter measurements, only 69% of well-differentiated carcinomas could be distinguished from atypical hyperplasia and it was concluded that these quantitative features did not have a role to play in this differential diagnosis.

4.4.3 Invasive breast carcinoma

Extent of invasive disease

The measurable size of a tumour is the usual gauge of the extent of disease and is a valuable determinant of prognosis [25]. It is a parameter that can be determined either from the gross specimen or the histological slides in the case of small or diffuse lesions. With the evolution of mammographic screening, more lesions will be encountered where the invasion is only detectable microscopically [26]. The concept of minimal invasive cancer was pioneered by Gallagher and Martin [27] and comprised non-invasive ductal and lobular lesions, along with invasive cases with a diameter no greater than 0.5 cm. These had been shown to have a likelihood of axillary metastases of less than 10% and high survival rates. In a subsequent American College of Surgeons survey of 1423 patients with cancers measuring less than 1 cm in diameter, Bedwani *et al.* [28] found that the 5-year survival figures for node-positive and node-negative patients were 53 and 70.3%, respectively. As in other organs, e.g., vulva and cervix, there remains debate as to what defines minimal invasive cancer and, although the original concept is sound [29], there is a need for standardization. Minimal invasive cancer has also to be distinguished from microinvasion, where the abnormality is limited to 1 mm.

Tumour grading and cellularity

It has been long recognized that tumour grade has an important influence on prognosis [30] but its designation is hampered by poor reproducibility [31]. In an attempt to achieve a degree of standardization in the UK, the National Health Service Breast Screening Programme [32] advocates the use of a grading system formed from tumour tubule formation, nuclear pleomorphism and mitoses. It is based on the work of Bloom and Richardson [33] and is shown in Table 4.1.

Thus, a grade I tumour shows tubule formation and relatively little cellular pleomorphism or mitotic activity. As with most grading systems, the greater number of lesions fall within the intermediate category (45%) and there is variation in applying what is a semiquantitative scheme. However, it does impart important, practical prognostic information. Bloom and Richardson [33] reported 5-year survival figures of 75, 53 and 31% for grade I, II and III cancers, respectively. More recently, Elston and Ellis [34] found differential survival figures using the modified grading system described above. Confirmation of the validity of a grading approach is gained from an interactive computerized morphometric study [35] on ductal breast cancer (not otherwise specified; NOS). This showed that textural parameters representing the numbers of large and dense chromatin clots and nuclear chromatin heterogeneity evolved in a continuous manner parallel with scores of 4–8 on the Bloom and Richardson scale. Similarly, a combination of mean nuclear area and the number of mitoses gave an 87.5% separation of grade I and II tumours in cytological aspirates. Adding in mean nuclear shape factor obtained an 83.3% classification of grade II and grade III cancers. It was concluded that 72.7% of

Table 4.1 National Health Service Breast Screening Programme grading system for breast carcinoma. Based on Bloom and Richardson [33]

Tubule formation	I $>$75% tumour	
	II 10–75% tumour	
	III $<$10% tumour	
Nuclear pleomorphism	I Regular, uniform	
	II Larger with variation	
	III Marked variation	
Mitoses	I 0–9	per 10 HPFs – field
	II 10–19	diameter 0.59 mm,
	III $>$20	area 274 mm^2

Grade I = score 3–5.
Grade II = score 6–7.
Grade III = score 8–9.
HPF, high-power field.

equivocally graded slides could be classified using morphometry with a high degree of accuracy [36].

Potential pitfalls and guidelines in applying a Bloom and Richardson-type scheme are well-reviewed elsewhere [37]. In a systematic morphometric approach Sharkey *et al.* [38] noted that patients were more likely to have recurrent disease if their tumours had a smaller proportion of *in situ* change (IN) and glandular differentiation (DI), i.e., higher-grade lesions. There were 24 recurrences in 33 patients with DI and IN $<$10% and none in 14 patients with DI and IN $>$10%. The method afforded systematic sampling of each lesion and was applied by a supervised technician. It was capable of assigning more cases to the grade 1 and 3 categories than the subjective method [33]. It also emphasized that grading should be performed on a sample that is representative of the entire tumour, rather than its least differentiated part [39] or relatively paucicellular centre [37].

The earliest morphometric studies have recommended a standard sampling pattern to account for this variation in cellularity in the different parts of a lesion [40]. Cellularity also bears a direct relation to the tumour subtype and connective-tissue fibroblastic response, e.g., medullary carcinoma is 64.5% composed of tumour cell volume and scirrhous carcinoma 21.5% [40]. Parham *et al.* [41] showed that the greater the tumour cell area/stroma ratio, the more prolonged was patient survival. It was also independent of histological grade and gave more prognostic information than the tumour diameter. Tumour cellularity was postulated to indicate greater cohesiveness and less ability to metastasize. However, others have found that the tumour cellularity index correlates with lymph node involvement and the number of mitotic figures per 10 HPFs [42]. These findings appear to be somewhat contrary to the benefits of tumour cellularity reported above.

The data in the preceding five studies was obtained by stereological techniques and ocular micrometers. More recently, breast cancer tissue sections have been assessed using immunochemistry with automatic image segmentation to determine percentage epithelial volume, similar to techniques used in gynaecological cancers [43].

Nuclear/nucleolar size and nodal metastases

Image cytometry of tumour cell nuclei has shown that it is possible to separate patients into node-positive and node-negative groups on the basis of nuclear area and descriptors of the chromatin structure [44]. Discriminant analysis proved quantitation to be a better predictor (73% efficient) of 5-year survival than histopathological grade (60.8%). Semi-automatic image analysis of a series of 90 cases showed that the mean nuclear area in lymph node metastases and in primary tumours with nodal involvement was significantly greater than in those without [45]. It was conjectured that the mean nuclear area is inversely related to prognosis. A further comparison of morphometry analysed three groups of tumour cells: (i) primary tumours without lymph node metastases; (ii) primary tumours with node metastases; and (iii) axillary lymph nodal deposits [46]. The mitotic index increased from group (i) to group (iii), and there was a reciprocal trend for tumour cellularity. Group (ii) had greater variation in nuclear measurements but the discrepancies from group (i) were not sufficient to allow them to be statistically separated. There was good correlation of morphometric features in primary tumours with lymph node disease and their metastatic deposits.

In a group of 65 patients with breast cancer and a follow-up period of at least 5 years, non-survivors had larger, more pleomorphic nucleoli with an SD value above 2.49 μm^2 [47]. This feature was of particular note, as several of these patients had a low mitotic activity index and small tumours, with some of them being node-negative. They might otherwise, therefore, have been included in a good-prognosis group. In cytological aspirates multivariate analysis isolated the total number of nucleoli per 100 nuclei as the best single prognostic variable [48], with the SD of nucleolar area also identified as superior to other nuclear parameters. Quantitation of nuclear morphology and fine chromatin structure have also been claimed to predict prognosis accurately [49], while the relevance of nucleolar topography has yet to be assessed [50].

A morphometric prognostic index

Nodal status, tumour size and histological grade in breast carcinoma have been used to form an index that gives valuable guidelines to prognosis and survival [51,52]. The virtues of a prognostic index are that it should be based on a number of features that are reliably identified, easily and reproducibly measured and a combination of which provides clinically useful prognostic information. They are derived by analysing detailed individual parameters in turn and then statistically determining the relative strength of their contribution to the prognosis.

This multiparameter approach was well-exemplified by Stenkvist *et al.* [53] who evaluated 22 cytometric features, the mitotic frequency and tritiated thymidine-labelling index in a range of 142 breast cancers. From this they derived a cytometric measure by combining the four features that most strongly correlated with mitotic frequency. Ultimately the variance of the nuclear area was identified as correlating most with mitoses and the recurrence rate. Subsequent to this, a detailed study compared the value of morphometry against classical prognosticators (tumour size, axillary nodal status) in 271 patients with follow-up periods varying between 5 and 12 years [54]. Univariate analysis showed the following features to be significant: lymph node status, tumour size, nuclear and histological grade, mitotic activity index, mean and SD of nuclear area and cellularity index. In summary, prognosis was worse with high nuclear and cytological grade, lymph node positivity, tumour size exceeding 3.0 cm, a mitotic activity index greater than 20 and mean nuclear area above 52 μm^2. Mitotic activity index (total number of sharply defined and unequivocal mitoses per 10 HPF) was identified as the most important feature but proved more powerful in a combination with tumour size and lymph node status. The morphometric prognostic index was therefore formulated as follows:

$$\text{MPI} = (0.3341 \cdot \sqrt{\text{MAI}}) + (0.2342 \cdot \text{tumour size (cm)}) - (0.7654 \cdot \text{lymph node status})$$

where MPI = morphometric prognostic index; MAI = mitotic activity index; and lymph node status: 1 = positive, 2 = negative.

Discriminant analysis calculated numerical probabilities based on the features in the prognostic index. Five-year survivals for lymph node-negative and -positive patients were 85 and 55% and these had improved prognostic index scores of 93 and 47%, respectively. The overall efficiency of the classification performance was assessed as 74.9%. The virtue of this approach was that it left considerably less prognostically uncertain cases (16%) than would be normally encountered in subjective grading, where many of the cases will fall. The index also performed well in a series of premenopausal patients [55]. The technique was commended for its simplicity, cheapness and more refined prognostic information (Fig. 4.6), also with the potential to identify responders/non-responders to chemotherapy [56].

A prospective evaluation of the system was carried out in 195 patients who had not received either chemotherapy or hormonal treatment [57]. Recurrence in 22% of the patients was more accurately determined by the prognostic index than by the presence of lymph node metastases (Table 4.2).

Mitotic activity index had the second strongest predictive prognostic value. The measurements were also carried out reliably, reproducibly and by different technicians. The relative weight of the mitotic activity index has also been emphasized by others [58]. Ten of nineteen patients with an index greater than 9 had recurrent disease within 18 months, whereas none of 9 patients with a low index (less than 9) had further problems. The prognostic index did not perform as well as in previous studies and this was attributed to blurring by lymph nodal status. Because of this it has been advocated that morphometry should be applied not only to the primary tumour but also to the nodal deposits, where available [59]. A combination of nuclear axis ratio of the primary tumour and a randomly selected lymph node metastasis afforded additional prognostic information. An enlarged tumour cell mean nuclear area and efferent vascular invasion in positive lymph nodes have also been regarded as unfavourable signs [60]. Van Diest *et al.* [61] have shown that a combination of parameters related to the variation in mitotic activity in lymph node metastases provided a satisfactory means of differentiating patients with a good (68% survival) and a poor (28% survival) prognosis. It also proved

Table 4.2 Actuarial recurrence-free rate for morphometric prognostic index in comparison to the presence of lymph node metastases

	Actuarial recurrence free rate (%)
Low prognostic index < 0.6	88*
High prognostic index > 0.6	50*
Node-positive	80†
Node-negative	62†

* $P < 0.001$.
† $P < 0.05$.

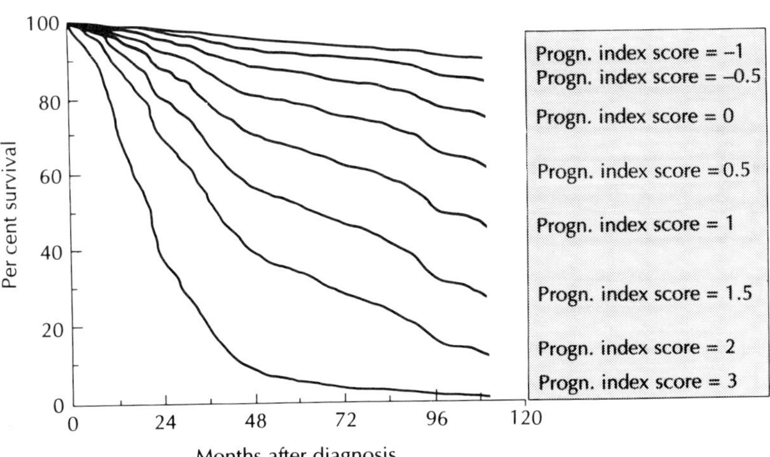

Fig. 4.6 Breast cancer patient survival in relation to tumour morphometric prognostic index score. From Baak *et al.* [54].

superior to the more usual morphometric prognosticators, e.g., volume percentage epithelium, nuclear/area and nuclear/axis ratio. However, it should be noted that there is potential for intrapatient variation of quantitative features in nodal metastases [62].

There have been direct comparisons between the morphometric prognostic index and DNA flow cytometry [63]. The index outperformed DNA ploidy in predicting distant recurrence. In individual parameter analysis, DNA ploidy was selected fourth after lymph node status, mitotic activity index and tumour size. As a result of this the DNA index incorporated in a linear combination with mitotic activity index and mean nuclear area achieved a high level of predictive accuracy, irrespective of nodal status [64]. This is envisaged as a useful additional criterion to the prognostic index. Syntactic structure analysis is also being assessed as an adjunctive prognosticator in invasive breast disease [65].

Baak and coworkers have studied many of these applications and also instigated a 10-year nationwide prospective study to assess the role of various quantitative parameters. It is to involve 3000 patients, 34 hospitals and 15 laboratories in the standardized acquisition and co-ordination of data relating to tumour size, nodal involvement, mitotic activity index, morphometric prognostic index, nuclear size, DNA and Ki-67 status and steroid content. Strict criteria have been laid down for the area of tumour selection, the number of nuclei to be measured, the definition of a mitosis and the number and size of the microscopic fields over which they are to be counted [66,67]. Initial work has found that mitosis counting can be highly reproducible if a strict protocol is carefully followed [68]. It is only through such an approach that the relative biological importance of individual facets of the disease will be elaborated.

Morphometry and DNA measurements

The application of DNA measurements is dealt with elsewhere and only alluded to here briefly. In a series of 65 patients there was no relation between DNA ploidy, lymph node status and tumour size [69], although tumours with a mitotic activity index above 10 were predominantly DNA aneuploid (61%). The morphometric prognostic index correlated with the DNA index in 63% of cases. Densitometry showed a wider variation in DNA content and nuclear size in short survival cases [70,71] while a combination of DNA content and the nucleolus/nucleus ratio assigned 100% of living and 81% of deceased cases to those exact categories [72]. In fine-needle aspirate specimens different subtypes of breast carcinomas vary in their DNA content and tumour cell nuclear area [73]. The feasibility of a malignancy grading system incorporating both cytometric and proliferation indices is addressed by Stenkvist *et al.* [74].

Cell markers

Present image analysis systems are capable of measuring both the distribution and intensity of stained elements and this has been used to effect in assaying a number of cell markers.

Proliferation antigens (Ki-67, PCNA)

Cell proliferation has traditionally been assessed by indirect and direct means, such as mitotic rate, incorporation of tritiated thymidine combined with autoradiography [75] and the S-phase fraction in flow cytometry [76]. More recent techniques involve the thymidine analogue bromodeoxyuridine and the immunodetection of the cell proliferation nuclear antigen Ki-67 [77]. Several of these studies have also been carried out in tandem with a comparison of steroid receptors. In brief they can be summarized as follows: Ki-67 expression is greater in malignant than benign breast disease [78,79]. Its level correlates with increasing tumour size [80], dedifferentiation, vascular invasion and lymph node involvement [78,81]. It is inversely related to oestrogen receptor status [78,80–82] and closely parallels the S-phase fraction [79,81]. It reflects tumour grade and mitotic count and is a better estimate of growth fraction than PCNA [83]. Thus it appears to identify a subset of cancers with more aggressive behaviour. It is applicable to frozen- and paraffin-section material but comparable results have been obtained with fine-needle aspirates [84,85]. Kuenen-Boumeester *et al.* [85] showed that Ki-67 was expressed stronger in the solid and comedo variants of NOS ductal cancer than in the mucinous or lobular types. However, there is not total agreement and one other study has noted no relationship between Ki-67 scores and the usual clinical and pathological parameters of breast cancer [86]. PCNA is being widely investigated as a marker of tumour proliferation, e.g., lung cancer [87] and a method of grading, e.g., glioma [88]. Reviews have recently expressed caution due to the possible resistance of epitopes to fixation and embedding, along with the multiplicity of epitopes and antibodies seen in PCNA [89].

Steroid receptors

The presence of oestrogen and progesterone receptors in breast cancer tissue is generally regarded as conferring a better overall prognosis and also assists in the selection of patients who may benefit from endocrine therapy. Assay has traditionally been either biochemically, by a dextran-coated charcoal radioligand-binding technique or manual assessment of tissue immunosections. The latter has the advantage of preserving morphology and recently it has been further refined by automatic image analysis. A number of authors have noted a close correlation between the techniques both in tissue sections [90,91] and fine-needle aspirates [92]. The benefits of a tissue technique are in being able to visualize intratumoural heterogeneity in steroid receptor status [93,94]. In a series of 49 cases, McClelland *et al.* [95] found that tamoxifen response rates of 0, 41 and 64% corresponded to steroid receptor scores of 0, 1–100 and >100, respectively, using a CAS 100 computer-assisted image analysis system. Previous quantitative studies have linked oestrogen receptor status to tumour elastosis [96,97] and inconsistently to cellularity [96,98]. Nuclear morphometric parameters have been found to be only weakly associated with oestrogen receptor positivity [97,99], which largely diminishes with increasing nuclear area. This has been confirmed stereologically with steroid-positive cases characterized as having smaller tumour cell volumes [100]. Oestrogen-negative tumours have also been found to have larger nuclei, greater DNA content and more condensed chromatin patterns [101].

Other markers

Semiquantitative scoring of carcinoembryonic antigen expression and peanut agglutinin binding in primary breast cancers and their nodal metastases failed to show correlation with any clinical, histopathological, biochemical or morphometric features [102]. Image analysis using a Quantimet system and visual assessment of a range of monoclonal antibodies gave comparable results and showed a negative correlation between tumour histological grade and breast carcinoma cell line antibody (BRST-1) and epithelial membrane antigen (EmA) antibody [103]. The quantitative assessment of C-*erb*B-2 oncogene expression has yet to be evaluated. In breast carcinoma the ratio of epithelial to stromal leucocytes is reversed due to a diminution in the former and an increase in the latter. In addition, the stromal lymphocytes show expression of activation markers [104], implying a local immunological reaction to the tumour. Diminished expression of the basement membrane antigens laminin and type IV collagen relates to a decrease in tumour steroid receptors and the presence of vascular and nodal involvement. This has been proposed as an indicator of metastatic potential [105], as has increased tumour angiogenesis [106].

4.4.4 Conclusion

Quantitation of fine-needle aspirates and breast tissue sections has shown differences between benign and malignant lesions, particularly in features such as cellularity, nuclear dimensions and texture and mitotic activity. They form a spectrum of abnormality in which the differences are not sufficiently distinctive to allow conclusively reliable separation of some lesions, e.g., intraduct carcinoma and atypical hyperplasia, benign breast disease and small-cell varieties of carcinoma such as infiltrating lobular. Cytological and histological grading systems are in effect subjective assessments of quantifiable parameters and their virtue in affording useful prognostic information has been confirmed by morphometry. Their application, along with derived multiparameter prognostic indices, has met with some success in established breast carcinoma where the importance of tumour size, mitotic activity and nodal status in disease recurrence and survival has been emphasized. Construction of a more comprehensive system inclusive of DNA and tumour marker measurements, e.g., Ki-67, awaits fuller evaluation. Well-organized, standardized and critically appraised studies will establish the role of these various parameters and determine a combination of them which is most adept at predicting prognosis and selecting subgroups of patients for appropriate treatment modalities.

References

1 Hutson SW, Cowen PN, Bird CC. Morphometric studies of age related changes in normal human breast and their significance for evolution of mammary cancer. *J Clin Pathol* 1985; 38: 281–287.

2 Pesce C, Colacino R. Morphometry of the breast fibroadenoma. *Pathol Res Pract* 1986; 181: 718–720.

3 Grenko RT, Lee KP, Lee KR. Fine needle aspiration cytology of lactating adenoma of the breast. A comparative light microscopic and morphometric study. *Acta Cytol* 1990; 34: 21–26.

4 Hart WR, Bauer RC, Oberman HA. *Cystosarcoma phyllodes.* A clinicopathological study of 26 hypercellular periductal stromal tumours of the breast. *Am J Clin Pathol* 1978; 70: 211–216.

5 Wolf B, Thompson J, Schwinde A. An ultrastructural morphometric analysis of normal mammary tissue and human breast cancer. *Anticancer Res* 1985; 5: 211–219.

6 Davies DH, Dance DR. Automatic computer detection of clustered calcifications in digital mammograms. *Phys Med Biol* 1990; 35: 1111–1118.

7 Schulte E, Wittekind C. The influence of the wet-fixed Papanicolaou and the air-dried Giemsa techniques on nuclear parameters in breast cancer cytology: a cytomorphometric study. *Diagn Cytopathol* 1987; 3: 256–261.

8 Duane GB, Kanter MH, Branigan T, Chang C. A morphologic and morphometric study of cells from colloid carcinoma of the breast obtained by fine needle aspiration. Distinction from other breast lesions. *Acta Cytol* 1987; 31: 742–750.

9 Hutchinson ML, Schultz DS, Stephenson RA, Wong KL, Harry T, Zahniser DJ. Computerised microscopic analysis of prostatic fine needle aspirates. Comparison with breast aspirates. *Anal Quant Cytol Histol* 1989; 11: 105–110.

10 Wittekind C, Schulte E. Computerized morphometric image analysis of cytologic nuclear parameters in breast cancer. *Anal Quant Cytol Histol* 1987; 9: 480–484.

11 Cornelisse CJ, De Koning HR, Arentz PW, Raatgever JW, van Heerde P. Quantitative analysis of the nuclear area variation in benign and malignant breast cytology specimens. *Anal Quant Cytol* 1981; 3: 128–134.

12 Mouriquand J, Gozlan-Fior M, Villemain D *et al.* Value of cytoprognostic classification in breast carcinomas. *J Clin Pathol* 1986; 39: 489–496.

13 Zajdela A, De Lariva LS, Ghossein NA. The relation of prognosis to the nuclear diameter of breast cancer cells obtained by cytologic aspiration. *Acta Cytol* 1979; 23: 75–80.

14 Kuenen-Boumeester V, Hop WCJ, Blonk DI, Boon ME. Prognostic scoring using cytophotometry and lymph node status of patients with breast carcinoma. *Eur J Cancer Clin Oncol* 1984; 20: 337–345.

15 Dziura BR, Bonfiglio TA. Needle cytology of the breast: a quantitative and qualitative study of the cells of benign and malignant ductal neoplasia. *Acta Cytol* 1979; 23: 332–340.

16 Mapstone NP, Zakhour HD. Morphometric analysis of fine needle aspirates from breast lesions. *Cytopathology* 1990; 1: 349–355.

17 Boon ME, Trott PA, van Kaam H, Kurver PJH, Leach A, Baak JPA. Morphometry and cytodiagnosis of breast lesions. *Virchows Arch Pathol Anat* 1982; 396: 9–18.

18 Beerman H, Veldhuizen RW, Blok RAP, Hermans J, Ooms ECM. Cytomorphometry as quality control for fine needle aspiration. A study in 321 breast lesions. *Anal Quant Cytol Histol* 1991; 13: 143–148.

19 Salmon I, Coibion M, Larsimont D *et al.* Comparison of fine needle aspirates of breast cancers to imprint smears by means of digital cell image analysis. *Anal Quant Cytol Histol* 1991; 13: 193–200.

20 Neal HJ, Hurst PR. The estimation of mean nuclear volume in the diagnosis of breast carcinoma. *Diagn Cytopathol* 1992; 8: 293–298.

21 van Bogaert L-J, DeMuylder C. Nuclear diameters of breast cancer cells in tissue sections. *Anal Quant Cytol* 1980; 2: 55–58.

22 Page DL, Anderson TJ. *Diagnostic Histopathology of the Breast.* Edinburgh: Churchill Livingstone, 1987.

23 Bhattacharjee DK, Harris M, Faragher EB. Nuclear morphometry of epitheliosis and intraduct carcinoma of the breast. *Histopathology* 1985; 9: 511–516.

24 Norris HJ, Bahr GF, Mikel UV. A comparative morphometric and cytophotometric study of intraductal hyperplasia and intraductal carcinoma of the breast. *Anal Quant Cytol Histol* 1988; 10: 1–9.

25 Koscielny S, Tubiana M, Le MG *et al.* Breast cancer: relationship between the size of the primary tumour and the probability of metastatic dissemination. *Br J Cancer* 1984; 49: 709–715.

26 Walker RA. Breast screening. In: O'Shea JP (ed.) *ACP Yearbook.* London: Stroudgate, 1991: 55–58.

27 Gallagher HS, Martin JE. An introduction to the concept of minimal breast cancer. *Cancer* 1971; 28: 1505–1507.
28 Bedwani R, Vana J, Rosner D, Schmitz RL, Murphy GP. Management and survival of female patients with 'minimal' breast cancer. As observed in the long term and short term surveys of the American College of Surgeons. *Cancer* 1981; 47: 2769–2778.
29 Hartmann WH. Minimal breast cancer: an update. *Cancer* 1984; 53: 681–684.
30 Patey DH, Scarff RW. The position of histology in the prognosis of carcinoma of the breast. *Lancet* 1928; 1: 801–804.
31 Stenkvist B, Westman-Naeser S, Vegelius J *et al.* Analysis of reproducibility of subjective grading systems for breast carcinoma. *J Clin Pathol* 1979; 32: 979–985.
32 NHS Breast Screening Programme. *Pathology Reporting in Breast Cancer Screening proposed by a Royal College of Pathologists Working Group.* London: Royal College of Pathologists, 1989.
33 Bloom HJG, Richardson WW. Histological grading and prognosis in breast cancer. A study of 1409 cases of which 359 have been followed for 15 years. *Br J Cancer* 1957; 11: 359–377.
34 Elston CW, Ellis IO. Pathological prognostic factors in breast cancer. I. The value of histological grade in breast cancer: experience from a large study with long-term follow-up. *Histopathology* 1991; 19: 403–410.
35 Larsimont D, Kiss R, D'Olne D *et al.* Relationship between computerised morphonuclear image analysis and histopathologic grading of breast cancer. *Anal Quant Cytol Histol* 1989; 11: 433–439.
36 van Diest PJ, Risse EKJ, Schipper NW, Baak JPA, Mouriquand J. Comparison of light microscopic grading and morphometric features in cytological breast cancer specimens. *Pathol Res Pract* 1989; 185: 612–616.
37 Elston CW. Grading of invasive carcinoma of the breast. In: Page DL, Anderson TJ (eds) *Diagnostic Histopathology of the Breast.* Edinburgh: Churchill Livingstone, 1987: 300–311.
38 Sharkey FE, Pavlak RJ, Greiner AS. Morphometric analysis of differentiation in human breast carcinoma. Tumor grading. *Arch Pathol Lab Med* 1983; 107: 406–410.
39 Sharkey FE. Morphometric analysis of differentiation in human breast carcinoma. Tumor heterogeneity. *Arch Pathol Lab Med* 1983; 107: 411–414.
40 Underwood JCE. A morphometric analysis of human breast carcinoma. *Br J Cancer* 1972; 26: 234–237.
41 Parham DM, Robertson AJ, Brown RA. Morphometric analysis of breast carcinoma: association with survival. *J Clin Pathol* 1988; 41: 173–177.
42 Ambros RA, Trost RC. Cellularity in breast carcinoma. *Am J Clin Pathol* 1990; 93: 98–100.
43 Schipper NW, Smeulders AWM, Baak JPA. Automated estimation of epithelial volume in breast cancer sections. A comparison with the image processing steps applied to gynecologic tumors. *Pathol Res Pract* 1990; 186: 737–744.
44 Kunze KD, Haroske G, Dimmer V, Meyer W, Theissig F. Grading and prognosis of invasive ductal mammary carcinoma by nuclear image analysis in tissue sections. *Pathol Res Pract* 1989; 185: 689–693.
45 Tosi P, Luzi P, Sforza V, Spina D, Miracco C, Santopietro R. Morphometrical assessment of mean nuclear area in breast cancer in comparison with that of lymph node metastases. *Pathol Res Pract* 1985; 180: 498–501.
46 van der Linden HC, Baak JPA, Smeulders AWM, Lindeman J, Meyer CJLM. Morphometry of breast cancer. I. Comparison of the primary tumours and the axillary lymph node metastases. *Pathol Res Pract* 1986; 181: 236–242.
47 Baak JPA. The relative prognostic significance of nucleolar morphometry in invasive ductal breast cancer. *Histopathology* 1985; 9: 437–444.
48 van Diest PJ, Mouriquand J, Schipper NW, Baak JP. Prognostic value of nucleolar morphometric variables in cytological breast cancer specimens. *J Clin Pathol* 1990; 43: 157–159.
49 Komitowski D, Janson C. Quantitative features of chromatin structure in the prognosis of breast cancer. *Cancer* 1990; 65: 2725–2730.
50 Lesty C, Raphael M, Chleq C, Binet JL. Nucleolar topography of nuclei in histologic sections. Application of a nonparametric approach to the study of breast cancer and non-Hodgkin's lymphoma. *Anal Quant Cytol Histol* 1990; 12: 242–250.
51 Haybittle JL, Blamey RW, Elston CW *et al.* A prognostic index in primary breast cancer. *Br J Cancer* 1982; 45: 361–366.
52 Todd JH, Dowle C, Williams MR *et al.* Confirmation of a prognostic index in primary breast cancer. *Br J Cancer* 1987; 56: 489–492.
53 Stenkvist B, Bengtsson E, Eriksson O, Jarkrans T, Nordin B, Westman-Naeser S. Correlation between cytometric features and mitotic frequency in human breast carcinoma. *Cytometry* 1981; 1: 287–291.
54 Baak JPA, van Dop H, Kurver PHJ, Hermans J. The value of morphometry to classic prognosticators in breast cancer. *Cancer* 1985; 56: 374–382.
55 van Diest PJ, Baak JPA. The morphometric prognostic index is the strongest prognosticator in premenopausal lymph node-negative and lymph node-positive breast cancer patients. *Hum Pathol* 1991; 22: 326–330.
56 van Diest PJ, Baak JPA, Matze-Cok P, Bacus SS. Prediction of response to adjuvant chemotherapy in premenopausal lymph node positive breast cancer patients with morphometry, DNA flow cytometry and Her-2/Neu oncoprotein expression. Preliminary

results. *Pathol Res Pract* 1992; 188: 344–349.

57 van der Linden JC, Baa JPA, Lindeman J, Hermans J, Meyer CJLM. Prospective evaluation of prognostic value of morphometry in patients with primary breast cancer. *J Clin Pathol* 1987; 40: 302–306.

58 Tosi P, Luzi P, Sforza V *et al.* Correlation between morphometrical parameters and disease-free survival in ductal breast cancer treated only by surgery. *Appl Pathol* 1986; 4: 33–42.

59 van der Linden JC, Baak JPA, Lindeman J, Hermans J, Meijer CJLM. Morphometry and breast cancer. II. Characterization of breast cancer cells with high malignant potential in patients with spread to lymph nodes: preliminary results. *J Clin Pathol* 1986; 39: 603–609.

60 Maehle BO, Skjaerven R. A prognostic index based on the mean nuclear area of breast cancer cells and efferent vascular invasion in the axillary nodes. *Diagn Histopathol* 1983; 6: 221–228.

61 van Diest PJ, Matze-Cok E, Baak JPA. Prognostic value of proliferative activity in lymph node metastases of patients with breast cancer. *J Clin Pathol* 1991; 44: 416–418.

62 van Diest PJ, Fleege JC, Matze-Cok E, Baak JPA. Intrapatient variation between breast cancer axillary lymph node metastases using quantifiable features. *Histopathology* 1992; 21: 257–262.

63 van der Linden JC, Lindeman JH, Baak JPA, Meijer CJLM, Herman CJ. The Multivariate Prognostic Index and nuclear DNA content are independent prognostic factors in primary breast cancer patients. *Cytometry* 1989; 10: 56–61.

64 Uyterlinde AM, Baak JP, Schipper NW, Peterse H, Matze E, Meijer CJL. Further evaluation of the prognostic value of morphometric and flow cytometric parameters in breast cancer patients with long follow-up. *Int J Cancer* 1990; 45: 1–7.

65 van Diest PJ, Fleege JC, Baak JPA. Syntactic structure analysis in invasive breast cancer: analysis of reproducibility, biologic background and prognostic value. *Hum Pathol* 1992; 23: 876–883.

66 Baak JPA, van Diest PJ, Stroet-Van Galen C *et al.* Data processing and analysis in the multicenter morphometric mammary carcinoma project (MMMCP). *Pathol Res Pract* 1989; 185: 657–663.

67 Baak JPA, van Diest PJ, Ariens AT *et al.* The multicenter morphometric mammary carcinoma project (MMMCP). A nationwide prospective study on reproducibility and prognostic power of routine quantitative assessments in The Netherlands. *Pathol Res Pract* 1989; 185: 664–670.

68 van Diest PJ, Baak JPA, Matze-Cok P *et al.* Reproducibility of mitosis counting in 2469 breast cancer specimens: results from the multicenter morphometric mammary carcinoma project. *Hum Pathol* 1992; 23: 603–607.

69 Uyterlinde AM, Schipper NW, Baak JPA. Comparison of extent of disease, morphometric and DNA flow cytometric prognostic factors in invasive ductal breast cancer. *J Clin Pathol* 1987; 40: 1432–1436.

70 Troncoso P, Dytch HE, Bibbo M, Wied GL, Dawson PJ. The significance of DNA measurements in a histologically defined subset of infiltrating ductal carcinomas of the breast with long-term follow-up. *Anal Quant Cytol Histol* 1989; 11: 166–172.

71 Tamura G, Masuda T, Sato HT, Satodate R, Ishida M, Saitoh K. Karyometric and DNA content analysis of cancer cells in stage III breast cancer with reference to prognosis. *Jpn J Clin Oncol* 1990; 20: 78–82.

72 Mariuzzi GM, Mambelli V, Criante P, Sisti S. Quantitative evaluation of morphological parameters for infiltrating ductal breast cancer prognosis. *Pathol Res Pract* 1989; 185: 698–700.

73 Boon ME, Auer GU, van Kaam H, Schwinghammer H. Classifying breast carcinomas with DNA measurements and morphometry. *Cytometry* 1984; 5: 469–472.

74 Stenkvist B, Bengtsson E, Eriksson O, Jarkrans T, Nordin B. Image cytometry in malignancy grading of breast cancer. Results in a prospective study with seven years of follow-up. *Anal Quant Cytol Histol* 1986; 8: 293–300.

75 Tubiana M, Pejovic MH, Chavaudra N, Contesso G, Malaise EP. The long-term prognostic significance of the thymidine labelling index in breast cancer. *Int J Cancer* 1984; 33: 441–445.

76 Haag D, Goerttler K, Tschahargane C. The proliferative index (PI) of human breast cancer as obtained by flow cytometry. *Pathol Res Pract* 1984; 178: 315–322.

77 Gerdes J, Lelle RJ, Pickartz H *et al.* Growth fractions in breast cancers determined *in situ* with monoclonal antibody Ki67. *J Clin Pathol* 1986; 39: 977–980.

78 Charpin C, Andrac L, Vacheret H *et al.* Multiparametric evaluation (SAMBA) of growth fraction (monoclonal Ki67) in breast carcinoma tissue sections. *Cancer Res* 1988; 48: 4368–4374.

79 Dawson AE, Norton JA, Weinberg DS. Comparative assessment of proliferation and DNA content in breast carcinoma by image analysis and flow cytometry. *Am J Pathol* 1990; 136: 1115–1124.

80 Veronese SM, Gambacorta M. Detection of Ki67 proliferation rate in breast cancer. Correlation with clinical and pathologic features. *Am J Clin Pathol* 1991; 95: 30–34.

81 Vielh P, Chevillard S, Mosseri V, Donatini B, Magdelenat H. Ki67 index and S-phase fraction in human breast carcinoma. Comparison and correlations with prognostic factors. *Am J Clin Pathol* 1990; 94: 681–686.

82 Bacus SS, Goldschmidt R, Chin D, Moran G, Weinberg D, Bacus JW. Biological grading of breast cancer using antibodies to proliferating cells and other markers. *Am J Pathol* 1989; 135: 783–792.

83 Leonardi E, Girlando S, Serio G *et al.* PCNA and Ki67 expression in breast carcinoma: correlations with clinical and biological variables. *J Clin Pathol* 1992; 45: 416–419.
84 Franklin WA, Bibbo M, Doria MI *et al.* Quantitation of estrogen receptor content and Ki-67 staining in breast carcinoma by the Micro TICAS image analysis system. *Anal Quant Cytol Histol* 1987; 9: 279–286.
85 Kuenen-Boumeester V, van der Kwast TH, van Laarhoven HAJ, Henzen-Logmans SC. Ki-67 staining in histological subtypes of breast carcinoma and fine needle aspiration smears. *J Clin Pathol* 1991; 44: 208–210.
86 Barnard NJ, Hall PA, Lemoine NR, Kadar N. Proliferative index in breast carcinoma determined *in situ* by Ki-67 immunostaining and its relationship to clinical and pathological variables. *J Pathol* 1987; 152: 287–295.
87 Theunissen PH, Leers MP, Bollen EC. Proliferating cell nuclear antigen (PCNA) expression in formalin-fixed tissue of non-small cell lung carcinoma. *Histopathology* 1992; 20: 251–255.
88 Allegranza A, Girlando S, Arrigoni GL *et al.* Proliferating cell nuclear antigen expression in central nervous system neoplasms. *Virchows Archiv-A, Pathol Anat* 1991; 419: 417–423.
89 McCormick D, Hall PA. The complexities of proliferating cell nuclear antigen. *Histopathology* 1992; 21: 591–594.
90 Bacus S, Flowers JL, Press MF, Bacus JW, McCarty KS Jr. The evaluation of estrogen receptor in primary breast carcinoma by computer-assisted image analysis. *Am J Clin Pathol* 1988; 90: 233–239.
91 Cohen O, Brugal G, Seigneurin D, Demongeot J. Image cytometry of estrogen receptors in breast carcinomas. *Cytometry* 1988; 9: 579–587.
92 Horsfall DJ, Jarvis LR, Grimbaldeston MA, Tilley WD, Orell SR. Immunocytochemical assay for oestrogen receptor in fine needle aspirates of breast cancer by video image analysis. *Br J Cancer* 1989; 59: 129–134.
93 Kommoss F, Bibbo M, Colley M *et al.* Assessment of hormone receptors in breast carcinoma by immunocytochemistry and image analysis. I. Progesterone receptors. *Anal Quant Cytol Histol* 1989; 11: 298–306.
94 Colley M, Kommoss F, Bibbo M *et al.* Assessment of hormone receptors in breast carcinoma by immunocytochemistry and image analysis. II. Estrogen receptors. *Anal Quant Cytol Histol* 1989; 11: 307–314.
95 McClelland RA, Finlay P, Walker KJ *et al.* Automated quantitation of immunocytochemically localized estrogen receptors in human breast cancer. *Cancer Res* 1990; 50: 3545–3550.
96 Underwood JC, Dangerfield VJM, Parsons MA. Oestrogen receptor assay of cryostat sections of human breast carcinomas with simultaneous quantitative histology. *J Clin Pathol* 1983; 36: 399–405.
97 Tosi P, Baak JPA, Luzi P, Sforza V, Santopietro R, Lio R. Correlation between immunohistochemically determined oestrogen receptor content, using monoclonal antibodies, and qualitative and quantitative tissue features in ductal breast cancer. *Histopathology* 1987; 11: 741–751.
98 Parham DM, Baker PR, Robertson AJ, Vasishta A, Baker PG, Smith G. Breast carcinoma cellularity and its relation to oestrogen receptor content. *J Clin Pathol* 1989; 42: 1166–1168.
99 Baak JP, Persijn JP. In search for the best qualitative microscopical or morphometrical predictor of oestrogen receptor in breast cancer. *Pathol Rest Pract* 1984; 178: 307–314.
100 Mattfeldt T, Neurohr W, Muller A, Klinga K. Stereologic correlates of steroid receptor concentration in invasive ductal breast cancer. *Anal Quant Cytol Histol* 1985; 7: 310–314.
101 Larsimont D, Kiss R, D'Olne D *et al.* Correlation between nuclear cytomorphometric parameters and estrogen receptor levels in breast cancer. *Cancer* 1989; 63: 2162–2168.
102 van der Linden JC, Baak JPA, Lindeman J, Smeulders AWM, Meyer CJLM. Carcinoembryonic antigen expression and peanut agglutinin binding in primary breast cancer and lymph node metastases: lack of correlation with clinical, histopathological, biochemical and morphometric features. *Histopathology* 1985; 9: 1051–1059.
103 Parham DM, Coghill G, Robertson AJ. Critical evaluation of monoclonal antibody staining in breast carcinoma. *J Clin Pathol* 1989; 42: 810–813.
104 Lwin KY, Zuccarini O, Sloane JP, Beverley PCL. An immunohistological study of leukocyte localisation in benign and malignant breast tissue. *Int J Cancer* 1985; 36: 433–438.
105 Charpin C, Andrac L, Habib MC *et al.* Correlation between laminin and type IV collagen distribution in breast carcinomas, and estrogen receptors expression, lymph node and vascular involvement. *Med Oncol Tumor Pharmacother* 1990; 7: 43–54.
106 Bosari S, Lee AKC, Delellis RA, Wiley BD, Heatley GJ, Silverman ML. Microvessel quantitation and prognosis in invasive breast carcinoma. *Hum Pathol* 1992; 23: 755–761.

4.5 TESTIS

4.5.1 Chromosomal disease

Standard stereological and histomorphometric techniques are easily applied to the testis and give information about tubule volume, cross-sectional area and length [1], as well as perimeter and surface area measurements [2]. This approach has shown that the ratio of tubular volume to interstitial cells is decreased in the following conditions: chromatin-negative del Castillo's syndrome, XXY Klinefelter's syndrome, ectopic, undescended and atrophic testes, maturation arrest and mild primary gonadal deficiency [3]. The atrophy of the del Castillo type results from a shortening of tubules proportional to their shrinkage in diameter and not from an actual tissue loss, which is the case in XXY Klinefelter's syndrome [4]. The hyperplasia of Leydig cells encountered in these conditions is only an apparent one due to the atrophy of other elements [5]. It has been shown that in patients with androgen insensitivity (testicular feminization) syndrome aged under 5 years, testicular histology is normal apart from slightly decreased mean tubule diameters. There was the usual number of germ cells, although after 7 years of age they showed increasingly abnormal morphology, including impaired tubular maturation and even carcinoma *in situ* [6]. Morphometry has also shown a significant reduction in the number and volume percentage of premeiotic germ cells correlating with the severity of chromosomal abnormalities in midterm aborted fetuses [7]. Trisomy 13 and 18 had values less than one-half those of control cases.

4.5.2 Physiology and infertility

Quantitation has given insights into the topographical arrangements and kinetics of spermatocytes within the normal testicular tubule [8] and shown the following age-related changes: increased basement membrane thickening, Leydig cell number and clusters, and decreased testicular volume and epididymal duct diameters. The morphological scoring also correlated with serum testosterone levels [9]. Semiquantitative evaluation of constituent tissue components also varies according to a range of testicular pathology [10].

Spermatogenic activity is gauged by the Johnsen index, which is the mean score of tubules on a scale in which complete inactivity counts as zero and maximal activity, with five or more free sperm in the lumen, equals 10. The mean normal score is 9.1, with 8 or less being abnormal and giving more information regarding oligospermia than the equivalent serum hormone concentrations or semen analysis [11]. High luteinizing hormone (LH) and follicle-stimulating hormone (FSH) levels correlate with germ-cell loss, tubular shrinkage, Johnsen score and interstitial fibrosis in oligo- or azoospermic patients with testes of normal size but are not related to plasma testosterone levels [12]. Thus it appears that carefully quantified testicular biosies are an accurate reflection of spermatogenic activity.

Image analysis of normal-sized testes in 42 infertile patients with sperm counts below 20 million/ml has shown hypercurvature of the tubules. This has been postulated to lead to internal obstruction and a failure of sperm discharge to the epididymis [2]. The histological features are figure-of-eight patterns caused either by the basement membranes of adjacent tubule cross-sections touching, or an hourglass-like constriction joining two circular sections in the one tube. This effects a tight U-turn in neighbouring tubules arranged in parallel and four or more of these configurations per 10 HPFs is considered diagnostic [13]. However, the significance of this hypercurvature syndrome remains controversial and awaits further validation [14,15]. Similar comment must be made about the condition of focal atrophy. It is characterized by clusters of tubule cross-sections, usually 3–8, all of which have undergone hyalinization and represent about 2% of the total tissue section area [4].

Morphometry of hypospermatogenesis in idiopathic male infertility and varicocele shows that vascular and interstitial fractions, as well as Leydig cell counts, are increased. This emphasizes that the predominant change is in the interstitium, with tubular damage being erratic and late [16] and also resulting in decreased germ-cell counts [17]. In contrast, postvasectomy patients have a marked increase in seminiferous tubular wall thickness and cross-sectional area, with significant reductions in Sertoli cell and spermatid numbers [18]. However, interstitial fibrosis was seen in a minority of patients (23%) and correlated strongly with infertility after surgically successful vasectomy reversal. Tubular mass and volume are inversely, and interstitial fibrosis directly, related to levels of chronic alcohol consumption and the presence of liver disease. This indicates that the germinal tissue is the most sensitive component in alcohol-based testicular atrophy while Leydig cells remained unchanged [19].

4.5.3 Germ-cell tumours

Carcinoma *in situ* of the adult testis is an entity with a recognized malignant potential and its features are well-described elsewhere [20]. It is proposed as an indicator for orchidectomy in unilateral disease and localized irradiation in bilateral disease. However, the average surgical pathologist is only likely to encounter it sporadically in association with an established germ-cell tumour and its diagnosis is dependent on factors such as optimal tissue fixation and subjectivity. The role of stereology is currently being assessed as a more objective means of attaining the diagnosis for therapeutic decisions. Sørensen and Müller [21] have determined unbiased stereological estimates of the volume-weighted mean nuclear volume (nuclear V_V) using the point-sampled intercept technique (Fig. 4.7) (see Section 1.6). Nuclear V_V is larger in testicular carcinoma *in situ* and its apparently normal adjacent ipsilateral and contralateral parenchyma than in the spermatogonia of normal adult controls (Fig. 4.8). However, the prognostic value of nuclear volume estimates requires further evaluation from larger series of patients. Morphometric quantitation has not been applied to any great extent in testicular germ-cell tumours. Analysis of the proliferative compartment in seminoma using thymidine autoradiography showed a homogeneous distribution of DNA-synthesizing seminoma cells in small-tumour foci. In tumours of > 2 cm diameter there were areas of cells with a high labelling index at the edge of the lesion and within it adjacent to vascular stroma [22]. The distribution of the proliferating compartment appeared to be related to tumour geometry and size rather than cytology, as an anaplastic seminoma had a comparable mean labelling index. Mitosis counting is subject to observer

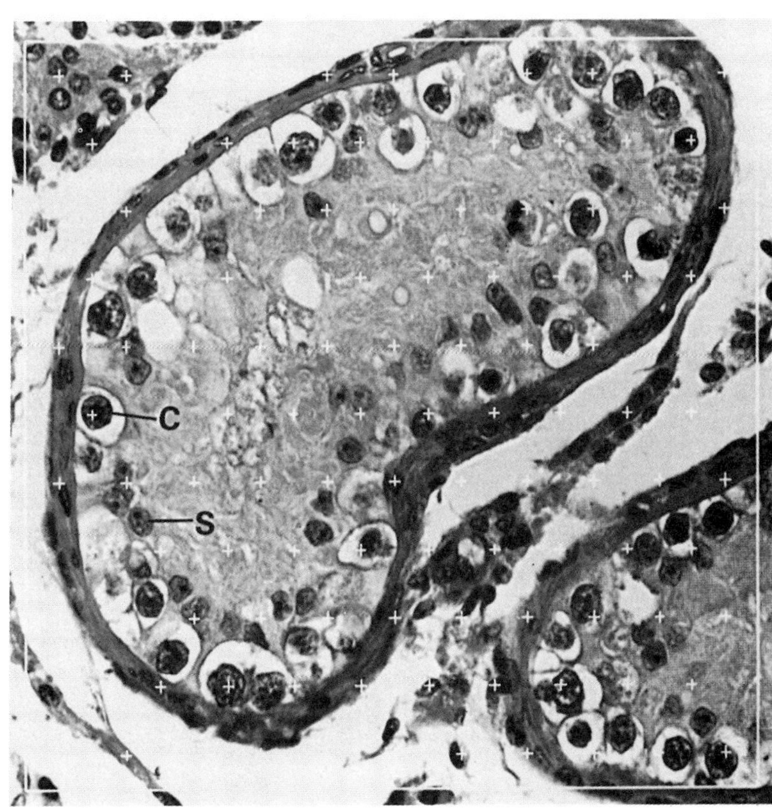

Fig. 4.7 Sampling grid superimposed on a field of seminiferous tubules showing germ-cell epithelium converted to carcinoma *in situ*. Only nuclei hit by points are sampled (see Section 1.6). C, carcinoma *in situ* cell; S, Sertoli cell. From Sørensen and Müller [21].

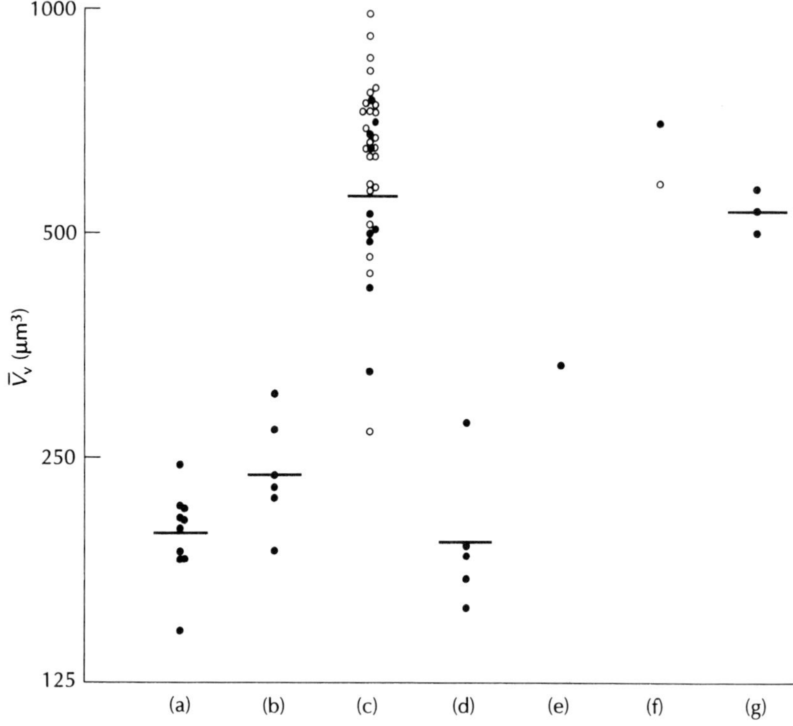

Fig. 4.8 Volume-weighted mean nuclear volume for: (a) spermatogonia in normal adult controls; (b) morphologically normal adult spermatogonia from either ipsi- or contralateral testis with coexisting carcinoma *in situ*; (c) testicular carcinoma *in situ* of the adult seminiferous epithelium; (d) spermatogonia in normal prepubertal controls; (e) morphologically normal prepubertal spermatogonia with coexisting contralateral carcinoma *in situ*; (f) testicular carcinoma *in situ* of the prepubertal testis; (g) adult cases of seminoma. (●) First diagnostic biopsies; (○) later biopsies. From Sørensen and Müller [21].

variation and, even when agreed, high-mitotic-rate seminomas do not appear to be of any worse prognosis than the more usual tumours [23]. Serum α-fetoprotein (AFP) levels correlate with the presence and quantity of endodermal sinus (yolk sac) tumour elements within primary germ-cell tumours or their metastases [24]. Seminoma and dysgerminoma had normal levels while pure embryonal carcinomas were slightly elevated. Endodermal sinus tumours had markedly raised AFP values in patients with active disease.

4.5.4 Conclusion

Quantitation in testicular disease can accurately assess spermatogenic activity and tubular morphology in the investigation of infertility. It may also have a role to play in defining carcinoma *in situ* as a guide to therapy.

References

1 Lennox B, Ahmad KN, Mack WS. Method for determining the relative total length of the tubules in the testis. *J Pathol* 1970; 102: 229–238.
2 Averback P, Wight DGD. Seminiferous tubule hypercurvature: a newly recognised common syndrome of human male infertility. *Lancet* 1979; 1: 181–183.
3 Dykes JRW. Histometric assessment of human testicular biopsies. *J Pathol* 1969; 97: 429–440.
4 Lennox B. The infertile testis. In: Anthony PP, MacSween RWM (eds) *Recent Advances in Histopathology*, vol. 11. Edinburgh: Churchill Livingstone, 1981: 135–148.
5 Ahmad KN, Dykes JRW, Ferguson-Smith MA, Lennox B, Mack WS. Leydig cell volume in chromatin-positive Klinefelter's syndrome. *J Clin Endocrinol Metab* 1971; 33: 517–520.
6 Muller J. Morphometry and histology of gonads from 12 children and adolescents with the androgen insensitivity (testicular feminization) syndrome. *J Clin Endocrinol Metab* 1984; 59: 785–789.
7 Coerdt W, Rehder H, Gausmann I, Johannisson R, Gropp A. Quantitative histology of human fetal testes in chromosomal disease. *Pediatr Pathol* 1985; 3: 245–259.
8 Schulze W, Rehder U. Organisation and morphogenesis of the human seminiferous epithelium. *Cell Tissue Res* 1984; 237: 395–407.
9 Oshima S, Okayasu I, Uchima H, Hatakeyama S. Histo-

pathological and morphometrical study of the human epididymis and testis. *Acta Pathol Jpn* 1984; 34: 1327–1342.

10 Meyer JM, Roos M, Rumpler Y. Statistical study of a semiquantitative evaluation of testicular biopsies. *Arch Androl* 1988; 20: 71–79.

11 Aafjes JH, Vijver JCM van der, Schenck PE. Value of a testicular biopsy rating for prognosis in oligozoospermia. *Br Med J* 1978; 1: 289–290.

12 Mikuz G, Leitner G, Scheiber K, Bartsch G. Correlation of hormone levels and quantitative histological findings in testicular biopsies. *Eur Urol* 1985; 11: 110–116.

13 Averback P. Histopathological diagnosis of hypercurved seminiferous tubules. *Histopathology* 1980; 4: 75–82.

14 Anonymous. A new cause for male sterility. *Lancet* 1979; i: 195–196.

15 Lennox B. A new cause for male sterility? *Lancet* 1979; i: 384.

16 Pesce CM, Reale A. Testis morphometry in varicocele. *Arch Androl* 1985; 15: 193–197.

17 Guarch R, Pesce C, Puras A, Lazaro J. A quantitative approach to the classification of hypospermatogenesis in testicular biopsies for infertility. *Hum Pathol* 1992; 23: 1032–1037.

18 Jarow JP, Budin RE, Dym M, Zirkin BR, Noren S, Marshall FF. Quantitative pathologic changes in the human testis after vasectomy. A controlled study. *N Engl J Med* 1985; 313: 1252–1256.

19 Karhunen PJ, Penttila A, Liesto K *et al.* Changes in germinal tissue and Leydig cells correlated with ethanol consumption in males with and without liver disease. *Arch Toxicol* 1984; (suppl 7): 155–158.

20 Shakkebaek NE, Berthelsen JG, Muller J. Histopathology of human testicular tumours: carcinoma *in situ* germ cells and invasive growth of different types of germ cell tumours. *INSERM* 1984; 123: 445–461.

21 Sørensen FB, Müller J. Stereological estimates of nuclear volume in normal germ cells and carcinoma *in situ* of the human testis. *Histopathology* 1990; 17: 327–334.

22 Rabes HM, Schmeller N, Hartman A, Rattenhuber U, Carl P, Staehler G. Analysis of proliferative compartments in human tumors. II. Seminoma. *Cancer* 1985; 55: 1758–1769.

23 Zuckman MH, Williams G, Levin HS. Mitosis counting in seminoma: an exercise of questionable significance. *Hum Pathol* 1988; 19: 329–335.

24 Talerman A, Haije WG, Baggermann L. Serum alphafetoprotein in patients with germ cell tumors of the gonads and extragonadal sites: correlation between endodermal sinus (yolk sac) tumor and raised AFP. *Cancer* 1980; 46: 380–385.

4.6 THYROID

4.6.1 Fine-needle aspiration

Boon *et al.* [1] quantified a series of 21 follicular adenomas, 13 follicular carcinomas and seven non-toxic goitres. They had mean nuclear areas and nuclear cytoplasmic ratios, as shown in Table 4.3.

These differences were statistically significant and a threshold value for nuclear area of 90 μm² correctly classified 100% of the adenomas and 76% of the carcinomas. In an extension of this work a comparison of follicular adenoma, carcinoma and their metastases prioritized, in decreasing order of importance, nuclear cytoplasmic ratio, nuclear size and nuclear perimeter as distinguishing variables [2]. A classification rule based on the first two of these parameters correctly placed 11 out of the 13 adenomas and 18 of the 20 carcinomas. The two misplaced adenomas were further sampled and the extra tissue blocks identified areas of invasive growth, establishing them as carcinoma. The calculation of probabilities from the quantitative data and the setting of numerical boundaries potentially allowed the use of threshold-based decision-making [3] as a means of determining preoperatively which thyroid nodules needed further intervention. The importance of nuclear area as a distinguishing feature in thyroid pathology has been emphasized elsewhere [4]. Montironi *et al.* [5] have also noted the number of nucleolated nuclei and percentage marginated nucleoli (touching the nuclear membrane) to separate follicular adenomas and carcinomas. Nucleolar features combined with nuclear area achieved an 87% accuracy in classifying these follicular lesions [6].

Intraoperative comparison of frozen sections and imprint preparations showed that the cytological features of note specific for carcinomas were: (i)

Table 4.3 Morphometric means for follicular lesions

	Nuclear area (μm) $\bar{x}$	Nuclear/cytoplasmic ratio $\bar{x}$
Goitre	25	0.41
Adenoma	74	0.48
Carcinoma	131	0.59

folding of the nuclear contour; (ii) density of the cytoplasmic matrix; and (iii) cell cluster size [7]. The image-processing routine allowed the size and frequency of cell clusters to be determined. Both follicular and papillary carcinoma had enlarged cell clusters with a significant component measuring > 300 μm in diameter. These did not occur in benign lesions. Variation in chromatin texture has also been useful in separating a range of benign and malignant lesions in touch imprints [8].

Form factor or nuclear shape does not differ between the various thyroid nodules [9,10], while indicators of nuclear size do [10], although this has been disputed to be limited to nuclear area in papillary carcinoma [9]. Several authors [9,11] have also commented on the technical difficulty of delineating well-defined cytoplasmic borders in the determination of nuclear cytoplasmic ratio. They have regarded morphometry as having only limited usefulness in separating benign and malignant lesions [9]. This is due to the wide variation that occurs, despite the significant differences that are found between features such as nuclear area and perimeter, in the spectrum of histological lesions [11] (Fig. 4.9).

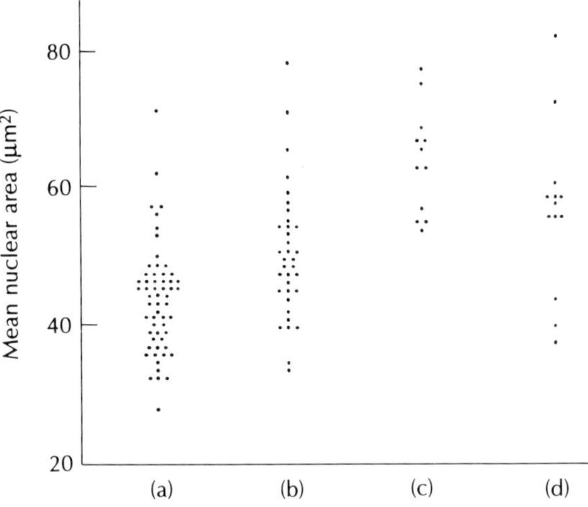

Fig. 4.9 Scatterplot showing mean nuclear area of papanicolaou (PAP) stained thyroid cell aspirates from (a) multinodular goitre, (b) follicular adenoma, (c) follicular carcinoma and (d) papillary carcinoma. Diagnoses were established by histology of subsequent resection specimens. From Wright *et al.* [11].

Oxyphilic or Hürthle cell lesions of the thyroid can be difficult to categorize as either benign or malignant and sometimes this designation is only retrospective once metastases have occurred. Morphometric estimations of nuclear area and its variation have not been found to be useful additional diagnostic criteria [12].

4.6.2 Tissue sections

The theme of nuclear size has also been investigated in histological sections. The diameters of 200 nuclei from each of 127 cases of thyroid carcinoma were significantly different among the four histological subtypes [13]. Undifferentiated carcinoma had the largest (8.7 μm) and medullary carcinoma the smallest (6.6 μm) mean nuclear diameters. It also significantly correlated with the degree of tumour differentiation, maximal tumour diameter, mitotic rate and the 5-year survival for all types of carcinoma. There was correlation for disease stage only in undifferentiated tumours. Ultrastructural stereology has shown the mean nuclear volume and surface area to increase, while the volume densities of rough endoplasmic reticulum and dense bodies decrease from normal thyroid through adenomas and follicular carcinomas to papillary carcinomas [14]. Interestingly, the diagnostic feature in papillary carcinoma of ground-glass nuclei was not associated with a lower volume density of heterochromatin. There were no striking differences in nuclear characteristics to allow the distinction between adenoma and well-differentiated follicular carcinoma to be made electron-microscopically. Various authors [15,16] have used computerized cell image analysis to assess morphometric, densitometric and textural parameters in a range of thyroid lesions. There was a statistically significant shift in DNA content from diploidy to aneuploidy, and increase in nuclear size and hyperchromatism from goitres through adenomas to carcinomas. The cell nuclei of papillary, follicular and medullary carcinomas displayed many similarities, although a subgroup of papillary carcinoma containing fewer chromatin clumps and hypochromatic nuclei was identified by cluster analysis.

Morphometry of papillary thyroid carcinoma has been specifically documented at light [17] and ultrastructural levels [18]. Ambros *et al.* [17] studied 28 patients with a mean follow-up period of 47 months, six of whom developed recurrent disease. The measurements were obtained by the use of an eyepiece graticule. Recurrence was most closely associated with the tumour size, SD of the estimated nuclear area (ENASD) and the cellularity mean index (CMI: defined as the percentage volume composed of tumour cells). Fifty-five per cent of patients with ENASD $>17\,\mu m^2$ and CMI $>40\%$ developed recurrence, as opposed to 5% of patients with lesser values. Morphometry was therefore advocated as a tool to provide prognostic information on the biological behaviour of papillary carcinoma. The quantitative nuclear and nucleolar characteristics of papillary carcinoma of the thyroid and ovary have been compared ultrastructurally by Payne *et al.* [18]. The thyroid carcinomas had smaller measurements of features related to nuclear and nucleolar size than ovarian carcinoma and these dimensions correlated with nuclear shape. The establishment of morphometric domains by three-dimensional cluster analysis showed that these were distinctly smaller in thyroid carcinoma and separate from ovarian carcinoma.

In a detailed study of follicular adenoma and well-differentiated follicular carcinoma stereology, flow cytometry and immunohistochemistry were carried out [19]. There were no significant differences in the stereological estimates of tumour-cell nuclear size and both groups contained comparable proportions of DNA diploid and DNA aneuploid neoplasms. Thyroglobulin, cytokeratin and vimentin antigens were also similarly expressed. Irrespective of their histological diagnosis, DNA aneuploid follicular lesions had greater nuclear area, perimeter and volume. Due to their similarities it was postulated, as reported by others [16], that some adenomas may in fact represent preinvasive carcinomas. It was also concluded that a definitive diagnosis cannot be made on the basis of quantitative cytological features and that capsular or vascular invasion is the only safe indicator of malignancy in the absence of metastases.

4.6.3 Conclusion

Goitres, adenomas and thyroid carcinomas have morphometric differences in aspirate cell cluster and nuclear size. However, these are not sufficiently distinctive to allow a reliable separation of all benign and malignant lesions (especially well-differentiated follicular carcinoma) and tissue architecture, e.g., capsular invasion, remains an important criterion for definitive diagnosis. Morphometry may have a role to play as a prognostic indicator in established carcinoma as nuclear size appears to relate to tumour DNA ploidy, recurrence rate and patient survival.

References

1 Boon ME, Löwhagan T, Willems JS. Planimetric studies on fine needle aspirates from follicular adenoma and follicular carcinoma of the thyroid. *Acta Cytol* 1980; 24: 145–148.

2 Boon ME, Lowhagen T, Cardozo PL, Blonk DI, Kurver PJH, Baak JPA. Computation of preoperative diagnosis probability for follicular adenoma and carcinoma of the thyroid on aspiration smears. *Anal Quant Cytol* 1982; 4: 1–5.

3 Pauker SG, Kassirer JP. The threshold approach to clinical decision making. *N Engl J Med* 1980; 302: 1109–1117.

4 De Santis M, Sciarrhetta F, Sudano L, Perronte Donnorso R. Morphometric evaluation of histological sections of the thyroid gland in benign and malignant follicular lesions. *Diagn Cytopathol* 1987; 3: 60–67.

5 Montironi R, Bracciscchi A, Scarpelli M, Matera G, Alberti R. Value of quantitative nucleolar features in the preoperative cytological diagnosis of follicular neoplasms of the thyroid. *J Clin Pathol* 1991; 44: 509–514.

6 Montironi R, Bracciscchi A, Scarpelli M, Sisti S, Alberti R. Well differentiated follicular neoplasms of the thyroid: reproducibility and validity of a 'decision tree' classification based on nucleolar and karyometric features. *Cytopathology* 1992; 3: 209–222.

7 Masuda T, Tezuka F, Konno H, Togashi A, Itoh Y, Sugawara T. Intraoperative imprint cytology of the thyroid gland with computer-assisted morphometric analysis of cell clusters. *Anal Quant Cytol Histol* 1988; 10: 294–298.

8 Kriete A, Schäffer R, Harms H, Aus HM. Computer-based cytophotometric classification of thyroid tumors in imprints. *J Cancer Res Clin Oncol* 1985; 109: 252–256.

9 Luck JB, Mumaw VR, Frable WJ. Fine needle aspiration biopsy of the thyroid – differential diagnosis by video image analysis. *Acta Cytol* 1982; 26: 793–796.

10 Sassi I, Mangilif F, Sironi M, Freschi M, Cantaboni A. Morphometric evaluation of fine needle biopsy of single thyroid nodules. *Pathol Res Pract* 1989; 185: 722–725.

11 Wright RG, Castles H, Mortimer RH. Morphometric analysis of thyroid cell aspirates. *J Clin Pathol* 1987; 40: 443–445.
12 Bondeson L, Bondeson AG, Lindholm K, Ljungrberg O, Tibblin S. Morphometric studies on nuclei in smears of fine needle aspirates from oxyphilic tumors of the thyroid. *Acta Cytol* 1983; 27: 437–440.
13 Lee TK, Myers RT, Bond MG, Marshall RB, Kardon B. The significance of nuclear diameter in the biologic behaviour of thyroid carcinomas: a retrospective study of 127 cases. *Hum Pathol* 1987; 18: 1252–1256.
14 Johannessen JV, Sobrinho-Simoes M, Finseth I, Pilstrom L. Ultrastructural morphometry of thyroid neoplasma. *Am J Clin Pathol* 1983; 79: 166–171.
15 Collin F, Salmon I, Rahier I, Pasteels J-L, Heimann R, Kiss R. Quantitative nuclear cell image analysis of thyroid tumors from archival material. *Hum Pathol* 1991; 22: 191–196.
16 Salmon I, Gasperin P, Pasteels JL, Heimann R, Kiss R. Relationship between histopathologic typing and morphonuclear assessments of 238 thyroid lesions: digital cell image analysis performed on Feulgen-stained nuclei from formalin-fixed paraffin embedded materials. *Am J Pathol* 1992; 97: 776–786.
17 Ambros RA, Trost RC, Campbell AY, Lambert WC. Prognostic value of morphometry in papillary thyroid carcinoma. *Hum Pathol* 1989; 20: 215–218.
18 Payne CM, Graham AR, Bjore CG Jr *et al.* Ultrastructural morphometric analysis of papillary neoplasms: biological and diagnostic relevance. *Hum Pathol* 1989; 20: 864–870.
19 Schürmann G, Mattfeldt T, Feichter G, Koretz K, Möller P, Buhr H. Stereology, flow cytometry and immunohistochemistry of follicular neoplasms of the thyroid gland. *Hum Pathol* 1991; 22: 179–184.

4.7 PARATHYROID

Mean nuclear diameter in 11 out of 18 parathyroid carcinomas was above the range [1] reported for parathyroid adenomas [2], where it also correlated with tumour weight and plasma calcium. The latter suggests that nuclear size may also be an index of functional activity. In chronic renal failure the size, cellular density and DNA content of the lower parathyroid glands were greater than in the upper, explaining the predilection of adenomas for this site [3].

References

1 Jacobi JM, Lloyd HM, Smith JF. Nuclear diameter in parathyroid carcinomas. *J Clin Pathol* 1986; 39: 1353–1354.
2 Lloyd HM, Jacobi JM, Cooke RA. Nuclear diameter in parathyroid adenomas. *J Clin Pathol* 1979; 32: 1278–1281.
3 Matsushita H. Different responses between the upper and lower parathyroid gland in a state of secondary hyperfunction. A study on chronic renal failure by morphometry and nuclear DNA analysis. *Virchows Arch A Pathol Anat Histol* 1989; 414: 331–337.

4.8 KIDNEY

Quantitative analysis of glomerular, tubular and vascular tissue components has been applied to a wide variety of renal disorders in an attempt to correlate alterations in morphology with dysfunction. A practical example of use at the bedside is the quantitative microscopy of first morning urine specimens as a predictor for the presence or absence of renal disease [1]. There is close correlation between the number of urinary renal casts and the presence and severity of renal disease on subsequent biopsy, with a positive predictive value of 93 and 100% based on first and second specimens. Morphometry has found a place in the elucidation of urinary tract disease [2] and initial renal studies concentrated on the normal and diseased glomerulus, using stereology [3] and point-counting [4]. Steffes *et al.* [3] established normative values for glomerular basement membrane width, relative volume of mesangium and its cellular and matrical components. Baak and Wehner [4] demonstrated the validity of a multivariate morphometric approach in achieving a 90.5% accurate classification of normal controls, minimal-change disease, mesangioproliferative glomerulonephritis and diabetic glomerulosclerosis. Parameters of importance were glomerular cellularity, mesangial and epithelial percentages and numbers of endothelial cells. Point-counting on biopsy and autopsy sections stained by an immunoperoxidase technique with antibodies to tubule cellular proteins (antisera to proximal tubule brush border, Tamm–Horsfall protein and epithelial membrane antigen) have demonstrated an association with renal function [5]. There was a correlation between the reciprocal of plasma creatinine concentration and the ratios of brush border and Tamm–Horsfall positive to negative tubules. In both the oligoanuric and polyuric phases of acute renal failure the peri- and intertubular capillary surface areas remain constant while Bowman's capsule, tubular epithelial tissue and microvascular lumina are all distended [6].

4.8.1 Vascular disease

Two groups of age- and sex-matched patients with either mild or severe systemic atherosclerosis had comparative autopsy measurements of glomerular area, percentage globally sclerotic glomeruli, arcuate/interlobular artery dimensions and interstitial fibrosis [7]. The patients with severe atherosclerosis had more sclerosed glomeruli, increased intrarenal arterial wall and glomerular areas. The latter occurred in non-sclerosed structures, suggesting compensatory hypertrophy. Interstitial fibrosis was similar and regression analysis identified age and intrarenal vascular disease as having highly significant independent associations with glomerulosclerosis. Fibroblastic intimal thickening and medial hyalinization characterize the changes in proximal arterial and distal arteriolar vessels in benign nephrosclerosis and they both evolve in a proportionate manner with increasing age and hypertension [8]. Morphometry suggests that it is the degree of arteriolar intimal thickening rather than hyaline change that causes renoparenchymal damage through ischaemia and leads to a deterioration in function [9]. It has also highlighted that the burden of damage in decompensated benign nephrosclerosis centres on postglomerular fibrosis and tubular atrophy. In contrast, the preglomerular vascular network is affected in malignant nephrosclerosis, with the resultant arteriolar stenosis protecting the supplied glomerulus [10].

Ultrastructural quantitation found subendothelial fibrinoid deposits to be a significant feature of renal biopsies in pre-eclamptic patients [11]. Glomerular capillary-wall reduplication, mesangial interposition and segmental hyalinosis were also noted, all of which regressed postnatally. An image analysis technique has been devised to plot the position of segmental lesions with reference to the glomerular hilum and its centre of gravity. In general they occur at three sites; the tip, the vascular pole and randomly, with the latter predominating in acute vasculitic-type glomerulonephritis [12].

4.8.2 Reflux nephropathy, diabetes, connective-tissue diseases

A digitizer was used to measure renal surface areas in intravenous pyelograms from 31 patients with reflux nephropathy who also had undergone biopsy [13]. There were positive correlations between renal size and function with inverse correlations between these and maximum glomerular size, the proportion of sclerosed glomeruli and vascular wall thickness. In addition the strongest morphological prognostic guide was the severity of segmental sclerosis. Ultrastructural analysis of the interstitium in reflux disease demonstrates an increase (24.7%) in its volume fraction to the detriment of tubular epithelial elements (40–50% reduction) [14].

The width of the peripheral glomerular basement membrane is normal at the onset of acute, juvenile IDDM but thickening is demonstrable by electron-microscopic quantitation as early as 2 years after disease onset [15]. Its functional significance is uncertain as stereology has shown it to progress at a different rate from mesangial expansion, and to be unrelated to either the duration of disease or the presence of nephropathy in diabetics [16]. It does relate to microalbuminuria [17] but the main factor dictating clinical nephropathy appears to be glomerular enlargement due to expansion in the mesangial matrix volume, and the percentage of sclerosed glomeruli [16–19]. It is hypothesized that this expansion leads to functional deterioration by restricting the glomerular capillary vasculature and its filtering surface [16]. Other workers have quantified more arteriolohyalinosis and glomerular subcapsular fibrosis in diabetics, along with mesangial increase in those patients with nephropathy. These two diabetic groups did not show any differences in vascular changes or the frequency of Kimmelstiel–Wilson or exudative lesions [20]. Glomerular basement membrane thickening and mesangial lesions may also develop in normal living related donor and cadaver kidneys transplanted into diabetic patients [21].

Standard morphometric, counting and grading methods in diffuse proliferative lupus glomerulonephritis identified a combination of serum creatinine, extent of extraglomerular deposits and intraglomerular monocytic infiltration to provide significant prognostic information about renal survival [22]. Point-counting was also used to determine the percentage of the cortical tubulointerstitial system occupied by mononuclear cell infiltrates (infiltrate index) and by interstitial connective tissue (interstitial index) [23]. Interstitial cell infiltrates and immune deposits were present in the majority of biopsies and there was significant correlation between the infiltrate and interstitial indices. Correlation with immune deposition was not significant and the findings suggested that tubulointerstitial damage is effected by inflammatory cell infiltrates and not immune deposits. Quantitation of serial biopsies during the treatment of diffuse lupus glomerulonephritis by total lymphoid irradiation and corticosteroids has shown a progressive reduction in glomerular inflammatory cells and immune deposits [24]. After 12 months there is a trend towards glomerulosclerosis, with the residual patent glomeruli undergoing adaptive enlargement.

Image analysis of renal tissue in systemic sclerosis confirms significantly increased intimal area in medium-sized and small arteries. The percentage vessel wall occupied by intima is increased and luminal occlusion is greatest in patients with diffuse disease and renal crisis [25].

4.8.3 Haematuria, glomerulonephritis

There is a group of patients who present with apparently idiopathic haematuria not due to lower urinary tract disorders, renal tumour or immune deposit glomerulonephritis. There may be an association with proteinuria and in a minority of cases progression to renal failure. Ultrastructural quantitation has shown the underlying lesion in a number of these patients to be an abnormally thin glomerular basement membrane (range 206–301 nm; control range 356–464 nm) [26]. It is characterized by diffuse but irregular attenuation, gaps or splits, occasional intramembranous lacunae and dense deposits, foot process fusion and endothelial swelling [26,27]. Thin membrane nephropathy (synonym: benign familial haematuria) may have a population incidence as high as 5% [28], present at any age and is a well-recognized cause of recurrent haematuria in childhood [29].

In membranous glomerulonephritis the degree of capillary basement membrane thickening, visceral epithelial cell numbers and area correlate with serum albumin levels, proteinuria, disease duration and the inverse of serum creatinine. In addition, capillary lumen and endothelial cell areas are decreased and this is exacerbated by hypertension [30]. High blood pressure also hastens the progression of IgA glomerulonephritis due to increased glomerular and vascular sclerosis, the latter being characterized by thicker, prominent vessels [31]. Further work on IgA nephritis has found that the width of cortical interstitial fibrosis, proximal tubular epithelial cell swelling and its decreased surface area correlate with serum creatinine and acute renal failure [32]. This emphasizes the influence of tubulointerstitial changes on glomerular function and prognosis, as found in a variety of glomerulopathies [33]. In children with minimal-change disease an increased mean glomerular tuft area correlates with progression to focal glomerulosclerosis and subsequent clinical deterioration [34].

4.8.4 Renal-cell carcinoma

Fuhrman *et al.* [35] have studied the prognostic significance of classical pathological features in renal-cell carcinoma. Stage of disease is the most important predictor of biological aggression and metastatic potential. Renal vein involvement is only significant in the presence of positive nodes or perinephric fat infiltration. Tumours under 3 cm in diameter generally do not metastasize, while the majority of those above 8 cm in diameter do. Lesions with a granular or sarcomatoid cell pattern are also more aggressive. In stage I disease the most significant prognostic criterion is nuclear cytological grade, which has an inverse relationship with 5-year survival rates. This has been confirmed by morphometry where short- and long-term survivors were well-separated by a nuclear area threshold value of $32\,\mu m^2$. Poor prognosis was associated with larger, non-elliptical nuclei [36]. González-Cámpora *et al.* [37] found a strong association between cytological grade and the nuclear parameters of area, major diameter and elongation. Adverse clinical outcome was associated with increased nuclear diameter and elongation. Multivariate analysis showed clinicopathological stage, major nuclear diameter, presence of anaplastic cells and nuclear area to be of predictive value. However, a discriminant function to separate nine so-called adenomas from the 64 carcinomas could not be successfully formulated. Others have also shown nuclear area to be a strong predictor of survival [38]. A further quantitative study emphasized the merits of assessing variables related to nuclear shape as a means of selecting a subgroup of stage I tumours with potentially aggressive disease for adjuvant therapy [39]. A similar approach is being explored in Wilms' tumour where, amongst others, factors such as nuclear roundness and ellipsoidicity can separate responders and non-responders [40].

Thymidine autoradiography has shown a higher labelling index in granular than clear cells, and in papillary and mixed solid/tubular growth patterns [41]. DNA cytophotometry demonstrates an increase in DNA aneuploidy content based on tumour size [42]. DNA aneuploidy also evolves in parallel with nuclear grade, mitotic rate, tumour stage, coexpression of cytokeratin and vimentin intermediate filaments and decreased survival [43].

4.8.5 Conclusion

Morphometry has given an insight into structure/function and glomerular/interstitial relationships in vascular, connective-tissue and diabetic renal disease and various glomerulopathies. In the latter it has been responsible for delineating the entity of thin basement membrane nephropathy. Quantitation of nuclear size and shape has a possible role in determining potential aggression and survival in stage I renal-cell carcinoma.

References

1 Gyory AZ, Hadfield C, Lauer CS. Value of urine microscopy in predicting histological changes in the kidney: double blind comparison. *Br Med J* 1984; 288: 819–822.

2 Wehner H. Urinary tract morphometry. An overview. *Anal Quant Cytol Histol* 1986; 8: 358–362.

3 Steffes MW, Barbosa J, Basgen JM, Sutherland DER, Najarian JS, Mauer SM. Quantitative glomerular morphology of the normal human kidney. *Lab Invest* 1983; 49: 82–86.

4 Baak JPA, Wehner H. A multivariate morphometric analysis of the glomeruli in the normal and pathologically changed human kidney. *Virchows Arch A Pathol Anat* 1983; 399: 105–114.

5 Howie AJ, Gunson BK, Sparke J. Morphometric correlates of renal excretory function. *J Pathol* 1990; 160: 245–253.

6 Klingebiel T, von Gise H, Bohle A. Morphometric studies on acute renal failure in humans during the oligoanuric and polyuric phases. *Clin Nephrol* 1983; 20: 1–10.

7 Kasiske BL. Relationship between vascular disease and age-associated changes in the human kidney. *Kidney Int* 1987; 31: 1153–1159.

8 Tracy RE, Velez-Duran M, Heigle T, Oalmann MC. Two variants of nephrosclerosis separately related to age and blood pressure. *Am J Pathol* 1988; 131: 270–282.

9 Katafuchi R, Takebayashi S. Morphometrical and functional correlations in benign nephrosclerosis. *Clin Nephrol* 1987; 28: 238–243.

10 Ratschek M, Ratschek E, Bohle A. Decompensated benign nephrosclerosis and secondary malignant nephrosclerosis. *Clin Nephrol* 1986; 25: 221–226.

11 Kincaid-Smith P. The renal lesion of pre-eclampsia revisited. *Am J Kidney Dis* 1991; 17: 144–148.

12 Newbold KM, Howie AJ. Analysis of the position of segmental lesions in glomeruli in vasculitis-type glomerulonephritis and other disorders. *J Pathol* 1990; 162: 149–155.

13 El-Khatib MT, Becker GJ, Kincaid-Smith PS. Morphometric aspects of reflux nephropathy. *Kidney Int* 1987; 32: 261–266.

14 Moler JC, Skriver E. Quantitative ultrastructure of human proximal tubules and cortical interstitium in chronic renal disease (hydronephrosis). *Virchows Arch A Pathol Anat Histol* 1985; 406: 389–406.

15 Osterby R. Morphometric studies of the peripheral glomerular basement membrane in early juvenile diabetes. I. Development of initial basement thickening. *Diabetologica* 1972; 8: 84–92.

16 Mauer SM, Steffes MW, Ellis EN, Sutherland DER, Brown GM, Goetz FC. Structural–functional relationships in diabetic nephropathy. *J Clin Invest* 1984; 74: 1143–1155.

17 Chavers BM, Bilous RW, Ellis EN, Steffes MW, Mauer SM. Glomerular lesions and urinary albuminin excretion in type I diabetes without overt proteinuria. *N Engl J Med* 1989; 320: 966–970.

18 Bilous RW, Mauer SM, Sutherland DL, Steffes MW. Mean glomerular volume and rate of development of diabetic nephropathy. *Diabetes* 1989; 38: 1142–1147.

19 Montironi R, Scarpelli M, Barbatelli G, Pisani E, Ansuini G, Mariuzzi GM. Diabetic glomerulosclerosis: computer aided quantitative microscopy. *Pathologica* 1986; 78: 219–226.

20 Thomsen OF, Andersen AR, Christiansen JS, Deckert T. Renal changes in long-term type I (insulin-dependent) diabetic patients with and without clinical nephro-

pathy: a light microscopic, morphometric study of autopsy material. *Diabetologia* 1984; 26: 361–365.
21 Mauer SM, Steffes MW, Connett J, Najarian JS, Sutherland DE, Barbosa J. The development of lesions in the glomerular basement membrane and mesangium after transplantation of normal kidneys to diabetic patients. *Diabetes* 1983; 32: 948–952.
22 Magil AB, Ballon HS, Chan V, Lirenman DS, Rae A, Sutton RAL. Diffuse proliferative lupus glomerulonephritis. Determination of prognostic significance of clinical, laboratory and pathologic factors. *Medicine* 1984; 63: 210–220.
23 Magil AB, Tyler M. Tubulo-interstitial disease in lupus nephritis. A morphometric study. *Histopathology* 1984; 8: 81–87.
24 Chagnac A, Kiberd BA, Farinas MC *et al.* Outcome of the acute glomerular injury in proliferative lupus nephritis. *J Clin Invest* 1989; 84: 922–930.
25 Trostle DC, Bedetti CD, Steen VD, Al-Sabbagh MR, Zee B, Medsger TA. Renal vascular histology and morphometry in systemic sclerosis. A case-control autopsy study. *Arthritis Rheum* 1988; 31: 393–400.
26 Dische FE, Weston MJ, Parons V. Abnormally thin glomerular basement membranes associated with hematuria, proteinuria or renal failure in adults. *Am J Nephrol* 1985; 5: 103–109.
27 Coleman M, Haynes WDG, Dimopoulos P, Barratt LJ, Jarvis LR. Glomerular basement membrane abnormalities associated with apparently idiopathic haematuria: ultrastructural morphometric analysis. *Hum Pathol* 1986; 17: 1022–1030.
28 Dische FE, Anderson VER, Keane SJ, Taube D, Bewick M, Parsons V. Incidence of thin membrane nephropathy: morphometric investigation of a population sample. *J Clin Pathol* 1990; 43: 457–460.
29 Lang S, Stevenson B, Risdon RA. Thin basement membrane nephropathy as a cause of recurrent haematuria in childhood. *Histopathology* 1990; 16: 331–337.
30 Aparicio SR, Woolgar AE, Aparicio SA, Watkins A, Davison AM. An ultrastructural morphometric study of membranous glomerulonephritis. *Nephrol, Dialysis, Transplant* 1986; 1: 22–30.
31 Katafuchi R, Vamvakas E, Neelakantappa J, Baldwin DS, Gallo GR. Microvascular disease and the progression of IgA nephropathy. *Am J Kidney Dis* 1990; 15: 72–79.
32 Mackensen-Haen S, Eissele R, Bohle A. Contribution on the correlation between morphometric parameters gained from the renal cortex and renal function in IgA nephritis. *Lab Invest* 1988; 59: 239–244.
33 Bohle A, Mackensen-Haen S, von Gise H *et al.* The consequences of tubulo-interstitial changes for renal function in glomerulopathies. A morphometric and cytological analysis. *Pathol Res Pract* 1990; 186: 135–144.
34 Fogo A, Hawkins EP, Berry PL *et al.* Glomerular hypertrophy in minimal change disease predicts subsequent progression focal glomerular sclerosis. *Kidney Int* 1990; 38: 115–123.
35 Fuhrman SA, Lasky LC, Limas C. Prognostic significance of morphologic parameters in renal cell carcinoma. *Am J Surg Pathol* 1982; 6: 655–663.
36 Tosi P, Luzi P, Baak JPA *et al.* Nuclear morphometry as an important prognostic factor in stage I renal cell carcinoma. *Cancer* 1986; 58: 2512–2518.
37 González-Cámpora R, Gonzalez De Chaves FJ, Mora-Marin J *et al.* Nuclear planimetry in renal-cell tumours. *Anal Quant Cytol Histol* 1991; 13: 54–60.
38 Gutierrez JL, Val-Bernal JF, Garijo MF, Buelta L, Portillo JA. Nuclear morphometry in prognosis of renal adenocarcinoma. *Urology* 1992; 39: 130–134.
39 Murphy GF, Partin AW, Maygarden SJ, Mohler JL. Nuclear shape analysis for assessment of prognosis in renal cell carcinoma. *J Urol* 1990; 143: 1103–1107.
40 Gearhart JP, Partin AW, Leventhal B, Beckwith JB, Epstein JI. The use of nuclear morphometry to predict response to therapy in Wilms' tumor. *Cancer* 1992; 69: 804–808.
41 Rabes HM, Carl P, Meister P, Rattenhumber U. Analysis of proliferative compartments in human tumors. I. Renal adenocarcinoma. *Cancer* 1979; 44: 799–813.
42 Banner BF, Brancazio L, Bahnson RR, Ernstoff MS, Taylor SR. DNA analysis of multiple synchronous renal cell carcinomas. *Cancer* 1990; 66: 2180–2185.
43 Dierick A-M, Praet M, Roels H, Verbeeck P, Robyns C, Oosterlinck W. Vimentin expression of renal cell carcinoma in relation to DNA content and histological grading: a combined light microscopic, immunocytochemical and cytophotometrical analysis. *Histopathology* 1991; 18: 315–322.

4.9 URINARY BLADDER

4.9.1 Urinary cytology

Initial work showed that the cellular and nuclear dimensions of normal voided urothelial cells vary from those derived from WHO grades I and II papillary transitional cell carcinoma of the bladder [1]. However, the morphometric differences were not sufficient to allow distinction of normal urothelium from grade I tumours and there was a degree of overlap between grade I and II lesions. For radio- and chemotherapeutic reasons it is important to discriminate between low-grade (I and II) and high-grade (III) carcinomas and this issue was further addressed in an extension of the original study [2]. A learning set of 20 cases was analysed morphometrically and the resultant classification rule applied to a new test set of a further 21 cases. Fifty cells were delineated by a semiautomatic technique in each instance and these results were directly compared with the histomorphometric and histological grading of their tissue samples. Some of the variables found to be statistically different between low- and high-grade lesions were mean nuclear area (76.6 vs 107.8 μm^2), mean nuclear perimeter (37.5 vs 43.5 μm) and mean nuclear cytoplasmic ratio (0.51 vs 0.58). Probability coefficients were calculated based on the morphometric classification rule to predict the likelihood of a lesion being low-grade. This showed excellent correlation between all three techniques in the test set. Interestingly, cytomorphometry correctly identified a case overlooked by histomorphometry of flat carcinoma *in situ*, which is characterized by more aggressive behaviour than exophytic papillary tumours [3]. This cytomorphometric technique was commended particularly in the follow-up of patients with transurethrally resected bladder cancers to detect possible recurrence. Later work also emphasized the value of the complementary information gained from a combined cyto- and histomorphometric approach [4].

Computerized semiautomated image analysis has been used to study cytology sample profiles in patients with bladder cancer [5] and the complex cell populations in the sediment of voided urine [6]. Application of a system of hierarchic classification to the digitized cell images allowed a triage procedure to extract from the analysis non-relevant data such as degenerate and inflammatory cell clusters. The cells accepted for final analysis were sufficient in number (only 200–300 required per case) and quality to allow construction of cytological profiles diagnostic of high-grade bladder carcinoma. There was particular emphasis on nuclear size, density and nuclear cytoplasmic ratio.

Densitometric analysis of polyomavirus-infected urothelial cells showed them to have aneuploid DNA values which could not be distinguished from exfoliated carcinoma cells [7]. On the other hand, image analysis of both the Papanicolaou- and Feulgen-stained preparations achieved good separation (misclassification rate approximately 4%). This was based on features related to nuclear texture and minimized the possibility of false-positive diagnosis occurring in this condition. Nuclear texture and geometric parameters also emerged as important variables in a study of urinary sediments from 119 patients with a wide variety of benign and neoplastic disorders of the urinary tract [8]. Discriminant analysis of the training set of 2442 cells identified nuclear area, nuclear cytoplasmic ratio, nuclear shape, nuclear texture and hyperchromasia as making most contribution to the data. The computer was preprogrammed to extract objects of no diagnostic value such as dirt, debris, inflammatory cell clusters and poorly preserved cells, and to focus on normal, atypical and malignant urothelium. Very few malignant or suspiciously atypical cells were classified as benign and vice versa. In the test set of 7050 images the computer classification correctly identified 16 out of 19 grade II papillary tumours and 13 out of 16 cases of carcinoma *in situ* – results comparable to the visual assessment. Low-grade tumours (grades I and II) were classified as abnormal and quantitation unexpectedly identified twice as many lesions as did subjective examination. It was speculated that the computer system was identifying cell features not yet perceptible to the eye and picking up early lesions. There was also a subgroup of false-positive samples from patients with prostatic carcinoma and benign hypertrophy, this finding in the latter being attributed to recent surgical instrumentation. Overall, the sensitivity of the image analysis system for the detection of documented urothelial carcinoma was 84% as opposed to 66% for visual cytodiagnosis.

Others have adopted a similar hierarchic decision-tree approach using statistical discriminant analysis to cull out of the data non-relevant images such as degenerate urothelium, squamous and white blood cells [9]. Papanicolaou-stained specimens obtained from routine screening and cell categories similar to those of Sherman *et al.* [8] were used. The image analysis system clustered positive specimens (49 cases of carcinoma grades II and III) separately from negative ones (26 benign samples; Fig. 4.10). This was based on the percentage occurrence rate of suspicious cells (atypical and malignant). The study illustrated the difficulty in designing a learning set of cells and a corresponding classifier without prior subjective knowledge of the samples. However, it did appear to be a useful technique for

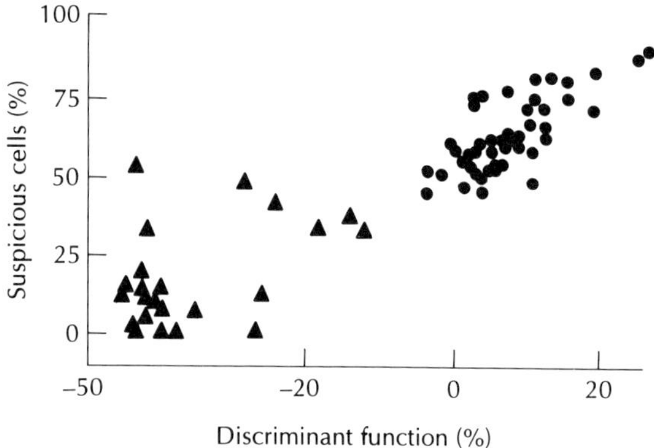

Fig. 4.10 Distribution of negative (▲) and positive (●) urinary sediment specimens on a testing set of 26 benign and 49 malignant (carcinoma grade II and higher) smears. From Brugal *et al.* [9].

sorting smear cell populations rather than designating individual cells.

It is accepted that the cytological and quantitative diagnosis of low-grade urothelial malignancy is difficult [10]. Quantitative fluorescence image analysis incorporates quantitation of DNA and morphometric analysis in a semiautomated system. It automatically scans the slide, images and quantifies the cells, but also allows individual event supervision by an observer. It has the advantage of being able to detect abnormalities in single cells whereas flow cytometry identifies cellular pattern distributions, that is the ratio of normal/abnormal cells. Acridine orange-stained samples were analysed in cohorts of 67 patients symptomatic for bladder cancer and 1385 people who were asymptomatic but had an occupational risk of exposure to aromatic amines [11]. In the symptomatic patients quantitative fluorescence image analysis had greater sensitivity (76 vs 33%) than routine cytopathology for detecting low-grade transitional cell carcinoma. It was recommended as an adjunct to flow cytometry and cytodiagnosis in the follow-up of bladder cancer patients and those in high-risk groups.

DNA cytophotometry has been assessed alongside cytological diagnosis and image analysis, with comparable results being achieved in the majority of cases [12]. In several instances altered DNA patterns were even detected in the absence of significant morphological abnormalities. A further comparison of DNA cytophotometry with flow cytometry emphasized the benefits of additional information conferred by the former technique [13]. In a series of washings from 50 patients with previous bladder tumours it was able to identify DNA aneuploidy in 14 cases classified as DNA diploid or equivocal by flow cytometry. In patients who had short-term current disease 15 had DNA aneuploidy patterns, but in six of these detection was by image cytophotometry alone. Routine cytology was noncontributory in eight of these cases, missing one carcinoma *in situ*, one invasive carcinoma and several low-grade tumours. The value of DNA aneuploidy as a marker of carcinoma *in situ*, high-grade or recurrent disease and these complementary quantitative techniques was confirmed.

4.9.2 Tissue sections

The well-recognized WHO system of grading papillary transitional-cell carcinomas of the bladder is based on multiple features such as numbers of cell layers, cell density, nuclear polarity, hyperchromatism, pleomorphism and mitoses [14]. As with all subjective systems, there is potential for marked intra- and interobserver variation. The high level to which this occurs has been highlighted in a study of 57 transurethrally resected bladder tumours [15]. The degree of inter- (correlation coefficient 0.51–0.67) and intraindividual (correlation coefficient 0.46) inconsistency was disturbing. The majority of pathologists assigned a different grade to the same lesion when it was reassessed in approximately 50% of cases. The same workers then selected 27 unequivocally graded carcinomas (six grade I, 10 grade II, 11 grade III) and applied to them a quantitative grading system [16]. The semiautomatic technique analysed three areas of tumour: (i) deep cells near the basement membrane; (ii) superficial cells near the bladder lumen; and (iii) cells with large nuclei, regardless of their location. An illustration of this was that the deep-cell nuclei in a grade I tumour ranged from 44 to 46 μm^2 and those in a grade III tumour from 69 to 77 μm^2. Similar differences between these two groups were also found for the other cell measurements. It was apparent that progression along the WHO spectrum was characterized by increased nuclear size affecting all cell layers. There was also anisokaryosis with bigger large nuclei showing greater variation with respect to their associated superficial and deep cells. The only significant difference between grade I and II tumours was in the size of the large nuclei, emphasizing the difficulty in distinguishing these on urinary cytology. Plots of mean nuclear area for the respective cell groups achieved reasonable separation of the three grades of lesion. Discriminant analysis generated a classification rule based on the mean nuclear area of the superficial cells and its SD, and calculated numerical probabilities for cases being low- or high-grade. No low-grade carcinomas were classified as high-grade, and vice versa, with the exception of four cases of carcinoma *in situ* where cytomorphometry and visual assessment proved superior. There was a minority of cases assigned as dubious but this is to be expected in what is a histological and cytological continuum. A reproducibility study showed excellent intra- and interindividual consistency with discrepancies always limited to no more than one grade and predominantly in the low-grade lesions [17]. The technique compared favourably with the corresponding histological assessment and was carried out by pathologists with varying morphometric expertise (Fig. 4.11). Further reproducibility studies favoured selective rather than a random nuclear sampling technique and gave a 93.2% agreement with histology based on low- (grades I and II) and high-grade (grade III) categories [18]. Morphometry correctly classified the low-grade tumours which had histological discrepancies and yielded better correlation with tumour stage and clinical follow-up in discrepant high-grade lesions.

Other authors have reported the use of computer-aided image analysis and multivariate classification systems in grading urothelial carcinoma. The classifiers are usually based on a number of variables related to nuclear size, shape, density and nucleolar characteristics [19–22] and increased values correlate with worse prognosis [23–25]. Stereological estimates showed that one of 35 patients with a mean nuclear volume below 300 μm³ died of bladder cancer, whereas 18 of 19 with a value of 500 μm³ or more developed invasive tumours or died from their disease [26]. Nuclear volume is also increased

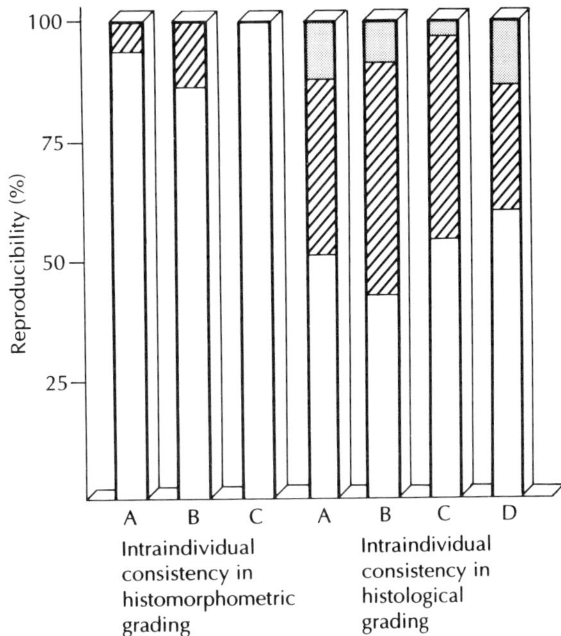

Fig. 4.11 Comparison of reproducibility between histomorphometric grading and previous histological grading of bladder cancer tissue sections. (□) Same grade allocated; (▨) difference of one grade allocated to a given lesion; (▒) difference of two grades. From Ooms *et al.* [17].

in flat carcinoma *in situ* but cannot distinguish those patients with coexisting invasive tumour or decreased survival [27]. Increasing nuclear area relates significantly to advancing tumour grade, depth of the invasion and survival [28]. A cut-off value of 95 μm² allowed categorization of conservatively treated grade II superficial (stages Ta, T1) carcinomas into two prognostic groups, with 5-year survival rates of 100 and 63.2%, respectively [29]. Lipponen *et al.* [30] calculated a 92% efficiency for quantitation in a three-tier (WHO I, II, III) grading system (nuclear area thresholds 50 μm², 75 μm²) and 96% in a two-tier (low-, high-grade) system (threshold 60 μm²). Nuclear area, its SD and the mean area of the 10 largest nuclei were good predictors of survival and yielded useful prognostic information when combined with clinical stage and histological grade [31]. Alterations in nuclear area were also paralleled by changes in the volume-corrected mitotic index [32], with higher values of the latter indicating increased likelihood of local tumour progression [33]. These quantitative techniques, in tandem with tumour stage and grade, closely reflected survival and were not strengthened any further by DNA flow cytometry [34].

A comparison of nuclear size, densitometric DNA content and chromatin pattern showed that grade III tumours had a much higher DNA content and proliferation index [35]. The morphonuclear parameters showed a continuous evolution along the histological spectrum. The databanks were set up as a preliminary exercise in creating an expert system of bladder malignancy diagnosis. Mulder *et al.* [36] found that mitotic counts and determination of growth fraction by Ki-67 were better indicators of disease progression in grade II tumours than DNA ploidy. The diversity in clinical course of these lesions is reflected in their wide range of proliferation indices, e.g., Ki-67, bromodeoxyuridine, factors that are elevated in grade III cases, invasion and carcinoma *in situ* [37].

Morphometry may be of use in identifying small-cell carcinoma of the bladder from poorly differentiated transitional-cell carcinoma [38]. Most of the lesions were DNA aneuploid but some DNA diploid cases also pursued a rapid, lethal clinical course. A comparative assessment of the value of morphometry, DNA flow cytometry and classic prognosticators has been carried out in superficial (stages Ta, T1) bladder carcinoma [39]. Eighty patients with at least 4 years' follow-up were studied and the quantitative techniques proved to be superior to histological grade as predictors of new tumour recurrence. The latter correlated significantly with large nuclei ($> 95\,\mu m^2$) and DNA aneuploidy, with both these parameters also reflecting progressive tumour grade and muscle invasion. Multivariate analysis selected DNA ploidy as the best individual discriminator. Enlarged nuclei and DNA aneuploidy also correlated with decreased 5-year survival rates but did not outperform tumour stage as the best overall indicator of survival [40].

4.9.3 Conclusion

There is wide variation in the cytological and histopathological assessment of papillary transitional carcinoma of the bladder, with particular problems in identifying low-grade lesions. Morphometric quantitation has shown an increased but continuous evolution of nuclear geometric features along the histological spectrum. However, it does appear to perform acceptably well in identifying high-grade lesions and correlates with the likelihood of local recurrence, extensive disease stage and cancer-related death occurring. Its ability to distinguish grade I and II tumours in combination with newer techniques such as fluorescence image analysis, cytometry and DNA flow cytometry awaits further evaluation, especially in the realms of creating diagnostic and prognostic expert systems. The determination of carcinoma *in situ* is more amenable to visual diagnosis or cytomorphometry.

References

1 Boon ME, Kurver PHJ, Baak JPA, Ooms ECM. Morphometric differences between urothelial cells in voided urine of patients with grade I and grade II bladder tumours. *J Clin Pathol* 1981; 34: 612–615.

2 Ooms ECM, Kurver PJH, Boon ME. Morphometrical analysis of urothelial cells in voided urine of patients with low and high grade bladder tumours. *J Clin Pathol* 1982; 35: 1063–1065.

3 Petersen RO. *Urologic Pathology*. Philadelphia: JB Lippincott, 1986.

4 van der Poel HG, Boon ME, Kok LP, Tolboom J, van der Meulen B, Ooms ECM. Can cytophotometry replace histomorphometry for grading of bladder tumours? *Virchows Arch A Pathol Anat Histol* 1988; 413: 249–255.

5 Koss LG, Bartels PH, Sychra JJ, Wied GL. Diagnostic cytologic sample profiles in patients with bladder cancer using TICAS system. *Acta Cytol* 1978; 22: 392–397.

6 Koss LG, Sherman AB, Adams SE. The use of hierarchic classification in the image analysis of a complex cell population. Experience with the sediment of voided urine. *Anal Quant Cytol* 1983; 5: 159–166.

7 Koss LG, Sherman AB, Eppich E. Image analysis and DNA content of urothelial cells infected with human polyomavirus. *Anal Quant Cytol* 1984; 6: 89–94.

8 Sherman AB, Koss LG, Wyschogrod D, Melder KH, Eppich EM, Bales CE. Bladder cancer diagnosis by computer image analysis of cells in the sediment of voided urine using a video scanning system. *Anal Quant Cytol Histol* 1986; 8: 177–186.

9 Brugal G, Quirion C, Vassilakos P. Detection of bladder cancers using a SAMBA 200 cell image processor. *Anal Quant Cytol Histol* 1986; 8: 187–194.

10 Murphy AW. Current status of urinary cytology in the evaluation of bladder neoplasms. *Hum Pathol* 1990; 21: 886–896.

11 Parry WL, Hemstreet GP. Cancer detection by quantitative fluorescence image analysis. *J Urol* 1988; 139: 270–274.

12 Koss LG, Eppich EM, Melder KH, Wersto R. DNA cytophotometry of voided urine sediment: comparison with results of cytologic diagnosis and image analysis. *Anal Quant Cytol Histol* 1987; 9: 398–404.

13 Koss LG, Wersto RP, Simmons DA, Deitch D, Herz F, Freed SZ. Predictive value of DNA measurements in bladder washings. Comparison of flow cytometry image cytophotometry and cytology in patients with a past history of urothelial tumours. *Cancer* 1989; 64: 916–924.

14 Mostofi FK, Sobin LH, Torloni H. Histological typing of urinary bladder tumours. In: *International Histological Classification of Tumours*, no. 10. Geneva: World Health Organization, 1973: 29–31.

15 Ooms ECM, Anderson WAD, Alons CL, Boon ME, Veldhuizen RW. Analysis of the performance of pathologists in the grading of bladder tumors. *Hum Pathol* 1983; 14: 140–143.

16 Ooms ECM, Kurver PHJ, Veldhuizen RW, Alons CL, Boon ME. Morphometric grading of bladder tumors in comparison with histologic grading by pathologists. *Hum Pathol* 1983; 14: 144–150.

17 Ooms ECM, Blok APR, Veldhuizen RW. The reproducibility of a quantitative grading system of bladder tumours. *Histopathology* 1985; 9: 501–509.

18 Blomjous CEM, Smeulders AWM, Baak JPA, Vos W, van Galen CM, Meijer CJLM. A comparative study in morphometric grading of transitional cell carcinoma of the urinary bladder. *Anal Quant Cytol Histol* 1989; 11: 426–432.

19 Mariuzzi GM, Montironi R, Scarpelli M, Pisani E, Ansuini G. Classification of non-invasive urothelial papillary lesions by the malignancy index. *Pathol Res Pract* 1985; 180: 294(A).

20 Hanai S, Kishi K, Watanabe S, Shimosato Y. Morphometry of bladder cancer cells in tissue sections according to histological grade of malignancy. *Jpn J Clin Oncol* 1985; 15: 671–678.

21 Montironi R, Scarpelli M, Pisani E *et al.* Multivariate classification of transitional cell tumors of the bladder: nuclear abnormality index and pattern recognition analysis. *Appl Pathol* 1986; 4: 48–54.

22 Shimazui T, Koiso K, Uchiyama Y. Morphometry of nucleoli as an indicator for grade of malignancy of bladder tumors. *Virchows Arch B Cell Pathol* 1990; 59: 179–183.

23 Nielsen K, Colstrup H, Nilsson T. Morphometric investigations on urinary bladder carcinomas, correlated to histological grading and to prognosis. *Pathol Res Pract* 1985; 180: 302(A).

24 Sowter C, Sowter G, Slavin G, Rosen D. Morphometry of bladder carcinoma: definition of a new variable. *Anal Cell Pathol* 1990; 2: 205–213.

25 Portillo JA, Val-Bernal JF, Garijo MI, Buelta L, Gutierrez JL. The value of nuclear area as a prognostic factor in T_1 papillary transitional cell carcinoma of the bladder. *Br J Urol* 1992; 70: 622–627.

26 Nielsen K, Colstrup H, Nilsson T, Gundersen HJG. Stereological estimates of nuclear volume correlated with histopathological grading and prognosis of bladder tumor. *Virchows Arch (Cell Pathol)* 1986; 52: 41–54.

27 Sørensen FB, Jacobsen F. Stereological estimates of nuclear volume in the prognostic evaluation of primary flat carcinoma *in situ* of the urinary bladder. *Histopathology* 1991; 18: 531–539.

28 Portillo JA, Val-Bernal JF, Garijo MF, Buelta L, Gutierrez JL. Prognostic correlation of morphometric values with survival in invasive transitional cell carcinoma of the bladder. *Br J Urol* 1992; 70: 628–633.

29 Blomjous CEM, Vos W, Schipper NW *et al.* The prognostic significance of selective nuclear morphometry in urinary bladder carcinoma. *Hum Pathol* 1990; 21: 409–413.

30 Lipponen P, Simpanen H, Pesonen E, Eskelinen M, Sotarauta M, Collan Y. Potential of morphometry in grading transitional cell carcinoma of the urinary bladder. *Pathol Res Pract* 1989; 185: 617–620.

31 Lipponen P, Eskelinen M. Nuclear morphometry in grading transitional cell bladder cancer compared with subjective histological grading. *Anticancer Res* 1990; 10: 1725–1730.

32 Lipponen PK, Kosma VM, Collan Y, Kulju T, Kosunen O, Eskelinen M. Potential of nuclear morphometry and volume-corrected mitotic index in grading transitional cell carcinoma of the urinary bladder. *Eur Urol* 1990; 17: 333–337.

33 Lipponen PK, Eskelinen MJ, Sotarauta M. Prediction of superficial bladder cancer by histoquantitative methods. *Eur J Cancer* 1990; 26: 1060–1063.

34 Lipponen PK, Collan Y, Eskelinen MJ, Pesonen E, Sotarauta M, Nordling S. Comparison of morphometry and DNA flow cytometry with standard prognostic factors in bladder cancer. *Br J Urol* 1990; 65: 589–597.

35 Deprez C, De Launoit Y, Kiss R. Computerized morphonuclear cell image analysis of malignant disease in bladder tissues. *J Urol* 1990; 143: 694–699.

36 Mulder AH, Van Hootegem JCSP, Sylvester R *et al.* Prognostic factors in bladder carcinoma: histologic parameters and expression of a cell cycle-related nuclear antigen (Ki-67). *J Pathol* 1992; 166: 37–43.

37 Limas C, Bigler A, Bair R, Bernhart P, Reddy P. Proliferative activity of urothelial neoplasms: comparison of BrdU incorporation, Ki67 expression, and nucleolar organiser regions. *J Clin Pathol* 1993; 46: 159–165.

38 Blomjous CEM, Vos W, Schipper NW, De Voogt HJ, Baak JPA, Meijer CJLM. Morphometric and flow cytometric analysis of small cell undifferentiated carcinoma of the bladder. *J Clin Pathol* 1989; 42: 1032–1039.

39 Blomjous ECM, Schipper NW, Baak JPA, Vos W, De Voogt HJ, Meijer CJLM. The value of morphometry

and DNA flow cytometry in addition to classic prognosticators in superficial urinary bladder carcinoma. *Am J Clin Pathol* 1989; 91: 243–248.

40 Blomjous CEM, Schipper NW, Vos W, Baak JPA, De Voogt HJ, Meijer CJLM. Comparison of quantitative and classic prognosticators in urinary bladder carcinoma. A multivariate analysis of DNA flow cytometric, nuclear morphometric and clinicopathological features. *Virchows Arch A Pathol Anat Histol* 1989; 415: 421–428.

4.10 PROSTATE GLAND

4.10.1 Benign nodular hyperplasia

Morphometry of benign prostatic hyperplasia has quantified its constituent tissue components and related them to glandular size [1]. In small transurethral resections glandular and stromal nodules comprised only 5% of the specimen, with bladder neck and anterior fibromuscular tissue predominating. In the majority of samples a proliferation of normal non-nodular connective tissue from the transitional zone was the main element. In larger specimens and enucleated glands, particularly those over 50 g, nodules were more evident and their increased epithelial stroma ratio formed a basis for the weight-related morphological evolution of benign hyperplasia. Quantitation has also identified two distinct anatomical zones in normal prostates (periurethral, peripheral) and three in benign hyperplasia (central hyperplasia, intermediate fibrous capsule, peripheral) – features which correlate with their magnetic resonance images [2].

4.10.2 Adenocarcinoma

Semiautomatic image analysis combined with cytophotometry found significant differences between benign (nodular hyperplasia, prostatitis) and malignant prostatic epithelium for the following variables: nucleoli (number, size and variability of size), regularity of nuclear arrangement, anisonucleosis, nuclear size, nuclear polymorphism and dissociation of cells [3]. The criteria nuclear/cytoplasmic ratio, hyperchromasia and anisochromasia were not contributory to the diagnosis. The latter was derived in individual cases by differing combinations of the altered parameters, emphasizing the heterogeneity in cell morphology and grade in prostatic cancer. Karyometric and ploidy estimates have shown a progressive derangement as benign nodular hyperplasia evolves through prostatic intraepithelial neoplasia (PIN) to adenocarcinoma. This is characterized by a shift from diploid to non-diploid values, increased nuclear size, diminished nuclear roundness [4] and nuclear size variation [5]. It has been suggested that cytological smear preparations are more suitable than tissue sections for the determination of DNA content and morphometric parameters such as nuclear shape, size and texture due to less overlap in cells [6]; others have noted differences in nuclear area measurements but similar nuclear shape values [7]. A 75% accurate prediction for well-differentiated adenocarcinoma was attained using mean nuclear area ($> 28\,\mu m^2$), mean nuclear diameter ($> 5\,\mu m$) and the presence of more than 5% of cells with a nuclear diameter greater than 6.15 μm [8]. Nuclear area, counts and optical density also emerged as important in distinguishing well-, moderately and poorly differentiated prostatic adenocarcinoma in a study where the images were segmented by an automated expert system [9].

One of the most popular methods of grading prostatic carcinoma has been the Gleason classification [10] which essentially mirrors the degree of architectural acinar formation and arrangement. It is the 'gold standard' against which quantitative studies have been compared and it remains a readily applicable prognostic tool [11]. Determination of relative nuclear roundness factor outperformed Gleason histological grade in predicting progression of disease, but was confined to those patients with stage A or B cancers [12]. Variance of nuclear roundness combined with clinical stage, Gleason score and age produced a prognostic score capable of stratifying patients with clinically localized cancers into three groups with different times to disease progression [13]. Ultrastructural stereological assessment of nucleolar surface area showed that progressive disease was always associated with a measurement greater than $2.4\,\mu m^2$. There was close correlation between nucleolar surface areas in the initial biopsy and subsequent prostatectomy specimen, whereas Gleason grade varied by more than 30% in 70% of cases. In addition, only nine of 16 patients with aggressive disease had Gleason scores above 6 [14]. A cytophotometric assessment of DNA content gave significant correlation with the following variables in decreasing order of importance: nuclear area variation, convex perimeter and mean maximum nuclear diameter [15]. A combined geometric/DNA nuclear grade of malignancy related more closely to clinical stage of disease ($r = 0.75$) than the visually assessed histological Gleason score ($r = 0.68$). However, in a further study Gleason grade and percentage tumour area were more important predictors of tumour progression than DNA ploidy [16]. Increased histological grade correlates with the degree of capsular penetration [17] and clinical stage [18]. In the latter study the percentage glandular differentiation determined by point-counting varied with stage (A 71%; D 28%) and showed significant differences between stages A, B and C, D. A combination of morphometrically derived percentage gland involvement by carcinoma and Gleason score were better indicators of pathological stage than tumour volume in clinical stage B cancers [19]. Tumour volume relates to the degree of capsular penetration and seminal vesicle involvement [20]. All six of 68 patients who developed lymph node or bone marrow secondaries had a tumour volume greater than 4 ml and this threshold separated those whose disease was confined to one lobe rather than having bilateral spread. McNeal [21] also found tumour volume to correlate closely with the extent of local spread and, when combined with percentage of high-grade tumour, to be strongly predictive of nodal metastases. Comparable estimates of tumour volume may be determined by computer planimetry or point-counting on marked histological slides [22]. It is also reflected in the serum prostate-specific antigen level in stage A carcinoma [23]. Quantitation helps to identify capsular penetration when perineural invasion involves more than one nerve, particularly if > 0.1 mm in diameter [24].

In incidentally detected prostatic carcinoma (stage O, A) the percentage of cancer in the tissue is a good predictor of subsequent disease progression [25]. Absolute area of carcinoma, percentage glandular involvement by tumour, Gleason grade and the percentage of diseased prostatic chippings are all independent prognostic indicators of survival [26]. The actual number of chips involved did not reach statistical significance and the percentage of affected chippings yielded as much information as the more time-consuming computer-assisted techniques. Previous work [27] had also shown the ratio of positive chips to be closely associated with tumour stage and the likelihood of cancer-related death. A review of image analysis in prostate cancer is given by Dalton [28].

4.10.3 Conclusion

Morphometry has shown the importance of cellular variables such as nuclear and nucleolar size in designating prostatic carcinoma. It has also validated the approach of histological grading based on glandular differentiation, as in the Gleason system, in imparting clinically useful information relating to the stage of disease and survival. The diagnostic surgical pathologist should note the necessity of reporting the percentage of transurethral resection chippings involved by carcinoma — a feature easily ascertained by direct visual assessment.

References

1 Prince H, McNeal JE, Stamey TA. Evolving patterns of tissue composition in benign prostatic hyperplasia as a function of specimen size. *Hum Pathol* 1990; 21: 578–585.

2 Hruban RH, Zerhouni EA, Dagher AP, Pessar ML, Hutchins GM. Morphologic basis of MR imaging of benign prostatic hyperplasia. *J Comput Assist Tomogr* 1987; 11: 1035–1041.

3 Bocking A, Auffermann W, Schwarz H, Bammert J, Dorrjer G, Vucicuja S. Cytology of prostatic carcinoma. Quantification and validation of diagnostic criteria. *J Anal Quant Cytol* 1984; 6: 74–88.

4 Montironi R, Scarpelli M, Sisti S *et al.* Quantitative analysis of prostatic intraepithelial neoplasia on tissue sections. *Anal Quant Cytol Histol* 1990; 12: 366–372.

5 Wang N, Stenkvist BG, Tribukait B. Morphometry of nuclei of the normal and malignant prostate in relation to DNA ploidy. *Anal Quant Cytol Histol* 1992; 14: 210–216.

6 Epstein JI, Christensen WN, Steinberg GD, Carter HB. Comparison of DNA ploidy and nuclear size, shape and chromatin irregularity in tissue sections and smears of prostatic carcinoma. *Anal Quant Cytol Histol* 1990; 12: 352–358.

7 Tardif CP, Partin AW, Qaqish B, Epstein JP, Mohler JL. Comparison of nuclear shape in aspirated and

histologic specimens of prostatic carcinoma. *Acta Cytol* 1993; 37: 105A.
8 Aragona F, Franco V, Rodolico V *et al.* Interactive computerized morphometric analysis for the differential diagnosis between dysplasia and well differentiated adenocarcinoma of the prostate. *Urol Res* 1989; 17: 35–40.
9 Bibbo M, Kim DH, Pfeifer T, Dytch HE, Galera-Davidson H, Bartels PH. Histometric features for the grading of prostatic carcinoma. *Anal Quant Cytol Histol* 1991; 13: 61–68.
10 Gleason DF. Classification of prostatic carcinomas. *Cancer Chemother Rep* 1966; 50: 125–128.
11 Gleason DF. Histologic grading of prostate cancer: a perspective. *Hum Pathol* 1992; 23: 273–279.
12 Clark TD, Askin FB, Bagnell CR. Nuclear roundness factor: a quantitative approach to grading in prostatic carcinoma, reliability of needle biopsy tissue, and the effect of tumor stage on usefulness. *Prostate* 1987; 10: 199–206.
13 Partin AW, Steinberg GD, Pitcock RV *et al.* Use of nuclear morphometry, Gleason histologic scoring, clinical stage, and age to predict disease-free survival among patients with prostate cancer. *Cancer* 1992; 70: 161–168.
14 Tannenbaum M, Tannenbaum S, De Sanctis PN, Olsson CA. Prognostic significance of nucleolar surface area in prostatic cancer. *Urology* 1982; 19: 546–551.
15 Robutti F, Pilato FP, Betta P-G. A new method of grading malignancy of prostate carcinomas using quantitative microscopic nuclear features. *Pathol Res Pract* 1989; 185: 701–703.
16 Humphrey PA, Walther PJ, Currin SM, Vollmer RT. Histologic grade, DNA ploidy and intraglandular tumor extent as indicators of tumor progression of clinical state B prostatic carcinoma. A direct comparison. *Am J Surg Pathol* 1991; 15: 1165–1170.
17 Miller GJ. Pathologic aspects of prostate cancer: prediction of malignant potential. *Urology* 1989; 34(suppl 4): 5–9.
18 Sharkey FE, Dusenbery DM, Moyer JE, Barry JD. Correlation between stage and grade in prostatic adenocarcinoma: a morphometric study. *J Urol* 1984; 132: 602–605.
19 Partin AW, Epstein JI, Cho KR, Gittelsohn AM, Walsh PC. Morphometric measurement of tumor volume and per cent of gland involvement as predictors of pathological stage in clinical stage B prostate cancer. *J Urol* 1989; 141: 341–345.
20 Stamey FA, McNeal JE, Freiha FS, Redwine E. Morphometric and clinical studies on 68 consecutive radial prostatectomies. *J Urol* 1988; 139: 1235–1241.
21 McNeal JE. Cancer volume and site of origin of adenocarcinoma in the prostate: relationship to local and distant spread. *Hum Pathol* 1992; 23: 258–266.
22 Schmid HP, McNeal JE. An abbreviated standard procedure for accurate tumor volume estimation in prostate cancer. *Am J Surg Pathol* 1992; 16: 184–191.
23 Carter HB, Partin AW, Epstein JI, Chan DW, Walsh PC. The relationship of prostate specific antigen levels and residual tumor volume in stage A prostate cancer. *J Urol* 1990; 144: 1167–1170.
24 Bastacky SI, Walsh PC, Epstein JI. Relationship between perineural tumor invasion on needle biopsy and radical prostatectomy capsular penetration in clinical stage B adenocarcinoma of the prostate. *Am J Surg Pathol* 1993; 17: 336–341.
25 Cantrell BB, De Klerk DP, Eggleston JC. Pathological factors that influence prognosis in stage A prostatic cancer: the influence of extent versus grade. *J Urol* 1981; 125: 516–520.
26 Foucar E, Haake G, Dalton L, Pathak DR, Lujan JP. The area of cancer in transurethral resection specimens as a prognostic indicator in carcinoma of the prostate: a computer-assisted morphometric study. *Hum Pathol* 1990; 21: 586–592.
27 Humphrey P, Vollmer RT. The ratio of prostate chips with cancer: a new measure of tumour extent and its relationship to grade and prognosis. *Hum Pathol* 1988; 19: 411–418.
28 Dalton LW. Computer-based image analysis of prostate cancer. Comments with emphasis on use of commercially available system. *Hum Pathol* 1992; 23: 280–286.

4.11 GYNAECOLOGICAL DISEASE

Quantitation in gynaecological disease has mainly centred on the following issues: (i) the morphology and progression of cervical intraepithelial neoplasia (CIN); (ii) early cervical squamous-cell carcinoma; (iii) the distinction between endometrial hyperplasia and adenocarcinoma; and (iv) prognosis in ovarian epithelial tumours.

4.11.1 Vulva, vagina

During the 1970s there were a number of reports noting that an absence of pelvic node metastases correlated with an early limited extent of invasion in vulval squamous-cell carcinoma. Wharton *et al.* [1] studied 45 patients with tumours <2 cm in diameter. In those with a depth of invasion <5 mm there were no nodal metastases, recurrences or cancer-related deaths. This contrasted to those with >5 mm tumour infiltration who had 25 and 15% rates for nodal disease and 5-year mortality, respectively. Others noted the possibility of infrequent metastases in these microcarcinomas and associated it with lymphovascular involvement, cellular anaplasia [2] and a confluent growth pattern [3]. The resultant controversy over the definition of the term microinvasive carcinoma has led to the recommendation that it be abandoned and replaced by stage Ia carcinoma, defined as a single lesion measuring 2 cm or less in diameter and invading no more than 1 mm in depth [4]. Quantitation has identified increased DNA content and nuclear cytoplasmic ratios in the cells of skin adjacent to vulval squamous carcinoma [5]. This emphasizes the associated field change that occurs and the need to assess resection margins in vulvectomy specimens. Survival in malignant melanoma of the vulva is directly related to the depth of invasion. Using eyepiece micrometer measurements taken from the granular layer and a levelling system (similar to that of Clark in cutaneous lesions), the most superficial primary tumour associated with a fatal disease course measured 1.4 mm deep [6]. Thinner lesions did not develop recurrent disease. Vulval smooth-muscle tumours are more likely to have aggressive behaviour and should be designated leiomyosarcoma if they meet the following criteria: >5 cm, infiltrating margins and more than 5 mitotic figures per 10 HPFs [7]. The latter feature in combination with cellular atypia are also prognostic indicators in vaginal leiomyomatous tumours [8].

4.11.2 Uterine cervix

CIN (or squamous intraepithelial lesion; SIL)

The cervical junctional squamous epithelium shows a range of abnormalities from those which lack any potential for evolving into a squamous-cell carcinoma to others that have a significant risk of progression. The term CIN was introduced for this premalignant lesion [9]. It has a postulated transit time to carcinoma *in situ* of 86 and 12 months from its mild and severe categories [10]. The latter may also evolve to invasive carcinoma over a 3–10-year period. It is subdivided into CIN grades I, II and III (corresponding to mild, moderate and severe dysplasia/carcinoma *in situ*) and its features are well-described elsewhere [11,12]. It forms a morphological spectrum of loss in cellular maturation characterized by cellular crowding, lack of stratification and differentiation, nuclear abnormalities (including enlargement, pleomorphism and hyperchromasia), increased [13] and abnormal [14] mitotic activity. These changes occur to varying degrees and levels throughout the epithelium depending on the severity of the lesion. Small- and large-cell non-keratinizing and large-cell keratinizing forms have been described. CIN affects both the surface epithelium and the endocervical crypts. In a series of 343 cervical conization specimens containing CIN III, 88.6% had some degree of crypt involvement [15]. The mean depth from the surface determined by a measuring graticule was 1.24 mm with a maximum of 5.22 mm. It was estimated that destruction of tissue to a depth of 2.92 mm (mean ± 1.96 SD) would eradicate involved crypts in 95% of patients and 3.80 mm (mean ± 3 SD), 99.7% of cases. The importance of removing this amount of tissue was emphasized to obviate the danger of leaving residual viable CIN from which an occult carcinoma could develop. Abdul-Karim *et al.* [16] found that the extent of surface and crypt involvement increased with worsening CIN grade and age. The mean crypt depths and surface linear dimensions for CIN I, II and III were 0.42 and 0.93 mm, 1.35 and 4.10 mm, and 5.84 and 7.60 mm, respectively. To eradicate CIN lesions, tissue destruction to a depth of 4.80 mm was recommended. The majority of lesions occupied the transformation zone but 9.7% were higher in the cervical canal and 3.1% were located in the ectocervix. This highlights the possibility of sampling error which exists in the assessment of CIN.

Quantitative histology has shown increases in nuclear volume [17], nuclear cytoplasmic ratio, the percentage of nuclei with nucleoli, nuclear area and perimeter on moving from normal epithelium and mild dysplasia towards infiltrating carcinoma [18,19]. The latter study also found alterations in stromal capillary dimensions; these biphasic epithelial/stromal derangements showed a continuous, gradual evolution with lesion severity. The values for moderate and severe dysplasia resembled carcinoma, reflecting their premalignant potential. This was mirrored in the estimates of DNA content with a parallel reduction in DNA diploidy and the appearance of DNA aneuploidy, as shown in other cytophotometry studies [20]. Interestingly, the development of microinvasion was associated with better differentiation and an increase in nuclear dimensions but a reduction in ploidy variation [19].

Semiautomated rapid DNA cytophotometry of cervical smears has been developed (e.g., Leitz TAS) to allow observer interaction with highly reproducible results [21]. It is faster than microspectrophotometry, allows operator cell selection that is missing in flow cytometry, and gives accurate altered measurements of DNA content in koilocytosis associated with CIN I [22] and malignancy [23]. Similar claims for high degrees of sensitivity in detecting CIN III and invasive carcinoma have also been made for quantitative fluorescent image analysis [24] and this awaits further evaluation.

Semiautomatic image analysis of cervical smear monolayers gives confirmation of a continuous progression of cellular changes along the spectrum from borderline dysplasia to carcinoma [25]. It is claimed that the geometric features of moderately dyskaryotic cells can be used to predict from what grade of parent CIN lesion they arise [26,27] and also in 80–90% of cases whether they will progress to more severe disease [28]. The discriminant analysis achieved this high degree of separation by identifying nuclear cytoplasmic ratio and nuclear texture (mean optical density) as the most important features [28,29]. At present, fully automated analysis systems are not as accurate as when an interactive operator-dependent step is included [30].

Cell counts linked to immunoperoxidase staining have shown increased human leucocyte antigen (HLA)-DR expression in human papillomavirus (HPV) infection, indicating participation of the cervical epithelium in local immune response [31]. In both HPV infection and CIN there is reversal of the helper/suppressor T-lymphocyte ratio, suggesting that there is also a localized acquired immune deficiency [32].

Endocervical intraepithelial neoplasia (EIN)

In a proportion of CIN lesions there is an associated abnormality of the endocervical epithelium ranging from mild atypia to adenocarcinoma *in situ*. In the author's experience designation of endocervical cell changes (especially in cervical smears) is a difficult and increasingly frequent practical problem. It is particularly important as adenocarcinoma *in situ* necessitates treatment by hysterectomy. There are marked similarities in the visual and quantitative nuclear changes in CIN and EIN [33], with early endocervical glandular neoplasia exhibiting an increase in nuclear size and nuclear cytoplasmic ratio. It has been claimed that measurement of these features can separate normal endocervical cells, adenocarcinoma *in situ* and microinvasive adenocarcinoma [34]. However the results did show overlap between disease categories and this needs further assessment.

In established cervical adenocarcinoma DNA content, the percentage of glandular lumen area, the mean and SD of nuclear area, as determined by image analysis of tissue sections, are useful predictors of tumour recurrence and survival in patients with stage I or II disease [35].

Cervical squamous-cell carcinoma

As in its vulval equivalent there is controversy over the definition of cervical microinvasive squamous carcinoma. It is a condition associated with a better prognosis and which may be treated by limited surgery. The International Federation of Gynaecology and Obstetrics (FIGO) defines stage Ia disease (microinvasive carcinoma) as those cases of epithelial abnormalities in which histological evidence of early stromal invasion is unambiguous. There is no attempt to specify maximum tumour size or depth of infiltration. This has led to diverse reports in the literature with extension into the stroma varying between 1 and 9 mm and measured from differing points of the epithelium. Burghardt [36] recognized the following disease phase: carcinoma *in situ*, early stromal invasion, microcarcinoma and clinical cancer. Microcarcinoma was recognized as those tumours where volume did not exceed 500 mm^3 and this correlated with no risk of metastatic spread provided that vascular invasion was absent [37]. Tumour volume was derived by graticule measurements of linear extent and depth, with an estimate of the third dimension from serial blocks and sections of known thickness. There is disagreement as to whether lymphatic channel involvement is [38] or is not [39] predictive of nodal metastases in carcinomas with a depth of invasion < 5 mm. What is clear is that the greater the tumour volume, the more likelihood there is of future consequences. In practical terms lesions should be categorized into those showing: (i) only early stromal invasion (cells not further than 1 mm from the nearest surface or crypt basement membrane); (ii) microinvasion (< 3 mm); and (iii) microcarcinoma (depth and largest dimension not exceeding 5 mm and 7 mm respectively, in the worst section) [12]. This should be supplemented by commenting on the presence or absence of vascular invasion as all of these features are helpful in selecting patients for treatment by cone biopsy, simple or extended Werdheim's hysterectomy.

Cytophotometry and stereology have shown marked heterogeneity of DNA content and nuclear volume in established squamous carcinoma cells [40]. Increased nuclear diameters and axes products also evolve in parallel with a shift from DNA diploidy to tetraploidy, and these factors were significant predictors of 10-year survival in patients treated with radiotherapy [41]. Immunodetection of the nuclear proliferation antigen Ki-67 does not correlate with any of the usual histological parameters and the establishment of its role in assessing cervical carcinoma requires further follow-up [42].

4.11.3 Uterine endometrium

Morphometry and stereology have been applied to both cytological and histological samples mainly in an attempt to characterize and distinguish normal, hyperplastic and neoplastic endometria. From a practical point of view it is not difficult to separate histologically benign and frankly carcinomatous endometrium. Hyperplasia, which is the subject of varying terminology and exhibits a spectrum of morphological change intermediate between those unequivocal states, is more difficult to define. Its evolution as a precursor of endometrial carcinoma is not well-characterized but its recognition is important due to the real possibility of subsequent or coexistent adenocarcinoma. Its histological features are well-described elsewhere [43–45]. In general there is simple or complex hyperplasia with or without cellular atypia. Simple hyperplasia equates to cystic change while complex hyperplasia shows varying degrees of architectural change. These are disorders of endometrial proliferation with no proven propensity for carcinoma formation. However, complex hyperplasia with atypia showing both marked architectural and cytological alterations does, in approximately 30% of cases, have a definite association with concurrent or subsequent adenocarcinoma. Adenocarcinoma *in situ* and intra-endometrial carcinoma merge with this severe atypical hyperplasia and difficulties arise in distinction from well-differentiated adenocarcinoma. The implications for the patient of hysterectomy are the same.

Cytomorphometry of epithelial abnormalities

Microspectrophotometry of nuclear area and extinction values were capable of distinguishing normal endometrial glandular cells, histiocytes and malignant tumour cells [46]. Planimetry of nuclear and cellular outlines has shown similarities in geometric dimensions between normals and simple hyperplasia and atypical hyperplasia and adenocarcinoma *in situ*, respectively [47]. In the latter conditions there were increases in the order of 10% in nuclear and cellular areas and prominent nucleoli were also evident. More recently morphometric analysis of nuclear size and shape in endometrial aspirates found significant differences in mean nuclear area for benign and malignant cells (38 vs 65 μm^2). However the range of normal values was so wide that it included over 70% of the malignant cases and with a threshold of 45 μm^2 there were 17% false-positive and 25% false-negative rates [48]. In a parallel study measurements in cystic and atypical hyperplasia tended towards the benign and malignant categories, respectively [49]. As previously there was marked group overlap and it was concluded that morphometry of nuclear size and shape was not contributory to the differential diagnosis of endometrial disease.

Histomorphometry of epithelial abnormalities

Eyepiece graticule determination of tubular volume and tubular surface to volume ratio showed significant changes between endometria at varying stages of the cycle, cystic and atypical hyperplasia [50]. Image analysis of nuclear texture and area resulted in a 60–70% separation of normal, atypical hyperplasia and carcinomatous uterine glands [51]. Thus it appeared that there was potential to separate various endometrial histologies by quantitation and this was studied subsequently, including its use in individual patient care [52]. Progression along the spectrum from hyperplasia to adenocarcinoma is associated with interobserver disagreement (12.1%) in categorization. This can be decreased by quantitation which is also superior to subjective assessment in correlating with the depth of myometrial wall infiltration in carcinoma [53]. Parameters that increase significantly with progression are volume percentage epithelium, inner surface density of glands, epithelial thickness and lumen diameter, factors which reflect glandular tortuosity and branching [54]. Nuclear variables such as area, long axis, SD of perimeter [54] and maximal diameter [55] are also altered. These studies serve to highlight the different features used in histological assessment and the greater weight attributed to architectural features by discriminant analysis in separating atypical hyperplasia from adenocarcinoma [56]. More recently a combination of cytological (SD of the shortest nuclear axis) and architectural (volume percentage stroma) morphometry has proven superior to nuclear quantitation alone in identifying cases of atypical hyperplasia that progressed and those that did not [57]. Determination of volume percentage epithelium and stroma has also been achieved by fully automated digital image analysis and gives excellent correlation with interactive methods [58].

Thymidine autoradiography [59] and flow cytometry [60] have found differences in the S-phase fractions and DNA content of normal, hyperplastic and malignant endometria. DNA microspectrophotometry is inferior to nuclear morphometry in separating benign and malignant endometrial disease, although excellent discrimination (97%) was achieved when both elements were combined [61]. The technique also has potential for specifically distinguishing between atypical hyperplasia and carcinoma.

In established uterine adenocarcinoma recurrence is related to histological grade and the depth of myometrial invasion [62]. The latter therefore acts as a basis for the selection of patients for adjuvant radiotherapy. It is usually expressed as the percentage of the myometrium infiltrated by tumour but is perhaps more accurately ascertained by the thickness of residual uninvaded tissue [63]. Histological grade is assessed by both architectural and cytological changes; these are somewhat inter-related as high-architectural-grade endometrial adenocarcinomas have greater mean shortest nuclear axis measurements and volume-weighted mean nuclear volumes [64].

Immunocytochemical assay by image analysis has been established for the assessment of oestrogen receptors, laminin, collagen and Ki-67 in various endometrial disorders [65].

Pure, mixed mesenchymal neoplasms

There are a number of pure and mixed uterine neoplasms where designation is based upon tumour size, cellularity, the character of the margin (pushing or infiltrating) and the number of mitoses per 10 HPFs. In general increased size, cellularity, mitoses and an invasive margin favour sarcoma in the following: endometrial stromal lesions (nodule, low- and high-grade sarcoma), leiomyomatous tumours [66], adenofibroma and adenosarcoma [67]. A review of this is presented by Clement [68].

4.11.4 Placenta

Clinically useful information can be gained from gross assessment of the placenta. Areas of infarction less than 5% of the villous parenchyma are common and of little consequence. However, extensive (> 10%) infarction is associated with a high incidence of fetal hypoxia, growth retardation and intrauterine death [69]. Systematic sampling and light microscopy with stereology and morphometry give a valuable insight into the physiology of placental function and fetal growth in various disorders [70]. The placental weight and parenchyma/non-parenchyma volume ratio is significantly reduced in small-for-gestational-age infants. The following are all diminished: parenchymal volume, intervillous space, total trophoblast, total villous capillaries and the number of syncytiovascular membranes. There are associated diminutions in the density of trophoblast, fibroblast and endothelial nuclei, with the peripheral villi being more affected than stem villi. All of these parameters indicate significantly less surface areas for gaseous exchange between mother and fetus. These reductions in functional placental tissue to the order of 45% correlate well with measurements of idiopathic intrauterine growth retardation [71]. Conversely, the placentae of diabetic mothers have increased values for the above features, enabling efficient support for the growth of the larger-than-normal fetus that occurs in this condition [72].

The placentae of smoking mothers have smaller villous capillary diameters, a decrease in vasculo-syncytial membranes and fetal vessel volume density, along with basement membrane thickening, all leading to lower birth weights [73]. The capillary lumen/diameter ratio is decreased in toxaemic pregnancies whether due to pre-eclampsia, essential hypertension or renal disease [74]. More recently, the value of perfusion fixation in morphometry of the placenta has been emphasized [75]. In molar pregnancy some investigations have centred on flow cytometry, although Franke *et al.* [76] found that increased nuclear area in the trophoblast of large villi correlated with subsequent persistent and progressive disease. Morphometric determination of villous size and trophoblast thickness has also been found to correlate with karyotypic abnormalities such as triploidy in first-trimester spontaneous abortions [77].

4.11.5 Ovary

Morphology of ovarian carcinoma has an undoubted influence on patient morbidity and mortality figures. This is reflected in the WHO classification [78] and the differing patient survival figures seen with the various histological types and nuclear grade of tumours [79]. These factors are outweighed by the importance of disease stage but are fundamental in the designation of lesions. An example of this is the distinction between benign, borderline and malignant ovarian epithelial tumours on the basis of mitotic activity, epithelial nuclear stratification, complexity and stromal invasion [80,81]. Mitotic activity greater than 5–10 per 10 HPFs and nuclear stratification of more than three or four layers associated with invasion characterize the progression from borderline to malignant categories in serous, mucinous, endometrioid and clear cell lesions. It is widely recognized that even amongst experienced gynaecological pathologists there is poor inter- and intraobserver agreement in histological assessment of tumour type and grade approximating to only 60–80% [82].

Quantitation has been claimed to achieve correct classification rates of more than 93% in categorizing benign, borderline and malignant mucinous tumours [83,84]. The best discriminator chose a combination of mean nuclear area, perimeter and short axis along with volume percentage epithelium and mitotic activity to minimize the degree of overlap between histologies for these individual features [83]. The morphometric technique was considered to have corrected histological assessment in two instances and was even subsequently applied in an individual case as a basis for decision-making regarding adjuvant chemotherapy [85]. It is reproducible and outperformed histological grading as a predictor of survival in patients with FIGO stage I disease [86]. A classifier based on mitotic index above 30 (mitotic figures per 25 fields, 400× magnification, 0.75 numerical aperture), volume percentage epithelium $>65\%$ and shortest nuclear axis greater than 1.1 μm indicated a poor prognosis in the common epithelial ovarian carcinomas. Furthermore, prediction of survival by morphometric categorization evolved in parallel with estimates of DNA content [87]. Together they identified a subset of aggressive DNA aneuploid tumours which also had geometric characteristics associated with an unfavourable outcome. It is recommended that a combination of morphometry with flow cytometry is comparable to histological grading in augmenting disease stage as important prognostic determinants [88].

In patients with late (stage III and IV) disease treated by cisplatin survival was linked to the following in decreasing order of importance: FIGO stage, bulky disease, SD and mean of nuclear area, DNA content, mitotic activity index and volume percentage epithelium [89]. Tumours with a mean nuclear area $>70\,\mu m^2$ were DNA aneuploid. Multivariate analysis chose nuclear area, disease bulk and FIGO stage to derive a function, a low value of which indicated a poor prognosis within 24 months.

The only favourable determinants were low-volume percentage epithelium and low mitotic activity. Other workers have used nuclear dimensions, density and mitoses to predict (with 79% accuracy) chemotherapy responders and non-responders [90]. Morphometry may also be able to distinguish chemoresponsive peritoneal tumour cells from mesothelial hyperplasia in second-look operations [91].

Multivariate analysis of mitotic activity, tumour volume fraction and measurements of nuclear size and shape have again emphasized clinical stage as the best predictor of prognosis. This was followed by the volume-corrected M/V index, which is the number of mitotic figures per square millimetre of neoplastic epithelium. This was true for all tumour subgroups and the M/V index was the only significantly independent prognosticator in stage I disease [92]. It is claimed that this gauge of proliferative activity is reproducible, and, superior to conventional histological grading and morphometry in estimating survival [93] (Fig. 4.12).

4.11.6 Conclusion

Quantitation in gynaecological disease has characterized the histological and cytological manifestations of CIN. Automated screening techniques are developing from this to augment the present labour-intensive manual methods. Depth of infiltration and tumour volume are important factors in the choice of therapy and prognosis in cervical and endometrial carcinoma. Architectural features outweigh cytological parameters in distinguishing endometrial hyperplasia from adenocarcinoma but perform better in a combined approach supplemented by estimates of DNA content. Morphometry of the placenta correlates with its disordered function in various diseases. Clinical stage remains the best indicator of survival in ovarian carcinoma. Additional information is provided by morphometry (volume percentage epithelium) and, in particular, mitotic activity.

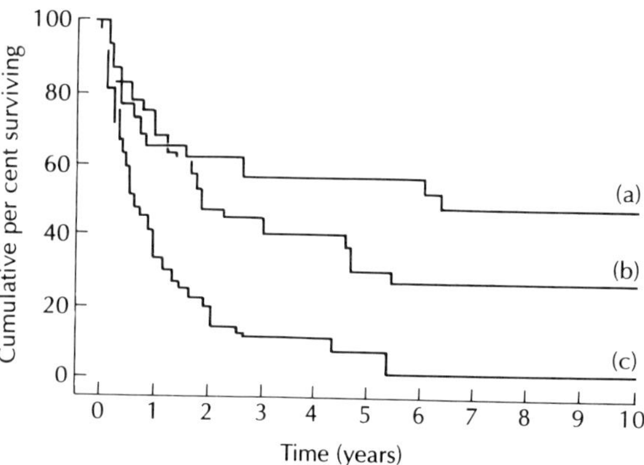

Fig. 4.12 Comparison of survival in 105 cases of ovarian carcinoma divided into three subclasses on the basis of the volume-corrected mitotic index (M/V index). Group (a) ($n = 29$): M/V index < 10 mitoses/mm^2; group (c) ($n = 44$): M/V index ≥ 20 mitoses/mm^2. From Haapasalo *et al.* [92].

References

1 Wharton JT, Gallagher S, Rutledge FN. Microinvasive carcinoma of the vulva. *Am J Obstet Gynecol* 1974; 118: 159–162.
2 Parker RT, Duncan I, Rampone J, Creasman W. Operative management of early invasive epidermoid carcinoma of the vulva. *Am J Obstet Gynecol* 1975; 123: 349–355.
3 Barnes AE, Crissman JD, Schellhas HF, Azoury RS. Microinvasive carcinoma of the vulva: a clinicopathologic evaluation. *Obstet Gynecol* 1980; 56: 234–238.
4 Kneale BL. Microinvasive cancer of the vulva: report of the ISSVD task force. *J Reprod Med* 1984; 29: 454–458.
5 Dalrymple JC, Brough AK, Monaghan JM. Morphometric analysis of nuclear/cytoplasmic ratios in normal and perineoplastic vulvar skin. *Histopathology* 1989; 14: 645–653.
6 Chung AF, Woodruff JM, Lewis JL. Malignant melanoma of the vulva: a report of 44 cases. *Obstet Gynecol* 1975; 45: 638–646.
7 Tavassoli FA, Norris HJ. Smooth muscle tumors of the vulva. *Obstet Gynecol* 1979; 53: 213–217.
8 Tavassoli FA, Norris HJ. Smooth muscle tumors of the vagina. *Obstet Gynecol* 1979; 53: 689–693.
9 Richart RM. Natural history of cervical intraepithelial neoplasia. *Clin Obstet Gynecol* 1967; 10: 748–784.
10 Richart RM, Barron BA. A follow-up study of patients with cervical dysplasia. *Am J Obstet Gynecol* 1969; 105: 386–393.
11 Buckley CH, Butler EB, Fox H. Cervical intraepithelial neoplasia. *J Clin Pathol* 1982; 35: 1–13.
12 Anderson MC. Premalignant and malignant disease of the cervix. In: Fox H (ed.) *Haines and Taylor Obstetrical and Gynaecological Pathology*, 3rd edn. Edinburgh: Churchill Livingstone, 1987: 255–301.
13 Chi CH, Rubio CA, Lagerlöf B. The frequency and

distribution of mitotic figures in dysplasia and carcinoma *in situ*. *Cancer* 1977; 39: 1218–1223.

14 Kirkland JA, Stanley MA, Cellier KM. Comparative study of histologic and chromosomal abnormalities in cervical neoplasia. *Cancer* 1967; 20: 1934–1952.

15 Anderson MC, Hartley RB. Cervical crypt involvement by intraepithelial neoplasia. *Obstet Gynecol* 1980; 55: 546–550.

16 Abdul-Karim FW, Fu YS, Reagan JW, Wentz WB. Morphometric study of intraepithelial neoplasia of uterine cervix. *Obstet Gynecol* 1982; 60: 210–214.

17 Sørensen FB, Bichel P, Jakobsen A. Stereological estimates of nuclear volume in squamous cell carcinoma of the uterine cervix and its precursors. *Virchows Arch A Pathol Anat* 1991; 418: 225–233.

18 Foraker AG, Reagan JW. Nuclear size and nuclear: cytoplasmic ratio in the delineation of atypical hyperplasia of the uterine cervix. *Cancer* 1956; 9: 470–479.

19 Mariuzzi GM, Montironi R, Di Loreto C, Sisti S. Multiparametric quantitation of the progression of uterine cervix preneoplasia towards neoplasia. *Pathol Res Pract* 1989; 185: 606–611.

20 Bohm N, Sandritter W. DNA in human tumours: a cytophotometric study. *Curr Top Pathol* 1975; 60: 151–219.

21 Aufferman W, Repges R, Bocking A. Rapid diagnostic DNA cytometry with an automatic microscope and a TV image-analysis system. *Anal Quant Cytol* 1984; 6: 179–188.

22 Watts KC, Husain OA, Campion MJ *et al.* Quantitative DNA analysis of low grade cervical intraepithelial neoplasia and human papillomavirus infection by static and flow cytometry. *Br Med J* 1987; 295: 1090–1092.

23 Chatelain R, Schunk T, Schindler EM, Schindler AE, Bocking A. Diagnosis of prospective malignancy in koilocytic dysplasias of the cervix with DNA cytometry. *J Reprod Med* 1989; 34: 505–510.

24 Smith JJ, Cowan L, Hemstreet G *et al.* Automated quantitative fluorescent image analysis of cervical cytology. *Gynecol Oncol* 1987; 28: 241–254.

25 Stern E, Rosenthal DL, McLatchie C, White BS, Castleman KR. An expanded cervical cell classification system validated by automated measurements. *Anal Quant Cytol* 1982; 4: 110–114.

26 Rosenthal DL, Suffin SC, Missirlian N, McLatchie C, Castleman KR. Cytomorphometric differences among individual 'moderate dysplasia' cells derived from cervical intraepithelial neoplasia. *Anal Quant Cytol* 1984; 6: 189–195.

27 Wheeler N, Suffin SC, Hall TL, Rosenthal DL. Prediction of cervical neoplasia diagnosis groups. Discriminant analysis on digitized cell images. *Anal Quant Cytol Histol* 1987; 9: 169–181.

28 Rosenthal DL, Philippe A, Hall TL, Harami S, Missirlian N, Suffin SC. Prognosis of moderate dysplasia. Predictive value of selected markers in routinely prepared cervical smears. *Anal Quant Cytol Histol* 1987; 9: 165–168.

29 Hall TL, Castleman KR, Rosenthal DL. Canonical analysis of cells in normal and abnormal cervical smears. *Anal Quant Cytol Histol* 1988; 10: 161–165.

30 Strohmeier R, Naujoks H, van Driel-Kulker AMJ, Ploem JS. Laboratory test of an automated cell analysis system for cervical screening. *Cytopathology* 1993; 4: 139–147.

31 Fais S, Delle Fratte F, Mancini F *et al.* Human cervical epithelial cells that express HLA-DR associated with viral infection and activated mononuclear cell infiltrate. *J Clin Pathol* 1991; 44: 290–292.

32 Tay SK, Jenkins D, Maddox P, Singer A. Lymphocytes phenotypes in cervical intraepithelial neoplasia and human papilloma virus infection. *Br J Obstet Gynaecol* 1987; 94: 16–21.

33 Rosenthal DL, McLatchie C, Stern E, White BS, Castleman KR. Endocervical columnar cell atypia coincident with cervical neoplasia characterized by digital image analysis. *Acta Cytol* 1982; 26: 115–120.

34 Clark AH, Betsill WL. Early Endocervical glandular neoplasm. II. Morphometric analysis of the cells. *Acta Cytol* 1986; 30: 127–134.

35 Fu YS, Hall TL, Berek JS, Hacker NF, Reagan JW. Prognostic significance of DNA ploidy and morphometric analyses of adenocarcinoma of the uterine cervix. *Anal Quant Cytol Histol* 1987; 9: 17–24.

36 Burghardt E. Diagnostic and prognostic criteria in cervical microcarcinoma. *Clin Oncol* 1982; 1: 323–333.

37 Burghardt E, Holzer E. Diagnosis and treatment of microinvasive carcinoma of the cervix uteri. *Obstet Gynecol* 1977; 49: 641–653.

38 Hasumi K, Sakamoto A, Sugano H. Microinvasive carcinoma of the uterine cervix. *Cancer* 1980; 45: 928–931.

39 Roche WD, Norris HJ. Microinvasive carcinoma of the cervix. The significance of lymphatic invasion and confluent patterns of stromal growth. *Cancer* 1975; 36: 180–186.

40 Valeri V, Cruz AR, Brandao HJS, Lison L. Relationship between cell nuclear volume and deoxyribonucleic acid of cells of normal epithelium, of carcinoma *in situ* and of invasive carcinoma of the uterine cervix. *Acta Cytol* 1967; 11: 488–496.

41 Atkins NB. Nuclear size in carcinoma of the cervix: its relation to DNA content and to prognosis. *Cancer* 1964; 17: 1391–1399.

42 Brown DC, Cole D, Gatter KC, Mason DY. Carcinoma of the cervix uteri: an assessment of tumour proliferation using the monoclonal antibody Ki-67. *Br J Cancer* 1988; 57: 178–181.

43 Fox H, Buckley CH. The endometrial hyperplasias and their relationship to endometrial neoplasia. *Histopathology* 1982; 6: 493–510.

44 Norris HJ, Tavassoli FA, Kurman RJ. Endometrial

hyperplasia and carcinoma: diagnostic considerations. *Am J Surg* 1983; 7: 839–847.
45 Hendrickson MR, Kempson RL. Endometrial hyperplasia, metaplasia and carcinoma. In: Fox H (ed.) *Haines and Taylor Obstetrical and Gynaecological Pathology*, 3rd edn. Edinburgh: Churchill Livingstone, 1987: 354–404.
46 Wied GL, Bahr GF, Oldfield DG, Bartels PH. Computer assisted identification of cells from uterine adenocarcinoma. A clinical feasibility study with TICAS. I. Measurements at a wavelength 530 nm. *Acta Cytol* 1968; 12: 357–370.
47 Ng ABP, Reagan JW, Cechner RL. The precursors of endometrial cancer: a study of their cellular manifestations. *Acta Cytol* 1973; 17: 439–448.
48 Skaarland E. Morphometric analysis of nuclei in epithelial structures from normal and neoplastic endometrium: a study using the Isaacs cell sampler and Endoscann instruments. *J Clin Pathol* 1985; 38: 496–501.
49 Skaarland E. Nuclear size and shape of epithelial cells from the endometrium: lack of value as a criterion for differentiation between normal, hyperplastic, and malignant conditions. *J Clin Pathol* 1985; 38: 502–506.
50 Biswas B, Finbow JA. Quantitative study of uterine curettage in the menstrual cycle. *J Clin Pathol* 1975; 28: 905–909.
51 Diegenbach PC, Baak JPA. Quantitative nuclear image analysis: differentiation between normal, hyperplastic and malignant appearing uterine glands in a paraffin section. II. Computer assisted recognition by discriminant analysis. *Eur J Obstet Gynaecol Reprod Biol* 1977; 7: 389–394.
52 Baak JPA, Diegenbach PC, Kurver PJH, Stolk HG, van der Harten J. An example of quantitative microscopy in individual patient care. *Mikroskopie (Wien)* 1980; 37(suppl): 305–307.
53 Baak JPA, Kurver PHJ, Boon ME. Computer-aided application of quantitative microscopy in diagnostic pathology. *Pathol Ann* 1982; 17: 287–306.
54 Baak JPA, Kurver PHJ, Diegenback PC, Delemarre JFM, Brekelmans ECM, Nieuwlaat JE. Discrimination of hyperplasia and carcinoma of endometrium by quantitative microscopy – a feasibility study. *Histopathology* 1981; 5: 61–68.
55 Colgan TJ, Norris HJ, Foster W, Kurman RJ, Fox CH. Predicting the outcome of endometrial hyperplasia by quantitative analysis of nuclear features using a linear discriminant function. *Int J Gynecol Pathol* 1983; 1: 347–352.
56 Baak JPA, Kurver PHJ, Overdiep SH *et al.* Quantitative, microscopical, computer-aided diagnosis of endometrial hyperplasia or carcinoma in individual patients. *Histopathology* 1981; 5: 689–695.
57 Baak JPA, Nauta JJP, Wisse-Brekelmans ECM, Bezemer DP. Architectural and nuclear morphometrical features together are more important prognosticators in endometrial hyperplasias than nuclear morphometrical features alone. *J Pathol* 1988; 154: 335–341.
58 Schipper NW, Smeulders AWM, de Lange JHM, Baak JPA. Quantification of epithelial area by image processing applied to endometrial-carcinomas: a comparison with ovarian tumors. *Hum Pathol* 1989; 20: 1125–1132.
59 Ferenczy A. The cytodynamics of endometrial hyperplasia and neoplasia. Part II: *in vitro* DNA histoautoradiography. *Hum Pathol* 1983; 14: 77–82.
60 Feichter GE, Hoffken H, Heep J *et al.* DNA-flow-cytometric measurements on the normal, atrophic, hyperplastic and neoplastic human endometrium. *Virchows Arch A Pathol Anat* 1982; 398: 53–65.
61 Norris HJ, Becker RL, Mikel UV. A comparative morphometric and cytophotometric study of endometrial hyperplasia, atypical hyperplasia and endometrial carcinoma. *Hum Pathol* 1989; 20: 219–223.
62 Hendrickson M, Ross J, Eifel PJ, Cox RS, Martinez A, Kempson R. Adenocarcinoma of the endometrium: analysis of 256 cases with carcinoma limited to the uterine corpus. Pathology review and analysis of prognostic variables. *Gynecol Oncol* 1982; 13: 373–392.
63 Templeton AC. Reporting of myometrial invasion by endometrial cancer. *Histopathology* 1982; 6: 733–737.
64 Nielsen AL, Nyholm HCJ. Stereological estimate of nuclear volume in endometrial adenocarcinoma of endometrioid type: reproducibility and intra-tumour variation. *Histopathology* 1993; 22: 17–24.
65 Charpin C, Andrac L, Habib MC *et al.* Immunocytochemical assays in human endometrial carcinomas: a multiparametric computerized analysis and comparison with non-malignant changes. *Gynecol Oncol* 1989; 33: 9–22.
66 Kempson RL, Hendrickson MR. Pure mesenchymal neoplasia of the uterine corpus. In: Fox H (ed.) *Haines And Taylor Obstetrical and Gynaecological Pathology*, 3rd edn. Edinburgh: Churchill Livingstone, 411–456.
67 Clement PB, Scully RE. Mullerian adenosarcoma of the uterus: a clinicopathologic analysis of 100 cases with a review of the literature. *Hum Pathol* 1990; 21: 363–381.
68 Clement PB. Pathology of the uterine corpus. *Hum Pathol* 1991; 22: 776–791.
69 Fox H. General pathology of the placenta. In: Fox H (ed.) *Haines and Taylor Obstetrical and Gynaecological Pathology*, 3rd edn, vol. 2. Edinburgh: Churchill Livingstone, 1987: 972–1000.
70 Teasdale F. Morphometric evaluation. *Contr Gynecol Obstet* 1982; 9: 17–28.
71 Teasdale F. Idiopathic intrauterine growth retardation: histomorphometry of the human placenta. *Placenta* 1984; 5: 83–92.
72 Teasdale F. Histomorphometry of the placenta of the diabetic woman: class A diabetes mellitus. *Placenta* 1981; 2: 241–252.

73 van der Velde WJ, Copius Peereboom-Stegeman JHJ, Treffers PE, James J. Structural changes in the placenta of smoking mothers: a quantitative study. *Placenta* 1983; 4: 231–240.
74 Las Heras J, Baskerville JC, Harding PG, Haust MD. Morphometric studies of fetal placental stem arteries in hypertensive disorders ('toxaemia') of pregnancy. *Placenta* 1985; 6: 217–227.
75 Jauniaux E, Moscoso JG, Vanesse M, Campbell S, Driver M. Perfusion fixation for placental morphologic investigation. *Hum Pathol* 1991; 22: 442–449.
76 Franke HR, Alons CL, Caron FJM. Quantitative morphology. A study of the trophoblast. *Virchows Arch (A)* 1985; 406: 323–331.
77 Rockelein G, Ulmer R, Schroder J. Karyotype and placental structure of first-trimester spontaneous abortions: a morphometrical study. *Eur J Obstet Gynaecol Reprod Biol* 1990; 38: 25–32.
78 Serov SF, Scully RE, Sobin LH. Histological typing of ovarian tumours. In: *International Histological Classifications of Tumours*, no. 9. Geneva: World Health Organization, 1973: 37–42.
79 Barber HRK, Sommers SC, Snyder R, Kwon TH. Histologic and nuclear grading and stromal reactions as indices for prognosis in ovarian cancer. *Am J Obstet Gynecol* 1975; 121: 795–805.
80 Hart WR, Norris HJ. Borderline and malignant mucinous tumors of the ovary. *Cancer* 1973; 31: 1031–1045.
81 Russell P. Common epithelial tumours of the ovary. In: Fox H (ed.) *Haines and Taylor Obstetrical and Gynaecological Pathology*, 3rd edn, vol. 1. Edinburgh: Churchill Livingstone, 1987: 556–622.
82 Baak JPA, Langley FA, Talerman A, Delemarre JFM. Intrapathologist and intrapathologist disagreement on ovarian tumor grading and typing. *Anal Quant Cytol Histol* 1986; 8: 354–357.
83 Baak JPA, Agrafojo Blanco A, Kurver PHJ *et al.* Quantitative analysis of borderline and malignant mucinous ovarian tumours. *Histopathology* 1981; 5: 353–360.
84 Baak JPA, Kurver PHJ, Boon ME. Experience with routine application of morphometry in diagnostic pathology. In: Collan Y, Romppanen T (eds) *Morphometry in Morphological Diagnosis*. Kuopia: Kuopio University Press, 1987: 97–107.
85 Baak JPA, van der Ley G. Borderline or malignant ovarian tumour? A case report of decision making with morphometry. *J Clin Pathol* 1984; 37: 1110–1113.
86 Baak JPA, Wisse-Brekelmans ECM, Langley FA, Talerman A, Delemarre JFM. Morphometric data to FIGO stage and histological type and grade for prognosis of ovarian tumours. *J Clin Pathol* 1986; 39: 1340–1346.
87 Baak JPA, Wisse-Brekelmans ECM, Uyterlinde AM, Schipper NW. Evaluation of the prognostic value of morphometric features and cellular DNA content in FIGO I ovarian cancer patients. *Anal Quant Cytol Histol* 1987; 9: 287–290.
88 Baak JPA, Chan KK, Stolk JG, Kenemans P. Prognostic factors in borderline and invasive ovarian tumors of the common epithelial type. *Pathol Res Pract* 1987; 182: 755–774.
89 Baak JPA, Schipper NW, Wiesse-Brekelmans ECM *et al.* The prognostic value of morphometrical features and cellular DNA content in *cis*-platin treated late ovarian cancer patients. *Br J Cancer* 1988; 57: 503–508.
90 Weger A-R, Ludescher C, Mikuz G *et al.* The value of morphometry to predict chemotherapy response in advanced ovarian cancer. *Pathol Res Pract* 1989; 185: 676–679.
91 Deligdisch L, Kerner H, Cohen CJ, Dargent E, Gil J. Morphometric differentiation between responsive tumor cells and mesothelial hyperplasia in second-look operations for ovarian cancer. *Hum Pathol* 1993; 24: 143–147.
92 Haapasalo H, Collan Y, Atkin NB, Pesonen E, Seppa A. Prognosis of ovarian carcinomas: prediction by histoquantitative methods. *Histopathology* 1989; 15: 167–178.
93 Haapasalo H, Collan Y, Seppa A, Gidlund A-L, Atkin NB, Pesonen E. Prognostic value of ovarian carcinoma grading methods – a method comparison study. *Histopathology* 1990; 16: 1–7.

4.12 RESPIRATORY DISEASE

In the upper respiratory tract a combined morphometry/stereology study of precancerous epithelium in nasal biopsies at light and electron microscopic levels has given a 91% agreement between the quantitative methods and histological assessment [1]. A change from metaplasia to dysplasia is characterized by an increase in nuclear, nucleolar, mitochondrial and cell sizes in the epithelial basal layer. Morphometry has also examined the use of nuclear parameters as a prognostic guide in the follow-up of squamous epithelial atypia in laryngeal biopsies [2]. In 10 patients who progressed to invasive carcinoma six were correctly identified (mean probability 94%) and four were misclassified. Previous morphological and photometric studies failed to highlight significant differences between laryngeal biopsies with dysplasia that progressed and those that did not [3]. Values for mean nuclear area $> 300\,\mu m^2$ and $< 250\,\mu m^2$ favour laryngeal verrucous carcinoma and squamous papilloma, respectively, although diagnosis should primarily be on histological grounds [4].

Quantitation has been applied to a wide variety

of lower respiratory tract disorders. Simple stereological techniques have established the number of alveoli in fetal life and childhood [5] and variables such as alveolar surface area, capillary surface and volume in adult normal and emphysematous lung [6]. In infants with bilateral lung hypoplasia, with or without oligohydramnios, morphometry has revealed decreased lung volumes, radial alveolar counts, alveolar numbers and surface area [7]. These parameters are all regarded as indicators of the lung diffusion capacity. Recently the range of studies has been augmented and expanded by computer-linked image analysis [8].

4.12.1 Cystic fibrosis

Chronic pulmonary disease is the most important cause of morbidity and mortality in cystic fibrosis, but its aetiology remains controversial. Despite clinical evidence of mucus hypersecretion, bronchial gland enlargement is only sometimes present [9]. There is also a marked similarity to controls in tracheobronchial gland numbers, activity and response to infection, and neutral/acid mucus content [10]. Pulmonary pathology in cystic fibrosis forms a heterogeneous group of postinflammatory destructive abnormalities which vary greatly from patient to patient and dictate the progression of disease. These include bronchiectasis, destructive/non-destructive emphysema, irregularity of small airways [9] and increased bronchial with decreased parenchymal volume proportions [11]. Lesions are also irregularly distributed throughout the lung with particular emphasis on the upper lobe [11]. This is also the preferential site for the range of bronchiectatic, interstitial and emphysematous bullous cysts that occur and are associated with a history of pneumothorax and abnormal chest radiology [12].

4.12.2 Smoking, chronic bronchitis and emphysema

A surprisingly small proportion of regular cigarette smokers develop clinically significant chronic airflow obstruction. Despite this, morphometry has shown a gradation of parenchymal and vascular changes from non-smokers through life-long smokers to those with airflow obstruction [13]. These include emphysema, narrowing of small airways and arterial muscularization and fibrosis, with the degree of emphysema relating to ventilatory function. The latter is worsened by the loss of alveolar attachments to small airways that occurs in smokers, a factor probably consequent upon bronchiolitis and responsible for early parenchymal destruction [14]. Interestingly, a pictorial grading system for pathological changes in the small airways gives comparable results to more formal morphometric analysis [15].

Excessive mucus secretion from the bronchial tree is accepted as the chief clinical hallmark of chronic bronchitis. Pathologically there is an elevated Reid index characterized by hypertrophy and hyperplasia of the bronchial mucus glands, resulting in an increased gland/wall thickness ratio [16]. This has been confirmed statistically but there is such a wide variation in individual cases that measurements should not be confined to one mucosal area [17]. In chronic bronchitis and emphysema, morphometric point-counting techniques have established the actual area and volume measurements of bronchial glands in microscopic sections, and emphysema in lung slices. This has been developed to ascertain baseline values against which individual cases may then be compared [18]. Immunolocalization of proteolytic neutrophil elastase also correlates with forced expiratory volume levels and linear intercept determination of emphysematous air space change, confirming its possible pathogenetic role [19].

4.12.3 Asbestosis

Cooke [20] recognized the association of pulmonary fibrosis with asbestos exposure. It is usually accompanied by pleural plaque formation and the degree of parenchymal fibrosis may be graded semi-quantitatively [21]. Its pathological diagnosis depends upon the demonstration of asbestos fibres (ferruginous bodies). It has become clear that identification of several bodies in the same microscopic field indicates very high exposure [22], with two in a 2 cm^2 standard-thickness section being equivalent to 200 per gram of wet fixed lung [23]. Calculations have been facilitated by the use of tissue digestion, electron diffraction and X-ray spectroscopy allied to scanning electron microscopy. These techniques increase the sensitivity of attributing lung fibrosis to asbestos inhalation and this has obvious medico-legal implications. However, they need to be examined in the context of a wider survey, establishing the prevalence of elevated fibre counts in non-asbestos-related cases.

Morphometry has also been applied to other dust diseases such as silicosis [24] and byssinosis [25].

4.12.4 Respiratory distress and sudden infant death syndromes

In bronchopulmonary dysplasia following infantile respiratory distress syndrome, morphometry has demonstrated diminished alveolar numbers and internal surface areas but normal small airway diameters [26]. There is also muscularization of intra-acinar arteries [27]. In adult respiratory distress syndrome there is a measurable progression from exudative alveolitis to sclerosing fibrosis [28]. This is associated with vascular damage consisting of tortuous vessels with fibrocellular intimal obliteration and muscularization of their walls [29]. Similar changes are also documented in oxygen toxicity [30]. Interactive image analysis has shown that bronchiolar wall thickness and cellularity are significantly greater in sudden infant death syndrome infants than in controls. This is predominantly due to widening of the adventitia which is infiltrated by excess numbers of both Schwann's and Langerhans' cells, presumably as a response to chronic or recurrent hypoxia [31].

4.12.5 Lung carcinoma

Cytomorphometry confirms that there is an increase in mean cellular and nuclear diameters, prominence of nucleoli and frequency of multinucleated forms as bronchial dysplasia progresses through *in situ* and early malignancy to frankly invasive squamous carcinoma [32]. The authors found the quantitative differences sufficient to allow separation of these lesions. Image analysis of Feulgen-stained sputa enabled DNA cytophotometry to identify, before cytological detection, 17 out of 19 cases that progressed to bronchial carcinoma. Of 11 cases classified as benign, nine were confirmed during follow-up investigations [33]. It is claimed that morphometry can separate well-differentiated pulmonary adenocarcinoma from atypical alveolar cuboidal cell hyperplasia on the basis of mean nuclear area and its SD [34]. Adenocarcinoma also has greater cellular and nuclear areas but smaller nucleoli than large-cell carcinoma of the lung [35].

In tissue sections measurement of tumour nuclear and cell diameters has shown a continuum of cell size from small- to large-cell undifferentiated lung carcinoma. In oat-cell carcinomas cell dimensions were partly dependent on the size of the biopsy and this study emphasized the difficulties in objective subclassification of lesions [36]. However, others have found discriminant analysis of multiple nuclear variables to give correct classification rates of 81.4, 93.2 and 74.7% for adenocarcinoma, small- and squamous-cell carcinomas [37]. Stereological estimates of mean nuclear volume emphasize a wide separation of small-cell carcinoma (152 μm^3) from non-small-cell tumours (736 μm^3) [38], a distinction that has important implications for surgery and adjuvant therapy. Morphometric, ultrastructural and immunohistochemical analyses of small-cell carcinoma show that it is a heterogeneous group of tumours and four subgroups have been proposed: oat, intermediate, combined oat and undifferentiated small-cell [39]. They overlap in their immunoexpression of markers (neuron-specific enolase), elaboration of neurosecretory granules and morphometric features such as nuclear area and nuclear cytoplasmic ratio. Its prognosis is poor and related to age, stage of disease and response to chemotherapy. Sforza *et al.* [40] have shown differences in mean nuclear area between the oat and intermediate-cell varieties (17.31 vs 25.75 μm^2) but similar form factor. None of the morphometric features correlated with survival, although others have found nuclear cytoplasmic ratio to be a strong predictor in neuroendocrine lung carcinoma [41]. Syntactic structure analysis suggests that patients suffering from tumours with smaller distances between neighbouring cells have a worse prognosis than those with larger distances [42]. When cytomorphometric parameters related to chromatin distribution and DNA ploidy are analysed there is a spectrum of change from classical carcinoids through atypical carcinoids to small-cell carcinomas. The latter have increased DNA content and hyperchromatism [43].

In bronchogenic carcinoma survival is strongly related to histological type, stage of disease and nodal metastases. Interestingly, an increased percentage of the total lymph node cut surface occupied by sinus histiocytosis is associated with an improved prognosis. This implies a local tumour–host reaction of the delayed hypersensitivity type. Conversely, hyperactivity of B-cell areas with the development of cortical follicles and germinal centres has a detrimental effect [44]. Stereology has derived a discriminant function analysis capable of classifying patients with epidermoid lung carcinoma as short- or long-term survivors [45] with an error rate of only 3.5%. The morphometric index was based on quantitation of tumour, stroma and necrosis components supplemented by the mitosis/necrobiosis ratio, reciprocal of cell count and number of apoptotic bodies. Tumours with greater epithelial volume, necrosis and mitoses did less well. Cagle *et al.* [46] found no correlation between nuclear morphometry and survival in stage I non-small-cell lung carcinoma. DNA cytophotometry indicates that there is a wider range and increased ploidy values in squamous-cell carcinoma than adenocarcinoma [47]. Incorporation of the antigen Ki-67 shows that these two subtypes vary widely in their proliferative stages, whilst small-cell carcinomas have consistently higher labelling [48].

4.12.6 Pleural effusions

Cells exfoliated from primary pleural mesotheliomas differ quantitatively from those of primary peritoneal lesions. They have larger nuclei, more anisokaryosis and higher nuclear cytoplasmic ratios. Peritoneal mesotheliomas also have a more pronounced degree of cytoplasmic vacuolation and nuclear compression [49]. A more common problem encountered by the practising pathologist is to distinguish between benign and malignant pleural mesothelial cells and secondary carcinoma. This issue has been addressed by a number of quantitative studies. In a series of 37 patients with malignant mesothelioma, 25 with benign pleural lesions and 25 with metastatic carcinoma, Kwee *et al.* found that a combination of histochemistry (diastase-periodic acid–Schiff stain) and immunochemistry (carcinoembryonic antigen reaction) was the best means of separating mesothelioma from metastases. This was not augmented by morphometry which was however able to distinguish between benign and malignant mesothelial cells on the basis of a nuclear area threshold value of 30 μm^2.

Separation of the latter diagnostic groups is also contributed to by the greater cytoplasmic area of mesothelioma [51] (Fig. 4.13) and the number, size and distribution of cytoplasmic lipid vacuoles. Benign cells have fewer, smaller vacuoles with a perinuclear arrangement as determined by vacuolar radii and centre of gravity topography [52]. Others have emphasized various geometric differences between benign and malignant mesothelial cells [53], including nuclear profile diameter [54], nuclear contour index, SD of nuclear area and nuclear perimeter [55]. The latter study, based on histological sections, used these variables to derive a classification rule which completely separated the

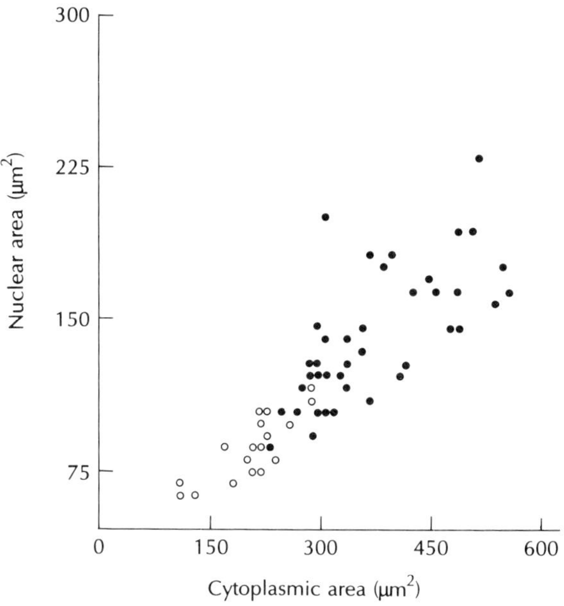

Fig. 4.13 Scattergram comparing nuclear area with cytoplasmic area for cases of primary pleural mesothelioma (•) and reactive mesothelial proliferation (○). From Kwee *et al.* [51].

diagnostic groups. Further factors claimed to assist in designation are nucleolar prominence and DNA content [56]. Misgivings have been expressed at both a light microscopic [57] and ultrastructural level [58] about the role of morphometry in distinguishing between benign pleural effusions and metastatic disease due to the wide range and overlap of geometric cellular features that occur.

4.12.7 Conclusion

Morphometry in respiratory disease has given insights into the pathogenesis and structure/function relationships in cystic fibrosis, chronic obstructive airways disease and smoking. Tissue quantitation of particulates is of importance in the pneumoconioses. In lung carcinoma it highlights the heterogeneity of lesions that exist and the prognostic importance of histological type and stage of disease. In pleural effusions it has a possible role in discriminating between benign and malignant mesothelial cells.

References

1 Reith A, Boysen M. A general model for the light and electron microscopic morphometry/stereology (M/S) of precancerous epithelial transformation using clinical biopsies. *Pathol Res Pract* 1984; 79: 210–215.

2 Olde Kalter P, Eelemarre JF, Alons CL, Meijer CJ, Snow GB. The prognostic significance of morphometry for squamous cell hyperplasia of the laryngeal epithelium. *Acta Oto-Laryngol* 1986; 102: 124–130.

3 Hellquist H, Olofsson J. Photometric evaluation of laryngeal epithelium exhibiting hyperplasia, keratosis and moderate dysplasia. *Acta Otolaryngol* 1981; 92: 157–165.

4 Cooper JR, Hellquist HB, Michaels L. Image analysis in the discrimination of verrucous carcinoma and squamous papilloma. *J Pathol* 1992; 166: 383–387.

5 Emery JL, Mithal A. The number of alveoli in the terminal respiratory unit of man during late intrauterine life and childhood. *Arch Dis Child* 1960; 35: 544–547.

6 Weibel ER. A simplified morphometry method for estimating diffusing capacity in normal and emphysematous human lungs. *Am Rev Respir Dis* 1973; 107: 579–588.

7 Wigglesworth JS, Hislop AA, Desai R. Biochemical and morphometric analyses in hypoplastic lungs. *Pediatr Pathol* 1991; 11: 537–549.

8 Gillooly M, Lamb D, Farrow ASJ. New automated technique for assessing emphysema on histological sections. *J Clin Pathol* 1991; 44: 1007–1011.

9 Sobonya RE, Taussig LM. Quantitative aspects of lung pathology in cystic fibrosis. *Am Rev Respir Dis* 1986; 134: 290–295.

10 Oppenheimer EH. Similarity of the tracheobronchial mucous glands and epithelium in infants with and without cystic fibrosis. *Hum Pathol* 1981; 12: 36–48.

11 Tomashefski JF, Bruce M, Goldberg HI, Dearborn DG. Regional distribution of macroscopic lung disease in cystic fibrosis. *Am Rev Respir Dis* 1986; 133: 535–540.

12 Tomashefski JF, Bruce M, Stern RC, Dearborn DG, Dahms B. Pulmonary air cysts in cystic fibrosis: relation of pathologic features to radiologic findings and history of pneumothorax. *Hum Pathol* 1985; 16: 253–261.

13 Hale KA, Ewing SL, Gosnell BA, Niewoehner DE. Lung disease in long-term cigarette smokers with and without chronic air-flow obstruction. *Am Rev Respir Dis* 1984; 130: 716–721.

14 Saetta M, Ghezzo H, Kim WD *et al.* Loss of alveolar attachments in smokers. A morphometric correlate of lung function impairment. *Am Rev Respir Dis* 1985; 132: 894–900.

15 Wright JL, Cosio M, Wiggs B, Hogg JC. A morphologic grading scheme for membranous and respiratory bronchioles. *Arch Pathol Lab Med* 1985; 109: 63–65.

16 Reid L. Measurement of the bronchial mucous gland layer: a diagnostic yardstick in chronic bronchitis. *Thorax* 1960; 15: 132–141.

17 Restrepo G, Heard BE. The size of the bronchial glands in chronic bronchitis. *J Pathol Bact* 1963; 85: 305–310.

18 Whimster WF. Diagnostic morphometry in emphysema and chronic bronchitis. *Anal Quant Cytol Histol* 1985; 7: 183–186.

19 Damiano VV, Tsang A, Kucich U *et al.* Immunolocalization of elastase in human emphysematous lungs. *J Clin Invest* 1986; 78: 482–493.

20 Cooke WE. Fibrosis of the lungs due to the inhalation of asbestos dust. *Br Med J* 1924; 2: 147.

21 Hinson KFW, Otto H, Webster I, Rossiter CE. Criteria for the diagnosis and grading of asbestosis. In: Bogovski P (ed.) *Biological Effects of Asbestos*. Lyons: IARC, 1973: 54–57.

22 Warnock ML, Prescott BT, Kuwahara TJ. Correlation of asbestos bodies and fibres in lungs of subjects with and without asbestosis. *Scann Elect Microsc* 1982; 2: 845–857.

23 Roggli VL, Pratt PC. Number of asbestos bodies on iron-stained tissue sections in relation to asbestos body counts in lung tissue digest. *Hum Pathol* 1983; 14: 355–361.

24 Siegesmund KA, Funahashi A, Yorde DE. Morphometric and elemental microanalytical studies of human lung in health and disease. *Br J Indust Med* 1985; 42: 36–42.

25 Edwards C, Carlile A, Rooke G. The larger bronchi in byssinosis: a morphometric study. *J Clin Pathol* 1984; 37: 20–22.

26 Sobonya RE, Logvinoff MM, Taussig LM, Theriault A. Morphometric analysis of the lung in prolonged bronchopulmonary dysplasia. *Pediatr Res* 1982; 16: 969–972.

27 Tomashefski JF, Oppermann HC, Vawter GF, Reid LM. Bronchopulmonary dysplasia: a morphometric study with emphasis on the pulmonary vasculature. *Pediatr Pathol* 1984; 2: 469–487.

28 Riede UN, Shah I. Diagnostic morphometry of the adult respiratory distress syndrome (shock lung). *Pathol Res Pract* 1984; 179: 204–206.

29 Tomashefski JF, Davies P, Boggis C, Greene R, Zapol WM, Reid LM. The pulmonary vascular lesions of the adult respiratory distress syndrome. *Am J Pathol* 1983; 112: 112–126.

30 Matsubara O, Takemura T, Nasu M *et al.* Pathological changes of the lungs after prolonged inhalation of high concentrations of oxygen. *Virchows Arch A Pathol Anat Histol* 1986; 408: 461–474.

31 Haque AK, Marcuso MG, Hokanson J, Nguyen ND, Nichols MM. Bronchiolar wall changes in sudden infant death syndrome: morphometric study of a new observation. *Pediatr Pathol* 1991; 11: 551–568.

32 Saito Y, Imai T, Nagamoto N *et al.* A quantitative cytologic study of sputum in early squamous cell bronchogenic carcinoma. *Anal Quant Cytol Histol* 1988; 10: 365–370.

33 Auffermann W, Bocking A. Early detection of precancerous lesions in dysplasias of the lung by rapid DNA image cytometry. *Anal Quant Cytol Histol* 1985; 7: 218–226.

34 Kodama T, Biyajima S, Watanabe S, Shimosato Y. Morphometric study of adenocarcinomas and hyperplasic epithelial lesions in the peripheral lung. *Am J Clin Pathol* 1986; 85: 146–151.

35 Burns TR, Underwood RD, Greenberg SD, Teasdale TA, Cartwright J. Cytomorphometry of large cell carcinoma of the lung. *Anal Quant Cytol Histol* 1989; 11: 48–52.

36 Vollmer RT. The effects of cell size on the pathologic diagnosis of small and large cell carcinomas of the lung. *Cancer* 1982; 50: 1380–1383.

37 Thunnissen EB, Diegenbach PC. Classification of lung carcinoma by means of digital nuclear image analysis. *Anal Quant Cytol Histol* 1986; 8: 301–304.

38 Aru A, Nielsen K. Stereological estimates of nuclear volume in primary lung cancer. *Pathol Res Pract* 1989; 185: 735–739.

39 Nomori H, Shimiosato Y, Kodama T, Morinaga S, Nakajima T, Watanabe S. Subtypes of small cell carcinoma of the lung: morphometric, ultrastructural and immunohistochemical analysis. *Hum Pathol* 1986; 17: 604–613.

40 Sforza V, Santopietro R, Bindi M, Tucci E, Pirtoli L, Tosi P. Clinical, histological and morphometrical parameters in small cell carcinoma of the lung: correlation with survival. *Appl Pathol* 1986; 4: 90–97.

41 Battlehner CN, Saldiva PHN, Carvalho CRR *et al.* Nuclear/cytoplasmic ratio correlates strongly with survival in non-disseminated neuroendocrine carcinoma of the lung. *Histopathology* 1993; 22: 31–34.

42 Kayser K, Fitzer M, Bulzebruck H, Bosslet K, Drings P. TNM stage, immunohistology, syntactic structure analysis and survival in patients with small cell anaplastic carcinoma of the lung. *J Cancer Res Clin Oncol* 1987; 113: 473–480.

43 Larsimont D, Kiss R, De Launoit Y, Melamed MR. Characterization of the morphonuclear features and DNA ploidy of typical and atypical carcinoids and small cell carcinomas of the lung. *Am J Clin Pathol* 1990; 94: 378–383.

44 Tosi P, Luzi P, Leoncini L, Mirracco C, Gambacorta M, Grossi A. Bronchogenic carcinoma: survival after surgical treatment according to stage, histologic type and immunomorphologic changes in regional lymph nodes. *Cancer* 1981; 48: 2288–2295.

45 Gerstl B, Wong S, Yesner R. Quantitative microscopy of epidermoid lung carcinoma: correlation with survival time. *J Natl Cancer Inst* 1976; 56: 463–469.

46 Cagle PT, Langston C, Fraire AE, Roggli VL, Greenberg SD. Absence of correlation between nuclear morphometry and survival in stage 1 non-small cell lung carcinoma. *Cancer* 1992; 69: 2454–2457.

47 Nishimiya K, Auer GU, Erhardt K, Wiman L-G, Kato H, Hayata Y. Nuclear DNA in histologic sections from squamous cell carcinoma and adenocarcinoma of the lung. *Anal Quant Cytol Histol* 1985; 7: 153–158.

48 Gatter KC, Dunnill MS, Gerdes J, Stein H, Mason DY. New approach to assessing lung tumours in man. *J Clin Pathol* 1986; 39: 590–593.

49 Boon ME, Kwee HS, Alons CL, Morawetz F, Veldhuizen RW. Discrimination between primary pleural and primary peritoneal mesotheliomas by morphometry and analysis of the vacuolization pattern of the exfoliated mesothelial cells. *Acta Cytol* 1982; 26: 103–108.

50 Kwee WS, Veldhuizen RW, Golding RP *et al.* Histologic distinction between malignant mesothelioma, benign pleural effusion and carcinoma metastasis. Evaluation of the application of morphometry combined with histochemistry and immunostaining. *Virchows Arch A Pathol Anat* 1982; 397: 287–299.

51 Kwee WS, Veldhuizen RW, Alons CA, Morawetz F, Boon ME. Quantitative and qualitative differences between benign and malignant mesothelial cells in pleural fluid. *Acta Cytol* 1982; 26: 401–406.

52 Boon ME, van Velzen D, Ruinaard C, Veldhuizen RW. Analysis of number, size and distribution patterns of lipid vacuoles in benign and malignant mesothelial cells. *Anal Quant Cytol Histol* 1984; 6: 221–226.

53 Scott N, Sutton J, Gray C. Morphometric diagnosis of serous effusions: refinement of differences between

benign and malignant cases by use of outlying values and larger sample size. *J Clin Pathol* 1989; 42: 607–612.
54 Marchevsky AM, Gil J, Caccamo D. Computerized interactive morphometry. A study of malignant mesothelioma and mesothelial hyperplasia in pleural biopsy specimens. *Arch Pathol Lab Med* 1985; 109: 1102–1105.
55 Robutti F, Betta P-G, Donna A, Pavesi M. A morphometrically-based classification rule for the diagnosis of primary mesothelial lesions. *J Pathol* 1990; 162: 57–60.
56 Ranaldi R, Marinelli F, Barbatelli G *et al.* Benign and malignant mesothelial lesions of the pleura: quantitative study. *Appl Pathol* 1986; 4: 55–64.
57 Christensen JA, Skaarland E. Nuclear and cell area measurements in the cytological evaluation of pleural effusions: a study of subjective assessments and morphometric measurements. *Diagn Cytopathol* 1987; 3: 50–54.
58 Dardick I, Butler EB, Dardick AM. Quantitative ultrastructural study of nuclei from exfoliated benign and malignant mesothelial cells and metastatic adenocarcinoma cells. *Acta Cytol* 1986; 30: 379–384.

4.13 CARDIOVASCULAR DISEASE

4.13.1 Atherosclerosis and blood vessels

This is one of the most important diseases in western society and quantitation has been employed to study the topography and morphology of its lesions with respect to dysfunction. In the thoracic and abdominal aortae of males aged 10–54 years, fatty streaks appear before raised plaque lesions and preferentially affect the intercostal ostia, aortic bifurcation and points of origin of the abdominal aorta branches [1]. Raised plaque lesions appear at the same sites of the intima affected by fatty streaks at younger ages. Ultrastructural stereology has shown atheromatous plaques to have a core which has depleted volume fractions of cells, ground substance and basement membrane, while extracellular lipid is increased by seven- to 10-fold [2]. Serum cholesterol promotes the progression of atherosclerosis as patients with high values have more florid lesions. Coronary artery luminal narrowing has also been linked to serum cholesterol and triglyceride levels and body mass index in failed human heart allografts [3]. Other major risk factors include diabetes and tobacco, which result in plaques with different proportions of constituent smooth-muscle and connective-tissue components [4]. In diabetics the cardiac arteriole and capillary numbers are decreased while the vessel diameters and wall thicknesses are increased, the latter by up to 50% [5]. Factors relating to the velocity and pressure of blood flow and luminal–endothelial events are fundamental to the pathogenesis of atherosclerosis. Susceptibility may in part be explained by the density of endothelial cells and their anchoring, folded cytoplasmic attachments [6] and the mural proportions of smooth-muscle cells [7], as shown ultrastructurally. Atheromatous intimal thickening is also inversely related to the fold-index of the internal elastic membrane, which may reflect the magnitude of tangential intimal tension [8]. Projection planimetry demonstrates that stenosis of coronary artery cross-sectional area must be >75% to be responsible for the development of collateral vessels or irreversible myocardial damage [9]. In practice the latter is determined by the presence of an acute intimal lesion, the grade of plaque and whether it is concentrically or eccentrically distributed [10]. It is also dictated by the site of the coronary artery lesion and the relative bulk of myocardium and vital structures that it supplies [11]. Viable and ischaemic myocardium have different affinities for various trichrome staining methods. This renders estimates of the percentage of ischaemic myocardium by use of point-counting on low-power histological sections relatively straightforward. Computer-assisted techniques have also been employed for the quantitation of myocardial fibrosis in subacute ischaemia [12].

Several techniques have been described for the morphometric analysis of arterial structure [13] and the main field of application has been in the lung [14] for the assessment of pulmonary hypertension [15]. Blood-vessel tumours are classified as benign, of intermediate malignancy or malignant. A quantitative feature that increases along this spectrum and that aids in lesion designation is mitotic activity, relevant examples being haemangiopericytoma, haemangioendothelioma and angiosarcoma [16].

4.13.2 Cardiac hypertrophy

Total heart weight varies according to age, body

build and weight [17]. A more accurate reflection of cardiac hypertrophy is obtained by ascertaining separately the septal, right and left ventricular weights. In hearts with left-sided hypertrophy ventricular wall thickness and total heart weight, which are usually above normal, are a good gauge of disease. Right ventricular hypertrophy, often occurring in hearts of normal weight, is masked by the disproportionate sizes of the respective chambers. Septal enlargement is commoner in left ventricular hypertrophy [18]. During physiological growth myocardial fibres enlarge, maintain a constant length/width ratio, number and capillary/fibre ratio. The left ventricle is heavier than the right because its fibres are thicker. In hypertrophy myofibres enlarge to a critical point when cardiac failure may ensue, and the resultant dilatation is characterized by excessive fibre-lengthening. However, this does not imply overstretching as architectural rearrangements enable the intersarcomere (Z-band) distance to be maintained [19]. Stereological studies have claimed that this is achieved by a true hyperplasia (cellular multiplication) beyond the critical stage [20]. Muscle fibre layers differ in orientation and number according to whether the heart is hypertrophied concentrically on the basis of pressure overload or eccentrically due to volume excess [21]. More recently, quantitation has employed morphometry in a range of cardiovascular diseases, including various valvular conditions [22] and the grading of pulmonary fat embolism [23]. In the former study the volume fraction of fibrous tissue was increased in valvular disease but did not correlate with the severity of the lesion. Myofibre hypertrophy was most marked in aortic stenosis and mitral incompetence, and fibre diameter correlated with left ventricular weight. Morphometry has also shown that the reduction in the outside diameter of the vessel wall in aortic coarctation is complicated by marked intimal thickening which causes further luminal stenosis [24].

4.13.3 Cardiomyopathy

Cardiomyopathy is diagnosed by the exclusion of ischaemic, valvular and hypertensive aetiologies. It is divided into dilated (congestive) and hypertrophic categories. The cause of dilated cardiomyopathy in many cases remains unknown, although there may well be a viral aetiology in a significant proportion. There are similarities in the thickness of the subendocardial hyaline layer [25] and atrial wall neuronal depopulation [26] between viral and idiopathic cases. The assessment of disease severity is dependent on right ventricular endomyocardial biopsy. Importantly, it has been shown that the percentage fibrosis is also related to biopsy site and biotome type [27] and this must be taken into account in comparative studies. Quantitation was carried out on 25 autopsy hearts for a series of cardiomyopathy patients with the following mean values: onset of heart failure 38 years, duration 5 years, age of death 43 years. The mean heart measurements were weight 513 g, left ventricle 89 ml, right ventricle 72 ml, right atrium 71 ml and left atrium 55 ml. Heart weight correlated with chamber volume, and atrial size with mitral and tricuspid valve ring dimensions [28]. Ultrastructural morphometry and stereology in paediatric cardiomyopathy has found an increase in mitochondrial size and number along with loss of contractile properties due to myofibrillar segregation on the basis of derangement and dislocation of thick and thin filaments [29].

Hypertrophic obstructive cardiomyopathy classically presents as a cause of angina or even sudden death in young to middle-aged males. There is asymmetrical interventricular septal hypertrophy with an increase above the normal value of unity for the septum : posterior ventricular wall thickness ratio. This may be associated with an abnormality of insertion of the anterior mitral valve cusp and subaortic stenosis leading to localized endocardial fibrosis [30]. Myofibre diameter is doubled to about 20 μm. A semiquantitative index based on histological features such as fibrosis, fibre diameter, muscle whorling, short interrupted fibres, nuclear enlargement and perinuclear haloes is increased [31]. Widespread ventricular septal disorganization of muscle is not specific for hypertrophic cardiomyopathy but has been shown by quantitation to be a sensitive marker for it [32]. It was detected in this study in 94% of patients and in over half of them in 25% of the tissue sections. Controls had fewer (26%) and localized areas restricted to 1.5% of the septum as opposed to 31%. Myocardial disarray is a natural phenomenon and can be exaggerated by block orientation and the sampling plane of section [33]. It must be regarded, therefore, as an important one of several clinicopathological facets contributing to the diagnosis of hypertrophic obstructive cardiomyopathy.

4.13.4 Cardiac transplantation

Quantitative birefringence measurement on endomyocardial biopsy specimens is a useful ancillary technique in addition to the number of circulating activated lymphocytes in the monitoring of cardiac allograft rejection [34]. It is an index of myocyte contractile function based on the ratio of its values before and after the addition of *in vitro* adenosine triphosphate and calcium. It correlates with grades 3 and 4 of the histological criteria for rejection. Image analysis has shown endomyocardial fibrosis in the donor heart shortly after transplantation and that its severity correlates with total ischaemic duration and transfer time, which is most marked in long-distance procurement [35]. In a proportion of these cases myocyte damage characterized by loss of birefringence was also seen.

4.13.5 Conclusion

Quantitation has given an insight into the pathogenesis and morphology of cardiac hypertrophy, atherosclerosis, pulmonary hypertension and cardiomyopathy. It is of use in the endomyocardial assessment of dilated cardiomyopathy and cardiac allograft rejection.

References

1 Ishii T, Malcolm GT, Osaka T *et al.* Variations with age and serum cholesterol level in the topographic distribution of macroscopic aortic atherosclerotic lesions as assessed by image analysis methods. *Modern Pathol* 1990; 3: 713–719.

2 Bocan TM, Schifani TA, Guyton JR. Ultrastructure of the human aortic fibrolipid lesion. Formation of the atherosclerotic lipid-rich core. *Am J Pathol* 1986; 123: 413–424.

3 Winters GL, Kendall TJ, Radio SJ *et al.* Post-transplant obesity and hyperlipidemia: major predictors of severity of coronary arteriopathy in failed human heart allografts. *J Heart Transplant* 1990; 9: 364–371.

4 Barbano EF, Newman GE, McCann RL *et al.* Correlation of clinical history with quantitative histology of lower extremity atheroma biopsies obtained with the Simpson atherectomy catheter. *Atherosclerosis* 1989; 78: 183–196.

5 Gherasim L, Tasca C, Havriliuc C, Vasilescu C. A morphological quantitative study of small vessels in diabetic cardiomyopathy. *Morphol Embryol* 1985; 31: 191–195.

6 Merrilees MJ, Shepphard AJ, Robinson MC. Structural features of saphenous vein and internal thoracic artery endothelium: correlates with susceptibility and resistance to graft atherosclerosis. *J Cardiovasc Surg* 1988; 29: 639–646.

7 Nikkari ST. Phenotype of smooth muscle cells in internal mammary arteries. *Artery* 1989; 16: 346–352.

8 Svendsen E, Dregelid E, Eide GE. Internal elastic membrane in the internal mammary and left anterior descending coronary arteries and its relationship to intimal thickening. *Atherosclerosis* 1990; 83: 239–249.

9 Falk E. Coronary artery narrowing without irreversible myocardial damage or development of collaterals. Assessment of 'critical' stenosis in a human model. *Br Heart J* 1982; 48: 265–271.

10 Davies MJ. The pathology of ischaemic heart disease. In: Anthony PP, MacSween RNM (eds) *Recent Advances in Histopathology*, vol. 13. Edinburgh: Churchill Livingstone, 1987: 85–201.

11 Kalbfleisch H, Hort W. Quantitative study on the size of coronary artery supplying areas postmortem. *Am Heart J* 1977; 94: 183–188.

12 Hoyt RH, Ericksen E, Collins SM. Computer-assisted quantitation of myocardial fibrosis in histologic sections. *Arch Pathol Lab Med* 1984; 108: 280–283.

13 Lowe L. Method for the morphometric analysis of arterial structure. *J Clin Pathol* 1984; 37: 1413–1415.

14 Puittinen J, Collan Y. Lung histomorphometry. In: Baak JPA, Oort J (eds) *A Manual of Morphometry in Diagnostic Pathology*. Berlin: Springer, 1983: 131–136.

15 Haworth SG, Reid L. A morphometric study of regional variation of lung structures in infants with pulmonary hypertension and congenital cardiac defect. A justification of lung biopsy. *Br Heart J* 1978; 40: 825–831.

16 Enzinger FM, Weiss SW. *Soft Tissue Tumours*. St Louis: Mosby, 1988: 545–580.

17 Zeek PM. Heart weight I. The weight of the normal heart. *Arch Pathol* 1942; 34: 820–830.

18 Fulton RM, Hutchinson EC, Jones AM. Ventricular weight in cardiac hypertrophy. *Br Heart J* 1952; 14: 413–420.

19 Linzbach AJ. Heart failure from the point of view of quantitative anatomy. *Am J Cardiol* 1960; 5: 370–382.

20 Astorri E, Chizzola A, Visioli O, Anversa P, Olivetti G, Vitali-Mazza L. Right ventricular hypertrophy — a cytometric study on 55 human hearts. *J Mol Cell Cardiol* 1971; 2: 99–110.

21 Tezuka F. Morphometric analysis of cardiac hypertrophy: left ventricular shape and number of muscle-fiber layers across left ventricular wall. *Tokoho J Exp Med* 1982; 138: 1–6.
22 Jantunen E, Halinen MO, Romppanen T, Kosma VM, Collan Y. Morphometric study of human myocardium in acquired valvular diseases. *Ann Med* 1989; 21: 435–440.
23 Bunai Y, Yoshimi N, Komoriya H, Iwasa M, Ohya I. An application of a quantitative analytical system for the grading of pulmonary fat embolism. *Forensic Sci Int* 1988; 39: 263–269.
24 Smith SH, Kelly DR. Coarctation of the abdominal aorta in a child: morphometric analysis of the arterial lesion. *Pediatr Pathol* 1986; 5: 363–371.
25 Olsen EGJ. Myocarditis — a case of mistaken identity? *Br Heart J* 1983; 50: 303–311.
26 Amorim DS, Olsen EGJ. Assessment of heart neurons in dilated (congestive) cardiomyopathy. *Br Heart J* 1982; 47: 11–18.
27 Meckel CR, Wilson JE, Sears TD, Rogers JG, Goaley TJ, McManus BM. Myocardial fibrosis in endomyocardial biopsy specimens: do different bioptomes affect estimation? *Am J Cardiovasc Pathol* 1989; 2: 309–313.
28 Tanaka M, Matsubara O, Kajita A, Hatakeyama S. Morphometrical analysis of autopsy hearts of congestive cardiomyopathy. *Bull Tokyo Med Dental Univ* 1983; 30: 73–94.
29 Bosman C, Boldrini R, Fusilli S. Dilated cardiomyopathy in infancy — ultrastructural image analysis for diagnostic purpose. *Pathol Res Pract* 1989; 185: 807–817.
30 Olsen EGT. The pathology of idiopathic hypertrophic subaortic stenosis (hypertrophic cardiomyopathy). A critical review. *Am Heart J* 1980; 100: 553–562.
31 van Noorden S, Olsen EGJ, Pearse AGE. Hypertrophic obstructive cardiomyopathy, a histological, histochemical, and ultrastructural study of biopsy material. *Cardiovasc Res* 1971; 5: 118–131.
32 Maron BJ, Roberts WC. Quantitative analysis of cardiac muscle cell disorganization in the ventricular septum of patients with hypertrophic cardiomyopathy. *Circulation* 1979; 59: 689–706.
33 Becker AE, Caruso G. Myocardial disarray. A critical review. *Br Heart J* 1982; 47: 527–538.
34 Wijngaard PLJ, Gimpel JA, Schuurman H-J, van der Meulen A, Gmelig Meyling FHJ, Jambroes G. Monitoring rejection after heart transplantation: cytoimmunological monitoring on blood cells and quantitative birefringence measurements on endomyocardial biopsy specimens. *J Clin Pathol* 1990; 43: 137–142.
35 Pickering JG, Boughner DR. Fibrosis in the transplanted heart and its relation to donor ischaemic time. Assessment with polarized light microscopy and digital image analysis. *Circulation* 1990; 81: 949–958.

4.14 NERVOUS SYSTEM DISEASE

4.14.1 Growth, ageing, alcohol, dementia

Morphometry has shown that normal cerebral cortex grows 25% faster than white matter during infancy. The normal adult size and cortex/white matter ratio of 1 : 1 is achieved by a prolonged period of white matter development [1]. Grey matter growth is accelerated in premature infants with intraventricular haemorrhage or periventricular leukomalacia due to perinatal stress. Quantitation also recognizes increased hydrocephalus and impaired white matter growth, respectively, in these conditions. Neuronal accumulation of lipofuscin is one of the best recognized microscopic alterations of the ageing brain. A computerized image analysis technique on aldehyde fuscin-stained tissue sections allows preservation of pigment topography and its reproducible quantitative assessment [2]. A detailed morphometric study of 20 μm tissue sections from the frontal, temporal and parietal lobes showed statistically significant age-related decrements in the following values: brain weight, cortical thickness in the mid frontal and superior temporal areas, large neurons ($> 90\,\mu m^2$) in all three areas, and the neurone/glia ratio in the mid frontal and inferior parietal regions [3]. Neuron numbers, density and percentage cell area were all unchanged but small neuron and glial cell numbers were increased. The conclusions were that ageing affects the frontal and parietal lobes more than the temporal, is characterized by shrinkage and loss of large neurons and an increase in glial tissue. Quantimet analysis has shown cerebral cortex neuronal shrinkage, along with neuronal loss and reduction in white matter volume at the rates of 1 and 0.8% per annum, respectively [4]. Ageing also leads to a reduction in Purkinje-cell densities in the cerebellum, particularly in its superior part, sufficient to give recognizable radiological and clinical changes in a number of cases [5]. White matter axonal degeneration is the major neurotoxic effect of chronic alcohol ingestion. It results in mild atrophy of the cerebral cortex (with a constant subcortical nuclear size), and moderate loss of cerebral white matter (up to 17.5%) accompanied by enlargement of the ventricular system (up to 71.9%) [6]. Purkinje-cell densities in the cerebellar vermis are also decreased by about 20% in alcholics, with the molecular layer being more susceptible than the granular or medullary layers [7].

Morphometry of brain specimens with Pick's disease, Alzheimer's disease and normal controls shows Pick's disease to have major reductions in brain weight, frontal and temporal cortical thickness and large neuron populations. There is no correlation with age of onset, disease duration or the number of histological Pick bodies. The changes were more marked than in Alzheimer's disease, particularly in the frontotemporal region [8], whereas only Alzheimer's disease had neuronal cell loss in the inferior parietal area. These differential changes in tissue patterns appear to be fairly characteristic of the different types of dementia [9]. Assessment of volumetric changes in coronal tissue slices shows that there is subcortical cerebral degeneration in both Parkinson's disease and Alzheimer's disease but that the latter also has superimposed lesions involving the cortical neurons and fibres of the white matter [10]. Image analysis allows a profile of neuronal distribution to be obtained in Alzheimer's disease [11]. This confirms a shift from large to small neurons with partial neuronal preservation, a feature which may be of relevance for neurotrophic drug therapy. Stereology has confirmed the presence of nerve cell shrinkage, with neurophil atrophy being of secondary importance [12]. Cortical amyloid deposition is a feature of Alzheimer's disease and is more amenable to quantitation when demonstrated by immunocytochemical than argyrophilic techniques [13]. Plaque amyloid deposition starts at the level of the capillary, from which there is a decreasing concentration gradient into the surrounding tissues [14]. Graticule counts have shown that the numbers of plaques and neurofibrillary tangles are increased, but pyramidal cell volume and numbers decreased, in the cerebral cortex of patients with dementia and Down's syndrome [15]. There is also a component of selective incomplete white matter infarction involving both axons and myelin in Alzheimer's disease [16].

Hippocampal pyramidal cell volume and density are decreased in schizophrenia [17]. Casanova *et al.* [18] critically review the use of quantitation in this disorder.

4.14.2 Meningioma

Meningioma is a benign tumour and recurrence, which is observed in only 2–3% of cases, is related to site, adequacy of surgical excision and a number of histological parameters. Varying degrees of importance are attributed to cellular atypia, mitoses, necrosis, hypercellularity and brain/meningeal infiltration. Morphometry did not identify any significant differences in cell counts, nuclear area fractions or mean nuclear area between cases that recurred and those that did not [19]. Histological type was of no relevance, although necrosis and bone invasion were. Similarly, Scarpelli *et al.* [20] found that cell density, nuclear area and perimeter and DNA content were of no predictive value. However, recurrent cases had prominent nucleoli and more nucleolar organizer regions (NORs) associated with a reduction in DNA diploidy and a slight shift to DNA polyploidy. AgNORs and mitotic counts gave better information than karyometric and DNA parameters. The proliferation and recurrence rates in meningioma may be more accurately reflected by bromodeoxyuridine estimates of the S-phase fraction [21] and analysis of nuclear antigen Ki-67 expression [22] rather than by classical histological features.

4.14.3 Glioma

Astrocytomas and oligodendrogliomas show a great deal of morphological variability in cellularity, pleomorphism, necrosis and mitotic activity. Automated morphometry and densitometry show that numerical nuclear density, deformation of nuclei and mitotic activity increase with advancing tumour grade. The SDs of nuclear size, shape and extinction values mirror the histological features and increase with grade progression, resulting in a 70–80% agreement between automated and histological classification [23]. It is claimed that a combination of morphometric–densitometric data of tumour cell nuclei with semiquantitative scoring of histological features gives a 94% agreement with subjective Kernohan grading [24]. Nuclear size and shape (roundness factor) have also been of use in separating patients with glioblastoma surviving less or more than 12 months [25] from those with glioblastoma multiforme and metastatic carcinoma [26]. Mitotic activity is a proven histological marker of survival in astrocytoma but identification of figures and count reproducibility necessitate expert guided field selection and sampling rules [27]. The frequency of mitoses also correlates with the proliferation rate, as assessed by Ki-67 staining, and recurrence [28].

4.14.4 Pituitary adenoma

The effects of pituitary adenomas are twofold: first, their endocrine activity, and second, they act as a localized space-occupying lesion. Hormonal secretion does lead to alterations in subcellular organelle numbers [29] but these are not specific to protein type [30]. Standard histological features do not reliably predict tumour growth but macroadenomas (> 1 cm diameter) tend to be more aggressive and locally destructive than microadenomas [31].

4.14.5 Uveal melanoma

Semiautomatic image analysis has shown features descriptive for nucleolar pleomorphism to correlate with mortality figures. A combination of the SD of nucleolar circumference with maximum tumour dimension correctly predicted the clinical course in 88% of cases [32]. SD of nucleolar area is also an important prognostic factor [33], which can be reproducibly measured by a technician [34] and correlates well with the mean diameter of the 10 largest nucleoli. The latter is easily obtained by using a simple eyepiece graticule which gives time and cost advantages over a computerized technique [35]. Stereological estimation of nucleolar volume offers superior prediction of clinical outcome compared to histomorphometric estimators of nucleolar size [36].

4.14.6 Peripheral nerve

It has long been recognized that micrometer measurements can demonstrate alterations in fibre diameters and internodal lengths in developing and regenerating nerves [37] as well as in ageing and pathological conditions [38]. The latter study showed variations in fascicle size, fibre diameter, density and distribution in the radial and sural nerves, whereas an ultrastructural approach allows assessment of axonal size and myelin sheath thickness [39]. Morphometry has become a widely applied method for the quantitative analysis of peripheral nerve diagnostic biopsies using either semiautomatic or automated techniques [40,41]. The system employed by Torch *et al.* [41] measures the axonal diameter, myelin sheath thickness and circularity in 1000 myelinated fibres per hour. It is designed to counteract the population heterogeneity and bimodal size distribution that occurs in peripheral nerve and to compile a morphometric database profile for peripheral neuropathies and normal controls.

4.14.7 Conclusion

Quantitation gives an insight into the pathogenesis and morphology of age- and alcohol-related brain changes, the various dementias and schizophrenia. Estimates of proliferation rates using Ki-67, bromodeoxyuridine and mitotic counts are useful in predicting recurrence in meningioma and glioma. In the latter histological grading may be supplemented by nuclear morphometry. Survival in uveal melanoma is related to maximal tumour diameter and the variation in nucleolar size. Morphometry is of use in determining nerve fibre profiles in peripheral neuropathies.

References

1 De La Monte SM, Hsu FI, Hedley-Whyte ET, Kupsky W. Morphometric analysis of the human infant brain: effects of intraventricular haemorrhage and periventricular leukomalacia. *J Child Neurol* 1990; 5: 101–110.

2 Casanova MF, Koliatsos V, Jengeleski CA. A method for the relative quantification of lipofuscin based on a computer image analysis system. *J Neurosci Methods* 1989; 30: 11–15.

3 Terry RD, De Teresa R, Hansen LA. Neocortical cell counts in normal human adult aging. *Ann Neurol* 1987; 21: 530–539.

4 Anderson JM, Hubbard BM, Coghill GR, Slidders W. The effect of advanced old age on the neurone content of the cerebral cortex. Observations with an automatic image analyser point counting method. *J Neurol Sci* 1983; 58: 235–246.

5 Torvik A, Torp S, Lindbone CF. Atrophy of the cer-

ebellar vermis in aging. A morphometric and histologic study. *J Neurol Sci* 1986; 76: 283–294.
6 De La Monte SM. Disproportionate atrophy of cerebral white matter in chronic alcoholics. *Arch Neurol* 1988; 45: 990–992.
7 Phillips SC, Harper CG, Kril J. A quantitative histological study of the cerebellar vermis in alcoholic patients. *Brain* 1987; 110: 301–314.
8 Hansen LA, De Teresa R, Tobias H, Alford M, Terry RD. Neocortical morphometry and cholinergic neurochemistry in Pick's disease. *Am J Pathol* 1988; 131: 507–518.
9 Dom R, Lammens M, Saedeller JD, Hauman H. Cytometrical and immunocytochemical investigation of brain nuclei in dementia. *Prog Clin Biol Res* 1989; 317: 375–381.
10 De La Monte SM, Wells SE, Hedley-Whyte T, Growdon JH. Neuropathological distinction between Parkinson's dementia and Parkinson's plus Alzheimer's disease. *Ann Neurol* 1989; 26: 309–320.
11 Allen SJ, Dawbarn D, Wilcock GK. Morphometric immunochemical analysis of neurons in the nucleus basalis of Meynert in Alzheimer's disease. *Brain Res* 1988; 454: 275–281.
12 Meier-Ruge W, Ulrich J, Stahelin HB. Morphometric investigation of nerve cells, neuropil and senile plaques in senile dementia of the Alzheimer type. *Arch Gerontol Geriatr* 1985; 4: 219–229.
13 Gentleman SM, Bruton C, Allsop D, Lewis SJ, Polak JM. A demonstration of the advantages of immunostaining in the quantification of amyloid plaque deposits. *Histochemistry* 1989; 92: 355–358.
14 Papolla MA. Image analysis microspectroscopy of senile plaque capillary amyloid in Alzheimer's disease. A preliminary study. *Arch Pathol Lab Med* 1989; 113: 866–871.
15 Mann DMA, Yates PO, Marcyniuk B. Some morphometric observations on the cerebral cortex and hippocampus in presenile Alzheimer's disease, senile dementia of Alzheimer type and Down's syndrome in middle age. *J Neurol Sci* 1985; 69: 139–159.
16 Englund E, Brun A. White matter changes in dementia of Alzheimer's type: the difference in vulnerability between cell compartments. *Histopathology* 1990; 16: 433–439.
17 Jeste DV, Lohr JB. Hippocampal pathologic findings in schizophrenia. A morphometric study. *Arch Gen Psychiatr* 1989; 46: 1019–1024.
18 Casanova MF, Kleinman JE. The neuropathology of schizophrenia: a critical assessment of research methodologies. *Biol Psychiatr* 1990; 27: 353–362.
19 Christensen D, Laursen H, Klinken L. Prediction of recurrence in meningiomas after surgical treatment. A quantitative approach. *Acta Neuropathol* 1983; 61: 130–134.
20 Scarpelli M, Montironi R, Sisti S *et al.* Quantitative evaluation of recurrent meningiomas. *Pathol Res Pract* 1989; 185: 746–751.
21 Hoshino T, Nagashima T, Murovic JA, Wilson CB, Davis RL. Proliferative potential of human meningiomas of the brain. A cell kinetics study with bromodeoxyuridine. *Cancer* 1986; 58: 1466–1472.
22 Roggendorf W, Schuster T, Peiffer J. Proliferative potential of meningiomas determined with the monoclonal antibody Ki-67. *Acta Neuropathol* 1987; 73: 361–364.
23 Martin H, Voss K, Hufnagl P, Frölich K. Automated image analysis of gliomas. An objective and reproducible method for tumor grading. *Acta Neuropathol* 1984; 63: 160–169.
24 Schad LR, Schmitt HP, Oberwittler C, Lorenz WJ. Numerical grading of astrocytomas. *Med Inf* 1987; 12: 11–22.
25 Scarpelli M, Montironi R, Collan Y *et al.* Malignant glial tumours: prognostic value of quantitative microscopy. *Neurochirurgia* 1989; 32: 135–140.
26 Giangaspero F, Muhlbaier LH, Burger PC. The glioblastoma multiforme and the metastatic carcinoma: a morphometric study of nuclear size and shape. *Appl Pathol* 1984; 2: 160–167.
27 Montironi R, Collan Y, Scarpelli M *et al.* Reproducibility of mitotic counts and identification of mitotic figures in malignant glial tumours. *Appl Pathol* 1988; 6: 258–265.
28 Patsouris E, Stocker U, Kallmeyer V, Keiditsch E, Mehraein P, Stavrou D. Relationship between Ki-67 positive cells, growth rate and histological type of human intracranial tumors. *Anticancer Res* 1988; 8: 537–544.
29 Dingemans KPI, Assies J, Jansen N, Diegenbach PC. Sparsely granulated prolactin cell adenomas of the pituitary gland. *Virchows Arch (A)* 1982; 396: 167–186.
30 Saeger W, Kant P, Caseliz J, Ludecke DK. Electron microscopical morphometry of pituitary adenomas: comparison of tumours in acromegaly and hyperprolactinaemia. *Pathol Res Pract* 1988; 183: 17–24.
31 Selman WR, Laws ER Jr, Scheithauer BW, Carpenter SM. The occurrence of dural invasion in pituitary adenomas. *J Neurosurg* 1986; 64: 402–407.
32 Gamel JW, McLean IW, Greenberg RA, Zimmerman LE, Lichtenstein SJ. Computerized histologic assessment of malignant potential: a method for determining the prognosis of uveal melanomas. *Hum Pathol* 1982; 13: 893–897.
33 Gamel JW, McLean IW. Computerized histopathologic assessment of malignant potential. II. A practical method for predicting survival following enucleation for uveal melanoma. *Cancer* 1983; 52: 1032–1038.
34 Gamel JW, Gleason J, Williams H, Greenberg R. Reproducibility of nucleolar measurements in human intraocular melanoma cells on standard histologic microslides. *Anal Quant Cytol* 1985; 7: 174–177.
35 Huntington A, Haugan P, Gamel J, McLean I. A simple cytologic method for predicting the malignant potential of intraocular melanoma. *Pathol Res Pract* 1989; 185: 631–634.

36 Sørensen FB, Gamel JW, McCurdy J. Stereologic estimation of nucleolar volume in ocular melanoma: a comparative study of size estimators with prognostic impact. *Hum Pathol* 1993; 24: 513–518.
37 Vizoso AD, Young JZ. Internode length and fibre diameter in developing and regenerating nerves. *J Anat* 1948; 82: 110–134.
38 O'Sullivan DJ, Swallow M. The fibre size and content of the radial and sural nerves. *J Neurol Neurosurg Psychiatr* 1968; 31: 464–470.
39 Bronson RT, Bishop Y, Hedley-White ET. A contribution to the electron microscopic morphometric analysis of peripheral nerve. *J Comp Neurol* 1978; 178: 177–186.
40 Selva J, Schoëvaërt-Brossault D, Said G. Automated morphometric analysis of cross sections of normal and pathological sural nerve biopsy specimens. *Biol Cell* 1981; 42: 57–64.
41 Torch S, Usson Y, Saxod R. Automated morphometric study of human peripheral nerves by image analysis. *Pathol Res Pract* 1989; 185: 567–571.

4.15 SKIN

Quantitation has been applied to a wide variety of dermatological disorders and some of these will be briefly reviewed.

4.15.1 Ageing

Morphometry of skin biopsies from the upper arm shows that there is an age-dependent decrease in skin thickness that is faster for the epidermis in men (7.2% of the original value/decade) than in women (5.7%) but equivalent for the dermis (6%) [1]. The values are lower than those usually obtained by physical methods of skin measurement. This may be related either to fixation artefact or overestimation by the latter techniques. The number of dermal elastic fibres does not vary with age but there is a continuous increase in the relative surface area and length of the elastic fibre system [2]. This is due to the apposition of glycoprotein, lipid and calcium-rich new elastin material to the pre-existing fibres by skin fibroblasts, and it accounts for the decrease in skin elasticity.

4.15.2 Connective-tissue disease

Quantitative assessment of dermal elastin in patients with systemic sclerosis shows that there is thickening, clumping and fragmentation similar to that seen in actinic damage and chronological ageing [3]. Stereological analysis has found that the relative volume of collagen fibres is decreased in the reticular dermis and that of elastin fibres increased in its upper layer in Ehlers–Danlos syndrome [4]. Dermal collagen fibre size is also significantly reduced.

4.15.3 Mast-cell disease

Mast cells are a normal cellular component of skin and their numbers may be altered in a variety of conditions. Adult mast cells are bigger and have larger granules than those in infants, while the nuclear size and granule numbers are comparable [5]. Mast-cell infiltrates in lesions such as basal-cell carcinoma and haemangioma are similar in character to those of normal adult controls. Those in mastocytosis have larger mean cell surface areas, nuclear areas and granule diameters and there are also proven quantitative differences between the cells in systemic and non-systemic disease [6]. The superficial dermis of lesional psoriatic skin contains more mast cells than normal or non-lesional psoriatic skin [7]. Mast-cell numbers and volume fractions are not reduced by either PUVA or steroid therapy, indicating that initial healing of psoriatic plaques is not correlated with mast-cell density.

4.15.4 Psoriasis

This common condition is characterized by epidermal hyperplasia with elongation of the rete pegs, acanthosis and parakeratosis. It is a hyperproliferative state with increased labelling and mitotic indices, growth fraction and reduced cell cycle times [8]. Cell counts illustrate the degree of hyperplasia, with estimates of 52 000 proliferating cells and 47 000 differentiating cells per square millimetre being approximately two to three times those of normal controls [9]. Weinstein *et al.* [9] give a good comprehensive review of cellular proliferation in psoriasis and its quantitation by a variety of techniques, such as tritiated thymidine autoradiography, enumeration of mitoses and flow cytometry. A number of the proven treatments for psoriasis such as dithranol, methotrexate and PUVA act by reducing the proliferative rate.

4.15.5 Tuberculosis, sarcoid, leprosy

Simple histometric cell counts have quantified the localization of immunocompetent cells within the tuberculin reaction [10] in normal controls and in patients with sarcoidosis [11]. The ratio of CD4/CD8-positive T cells is increased and there are significant numbers of infiltrating mononuclear cells, even in clinically negative reactions. Tosi *et al.* [12] found epithelioid cell nuclear profiles in sarcoidosis to have more plump, elliptical shapes than in tuberculous granulomas.

There is evidence linking mast cells to the development of delayed hypersensitivity reactions. They are increased in the unaffected skin, skin appendage structures and granulomatous lesions of leprosy where it is postulated that release of mediators causes tissue damage [13]. In both tuberculoid and lepromatous leprosy, quantitation shows a common mechanism of nerve damage in the early stages and more diffuse involvement than is expected inclusive of non-lesional skin [14].

4.15.6 Cutaneous mononuclear infiltrates

There are a number of benign and malignant cutaneous diseases that are in part characterized by epidermal/dermal lymphocytic and/or histiocytic infiltration.

Systemic and discoid lupus erythematosus, Jessner's infiltrate, dermatoses

Histochemical quantitation of T-lymphocyte and macrophage numbers is not of diagnostic help in the differential diagnosis of systemic and discoid lupus erythematosus and Jessner's lymphocytic infiltrate. The majority of cells are T lymphocytes and macrophages are also increased in all three conditions [15]. Smolle [16] used image analysis to count the numbers of mononuclear cells staining positively with various monoclonal antibodies in a wide range of inflammatory dermatoses and skin tumours. He found that cutaneous mononuclear cells are arranged in T, B and monocyte compartments which reiterate normal lymphoid tissue and give a limited range of distinct patterns. Similar patterns were found in markedly different clinical and histological conditions, indicating that they are not disease-specific but rather reflect general anatomical and functional relationships of inflammatory cells and the skin. T cells were the predominant lymphocytes in normal skin and this component was uniformly expanded in peritumoural infiltrates and dermatoses. They showed minor quantitative differences which were not sufficiently distinctive to be diagnostic. For example, there was an increase in intraepidermal helper–inducer T cells in allergic contact dermatitis and psoriasis. The former is associated with greater numbers of antigen-presenting Langerhans' cells, and the latter may represent a cytotoxic immune response to stratum corneum antigens. Langerhans' cells were reduced in lichen planus and discoid lupus erythematosus and increased in sarcoidosis, the granulomatous reaction indicating persistent helper-cell activation in this particular disease. Suppressor–cytotoxic T cells were increased in keratoses, squamous carcinoma, naevi, malignant melanoma and mycosis fungoides. The infiltrate of low-grade B-cell lymphoma was surrounded by T-cell compartments and the only skin lesion predominated by aggregates of B cells without a T-cell component was high-grade B-cell lymphoma. The epidermis is not normally a lymphoid compartment but may become so in diseased skin. In various dermatoses keratinocyte expression of HLA-DR positivity is associated with T-lymphocyte epidermotrophism. In particular the number of HLA-DR-positive keratinocytes correlates with the proportion of epidermotropic T suppressor–cytotoxic cells, suggesting that a close pathophysiological interaction exists [17].

Lymphomatoid papulosis, lymphomatoid granulomatosis

Lymphomatoid papulosis consists of a persistent, intermittent and self-healing papular eruption which appears clinically benign but has a malignant histological appearance. The wedge-shaped dermal infiltrate is composed of lymphocytes, histiocytes, polymorphs and atypical mononuclear cells. These are present as small or large (up to 35 μm) hyperconvoluted cells, with their relative proportions dictating clinical behaviour. Type A lesions with predominantly large atypical cells showing a shift from diploid to aneuploid DNA content have a worse prognosis [18] and a minority may progress to malignant lymphoma. Another progressive condition (12% of cases) that has a high mortality (median survival 14 months) is lymphomatoid granulomatosis [19]. This angiocentric and destructive lymphohistiocytic infiltrate involves the lungs, nervous system, kidney and skin. Prognosis worsens with greater proportions of atypical lymphoreticular cells in the infiltrate: 81% of 26 patients with > 50% atypical cells died, compared to only 48% of 23 patients with no such constituent cells. Higher percentages of small lymphocytes, histiocytes, plasma cells and fibrosis improve the clinical outlook.

Cutaneous T-cell lymphoma (mycosis fungoides, Sézary's syndrome)

A discussion of lymphoproliferative conditions of the skin is given by Slater [20]. Both B-cell and T-cell non-Hodgkin's lymphoma may involve the skin and are characterized by somewhat differing histological patterns of infiltration. T-cell lymphoma shows disproportionately frequent epidermotrophic cutaneous involvement, with its most widely recognized forms being mycosis fungoides and Sézary's syndrome. Cutaneous mycosis fungoides is divided into erythematous patch, plaque and tumour stages which may then evolve to visceral disease. Its leukaemic variant, Sézary's syndrome, is also associated with peripheral blood involvement and lymphadenopathy. These conditions are characterized by the presence of enlarged, atypical hyperconvoluted cells in the blood and cutaneous infiltrate. These Sézary or mycosis cells are large (15–30 μm), hyperchromatic, irregularly convoluted or cerebriform in outline, with marginated chromatin and a high nuclear cytoplasmic ratio [21]. A smaller cell variant, termed the Lutzner cell, has also been described and cytophotometry has shown both these cell populations to have a shift in DNA content towards triploidy and tetraploidy [22]. Schmoeckel *et al.* [23] quantified the lymphoid cellular infiltrate in mycosis fungoides, Sézary's syndrome, parapsoriasis en plaques, contact dermatitis and psoriasis. The numbers of Lutzner cells (defined as lymphoid cells with at least three deep nuclear indentations) were doubled in mycosis, quadrupled in parapsoriasis and increased by a factor of seven in Sézary's syndrome. The proportions of lymphoplasmacytoid and immunoblastic forms were also greater in the malignant cases. Similarly, computer-assisted planimetry separated 95% of benign lesions from 12 cases of mycosis/Sézary's syndrome by discriminant analysis based on the frequency distribution of an ultrastructural nuclear shape parameter – nuclear contour index (NCI) [24]. Most of the malignant cases had lymphoid infiltrates with an NCI of more than 11.5 and there was good correlation in these cells with cytophotometrically determined DNA abnormalities such as triploidy and tetraploidy. Prospective use of the morphometric predictions showed that five of seven cases classified as malignant progressed to mycosis fungoides, whilst benign lesions remained so. In a subsequent study analysis of the NCI frequency histograms separated 20 T-cell lymphomas from 14 benign infiltrates (psoriasis, Jessner's, atopic dermatitis) with a probability of more than 95%. Clinical follow-up of the 20 patients classified as malignant showed that 17 developed mycosis fungoides and two lymphomatoid papulosis [25]. Subsequently, Shum *et al.* [26] used the criteria established by McNutt *et al.* [27] of mean NCI, percentage of lymphoid cells with NCI > 7 and nuclear profile area > 30 μm^2 to study 43 cases of mycosis fungoides and 28 non-mycosis lymphoid skin infiltrates. The sensitivity for separating benign and malignant lesions was only 47% but there were no false-positives. Despite these discrepancies, a number of which may be explained by differing methodologies, it is recognized that morphometric analysis has a potential role to play in the diagnosis of cutaneous T-cell lymphoma. This may also be improved by confining the measurements to PCNA-positive cells [28]. Immunochemistry is useful in establishing whether a lymphoid infiltrate is of T- or B-cell lineage. Thus Payne *et al.* [29] were able to distinguish mycosis fungoides from convoluted B-cell lymphomas by combining immunochemistry with ultrastructural morphometric dual-parameter analysis of mean nuclear form factor and perimeter. Rather than formally measure the NCI they separated mycosis fungoides from benign lymphoid infiltrates by its low percentage of cells with no sharply angled nuclear indentations as determined by visual inspection of the electron micrographs. Planimetry has also identified a component of Langerhans' cells within the infiltrate of mycosis fungoides and this interaction may help to explain its dermal/epidermal distribution [30].

Circulating Sézary-like mononuclear cells have also been found in patients with contact dermatitis, atopic dermatosis and exfoliative psoriasis [31]. In these benign dermatoses they invariably have an absence of mitotic figures and are smaller (6–12 μm diameter) than in mycosis fungoides or Sézary's syndrome [32]. More recently, ultrastructural morphometry and quantitative immunohistochemistry have demonstrated in benign lymphoid infiltrates a skin-associated T cell with increased nuclear contour irregularity [33]. It is strongly Leu-8- and Leu-9-positive and is speculated to be the normal counterpart to the malignant clonally expanded T cell found in mycosis fungoides and Sézary's syndrome.

Immunohistochemical analysis of involved lymph nodes [34] and skin [35] in cutaneous T-cell lymphoma shows that the constituent cells are of the helper–inducer subset with the helper/suppressor ratio in the dermal infiltrate significantly exceeding that of normal blood [36]. There are also increased numbers of Langerhans' cells in contact with these T-helper lymphocytes [37] and their complex interaction with keratinocytes suggests that mycosis fungoides may in part be a disease activated by antigen persistence [38]. Note that helper/suppressor lymphocyte ratios vary 68-fold in benign cutaneous infiltrates and are of no use as a diagnostic tool in defining T-cell malignancy [33].

4.15.7 Basal-cell carcinoma, schwannoma

Basal-cell carcinoma is a slowly growing tumour despite its high mitotic rate and this can be accounted for by the prominent degree of single-cell apoptotic necrosis [39]. Aggressive recurrent and metastasizing basal-cell carcinoma has been compared morphometrically with the more usual variant. There are significant differences in nuclear area, perimeter, maximum diameter and polarity between the two categories which can be separated by discriminant analysis [40].

The mitotic index is increased in malignant schwannoma (mean 6.0) compared to benign lesions (mean 0.32) [41], a feature that is found in most cutaneous or subcutaneous sarcomas.

4.15.8 Melanocytic naevi, malignant melanoma

Cell size

Maturation towards the base of a cutaneous melanocytic lesion is a useful histological sign in designating it as benign. This takes several forms, such as adipocytic or neural differentiation or simply a decrease in cell size. The latter has been confirmed by light and ultrastructural morphometry as an atrophy of all cellular constituents except for mitochondria and microfilaments [42]. Spitz naevus (synonym: juvenile melanoma) is a benign naevus occurring in children, teenagers and young adults and which has a number of histological features similar to malignant melanoma. The age at presentation, its symmetry, telangiectasia, lack of pigmentation, lymphocytic infiltrate and cell type are all helpful in making the diagnosis. Immunohistochemical quantitation shows that its staining intensity for S-100 protein and neuron-specific enolase is significantly less than in malignant melanoma and comparable to that of usual benign naevi. In addition, the majority of Spitz naevi have a normal densitometrically determined diploid DNA content [43]. Semiautomatic image analysis has also been used to study the nuclear features in 40 cases each of benign naevi, Spitz naevi and malignant melanoma [44]. A maturation parameter (MP) was determined by calculating the ratio of the nuclear areas in the deep and superficial portions of the lesion. The mean MP values were as follows: dermal naevi 0.720, Spitz naevi 0.725 and malignant melanoma 1.125 (melanoma vs benign lesions $P < 0.01$; Fig. 4.14). The efficiency for the MP in distinguishing melanoma from dermal naevi and Spitz naevi was 0.95 and 0.97, respectively. Measurements confined to the superficial portion only were less efficient and better discrimination was achieved by studying the deep aspect where mean nuclear areas were dermal naevi 18 μm^2, Spitz naevi 27.6 μm^2 and melanoma 38.3 μm^2.

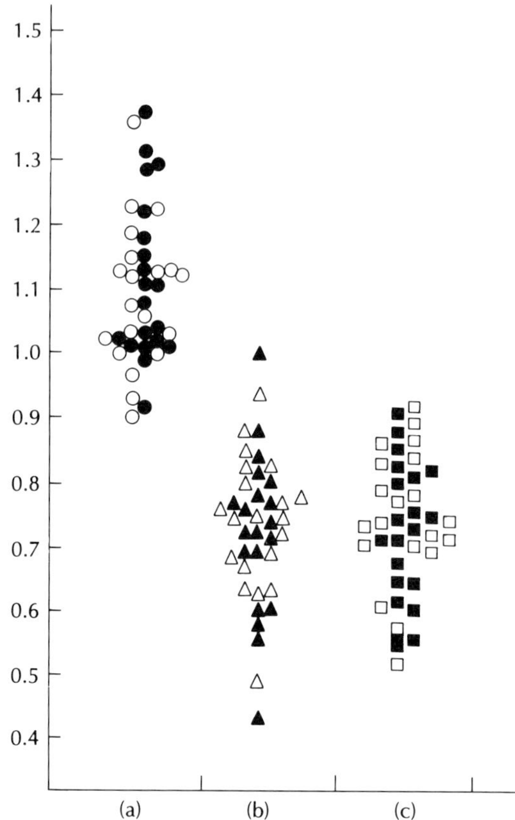

Fig. 4.14 Maturation parameter (r = ratio of deep nuclear area/superficial nuclear area) in melanocytic lesions. (a) Malignant melanoma; (b) dermal naevus; (c) Spitz naevus. Open symbols = training set; closed symbols = test set. From Smolle *et al.* [44].

Nuclear volume

Stereological estimates indicate that the volume-weighted mean nuclear volume (V_v) is increased in malignant melanoma by a factor of two or three over benign naevi [45]. Sørensen [46] found mean V_v of 122 and 245 μm³ for benign and invasive lesions, respectively. Patients with melanoma whose nuclear V_v values overlapped with the benign range had a favourable prognosis. Nuclear V_v did not show significant heterogeneity in naevi or melanoma and was more efficient and sensitive than two-dimensional morphometry (nuclear area, density, mitotic index) in distinguishing between the same series of benign and malignant cases. Mean nuclear V_v does not differ significantly between primary cutaneous melanoma and their equivalent metastases, although the latter show increased variability of this parameter [47]. The metastases also have greater heterogeneity in flow cytometrically determined DNA content, although DNA aneuploidy does not directly correlate with increased nuclear volume. Nuclear volume is also capable of predicting thin melanomas with potential for metastases and it may be used as a tool for selective adjuvant chemotherapy in these patients [48].

Vascularity

Computerized morphometry of frozen sections stained with antibodies to endothelial cells has shown marked differences in vascular distribution in the connective tissue at the base of benign naevi, primary and metastatic malignant melanoma [49]. The mean area occupied by small vessels (minimum diameter less than 20 μm) was 0.3 μm^2 in benign naevi, 0.6 μm^2 in primary melanoma and 1.2 μm^2 in metastases ($P < 0.05$). There was also strong correlation between the number of small vessels and the Ki-67 proliferative activity. These findings illustrate the close interaction that exists between tumour proliferation and neovascularization in the host dermis. This is also highlighted by a further immunohistochemical quantitative study that examined tumour-base vascularity in two groups of melanoma (0.76–4.0 mm thick) matched for age, sex, Breslow thickness and Clark level of invasion [50]. The percentage vascular area at the tumour base was more than twice that in patients who developed locoregional or systemic metastases than in those with no evidence of recurrence.

Dysplastic naevi, *in situ* melanoma

Dysplastic naevi occur either as multiple lesions in a small group of patients with a family history of propensity for the development of melanoma, or sporadically in individuals who may or may not have a concurrent or subsequent melanoma lesion. They are defined by both cytological and architectural alterations and there remains considerable variation in their reported frequency, assessment and importance [51,52]. Computerized image analysis has found that they have significantly greater values over compound naevi for the following variables: SD of nuclear area, mean nuclear roundness, mean and SD of DNA content [53]. No dysplastic naevi were DNA aneuploid but they did have hyperdiploid values. There were no significant differences in the measured parameters within a lesion or between those in patients with single or multiple naevi. In contrast, malignant melanomas were DNA aneuploid with greater nuclear area and variability. Superficial spreading malignant melanoma is usually surrounded by a horizontal intraepidermal component (or *in situ* change) measuring a variable length of three to four rete pegs or more. Schmiegelow *et al.* [54] have assessed nuclear area and DNA content in the invasive nodule of malignant melanomas, their surrounding intraepidermal component and metastases. This showed an incremental gradation of change in nuclear size, DNA content (and their variability) and mitotic index along the spectrum of lesions from *in situ* change to primary melanoma and metastases. There was also considerable heterogeneity between individual tumours and their metastases. This study therefore confirmed the malignant potential of melanoma *in situ*.

Depth of melanoma invasion – Clark level, Breslow thickness

One of the most commonly used measurements in diagnostic histopathology is the depth of invasion in malignant melanoma as this is a strong indicator of prognosis and influence on therapy. Clark *et al.* [55] described three variants of malignant melanoma; superficial spreading melanoma, lentigo maligna melanoma (Hutchinson's melanotic freckle) and nodular melanoma. The former two variants are characterized by a relatively long period of centrifugally spreading, horizontal, superficial growth before a more aggressive invasive (vertical) component develops. Nodular melanoma exhibits a tendency for early and uniform vertical invasion. It is the extent of this invasion that influences prognosis so much and these authors defined it according to five different anatomical levels (Table 4.4).

The data for all 208 cases studied showed median survival times for patients with levels II, III, IV and V lesions to be 6.83, 6.38, 5.21 and 3.50 years, respectively. The comparative mortality rates for the various subtypes were superficial spreading melanoma 31.5%, nodular melanoma 56.1% and lentigo maligna melanoma 10.3%. In addition, superficial spreading melanoma showed a better survival than nodular melanoma for equivalent anatomical levels of invasion. Breslow [56] published the second key paper in the assessment of invasion in melanoma. By means of an ocular micrometer the maximal thickness of the lesion was measured from either the top of the epidermal granular layer or the base of the ulcerated skin surface to its deepest point of invasion. Maximal cross-sectional area was also calculated by multiplying thickness by maximal diameter and the measurements were compared to Clark's anatomical levels. It was found that no patient with a lesion less than 5 mm in diameter, 0.76 mm in thickness or 6.01 mm^2 in maximal cross-sectional area developed recurrent or metastatic disease. The smallest melanoma to recur or metastasize was 0.88 mm thick, and there was subsequent disease in 100% of lesions >5 mm in thickness. Tumour thickness was the most useful parameter and it identified 38 out of the 71 patients who remained free of disease. There was good correlation between tumour thickness and Clark staging. Of the six level III lesions that recurred, all were >0.76 mm in thickness while thinner level III lesions survived 5 years or more disease-free. It is necessary to take into account the variation in thickness within a lesion and the difficulty in defining the deepest malignant cell. Despite this, the

Table 4.4 Anatomical Clark levels of invasion in melanoma

Level	Anatomical structure
I	Epidermis (melanoma *in situ*)
II	Papillary dermis
III	Papillary/reticular dermis interface
IV	Reticular dermis
V	Subcutaneous tissue

Breslow thickness has become regarded as the most important prognostic indicator, and the width of surgical margins is based on this measurement [57, 58]. It has now become accepted practice to define malignant melanoma as being thin (< 0.76 mm), of intermediate thickness (0.76–1.5 mm) or thick (> 1.5 mm). This can also be augmented by combining it with Clark level. Schmoeckel and Braun-Falco [59] found that a prognostic index calculated from the product of tumour thickness and the number of mitoses per square millimetre was the most accurate method of predicting which patients would remain recurrence- or metastasis-free. Mitotic rate proved nearly as good as the prognostic index and these parameters outperformed tumour thickness and level of invasion. Breslow depth was also inferior to the prognostic index in melanoma of intermediate thickness where the latter identified a subgroup with a worse than anticipated prognosis (57.5 vs 84.1% 5-year survival) [60]. Depth of invasion remained the measurement of choice in thin and thick lesions. There is a minority of patients with thick melanoma who have reasonably long disease-free survival periods. Blessing *et al.* [61] identified 41 such patients with no evidence of metastases after a minimum of 6 years. They had the following features in common: (i) sited on the head, neck and arm rather than the trunk; (ii) an absence of vascular invasion; and (iii) a pushing rather than an irregularly infiltrating base. In a similar study of 13 patients with 10-year survival periods compared to 13 short-term survivors, none of the classical prognostic factors were capable of separating the groups. These included level of invasion, ulceration, mitotic rate, inflammatory response, tumour regression, necrosis, vascular invasion, satellitosis, depth of invasion, cell or lesion type, borders, DNA content or cytomorphometrically derived nuclear area [62].

Nuclear shape and area

Multivariate analysis found that in addition to tumour thickness the only other variable of prognostic significance was the nuclear correlation coefficient (NCC) [63]. This morphometric parameter is a measure of roundness versus ellipsoidicity, regularity and homogeneity of nuclear shape and it is correlated to the nuclear axes ratio (long axis divided by the short axis). Lesions with a low NCC value (ellipsoid spindle-shaped nuclei) had better prognosis irrespective of tumour thickness. Mean tumour-cell nuclear area has also emerged as being significantly greater in non-survivors than survivors in both the superficial (51.1 vs 43.7 μm^2) and deep layers (42.9 vs 36.4 μm^2) of malignant melanoma [64]. This is due to a uniform increase in tumour cell size and not to a clonal proliferation of any particular cell subset.

Nodal disease

The number of involved lymph nodes in clinical stage II melanoma has an overall survival/mortality predictive capability of 61%. This is improved to 86% when a combination of the number of positive nodes is used with a micrometer estimate of the percentage of the nodal diameter that is involved [65].

4.15.9 Conclusion

Quantitation in skin disease has identified changes in dermal elastin with age and in connective-tissue disease. Mast cell size and granule diameter are greater in urticaria pigmentosa and psoriasis has been characterized as an epidermal hyperproliferative stage. Immune cell counts are not of use in differentiating various dermatoses. The numbers of atypical lymphoid cells influences the prognosis in lymphomatoid papulosis and granulomatosis. Their presence aids the diagnosis of mycosis fungoides and Sézary's syndrome where they are enlarged and have sharp nuclear indentations (increased nuclear contour index). Cell and nuclear size are smaller in benign naevi than in malignant melanoma where there is also a loss of progressive maturation towards the lesion base. Stereologically derived nuclear volume outperforms two-dimensional morphometry in separating benign and malignant melanocytic lesions. Tumour base vascularity is greater in melanoma and those that subsequently recur. Quantitation confirms the premalignant nature of intraepidermal melanoma *in situ*. In established malignant melanoma the most important measurement in assessing prognosis and influencing therapy is the Breslow thickness or depth of invasion. On the basis of this, melanomas can be defined as thin, of intermediate thickness or thick, each with differing outlooks. Increased nuclear area, number and percentage area of nodes involved also worsen prognosis.

References

1 Branchet MC, Boisnic S, Frances C, Robert AM. Skin thickness changes in normal aging skin. *Gerontology* 1990; 36: 28–35.

2 Robert C, Lesty C, Robert AM. Ageing of the skin: study of elastic fiber network modifications by computerized image analysis. *Gerontology* 1988; 34: 291–296.

3 Rustin MH, Papadaki L, Rode J, Dowd PM. Elastic fibres in patients with systemic sclerosis. A morphological study. *Virchows Arch A* 1989; 416: 115–120.

4 Vitellaro-Zuccarello L, Dyne K, Cetta G. Biochemical, morphological and stereological study of the dermis in three members of a large family with type IV Ehlers–Danlos syndrome. *Connect Tissue Res* 1989; 23: 1–17.

5 Tharp MD, Glass MJ, Seelig LL Jr. Ultrastructural morphometric analysis of human mast cells in normal skin and pathological cutaneous lesions. *J Cutan Pathol* 1988; 15: 78–83.

6 Tharp MD, Glass MJ, Seelig LL Jr. Ultrastructural morphometric analysis of lesional skin: mast cells from patients with systemic and nonsystemic mastocytosis. *J Am Acad Dermatol* 1988; 18: 298–306.

7 Toyry S, Fraki J, Tammi R. Mast cell density in psoriatic skin. The effect of PUVA and corticosteroid therapy. *Arch Dermatol Res* 1988; 280: 282–285.

8 Wright N. Cell proliferation in health and disease. In: Anthony PP, MacSween RNM (eds) *Recent Advances in Histopathology*, vol. 12, Edinburgh: Churchill Livingstone, 1984: 17–33.

9 Weinstein GD, Ross P, McCullough JL, Colton A. Proliferative defects in psoriasis. In: Wright NA, Camplejohn RS (eds) *Psoriasis: Cell Proliferation*. Edinburgh: Churchill Livingstone, 1983: 189–208.

10 Gibbs JH, Ferguson J, Brown RA. Histometric study of the localisation of lymphocyte subsets and accessory cells in human Mantoux reactions. *J Clin Pathol* 1984; 37: 1227–1234.

11 Lowe JG, Gibbs JH, Potts RC, Standord JL, Swanson Beck JS. Histometric studies on cellular infiltrates of tuberculin tests in patients with sarcoidosis. *J Clin Pathol* 1991; 44: 219–223.

12 Tosi P, Miracco C, Luzi P. Morphometric distinction of granulomas in tuberculosis and sarcoidosis. *Anal Quant Cytol Histol* 1986; 8: 233–240.

13 Cree IA, Coghill G, Beck JS. Mast cells in leprosy skin lesions. *J Clin Pathol* 1990; 43: 196–200.

14 Shetty VP, Antia NH, Jacobs JM. The pathology of early leprous neuropathy. *J Neurol Sci* 1988; 88: 115–131.

15 Konttinen YT, Reitamo S, Ranki A, Segerberg-Konttinen M. T-lymphocytes and mononuclear phagocytes in the skin infiltrate of systemic and discoid lupus erythematosus and Jessner's lymphocytic infiltrate. *Br J Dermatol* 1981; 104: 141–145.

16 Smolle J. Mononuclear cell patterns in the skin. An immunohistological and morphometrical analysis. *Am J Dermatopathol* 1988; 10: 36–46.

17 Smolle J, Soyer HP, Juettner FM, Torne R, Stetiner H, Kerl H. HLA-DR-positive keratinocytes are associated with suppressor lymphocyte epidermotropism. A biomathematical study. *Am J Dermatopathol* 1988; 10: 128–132.

18 Willemze R, Meyer CJLM, van Vloten WA, Scheffer E. The clinical and histological spectrum of lymphomatoid papulosis. *Br J Dermatol* 1982; 107: 131–144.

19 Katzenstein A-LA, Carrington CB, Leibow AA. Lymphomatoid granulomatosis. A clinicopathologic study of 152 cases. *Cancer* 1979; 43: 360–373.

20 Slater DN. Lymphoproliferative conditions of the skin. In: Anthony PP, MacSween RNM (eds) *Advances in Histopathology*, vol. 12, Edinburgh: Churchill Livingstone, 1984: 83–110.

21 Lutzner MA, Jordan HW. Ultrastructure of an abnormal cell in Sézary's syndrome. *Blood* 1968; 31: 719–726.

22 Lutzner MA, Emerit I, Durepaire R, Flandrin G, Grupper C, Prunieras M. Cytogenetic, cytophotometric and ultrastructural study of large cerebriform cells of the Sézary syndrome and description of a small cell variant. *J Natl Cancer Inst* 1973; 50: 1145–1162.

23 Schmoeckel C, Burg G, Braun-Falco O. Quantitative analysis of lymphoid cells in mycosis fungoides, Sézary's syndrome and parapsoriasis en plaques. *Arch Dermatol Res* 1979; 264: 17–28.

24 Meijer CJLM, van Der Loo EM, van Vloten WA, van der Velde EA, Scheffer E, Cornelisse CJ. Early diagnosis of mycosis fungoides and Sézary's syndrome by morphometric analysis of lymphoid cells in the skin. *Cancer* 1980; 45: 2864–2871.

25 van der Loo EM, van Vloten WA, Cornelisse CJ, Scheffer E, Meijer CJLM. The relevance of morphometry in the differential diagnosis of cutaneous T cell lymphomas. *Br J Dermatol* 1981; 104: 257–269.

26 Shum DT, Roberts JT, Smout MS, Wells GA, Simon GT. The value of nuclear contour index in the diagnosis of mycosis fungoides. An assessment of current ultrastructural morphometric diagnostic criteria. *Cancer* 1986; 57: 298–304.

27 McNutt NS, Heilbron DC, Crain WR. Mycosis fungoides: diagnostic criteria based on quantitative electron microscopy. *Lab Invest* 1981; 44: 466–474.

28 Clarke AMT, Reid WA, Jack AS. Combined proliferating cell nuclear antigen and morphometric analysis

in the diagnosis of cutaneous lymphoid infiltrates. *J Clin Pathol* 1993; 46: 129–134.
29 Payne CM, Grogan TM, Lynch PJ. An ultrastructural morphometric and immunohistochemical analysis of cutaneous lymphomas and benign, lymphocytic infiltrates of skin: useful criteria for diagnosis. *Arch Dermatol* 1986; 122: 1139–1154.
30 Caorsi I, Figueroa CD, Rodriguez EM. Morphologic and morphometric study of the two main cell lineages involved in mycosis fungoides: the lymphoid cells and the Langerhans' cells. *Ultrastruct Pathol* 1982; 3: 119–136.
31 Duncan SC, Winkelmann RK. Circulating Sézary cells in hospitalised dermatology patients. *Br J Dermatol* 1978; 99: 171–178.
32 Meyer CJIM, van Leeuwen AWFM, van der Loo EM, van de Putte LBA, van Vloten WA. Cerebriform (Sézary-like) mononuclear cells in healthy individuals: a morphologically distinct population of T cells. Relationship with mycosis fungoides and Sézary's syndrome. *Virchows Arch B Cell Pathol* 1977; 25: 95–104.
33 Payne CM, Spier CM, Grogan TM *et al.* Nuclear contour irregularity correlates with Leu-9, Leu-8 cells in benign lymphoid infiltrates of skin. An ultrastructural morphometric and quantitative immunophenotypic analysis suggesting the normal T-cell counterpart to the malignant mycosis fungoides/Sézary cell. *Am J Dermatopathol* 1988; 10: 377–389.
34 Kung PC, Berger CL, Goldstein G, Logerfo P, Edelson RL. Cutaneous T cell lymphoma: characterisation by monoclonal antibodies. *Blood* 1981; 57: 261–266.
35 Thomas JA, Janossy G, Graham-Brown RAC, Kung PC, Goldstein G. The relationship between T lymphocyte subsets and Ia-like antigen positive non-lymphoid cells in early stages of cutaneous T cell lymphoma. *J Invest Dermatol* 1982; 78: 169–176.
36 Holden CA, Morgan EW, MacDonald DM. The cell population in the cutaneous infiltrate of mycosis fungoides: *in situ* studies using monoclonal antisera. *Br J Dermatol* 1982; 106: 385–392.
37 Mackie RM, Turbitt ML. The use of a double-label immunoperoxidase monoclonal antibody technique in the investigation of patients with mycosis fungoides. *Br J Dermatol* 1982; 106: 379–384.
38 Chu B, Berger CL, Lynfield Y, Essesse I, Edelson RL. Pathogenesis of cutaneous T cell lymphoma. In: Goos M, Christophers E (eds) *Lymphoproliferative Disease of the Skin.* Berlin: Springer-Verlag, 1981: 57–64.
39 Kerr JFR, Searle J. A suggested explanation for the paradoxically slow growth rate of basal-cell carcinoma that contain numerous mitotic figures. *J Pathol* 1972; 107: 41–44.
40 De Rosa G, Vetrani A, Zeppa P *et al.* Comparative morphometric analysis of aggressive and ordinary basal cell carcinoma of the skin. *Cancer* 1990; 65: 544–549.
41 Pesce CM, Sanguineti G, Reale A. Mitotic activity of schwannomas. *Clin Neuropathol* 1984; 3: 153–154.
42 Goovaerts G, Buyssens N. Nevus cell maturation or atrophy? *Am J Dermatopathol* 1988; 10: 20–27.
43 Rode J, Williams RA, Jarvis LR, Dhillon AP, Jamal O. S100 protein, neurone specific enolase, and nuclear DNA content in Spitz naevus. *J Pathol* 1990; 161: 41–45.
44 Smolle J, Soyer HP, Juettner FM, Hoedl S, Kerl H. Nuclear parameters in the superficial and deep portion of melanocytic lesions. A morphometrical investigation. *Pathol Res Pract* 1988; 183: 266–270.
45 Brüngger A, Cruz-Orive LM. Nuclear morphometry of nodular malignant melanomas and benign nevocytic nevi. *Arch Dermatol Res* 1987; 279: 412–414.
46 Sørensen FB. Stereological estimation of nuclear volume in benign melanocytic lessons and cutaneous malignant melanomas. *Am J Dermatopathol* 1989; 11: 517–527.
47 Sørensen FB, Kristensen IB, Grymer F, Jakobsen A. DNA-index and stereological estimation of nuclear volume in primary and metastatic malignant melanomas: a comparative study with analysis of heterogeneity. *APMIS* 1990; 98: 61–70.
48 Binder M, Dolezal I, Wolff K, Pehamberger H. Stereologic estimation of volume-weighted mean nuclear volume as a predictor of prognosis in 'thin' malignant melanoma. *J Invest Dermatol* 1992; 99: 180–183.
49 Smolle J, Soyer H-P, Hofmann-Wellenhof R, Smolle-Juettner F-M, Kerl H. Vascular architecture of melanocytic skin tumors. A quantitative immunohistochemical study using automated image analysis. *Pathol Res Pract* 1989; 185: 740–745.
50 Srivastava A, Laidler P, Davies RP, Horgan K, Hughes LE. The prognostic significance of tumor vascularity in intermediate-thickness (0.76–0.4 thick) skin melanoma. A quantitative histologic study. *Am J Pathol* 1988; 133: 419–423.
51 Clemente C, Cochran AJ, Elder DE *et al.* Histopathologic diagnosis of dysplastic nevi: concordance among pathologists convened by the World Health Organization melanoma programme. *Hum Pathol* 1991; 22: 313–319.
52 Ackerman AB. What naevus is dysplastic, a syndrome and the commonest precursor of malignant melanoma? A riddle and an answer. *Histopathology* 1988; 13: 241–256.
53 Fleming MG, Wied GL, Dytch HE. Image analysis cytometry of dysplastic nevi. *J Invest Dermatol* 1990; 95: 287–291.
54 Schmiegelow P, Oppermann T, Nussgen A, Schroiff R, Janner M, Breitbart EW. Melanoma *in situ* (MIS) adjacent to an invasive nodular melanoma ('SSM/NM') and its metastases – DNA-cytophotometry, mitotic index, and anisokaryosis. *Virchows Arch A* 1987; 411: 213–221.
55 Clark WH, From L, Bernardino EA, Mihm MC. The histogenesis and biological behaviour of primary

human malignant melanomas of the skin. *Cancer Res* 1969; 29: 705–727.
56 Breslow A. Thickness, cross-sectional areas and depth of invasion in the prognosis of cutaneous melanoma. *Ann Surg* 1970; 172: 902–908.
57 Breslow A. Prognosis in cutaneous melanoma: tumor thickness as a guide to treatment. *Pathol Ann* 1980; 15: 1–22.
58 Veronesi U, Cascinelli N, Adamus J *et al.* This stage I primary cutaneous malignant melanoma. Comparison of excision with margins of 1 or 3 cm. *N Engl J Med* 1988; 318: 1159–1162.
59 Schmoeckel C, Braun-Falco O. Prognostic index in malignant melanoma. *Arch Dermatol* 1978; 114: 871–873.
60 Kopf AW, Gross DF, Rogers GS *et al.* Prognostic index for malignant melanoma. *Cancer* 1987; 59: 1236–1241.
61 Blessing K, McLaren KM, McLean A, Davidson P. Thick malignant melanomas (> 3.0 mm Breslow) with good clinical outcome: a histological study and survival analysis. *Histopathology* 1991; 18: 143–148.
62 Rivers JK, McCarthy SW, Shaw HM *et al.* Patients with thick melanomas surviving at least 10 years: histological, cytometric and HLA analysis. *Histopathology* 1991; 18: 339–346.
63 Baak JPA, Tan GJKH. The adjuvant prognostic value of nuclear morphometry in stage I malignant melanoma of the skin. A multivariate analysis. *Anal Quant Cytol Histol* 1986; 8: 241–244.
64 Tosi P, Luzi P, Sforza V *et al.* The nuclei in cutaneous malignant melanoma, stage I, are smaller in survivors than in non-survivors. *Pathol Res Pract* 1989; 185: 625–630.
65 Cochran AJ, Lana AM, Wen DR. Histomorphometry in the assessment of prognosis in stage II malignant melanoma. *Am J Surg Pathol* 1989; 13: 600–604.

4.16 LYMPH NODE, THYMUS AND SPLEEN

Morphological evidence of cell-mediated immunity characterized by increased counts of paracortical immunoblasts and sinus histiocytes in regional lymph nodes draining carcinoma of the sigmoid colon is claimed to confer increased survival [1]. Morphometry has also postulated delayed immunity manifested by paracortical transformation as a barrier to nodal metastases in laryngeal carcinoma [2]. Ultrastructural quantitation of lymph node cell suspensions based on the parameter NCI separates involved from non-involved dermatopathic lymphadenopathy in patients with mycosis fungoides [3]. Cytocentrifuge smears have been recommended over nodal imprints when determining variables such as nuclear area by morphometry, as better definition is obtained [4]. Quantitation of fine-needle aspirates shows marked heterogeneity of nuclear area in both reactive nodes and diffuse large-cell lymphoma, contrasting with the homogeneity of small-cell lymphoma [5]. In the latter and nodal involvement by chronic lymphocytic leukaemia, cases with a morphometrically determined large-cell component have a worse prognosis [6]. Semiautomatic image analysis of reactive nodal, splenic and tonsillar lymphoid tissue reveals relationships in cellular dimensions not wholly appreciable to the eye [7]. Mantle zone and paracortical lymphocytes are significantly smaller and have a more regular, rounded contour than small untransformed germinal centre cells. The latter bear a constant relationship to their larger transformed follicle-centre equivalents, despite wide variations in nuclear size between lymph node samples. This study acts as a suitable baseline against which to compare the quantitative features of malignant lymphoma, the subject of the majority of such studies in nodal tissue, and a review of which is given by Crocker [8].

4.16.1 Non-Hodgkin's lymphoma (NHL)

Initial semiautomatic image analyses showed that nuclear size, size distribution and density corresponded closely to histological classification [9]. However, these parameters were not able to define morphometric subtypes of NHL, although the case numbers were small and it was felt that the technique could be of potential use in this area. Following earlier work on lymph node imprints [10], Crocker *et al.* [11] found that measurements of mean nuclear maximum diameter were considerably greater in high-grade than in low-grade NHL. Mean maximum nuclear diameter increased in the following order: centrocytic, centrocytic/centroblastic, centroblastic and immunoblastic lymphoma. In addition each lymphoma comprised two cell populations, small and large cells, in a variety of proportions relating to the histological cell type. Stereology has also found significant geometric cellular differences between low- and high-grade malignant lymphoma [12] and this is confirmed by morphometry for a range of B-cell NHLs measured on both semithin plastic sections [13] and cytological aspirates [14].

Follicular lymphoma can be difficult to distinguish from florid reactive hyperplasia. Morphometry has shown follicle size and variation in shape to be greater in reactive hyperplasia than the somewhat uniform pattern of follicular lymphoma. In the latter there is an absence of the mantle zone which constitutes up to 65.5% of the follicle area in reactive hyperplasia [15]. In follicular lymphoma the tumour cells may be of a similar size to unstimulated (mature) mantle-zone lymphocytes but are more irregular in shape with invagination of their nuclear profiles [16]. This feature is underestimated – the 4–5% of nuclear profiles with clefts appreciable in histological sections actually represent 25–30% of the lymphocyte population. Tosi *et al.* [17] found nuclear area to be larger in follicular lymphoma than in reactive germinal-centre cells, and profile invaginations to decrease in depth and increase in angle as the nucleus enlarged. This morphometric study did not find any correspondence between neoplastic and non-neoplastic nuclei with regard to the symmetry and angle of the invaginations. Ultrastructural morphometric studies of benign reactive hyperplasia have shown that there is a gradual increase in nuclear size from the mantle zone to the reactive germinal centre but that nuclear shape shows greater heterogeneity in both areas [18]. This surprising degree of irregularity in small mature mantle-zone lymphocytes was also confirmed by their distribution of nuclear invagination frequency and depth, comparable to that of centrocytes and centroblasts [19]. The main difference therefore between the physiological range of benign lymphoid cells and those of NHL lies not in irregularity of nuclear shape but in nuclear area. Evidence now exists to suggest that this is in part determined by the distribution of condensed (hetero-) chromatin and the arrangement of the interchromatinic (euchromatin) nuclear compartment [20]. Tosi *et al.* [21] support the finding of nuclear irregularity in the different zones of reactive follicles and NHL. There were significant differences in the proportions of various subtypes of nuclear shape characterizing mantle zone, centrocytic and immunocytic lymphomas, confirming them as distinct entities.

Analysis of centroblastic and immunoblastic NHL shows a wide range of values for mean nuclear area within a given tumour, emphasizing the heterogeneity and interobserver variation that is seen in their classification [22]. The majority of tumours had a mean nuclear size more characteristic of partially transformed germinal-centre lymphocytes. This variation and identification of three constituent cell populations showed the lack of a constant relationship to a counterpart transformed cell in benign nodes. As in previous studies of reactive hyperplasia, follicular lymphoma, mantle zone and centrocytic lymphoma [16–19,21], these workers questioned the validity of the Lukes–Collins and Kiel concept of NHL classification being based and modelled on their benign cell equivalents in an actively transforming follicle. However, these high-grade lesions undoubtedly had larger, more irregularly shaped nuclei, and nuclear shape (NCI) combined with immunochemistry has proven helpful in distinguishing histiocytic from centroblastic and immunoblastic NHL [23]. Morphometry also achieved an 88% separation of centroblastic and immunoblastic NHL using discriminant analysis based on the following parameters: nucleolar area, cytoplasm/nucleus ratio, number of nucleoli per cross-section, relative nucleolar eccentricity (rNE) and the percentage of immunoblasts [24]. Immunoblasts were defined morphometrically as being $>28\ \mu m^2$, with one nucleolus and an rNE of <0.45. Immunoblast percentage was the most important distinguishing feature, followed by nucleolar number and eccentricity. Centroblastic lymphomas had a greater number of small nucleoli which were variably sited, especially towards the periphery of the nucleus (Fig. 4.15). Complete group separation was not achieved and it was observed that these lesions form a morphological spectrum with transitional cases. The clinical relevance of the definition of these tumour cell types was emphasized, as pure centroblastic lymphomas (with a nodular low-power architecture) are large-cell NHLs with a relatively good prognosis. Broadly similar results and conclusions were obtained by the same workers using cytological preparations where mean nucleolar area and the percentage of immunoblasts emerged strongly from the discriminant analysis

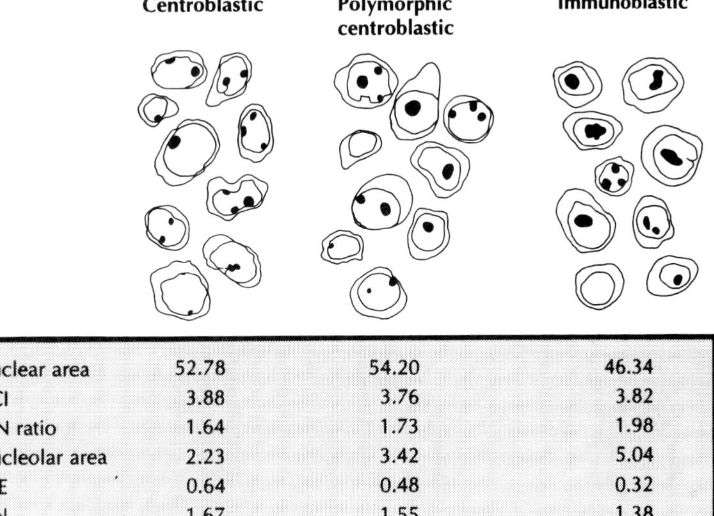

	Centroblastic	Polymorphic centroblastic	Immunoblastic
Nuclear area	52.78	54.20	46.34
NCI	3.88	3.76	3.82
C/N ratio	1.64	1.73	1.98
Nucleolar area	2.23	3.42	5.04
rNE	0.64	0.48	0.32
n/N	1.67	1.55	1.38

Fig. 4.15 Graphic examples of morphometric data derived from the spectrum of large-cell (centroblastic, immunoblastic) non-Hodgkin's lymphoma. The equivalent data are listed below each example. NCI, nuclear contour index; rNE, relative nucleolar eccentricity. From van der Valk *et al.* [24].

[25]. Shape analytical morphometry of nuclear and nucleolar contours in tissue sections also discriminates between centroblastic and immunoblastic lymphoma with a claimed 97% efficiency [26].

One of the characteristic features of T-cell lymphoma is its cellular heterogeneity and pleomorphism. Morphometry has confirmed marked variation in nuclear area and shape. This is particularly so in nuclei $>25\,\mu m^2$ where this variability contrasts with the greater degree of regularity that reactive paracortical lymphocytes show as they progressively enlarge [27]. However, it should be noted that there was considerable overlap in cellular measurements between reactive nodes and T-zone lymphomas. Sigaux *et al.* [28] found that nuclear area, its coefficient of variation and nuclear irregularity differed with the various distinct subclasses of peripheral T-cell NHL. Morphometry has also been suggested as a means of distinguishing Burkitt-like lymphoma from neuroendocrine carcinoma of the nasal cavity [29].

Immunoassay of the nuclear proliferation antigen Ki-67 shows its cell count index to correlate with NHL grade [30]. In addition, the minority of low-grade lymphomas with a high index had worse survival than the majority with a low score. Interestingly, high-grade lesions with a very high index survived longer than other equivalent lesions due to an increased response to therapy achieving either a complete or partial remission [31]. Comparable results for Ki-67 staining are achieved in tissue sections and fine-needle aspirate material [32]. A parallel study of tritiated thymidine uptake, volume spectroscopy and flow cytometry in NHL cell suspensions separated them from reactive nodal populations [33]. There was marked heterogeneity in ^{3}H-thymidine uptake, especially in low-grade centrocytic/centroblastic and lymphoplasmacytoid lymphoma. High-grade centroblastic and immunoblastic lymphomas had significantly increased ^{3}H-thymidine uptake, nuclear and cell volumes, DNA index and aneuploid cell components. In addition, patients with localized disease (stage I and II) and constitutional (B) symptoms had greater uptake. This is presumably due to the cell type being more frequently of the high-grade variety, leading to earlier clinical presentation and more restricted disease bulk at the time of biopsy. Morphometric measures of nuclear size also correlate with PCNA staining [34].

4.16.2 Hodgkin's lymphoma

The wide range of constituent cell types forms the basis of the Rye classification of Hodgkin's disease [35], but is also the reason why there is considerable interobserver variation in its application, with only nodular sclerosis being designated with any degree of consistency [36]. In general differential cell counts support the classification, although they illustrate minor discrepancies between subjective and objective appraisal of lymphoid and mononuclear cell distribution in the various categories [37]. The proportions of macrophage numbers are lymphocyte-predominant (1.8–16%), nodular sclerosis (13.6–22.1%) and mixed cellularity (6.5–14.6%) and there is a marked increase in lymphocyte-depleted Hodgkin's disease (39.8–47.7%). In the lymphocyte-predominant group they have a bimodal distribution with the second peak attributed to the lymphocytic and histiocytic variant [38].

The numbers of eosinophil polymorphonuclear leucocytes are increased and cell counts show variation with Rye classification histological subtype as follows: lymphocyte-predominant 0.24%, nodular sclerosis 13.2%, mixed cellularity 5.35%, lymphocyte depletion 22.6% [39]. Mast cells are few in number in lymphocyte-predominant, depleted and mixed cellularity Hodgkin's disease but much more prevalent in nodular sclerosis [40]. The biological significance of these findings is uncertain but they serve to emphasize one aspect of the heterogeneity of cellular composition upon which the histological diagnosis is based. Semiautomatic image analysis of Hodgkin's Reed–Sternberg cells and anaplastic large-cell lymphoma shows a continuous spectrum of nuclear and nucleolar areas and circularity as well as immunoexpression [41]. There is considerable intercase and intergroup variability in nuclear and nucleolar size and profile. Interestingly, the most significant features capable of separating the two groups are the numbers of granulocytes and lymphocytes which are depleted in anaplastic large-cell lymphoma. Freeman *et al.* [42] regard Hodgkin's disease as a high-grade lymphoma with the mononuclear Hodgkin's and Reed–Sternberg cells the neoplastic element: they are highly proliferative, being PCNA-positive and AgNOR-rich.

4.16.3 Thymus

Image analysis of thymic germinal centres in patients with myasthenia gravis shows that there is an inverse correlation between mean area, perimeter and diameter and signs of clinical improvement [43]. Morphometry reveals nuclear area of epithelial cells in thymoma to be greater than those of thymic hyperplasia and normal thymus [44]. The nuclei of invasive thymomas are also larger than non-invasive lesions. In addition the values for thymoma associated with myasthenia gravis are similar to those of invasive cases, suggesting that they might have premalignant potential.

4.16.4 Spleen

Eyepiece graticule point-counting has shown that infants dying from sudden infant death syndrome or cot death have more splenic lymphoid and germinal-centre tissue than controls, indicating a greater amount of postnatal antigenic stimulation [45]. Cell suspensions of lymph nodes and spleen involved by Hodgkin's disease have increased numbers of T cells, while the splenic percentage of B cells is reduced [46]. The white pulp, B-cell and germinal-centre areas are unchanged. The red pulp has a marked increase in the number of capillaries [47], whereas the pulp cords and sinuses are expanded in hairy-cell leukaemia [48]. Morphometry has also shown hairy cells to be quantitatively different from other small-cell lymphomas [49].

4.16.5 Conclusion

Quantitation illustrates the range of cellular geometric dimensions and composition that act as a basis for the histological classification of both Hodgkin's disease and NHL. Nuclear size and shape give some insight into the cellular antecedents of NHL and serve to distinguish low-grade from high-grade malignancy. The latter have larger cells with greater DNA content and can be characterized as centroblastic or immunoblastic by their nucleolar size and distribution characteristics. These various morphological subtypes confer differing prognoses and survival, although this is outweighed by clinical stage of disease. Nuclear size may act as a guide to malignancy in thymomas.

References

1 Patt DJ, Brynes RK, Vardiman JW, Coppleson LW. Mesocolic lymph node histology is an important prognostic indicator for patients with carcinoma of the sigmoid colon: an immunomorphologic study. *Cancer* 1975; 35: 1388–1397.

2 Resta L, Cimmino A, Facilone F, Santangelo A. Computer-aided morphometric analysis of lymph nodes draining laryngeal carcinomas. *Appl Pathol* 1986; 4: 108–112.

3 van der Loo EM, Cornelisse CJ, van Vloten WA, van der Velde EA, Scheffer E, Meijer CJLM. Diagnostic morphometry of isolated lymph node cells from patients with mycosis fungoides and Sézary's syndrome. *Virchows Arch B, Cell Pathol* 1980; 33: 107–116.

4 Stevens MWI, Fazzalari NL, Crisp DJ. Lymph node cellular morphology: comparative study of imprints and cytocentrifuge smears. *J Clin Pathol* 1987; 40: 751–755.

5 Dawsey SM, Korn EL, Layfield LJ. Morphometric analysis of the homogeneity of lymphoid cell populations in fine needle aspiration cytology smears. *Am J Clin Pathol* 1989; 92: 458–464.

6 Guigui B, Raphael M, Nonnenmacher L, Boisnic S, Binet JL. Prognostic significance of a morphometric study of lymph node biopsies in chronic lymphocytic leukaemia. *Scand J Haematol* 1986; 37: 371–379.

7 Dardick I, Dardick AM. Morphometry of normal human lymphoid tissues. Nuclear parameters for comparative studies of lymphoma. *Arch Pathol Lab Med* 1984; 108: 190–196.

8 Crocker J. Morphometric and related quantitative techniques in the study of lymphoid neoplasms. *J Pathol* 1984; 143: 69–80.

9 Abbott CR, Blewitt RW, Bird CC. Quantitative analysis of non-Hodgkin's lymphoma. *J Clin Pathol* 1982; 35: 135–138.

10 Crocker J, Curran RC. A study of nuclear diameters in lymph node imprints using the Zeiss Microvideomat. *J Clin Pathol* 1979; 32: 670–674.

11 Crocker J, Jones EL, Curran RC. Study of nuclear diameters in non-Hodgkin's lymphomas. *J Clin Pathol* 1982; 35: 954–958.

12 Zardawi IM, Firman DW, Sims TA. Stereological analysis of non-Hodgkin's lymphomas. *Pathology* 1984; 16: 387–392.

13 van der Valk P, Mosch A, Kurver PJ. Morphometric characterisation of 52 B cell non-Hodgkin's lymphomas. *J Clin Pathol* 1983; 36: 289–297.

14 Stevens MW, Crowley KS, Fazzalari NL. Use of morphometry cytological preparations for diagnosing follicular non-Hodgkin's lymphomas. *J Clin Pathol* 1988; 41: 370–377.

15 Crocker J, Jones EL, Curran RC. A quantitative study of the size of benign and malignant lymphoid collicles. *J Clin Pathol* 1983; 36: 1055–1061.

16 Dardick I, Caldwell DR, Bailey DB, Dardick AM, Jeans MTD. Nuclear morphologic and morphometric analyses of nodular poorly differentiated lymphocytic lymphoma. Assessment of small cleaved nuclei. *Hum Pathol* 1985; 16: 1187–1199.

17 Tosi P, Leoncini L, Spina D, Del Vecchio MT. Morphometric nuclear analysis of lymphoid cells in center cell lymphomas and in reactive germinal centers. *Am J Pathol* 1984; 117: 12–17.

18 Dardick I, Cavell S, Moher D, Seely P, Dardick A, Burns BF. Ultrastructural morphometric study of follicular center lymphocytes. I. Nuclear characteristics and the Lukes-Collins concept. *Ultrastruct Pathol* 1989; 13: 373–391.

19 Dardick I, Cavell S, Moher D *et al.* Ultrastructural morphometric study of follicular center lymphocytes. II. Analyses of cleaved-cell populations do not support the Lukes-Collins concept. *Ultrastruct Pathol* 1989; 13: 393–404.

20 Dardick I, Moher D, Cavell S *et al.* An ultrastructural morphometric study of follicular center lymphocytes: III. The control of lymphocyte nuclear size in reactive hyperplasia and non-Hodgkin's lymphoma. *Mod Pathol* 1990; 3: 176–185.

21 Tosi P, Luzi P, Leoncini L, Rivano MT, Barbini P, Pileri S. Mantle zone lymphoma: a morphometric comparison with centrocytic and immunocytic lymphomas and reactive secondary follicles. *Hum Pathol* 1988; 9: 1293–1300.

22 Dardick I, Caldwell DR, McCaughey WTE, Al-Jabi M. Nuclear morphologic and morphometric analyses of large non-cleaved cell and immunoblastic non-Hodgkin's lymphomas. *Hum Pathol* 1984; 15: 965–972.

23 van der Valk P, Herman SJ, Brand R, Cornelisse CJ, Spaander PJ, Meijer CJLM. Morphometric characterisation of diffuse large cell (histiocytic) lymphomas. *Am J Pathol* 1982; 107: 327–335.

24 van der Valk P, Ball P, Mosch A, Meijer CJLM. Large cell lymphomas. I. Differential diagnosis of centroblastic and B-immunoblastic subtypes by morphometry on histologic preparations. *Cancer* 1984; 54: 2082–2087.

25 Ball PJ, van der Valk P, Kurver PHJ, Lindeman J, Meijer CJLM. Large cell lymphoma. II. Differential diagnosis of centroblastic and B-immunoblastic subtypes by morphometry on cytologic preparations. *Cancer* 1985; 55: 486–492.

26 Ricco R, De Benedictis G, Lettini T *et al.* Non-Hodgkin's lymphoma diagnosis aided by the SAM system. *Pathol Res Pract* 1989; 185: 719–721.

27 Tosi P, Leoncini L, Baak JPA, Luzi P, Cintorino M, Barbini P. Comparative morphometric analysis of nuclear area and shape in peripheral T-zone lymphomas and in paracortical areas of normal and reactive lymph nodes. *Anal Quant Cytol Histol* 1988; 10: 285–293.

28 Sigaux F, Flandrin G, Valensi F. Can peripheral T-cell

lymphomas be morphologically subclassified? A morphometric approach to 21 cases. *Cytometry* 1986; 7: 371–377.
29 Payne CM, Smith WL, Grogan TM, Nagle RB, Paplanus SH, Palmer T. Ultrastructural morphometry distinguishes Burkitt's-like lymphomas from neuroendocrine neoplasms: useful criteria applied to the evaluation of a poorly differentiated neuroendocrine neoplasm of the nasal cavity masquerading as Burkitt's-like lymphoma. *Mod Pathol* 1989; 2: 35–45.
30 Houmand A, Abrahamsen B, Tinggaard Pedersen N. Relevance of Ki-67 expression in the classification of non-Hodgkin's lymphomas: a morphometric and double-immunostaining study. *Histopathology* 1992; 20: 13–20.
31 Hall PA, Richards MA, Grehory WM, d'Ardenne AJ, Lister TA, Stansfeld AG. The prognostic value of Ki-67 immunostaining in non-Hodgkin's lymphoma. *J Pathol* 1988; 154: 223–235.
32 Brown DC, Gatter KC, Mason DY. Proliferation in non-Hodgkin's lymphoma: a comparison of Ki-67 staining on fine needle aspiration and cryostat sections. *J Clin Pathol* 1990; 43: 325–328.
33 Kvaloy S, Godal T, Marton PF, Steen H, Brennhovd IO, Abrahamsen AF. Spontaneous [^{3}H]-thymidine uptake in histological subgroups of human B cell lymphomas. *Scand J Haematol* 1981; 26: 221–234.
34 Swerdlow SH, Westermann CD, Pelstring RJ, Saboorian MH, Williams ME. Growth fraction in centrocytic and follicular centre cell lymphomas: assessment in paraffin sections with a proliferating cell nuclear antigen antibody and morphometric correlates. *Hum Pathol* 1993; 24: 540–546.
35 Lukes RJ, Craver LH, Hall TC, Rappaport H, Ruben P. Report of the Nomenclature Committee. *Cancer Res* 1966; 26: 1311.
36 Holman CDJ, Matz LR, Finlay-Jones LR *et al.* Interobserver variation in the histopathological reporting of Hodgkin's disease and analysis of diagnostic subcomponents using Kappa statistics. *Histopathology* 1983; 7: 399–407.
37 Livesey AE, Sutherland FI, Brown RA, Beck JS, Macgillivray JB, Slidders W. Cytological basis of histological typing of diffuse Hodgkin's disease. Demonstration of an implied misnomer in the terminology of the Rye classification. *J Clin Pathol* 1978; 31: 551–559.
38 Crocker J, Jones EL, Curran RC. A quantitative study of a-naphthyl acetate esterase-positive cells in Hodgkin's disease. *J Clin Pathol* 1982; 35: 1301–1306.
39 Fuggle WJ, Crocker J, Smith PJ. A quantitative study of eosinophil polymorphs in Hodgkin's disease. *J Clin Pathol* 1984; 37: 267–271.
40 Crocker J, Smith PJ. A quantitative study of mast cells in Hodgkin's disease. *J Clin Pathol* 1984; 37: 519–522.
41 Leoncini L, Del Vecchio MT, Kraft R *et al.* Hodgkin's disease and CD30-positive anaplastic large cell lymphomas – a continuous spectrum of malignant disorders. A quantitative morphometric and immunohistologic study. *Am J Pathol* 1990; 137: 1047–1057.
42 Freeman J, Kellock DB, Yu C-WC, Crocker J, Levison DA, Hall PA. Proliferating cell nuclear antigen (PCNA) and nucleolar organiser regions in Hodgkin's disease: correlation with morphology. *J Clin Pathol* 1993; 46: 446–449.
43 Moran CA, Suster S, Gil J, Jagirdar M. Morphometric analysis of germinal centers in non-thymomatous patients with myasthenia gravis. *Arch Pathol Lab Med* 1990; 114: 689–691.
44 Nomori H, Horinouchi H, Kaseda S, Ishihara T, Torikata C. Evaluation of the malignant grade of thymoma by morphometric analysis. *Cancer* 1988; 61: 982–988.
45 Barzanji AJ, Emergy JL. Quantitative study of the lymphatic tissue and germinal centres in the spleen in infants dying from expected and unexpected causes (cot deaths). *Histopathology* 1977; 1: 445–449.
46 Pinkus GS, Barbuto D, Said JW. Lymphocyte subpopulations of lymph nodes and spleens in Hodgkin's disease. *Cancer* 1978; 42: 1270–1279.
47 van Krieken JHJM, Te Velde J, Hermans J, Welvaart K. The splenic red pulp; a histomorphometrical study in splenectomy specimens embedded in methylmethacrylate. *Histopathology* 1985; 9: 401–416.
48 Re G, Pileri S, Cau R, Bucchi ML, Casali AM, Cavelli G. Histometry of splenic microvascular architecture in hairy cell leukaemia. *Histopathology* 1988; 13: 425–434.
49 Meijer CJLM, van der Valk P, Jansen J. Hairy cell leukaemia: an immunohistochemic and morphometric study. *Semin Oncol* 1984; 11: 347–352.

4.17 BONE MARROW

Morphometry has been applied to both bone marrow aspirate and trephine biopsy samples. Differential white cell counts on paired specimens show that trephines yield relatively more immature myeloid forms and aspirates more lymphocytes and polymorphs [1]. Image cytometry of marrow aspirates has characterized normal erythropoiesis [2], granulopoiesis [3] and blast cells in refractory anaemia [4]. This showed that haemopoietic maturation is associated with changes in nuclear area, nuclear outline and cytoplasmic hue. Aspirates and trephines are complementary techniques, each capable of affording valuable clinical information. Aspirate material gives better morphological and immunological preservation for the detailed subtyping of leukaemia and lymphoma. Trephines are particularly useful in estimating disease bulk and pattern of infiltration, e.g., focal, interstitial or diffuse. The nature of a dry tap becomes evident as to whether it is on the basis of aplasia or a packed marrow. Trephines are also better at establishing the presence of fibrosis and secondary carcinoma. Use of plastic embedded semithin sections has been advocated but current practice finds that routinely processed high-quality paraffin sections yield good cytological detail sufficient for diagnostic purposes [5].

4.17.1 Lymphoblastic leukaemia

Aspirate samples from a series of 21 children with acute lymphoblastic leukaemia (ALL) were studied by semiautomatic image analysis [6]. Cell area was larger and nuclear/cell area ratio smaller in short-term survivors than in those who died. Bivariate graphs of these two parameters gave reasonable group separation, although there was a degree of overlap. This is indicative of the morphological continuum that exists and the difficulties that are encountered in attempting to apply a subjective classification, such as the three-tier French–American–British system. It is based on semiquantitative estimates of nuclear cytoplasmic ratio, number and prominence of nucleoli, nuclear membrane outline and cell size [7]. Quantitation has shown that the two features usually given most weight (nuclear/cell area ratio and prominence of nucleoli) are in fact the most subjective and instrumental in the variation in concordance [8]. All cells have measurably larger nuclei with more heterochromatin and less cytoplasm than those of acute myeloid leukaemia [9] and this may be helpful in making this important clinical distinction.

4.17.2 Megakaryocytes, myeloproliferative disease

In thrombocytopenia it is important to know the marrow content of megakaryocytes. Decreased numbers indicate a central failure of production, whilst a normal or increased value implies peripheral destruction. Simple cell counts over 50 HPFs of 5 μm paraffin sections of normal marrow showed overall haemopoietic cellularity to be about 72%. The mean number of megakaryocytes per HPF was 1.5 and this did not vary with age or sex [10]. More recently, normal marrow trephine biopsies have been studied using morphometry and immunochemistry (monoclonal antibody against a platelet glycoprotein) to identify and define the range of precursors in megakaryocyte production [11]. For example, promegakaryoblasts had a frequency of 140/mm^3 and constituted 8% of positively stained megakaryocytic elements. They were characterized by a size of 41.5 μm^2, a diameter of 7.7 μm, a high nuclear cytoplasmic ratio (0.32) and nearly circular outlines of their nuclear and cellular perimeters. A note of caution was sounded about using morphometry on aspirate samples as megakaryocyte size increased, probably due to flattening.

Thiele and others have studied a wide range of myeloproliferative disorders using morphometry on bone marrow trephines. Quantitative estimates of marrow megakaryopoiesis and elevated peripheral blood platelet counts separated various myeloproliferative disorders into two major categories as follows: (i) controls, chronic granulocytic leukaemia and myelitis; and (ii) agnogenic myeloid metaplasia, osteomyelofibrosis/sclerosis, polycythaemia vera, reactive thrombocytosis and primary thrombocythaemia [12]. In particular primary thrombocythaemia showed a combination of normal megakaryocytic maturation and nuclear polyploidy as in polycythaemia vera. This suggested that it represents a monolinear growth of megakaryopoiesis similar to that of granulopoiesis in chronic myeloid leukaemia, and contrasting with the atypia and mixed cellularity of myeloid metaplasia and osteomyolofibrosis. This study was based on enumeration of megakaryocytes, their density, cellular and nuclear dimensions and outline. As mentioned previously, this group of workers have employed a combined morphometric and immunohistochemical approach better to define marrow megakaryopoiesis. They have found significant differences in several megakaryocytic parameters (frequency, size, shape of nuclei) between osteomyelofibrosis/sclerosis and chronic myeloid leukaemia [13]. The numbers of megakaryocytes and promegakaryoblasts are also increased in the various subtypes of the myelodysplastic syndrome and there is a predominance of small forms. Their morphometrically determined nuclear features and nuclear cytoplasmic ratio are more pleomorphic than in chronic myeloid leukaemia, indicative of the severe haemopoietic defect that is present in myelodysplasia [14]. Interestingly, megakaryopoiesis was found to be decreased postchemotherapy. In chronic myeloid leukaemia megakaryopoiesis shows a non-disorderly expansion allied to a proportional increase in the platelet count. As in myelodysplasia there is also significant nuclear size reduction [15]. A cohort of 65 patients with chronic myeloid leukaemia was separated into two groups with differing survivals as follows: group I (24 months' survival, megakaryocytic subtype, with fibrosis) and group II (36 months' survival, granulocytic subtype). Histological variables that showed significant correlation with prognosis were density of neutrophils and reticulin fibres, and the ratio of granulopoiesis to megakaryopoiesis [16]. Further regression analysis of histomorphometric and clinical data such as peripheral blood neutrophil and myeloblast percentages, liver size, the amount of granulopoiesis and marrow reticulin density identified two groups with survival periods of 14 and 41 months respectively. Two of the histomorphometric marrow parameters, namely the amount of granulopoiesis and reticulin fibre density, had significant correlation with prognosis.

In acute non-lymphatic leukaemia the presence of fibrosis does not correlate with survival [17], whereas better remission and prognosis are achieved in those cases with greater median megakaryocyte diameters [18]. Assay of PCNA-labelling index and Ki-67 staining shows proliferation to be markedly increased in polycythaemia rubra vera [19]. Enhanced PCNA staining may also help to identify cases of myelodysplastic syndrome evolving into overt leukaemia [20].

4.17.3 Myeloma

Multiple myeloma is a clinicopathological diagnosis comprising anaemia, painful osteolytic bone lesions, an IgM monoclonal paraprotein, Bence-Jones protein in the urine and bone marrow plasmacytosis. Morphometry demonstrates significant correlations between the number of osteoblasts, lytic bone lesions, serum IgM titre and marrow plasma cell density [21]. The latter separated myeloma of the plasmacytic type from reactive plasmacytosis but did not discriminate it from benign monoclonal gammopathy of uncertain significance. However, van der Sandt *et al.* [22] have claimed that this distinction can be made by assessing nuclear eccentricity, area, cytoplasmic area and their ratios.

4.17.4 Conclusion

Quantitation in bone marrow disease varies greatly in its sophistication. Simple semiquantitative estimates such as whether the blast or plasma cell percentage is less or more than 30% are the most frequently used in everyday practice for the diagnosis of acute leukaemia and myeloma. Morphometry has identified that increased cell size is of better prognosis in lymphoblastic leukaemia of childhood. It has established a range of values for megakaryopoiesis in normal marrow and chronic myeloproliferative disorders. It can predict differing survival rates in chronic myeloid leukaemia on the basis of the proportions of granulopoiesis, megakaryopoiesis and reticulin content.

References

1 Wilkins BS, O'Brien CJ. Techniques for obtaining differential cell counts from bone marrow trephine biopsy specimens. *J Clin Pathol* 1988; 41: 558–561.
2 Gauvain C, Seigneurin D, Brugal G. A quantitative analysis of the human bone marrow erythroblastic cell lineage using the SAMBA 200 cell image processor. I. The normal maturation sequence. *Anal Quant Cytol Histol* 1987; 9: 253–262.
3 Seigneurin D, Gauvain C, Brugal G. A quantitative analysis of the human bone marrow granulocytic cell lineage using the SAMBA 200 cell image processor. I. The normal maturation sequence. *Anal Quant Cytol* 1984; 6: 168–178.
4 Seigneurin D, Brugal G, Payard D, Gauvain C. A quantitative analysis of the human bone marrow granulocytic cell lineage using the SAMBA 200 cell image processor. II. The blast cells in refractory anaemia with an excess of blasts. *Anal Quant Cytol Histol* 1986; 8: 281–292.
5 Gatter KC, Heryet A, Brown DC, Mason DY. Is it necessary to embed bone marrow biopsies in plastic for haematological diagnosis? *Histopathology* 1987; 1: 1–7.
6 Tosi P, Luzi P, Miracco C *et al.* Morphometry for the prognosis of acute lymphoblastic leukemia in child-

hood. *Pathol Res Pract* 1987; 416–420.

7 Bennett JM, Catovsky D, Daniel MT *et al.* French–American–British (FAB) co-operative group. Proposals for the classification of the acute leukaemia. *Br J Haematol* 1976; 33: 451–458.

8 Childs CC, Stass SA, Bennett JM. The morphologic classification of acute lymphoblastic leukemia in childhood. Observations on concordance using a simple scoring system. *Am J Clin Pathol* 1986; 86: 503–506.

9 Ochiai F, Eguchi M. Morphometrical evaluation of acute leukemic cells by electron microscopy. Discrepancy between morphological characteristics in FAB classification and electron microscopic morphometry. *Virchows Arch (B)* 1987; 52: 403–411.

10 Singal R, Belliveau RR. Quantitation of megakaryocytes in normal bone marrow. *Anal Quant Cytol Histol* 1988; 10: 33–36.

11 Thiele J, Wagner S, Dienemann D, Weinhold S, Fischer R, Stein H. Megakaryocyte precursors (promegakaryoblasts and megakaryoblasts) in the normal human bone marrow. An immunohistochemical and morphometric study on routinely processed trephine biopsies. *Anal Quant Cytol Histol* 1990; 12: 285–289.

12 Thiele J, Funke S, Holgado S, Choritz H, Georgii A. Megakaryopoiesis in chronic myeloproliferative diseases. A morphometric evaluation with special emphasis on primary thrombocythemia. *Anal Quant Cytol* 1984; 6: 155–167.

13 Thiele J, Steinberg T, Hoeppner B *et al.* Histo- and immunomorphometry of megakaryopoiesis in chronic myeloid leukaemia with myelofibrosis and so-called (idiopathic) osteo-myelofibrosis/-sclerosis. *Anal Cell Pathol* 1990; 2: 215–227.

14 Thiele J, Quitmann H, Wagner S, Fischer R. Dysmegakaryopoiesis in myelodysplastic syndromes (MDS): an immunomorphometric study of bone marrow trephine biopsy specimens. *J Clin Pathol* 1991; 44: 300–305.

15 Thiele J, Wagner S, Weuste R *et al.* An immunomorphometric study on megakaryocyte precursor cells in bone marrow tissue from patients with chronic myeloid leukemia (CML). *Eur J Haematol* 1990; 44: 63–70.

16 Thiele J, Wienhold S, Zankovich R, Fischer R. A histomorphometric analysis of trephine biopsies of bone marrow from 65 patients with chronic myeloid leukaemia. Classification of patients into subgroups with different survival patterns. *Anal Quant Cytol Histol* 1990; 12: 103–116.

17 Fohlmeister I, Klein H, Thiele J. Morphometric assessment of bone marrow fiber content in acute nonlymphatic leukaemia at presentation. *Anal Quant Cytol Histol* 1988; 10: 110–114.

18 Brody JP, Krause JR. Morphometric study of megakaryocytes size and prognosis in adults with acute non-lymphatic leukaemia. *Leuk Res* 1986; 10: 475–480.

19 Thiele J, Meuter RB, Titius RB, Zankovich R, Fisher R. Proliferating cell nuclear antigen expression by erythroid precursors in normal bone marrow, in reactive lesions and in polycythaemia rubra vera. *Histopathology* 1993; 22: 429–435.

20 Kitagawa N, Kamiyama R, Kasuga T. Expression of the proliferating cell nuclear antigen in bone marrow cells from patients with myelodysplastic syndromes and aplastic anaemia. *Hum Pathol* 1993; 24: 359–363.

21 Thiele J, Arenz B, Klein H. Differentiation of plasma cell infiltrates in the bone marrow. A clinicopathological study on 80 patients including immunohistochemistry and morphometry. *Virchows Arch [A]* 1988; 412: 553–562.

22 van Der Sandt MM, Lindeman J, Herman CJ. Morphometry of plasma cell dyscrasias. *Lab Invest* 1985; 52: 72–75.

4.18 SYNOVIUM, SOFT TISSUES AND MUSCLE

4.18.1 Synovium and soft tissues

There has been relatively little use of tissue morphometry in the study of synovial disease. Most papers have adopted a semiquantitative approach and in only a minority have cell numbers been counted, unlike joint fluid where this is standard. Despite this, these studies provide some diagnostically useful information. In rheumatoid arthritis, gout, pseudogout, systemic lupus erythematosus, infectious arthritis and degenerative joint disease the main specific characteristics are bacteria (infection), crystals (gout/pseudogout) and lymphoid follicles (rheumatoid arthritis). There is wide variation in the total cellularity, differential leucocyte counts and correlation of cell types between the synovial lining and joint fluid content [1]. For example, degenerative joint disease is paucicellular and infective arthritis polymorph-rich, whilst rheumatoid disease joint fluid contains numerous polymorphs but its synovial lining is significantly hyperplastic, covered by fibrin and infiltrated by mononuclear cells.

Cooper *et al.* [2] used semiquantitative scoring of multiple histological parameters to create a synovial biopsy profile for each clinical diagnostic group. From this databank they could statistically determine the likelihood of any particular synovial biopsy belonging to one of paired clinical groups. Agreement between the clinical and discriminant function diagnoses ranged from 54 to 78% and was best for differentiating osteoarthritis and rheumatoid arthritis. Morphometry has shown that there is a marked increase in synovial mononuclear cell density in rheumatoid disease over osteoarthritis and differences in lymphocyte subsets [3]. In rheumatoid arthritis there are increased numbers of plasma cells staining for immunoglobulins in the following order: IgM, IgA and IgG [4]. There is a preferential increase in IgM-containing cells, reflecting localized production of IgM rheumatoid factor by the inflamed synovium. Cell counts in rheumatoid disease show increased expression of HLA-DR macrophage-like interdigitating cells, forming close links with helper T cells. This is interpreted as indicating a disease of T-lymphocyte/macrophage immunoregulation [5,6] and the interaction is instrumental in determining the ultimate architecture of the inflammatory infiltrate in the rheumatoid synovium [7].

For a concise overview of synovial biopsy pathology, the reader is directed to Revell [8].

Quantitation of soft-tissue tumours has concentrated mainly on indices of proliferation, such as mitoses and DNA content, as a guide to designation and prognosis. The reader is referred to a standard text [9]. One example where systematic quantitation has been applied is malignant fibrous histiocytoma [10]. Disease-free survival is related to DNA index and overall survival to a nuclear shape factor.

4.18.2 Muscle

R. W. LYNESS (co-author)

The role of muscle biopsy in the diagnosis of muscle disease is well reviewed by Weller [11]. It is crucial to interpret it in tandem with family history, age of the patient, clinical features and other investigations such as electromyography and serum creatinine phosphokinase. This integrated approach allows appropriate diagnosis, treatment, prognostication and genetic counselling for relatives, with classification into categories of neurogenic muscle disease, disorders of neuromuscular transmission and primary myopathies. There are a number of characteristic histological and histochemical appearances in congenital, metabolic and destructive myopathies (e.g., polymyositis) and muscular dystrophy. Being an invasive technique, it is essential to optimize the information derived from it.

Histological examination of skeletal muscle is usually carried out on a biopy from a limb muscle. The selection of muscle and site for biopsy is important as the distribution of fibre types varies and may be of one predominant kind in a particular muscle group, e.g., deltoid or calf muscles. The belly of the muscle also yields more diagnostic clues than its insertions. The main aim is to determine whether the muscular abnormality is part of a systemic condition (e.g., polyarteritis nodosa, amyloidosis, drugs, cystocercosis); secondary to disease affecting the muscle nerve supply (e.g., infantile spinal muscular atrophy, amyotrophic lateral sclerosis, diabetic neuropathy); or a primary myopathy (e.g., Duchenne muscular dystrophy, myotonica dystrophica) which is usually congenital. Longitudinal and transverse sections are both necessary for examination, morphometry being performed on the latter. Histological assessment includes the presence, site and nature of any inflammatory process, the quality of intermuscular connective tissue, the size of muscle fascicles and uniformity of fibres within them. Contiguous fibre groups are examined for signs of group atrophy or hypertrophy and the site of these changes within the fascicles. Atrophy, hypertrophy, fibre-splitting, central nuclei, nuclear-clumping and phagocytosis by monocytes of individual fibres are noted [12]. The information derived has been greatly enhanced by the ability to define different fibre subtypes, their number, size and distribution within normal and diseased muscle. Preincubation of frozen sections with myofibrillar adenosine triphosphatase (ATPase) at pH 4.3, 4.6 and 9.4 differentiates a black/white chequerboard pattern of type 1 (slow-twitch) and types 2A, 2B, 2C (fast-twitch) fibres normally present in a ratio type 1/type 2 of 1 : 2. Fibre-type enumeration, distribution and measurement of shortest cross-sectional diameter (least affected by the plane of section) are facilitated, these factors varying with age, sex, physique, anatomical site and disease category.

Evidence is sought for loss of the normal myofibrillar ATPase pattern. Muscle fibre-type grouping denotes a process of denervation/reinnervation [13,14]. Predominance of one fibre type (e.g., type I myopathy >55%) may either be real or apparent, due to loss of other types, and can only be established by fibre counts in comparison with normal controls. Both fibre types may be atrophic or hypertrophic and this is determined by morphometry of fibre transverse diameters and histographic techniques [15]. Atrophy and compensatory hypertrophy may coexist in the same biopsy. Selective type 1 atrophy is diagnostic of myotonica dystrophica and type 2 atrophy a non-specific change in ageing, general debility, prolonged steroid therapy and neurogenic abnormalities [16]. Varying degrees of fibre atrophy, grouping, angulation and compensatory hypertrophy suggest a neurogenic aetiology. Myopathic patterns are characterized by absence of small angular fibres, differing combinations of atrophy or hypertrophy in one or both fibre types and absolute or relative fibre-type deficiency. The dystrophies show severe myofibre hypertrophy.

Morphometric quantitation, in addition to the histological appearance of a muscle biopsy, is therefore crucial in its assessment [17,18]. Fibre-type transverse diameters may be determined by a simple eyepiece micrometer calibrated against a graduated scale, linear measurement of photographic enlargement, semiautomated or automated image analysis computerized techniques. The latter methods enable more rapid fibre-type enumeration and construction of fibre-size distribution histograms, giving visual comparison with the range of fibres in normal biopsies and direct assessment of atrophy or hypertrophy. Reports may include fibre-type means, SDs and coefficients of variation in transverse diameter. The computer software also allows assimilation of various other morphometric variables (e.g., shape, percentage of internal nuclei) and statistical and distribution data from the measurements. Quantitation can potentially detect early, mild pathological changes or where the sampled muscle is focally involved and chart the severity, progression or regression of disease in serial biopsies. It is important that a representative sample is obtained and usually all the fibres in an arbitrary number of fields (not fewer than five) chosen at random are measured. Standard practice is for at least 100 fibres of each type (200 in total) to be assessed and most needle biopsies have sufficient material for quantitation [18]. Semiautomated computerized techniques compare favourably with manual methods for accuracy, reproducibility and ease of acquisition of data and are now routinely used in diagnostic laboratories [19]. No doubt muscle histochemistry will become amenable to the segmentation capabilities of automated systems and lend itself to developments such as HOME (Highly Optimized Microscope Environment) [20].

4.18.3 Conclusion

Quantitation has given some insight into the pathogenesis of synovial disease and assessment of proliferation factors has a role to play in the prognostication of soft-tissue tumours. Morphometry is crucial in evaluating a muscle biopsy but must be viewed in comparison with normal controls matched for age, sex and anatomical site.

References

1 Goldenberg DL, Cohen AS. Synovial membrane histopathology in the differential diagnosis of rheumatoid arthritis, gout, pseudogout, systemic lupus erythematosus, infectious arthritis and degenerative joint disease. *Medicine (Baltimore)* 1978; 57: 239–252.

2 Cooper NS, Soren A, McEwen C, Rosenberger JL. Diagnostic specificity of synovial lesions. *Hum Pathol* 1981; 12: 314–328.

3 Kennedy TD, Plater-Zyberk C, Partridge TA, Woodrow DF, Maini RN. Morphometric comparison of synovium from patients with osteoarthritis and rheumatoid arthritis. *J Clin Pathol* 1988; B: 847–852.

4 Revell PA, Mayston V. Histopathology of the synovial membrane of peripheral joints in ankylosing spondylitis. *Ann Rheum Dis* 1982; 41: 579–586.

5 Poulter LW, Duke O, Hobbs S, Janossy G, Panayi G. Histochemical discrimination of HLA-DR positive cell populations in the normal and arthritic synovial lining. *Clin Exp Immunol* 1982; 48: 381–388.

6 Janossy G, Duke O, Poulter LW *et al.* Rheumatoid arthritis — a disease of T-lymphocyte/macrophage immunoregulation. *Lancet* 1981; ii: 839–842.

7 Meijer CJLM, De Graaf-Reitsma CB, Lafeber GJM, Cats A. *In situ* localisation of lymphocyte subsets in synovial membranes of patients with rheumatoid arthritis with monoclonal antibodies. *J Rheumatol* 1982; 9: 359–365.

8 Revell PA. The synovial biopsy. In: Anthony PP, MacSween RNM (eds) *Recent Advances in Histopathology*, vol. 13. Edinburgh: Churchill Livingstone, 1987: 79–93.

9 Enzinger FM, Weiss SW. *Soft Tissue Tumours.* St

Louis: Mosby, 1988: 545–580.

10 Becker RL, Venzon D, Lack EE *et al.* Cytometry and morphometry of malignant fibrous histiocytoma of the extremities. Prediction of metastasis and mortality. *Am J Surg Pathol* 1991; 15: 957–964.

11 Weller RO. Muscle biopsy and the diagnosis of muscle disease. In: Anthony PP, MacSween RNM (eds) *Recent Advances in Histopathology*, vol. 12. Edinburgh: Churchill Livingstone, 1984: 259–288.

12 Dubowitz V. *Muscle biopsy. A Practical Approach.* London: Baillière Tindall, 1985.

13 Romanul FCA, Van der Meulen JD. Reversal of the enzyme profiles of muscle fibres in fast and slow muscles by cross-innervation. *Nature* 1966; 212: 1369.

14 Dubowitz V. Cross-innervated mammalian skeletal muscle: histochemical, physiological and biochemical observations. *J Physiol* 1967; 193: 481.

15 Brooke MH, Engel WK. The histographic analysis of human muscle biopsies with regard to fibre types — Part 1 (adult male and female). *Neurology* 1969; 19: 221.

16 Engel WK. Selective and non-selective susceptibility of muscle fibre types. *Arch Neurol* 1970; 22: 97.

17 Bennington JL, Krupp M. Morphometric analysis of muscle. In: *Heffner RR (ed.) Contemporary Issue in Surgical Pathology*, vol. 3. *Muscle Pathology*. New York: Churchill Livingstone, 1984: 43–71.

18 Swash M, Swartz MS. *Biopsy Pathology of Muscle*, end edn. London: Chapman and Hall Medical, 1991: 38–52.

19 Slavin G, Sowter C, Ward P, Paton K. Measurement of striated muscle fibre diameters using interactive computer-aided microscopy. *J Clin Pathol* 1982; 35: 1268–1271.

20 Sowter C, Slavin G. D-I-Y at home. *The Association of Clinical Pathologists Yearbook* 1994: 47–48.

4.19 BONE HISTOMORPHOMETRY

J. McCLURE

Bone histomorphometry is rarely undertaken in general histopathology laboratories. Undoubtedly specialized preparative techniques and skills are required as well as a significant capital investment. It is logical to have economics of scale and a particular clinical interest in bone metabolic problems is needed to produce an efficient clinicopathological synergy. Given the value of the information which may be abstracted from bone biopsies and the incidence of metabolic bone disorders it would be appropriate for each UK health-care region to have a unit capable of performing bone histomorphometry.

Almost universally bone biopsies are taken from the iliac crest 2.5 cm below and 2.5 cm behind the anterior superior iliac spine. It is now conventional practice to take a transiliac biopsy which results in a core of trabecular bone with plates of external and internal cortical bone. The volume of trabecular bone is, therefore, determined in part by the separation of the cortices. The technique of taking a core vertically through the iliac crest between the cortical plates produces an unpredictable length of trabecular core and has largely been abandoned. The practice of taking a large wedge of bone under general anaesthesia is also unsatisfactory. It is important that the individual taking the biopsy is experienced and some bone histomorphometrists are biopsy-takers. Good internal and external periosteal local anaesthesia is important. The taking of the biopsy is variably uncomfortable but postoperative complications are rare and are usually local haematomas. The defect at the biopsy site is commonly repaired by fibrous tissue and is detectable by X-ray for a long time after the event.

There are several biopsy tools available and some are motorized [1]. The cutting edge is serrated and the internal diameter is between 7 and 10 mm. Small fragments of trabecular bone (bone dust) are created by the movement of the trephine and these are forced into the core of tissue. These fragments are important in that they must be recognized and excluded from the histomorphometric process. In osteoporotic cases the trabecular bone may fragment and detach from the inner cortical plate, which may remain *in situ*. Care must be taken when extruding the bone core from the trephine to avoid impaction of the tissue.

If the bone tissue has been labelled *in vivo* with tetracycline (250 mg four times daily for 3 days repeated after 10 days — biopsy taken 3 days after the last dose) then the biopsy is fixed in absolute alcohol for 48 h. If the patient has not been labelled then the biopsy should be fixed in 10% buffered formalin (pH 7.2) for the same time period. Since the essence of bone histomorphometry is the assessment of undecalcified sections, these must be prepared by embedding in a resin and cutting the sections with a motorized heavy-duty microtome. Different laboratories use different resins (methyl methacrylate, LR white, Araldite). Although the microtome represents a significant capital investment, it can be used for other purposes, such as the cutting of large decalcified or soft-tissue blocks.

It is usual to cut sections at between 7 and 10 μm and at 20 μm (these are examined in ultraviolet light for tetracycline fluorescence). Particular attention must be given to flattening the sections on glass slides prior to staining. Various stains may be applied depending on the particular combination of features which it is desired to demonstrate. The important distinction is between mineralized and non-mineralized (osteoid) tissue, although nuclear/cytoplasmic detail may be required. Goldner's trichrome stain is popular, alkaline toluidine blue provides a lot of cellular detail and the von Kossa technique with a safranin counterstain [2] is particularly useful for semiautomatic/automatic image analysis.

Histomorphometric analysis of bone is usually carried out only on undecalcified sections and microscopy with transmitted, crossed polarized and ultraviolet light is necessary. Quantification of the surface features of trabecular structures and the volume of bone matrix and osteoid can be done by line intersect and point-counting techniques using one of several eyepiece graticules in transmitted light. All graticules have lines and points. Osteoid and eroded surfaces can be measured by counting the number of graticular line intersections with osteoid or eroded surfaces and results expressed as a percentage of the total number of intersections with the bone surface. Osteoid and total bone volumes are measured by counting the number of graticular points lying on osteoid or total matrix and expressing the result as a percentage of the total number of points in the graticule array. Fields for examination must be picked at random and examined at a fixed magnification. The number of fields studied depends on the precise reason for the study and statistical advice is useful. A convenient way of reaching an acceptable figure is the drawing of a damping curve (Fig. 4.16). The cumulative mean for the fields studied is plotted until a constant value is obtained. The mineral apposition rate (MAR) is estimated from 20 μm thick unstained sections seen in ultraviolet light [3]. The distance between time-spaced tetracycline labels is measured at four equidistant points along randomly selected labels. The mean distance of separation is multiplied by Frost's correction factor (0.74) to give a

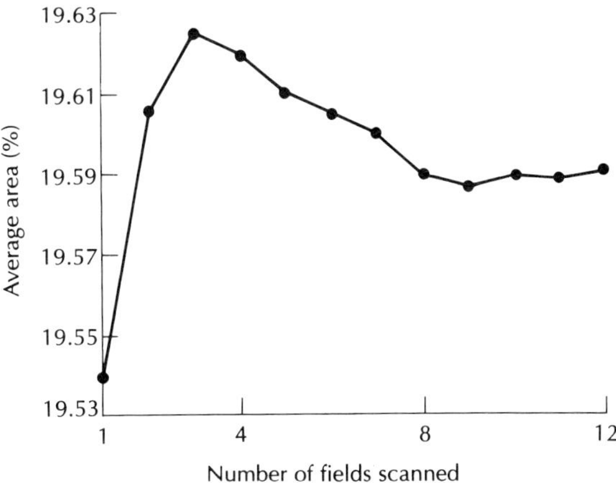

Fig. 4.16 This illustrates a damping curve. The plotting of cumulative means of an area within a field leads to a steady value at 19.59%.

result in microns per day. This parameter is useful in distinguishing hyperosteoidosis due to impaired mineralization (osteomalacia) from that due to high turnover (e.g., in hyperparathyroidism).

The use of eyepiece graticules is available to all microscopists and it can be an efficient way of doing histomorphometry. Semiautomatic and automatic image analysis systems might seem, at first sight, to offer less labour-intensive approaches. However, such systems are expensive and often require a significant amount of user input, especially to edit out processing blemishes and imperfections.

Morphometry as applied here is concerned with obtaining information about three-dimensional (3D) structures from two-dimensional (2D) flat images. Methods used derive 2D numerical data from cut surfaces [4,5] and the data interpreted with a view to quantifying geometric form in complex 3D structures. This is often termed 'stereology' (see Chapter 1). A basic principle of such interpretation is that of the geologist Delesse [6], which states that in an infinitely thin section, the area fraction of sectioned profiles is proportional to the volume fraction in 3D space and it has demonstrated that the theorem is valid if structural components are randomly distributed and chosen for study at random. Since bone tissue sections are 'infinitely' thin compared to the whole skeleton, the measurement of area is a legitimate proxy for volume.

A useful eyepiece graticule is that devised by Merz and Schenk [7]. The test lattice consists of alternating confluent semicircles producing a parallel grid of sigmoid curves (Fig. 4.17). These are enclosed within a square demarcated boundary and superimposed on the sigmoid lines are 36 points, each at a corner of a smaller square. This graticule is designed to eliminate the effect on non-random distribution of the feature of interest within the section.

Tetracycline fluorescence of bones, first described by Milch *et al.* [8], is due to the chelation of amorphous calcium phosphate in stoichiometrical binding [9] and the reaction takes place only at sites of active calcification. The MAR is commonly derived by dividing the distance (microns) between time-spaced labels by time between tetracycline label administration (days) and correcting for geometrical error by applying the Frost correction factor.

A number of histomorphometric parameters and their typical values are given in Table 4.5.

The question of uniformity and reproducibility of results has been addressed by various authors and a number of factors have been studied with regard to these variables. These include inter- and intraobserver variation, variability in biopsy location, homogeneity of different sections, errors arising from changes in magnification and errors related to the use of different stains. Studies of inter- and intraobserver variation have shown that extensive observer experience is not necessary when considering volume and surface measurements and good correlations have been obtained between different observers and between different study centres [10].

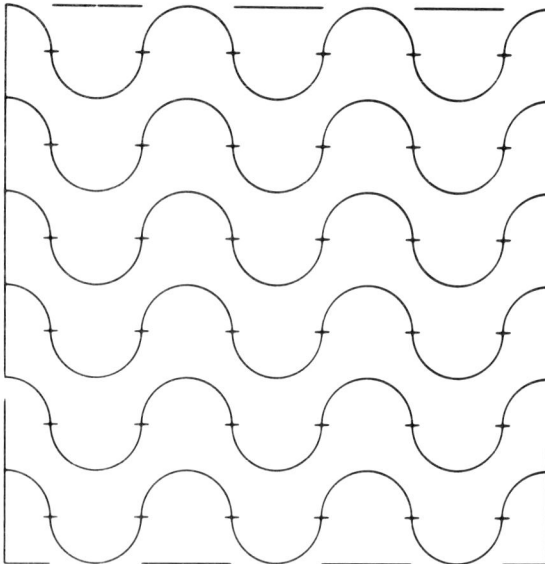

Fig. 4.17 This illustrates the configuration of the Merz graticule. At the points of alternation of the semicircles are short horizontal bars. The intersects of the bars and the sinusoidal curve are the points used in point-counting.

Table 4.5 Histomorphometric bone parameters and their typical values. These values have been culled from a number of published series of 'normal' values. Strictly speaking, a local reference range should be developed but it may take some time to acquire material. However, the effort is ultimately worthwhile

Parameter	Age	Value
1 Bone volume	< 50 years	18–28%
	> 50 years	12–18%
2 Osteoid volume		< 0.2%
3 Osteoid surface	< 50 years	5–20%
	< 50 years	5–40%
4 Osteoid thickness		9 + 3.5 μm
5 Eroded surface		< 16.5%
6 Osteoclast surface		< 1.5%
7 Osteoclast number		$5.6 \times 10^{-2}/\text{mm}^{-2}$
8 Mineralizing surface		> 70%
9 Mineral apposition rate		1 μm/day

The variation produced by sampling different biopsy sites can be significant [11,12]. However, several studies have shown that there is no appreciable difference in values derived from sections of adjacent biopsy sites from a standard location [12–15] or from biopsies taken in a similar position from the opposite iliac crest [12,16–19]. There are, however, differences in reproducibility if biopsies are taken from regions away from the standard site [12]. It has also been shown that results from vertical iliac crest biopsies are not as reproducible as those from transiliac trephine cores taken 2.5 cm below and behind the anterior superior iliac spine [12,20].

Studies of intrasectional variation have shown that reproducibility of results is good [21]. One study [22] claims significant variation but this is based on low point counts in osteopenic patients, which is a likely source to error [5]. Increases in magnification may be accompanied by an increase in the calculated surface density of osteoid [23], although changes in the range 25× to 400× have no discernible effect on the estimation of bone volume. In any study the use of a constant magnification is advised. Different staining methods do not produce significant errors in bone volume or surface osteoid measurements [24]. Reproducibility in measuring MAR is good. A high dose of tetracycline must be avoided as it may inhibit mineralization. Biopsy should be avoided until 24 h after the last tetracyline dose to avoid undue leaching of tetracyline by the tissue fixative [25].

4.19.1 Conclusion

The abstraction of histomorphometric data is key to the accurate diagnosis of metabolic bone disease. Some capital investment and the development of technical expertise are required to establish a laboratory capable of producing undecalcified bone tissue sections. The application of relatively straightforward histomorphometric techniques will be diagnostically rewarding.

References

1 Lalor B, Freemont A, Carlisle S. An improved transiliac crest biopsy drill for quantitative histomorphometry. *Bone* 1986; 7: 273–276.

2 Pearse AGE. Inorganic constituents and foreign substances. In: Pearse AGE (ed.) *Histochemistry: Theoretical and Applied*, vol. 2. London: Churchill Livingstone, 1985: 982–983.

3 Frost HM. *Mathematical Elements of Bone Remodelling*. Springfield: Charles C Thomas, 1964.

4 Underwood JCE. *Introduction to Biopsy Interpretation and Surgical Pathology*. Berlin: Springer Verlag, 1981.

5 Atherne WA, Dunnil MS. *Morphometry*. London: Edward Arnold, 1982.

6 Delesse MA. Procédé mécanique pour déterminer la composition des roches. *Proc Acad Sci Paris* 1847; 25: 544–552.

7 Merz WA, Schenk RK. A quantitative histological study on bone formation in human cancellous bone. *Acta Anat* 1970; 76: 1–15.

8 Milch RA, Rall DP, Tobhe JE. Bone localisation of tetracycline. *J Natl Cancer Inst USA* 1957; 19: 87–90.

9 Urist MR, Ibsen KH. Chemical reactivity of mineralisation tissue with oxytetracycline. *Arch Pathol* 1963; 76: 484–496.

10 Delling G, Luchmann H, Baron R, Matthews CHE, Olah A. Investigation of intra- and inter-reader reproducibility. In: Jee WSS, Parfitt AM (eds) *Bone Histomorphometry: Third International Workshop*. Paris: Armour Montague, 1981: 419–427.

11 Ellis HA, Peart KM. Quantitative observations on mineralised and non-mineralised bone in the iliac crest. *J Clin Pathol* 1972; 25: 277–286.

12 Melsen F, Melsen B, Moskilde L. An evaluation of the quantitative parameters applied in bone histology. *Acta Pathol Microbiol Scand* 1978; 86: 63–69.

13 Beck JS, Nordin BEC. Histological assessment of osteoporosis by iliac crest biopsy. *J Pathol Bact* 1960; 80: 391–397.

14 Garner A, Ball J. Quantitative observations on mineralised and unmineralised bone in chronic renal azotaemia and intestinal malabsorption syndrome. *J Pathol Bact* 1966; 91: 545–561.

15 Chevassieux PM, Arlet ME, Meunier PJ. Intersample variation in bone histomorphometry: comparison between parameter values measured on two contiguous transiliac bone biopsies. *Calcif Tissue Int* 1985; 37: 345–350.

16 Ritz E, Krempien B, Mehls O, Malluche H. Skeletal abnormalities in chronic renal insufficiency before and during maintenance haemodialysis. *Kidney Int* 1973; 4: 116–127.

17 Coupron P, Meunier PJ, Bresset C, Giroux GM. Amount of bone in iliac crest biopsy. Significance of the trabecular bone volume: its values in normal and pathological conditions. In: Meunier PD (ed.) *Bone Histomorphometry, Second International Workshop*. Paris: Armour Montague, 1976: 39.

18 Visser WJ, Neirmans HJ, Roelofs JMM, Raymaker JA, Duursma SA. Comparative morphometry of bone biopsies obtained by two different methods from the left and right crest. In: Meunier PJ (ed.) *Bon Histomorphometry, Second International Workshop*. Paris: Armour Montague, 1976: 79.

19 Visser WJ, Roelofs JMM, Duursma SA. Bone density in the iliac crest. *Metab Bone Dis Rel Res* 1981; 3: 187–190.

20 Wakamatzu E, Sissons HA. The cancellous bone of the iliac crest. *Calcif Tissue Res* 1969; 4: 147–161.

21 Malluche HH, Merger W, Sherman D, Massry SG. Quantitative bone histology in 84 normal American subjects. Morphometric analysis and analysis of variance in iliac bone. *Calcif Tissue Int* 1982; 34: 449–455.

22 Podenphant J, Gotfredsen A, Nilas L, Norgard H, Brendstrup O, Christiansen C. Iliac crest biopsy: an investigation on certain aspects of precision and

accuracy. *Bone Mineral* 1986; 1: 279–287.
23 Woods CG, Morgan DB, Paterson CR, Gossman HH. Measurement of osteoid in bone biopsy. *J Pathol Bact* 1968; 95: 441–447.
24 Meunier PJ, Edouard C. Quantification of osteoid tissue in trabecular bone. Methodology and results in normal iliac bone. In: *Proceedings of the First International Workshop on Bone Morphometry*. Ottawa: Ottawa University Press, 1973: 191–196.
25 Revell PA. Normal bone. In: *Pathology of Bone*. Berlin: Springer Verlag, 1986: 1–30.

5

NUCLEOLAR ORGANIZER REGIONS

P. W. HAMILTON

Nucleolar organizer regions (NORs) are loops of DNA containing the genes which transcribe ribosomal RNA (rRNA). rRNA is an important component of the ribosome and so the transcription of NOR genes is vital to the synthesis of cell protein. The normal human genome possesses 10 NORs, positioned in pairs on the short arms of the five acrocentric chromosomes (chromosomes 13, 14, 15, 21, 22). The location of NORs can be visualized by *in vitro* hybridization with radiolabelled rRNA [1,2] or by silver-binding argyrophilic techniques [3,4]. Both these methods have been used for some time by cytogeneticists to identify NORs on metaphase chromosome spreads but it is only relatively recently that they have been assessed in histological material, particularly using the silver-binding technique. In this method, the silver does not bind to the NORs themselves but to proteins which are in close association with them. Due to their argyrophilia these stained proteins are commonly referred to as AgNORs. While the method does not identify NORs directly, studies have demonstrated a correlation between the position of AgNORs and rRNA hybridization sites [5]. However, the *numbers* of AgNOR staining and NOR hybridization sites are often not correlated [6,7] and it has been concluded that only transcriptionally active NORs are argyrophilic [8].

The NOR-associated proteins have been shown to include RNA polymerase [9], nucleolin (C_{23} protein) [10,11], B_{23} protein [12], pp135 and pp105 [13], and unnamed proteins with a molecular weight of 100 kDa [14] and 80 kDa [15]. The role of these proteins is not fully known. While RNA polymerase I, nucleolin and B_{23} are known to be involved in transcription, they may in association with the other recognized proteins have a structural role in maintaining the chromatin in an extended form [16].

AgNORs can now be identified on formalin-fixed paraffin-embedded tissue sections, cytological smears and plastic sections [17]. This has been facilitated by the introduction of a simple one-step technical procedure [18] carried out at 20°C [17]. Other improvements to the technique have been subsequently reported [19]. AgNORs are recognized as small black intranuclear dots (Fig. 5.1) of varying number and size which do not represent, but may be seen as an integral part of, nucleoli [17,20]. As NORs are crucial to the synthesis of proteins, it was suggested that, like nucleoli, their numbers might reflect increased cell activity [17]. This association is made more specific by the fact that the AgNOR technique only identifies NORs which are actively transcribing [8]. As cell activity is altered in neoplasia, it was a natural step to examine the role of AgNORs in the morphological evaluation of neoplasia [17,20]. Not only have their numbers been considered but also the size of AgNOR bodies have been measured using morphometric techniques. Such studies have permitted quantitative comparisons between histopathological and clinical entities and have shown that AgNOR assessment may have a positive role in the diagnosis, grading and prognosis of malignancy.

Before a review of the histopathological applications of AgNOR quantitation, it is important to examine what an increase in AgNOR number and

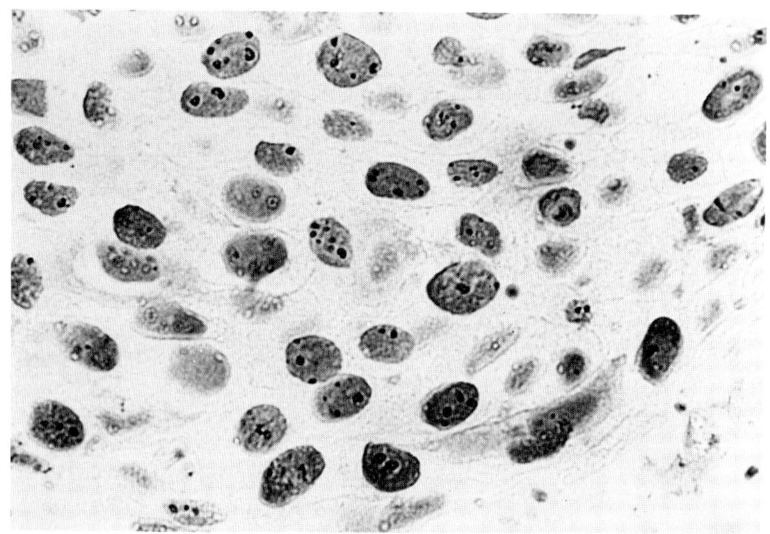

Fig. 5.1 Photomicrograph of AgNORs in cervical dysplasia (cervical intraepithelial neoplasia; CIN III). Courtesy of Dr H. Bharucha.

size indicates in biological terms. It is also important to recognize the problems associated with the identification and counting of AgNORs on histological sections or cytological smears.

5.1 POSSIBLE INTERPRETATIONS OF AN INCREASE IN AgNOR NUMBER AND SIZE

5.1.1 RNA transcription or cell proliferation?

As the silver colloid technique only stains the proteins associated with transcriptionally active NORs, it is thought that the AgNOR number should directly indicate rRNA gene activity. This has been demonstrated by de Capoa *et al.* [21], who showed that cells incubated with certain hormones known to increase rRNA synthesis also had increased AgNOR numbers. This assumption would be true if the NORs were in a state of continual dispersion within the nucleus. However, it is well-documented that during the normal cell cycle, NORs undergo a process of aggregation and dispersion [22–24]. Generally, in the G_0/G_1 stage, AgNORs are in close association forming clearly defined nucleoli. Increased AgNOR dispersion is seen in S phase and mitosis due to chromosomal disorganization with the reorganization of the nucleolus in telophase and cell re-entry into the G_0/G_1 phase. Therefore, what is counted as a single AgNOR may in fact be an aggregation of several AgNORs, all of which are transcriptionally active. Although there is no doubt that the actual number of active NORs should increase in accordance with cell activity and demand for protein [25,26], AgNOR number as measured histologically may not be an absolute indication of rRNA transcription. This has been confirmed by Derenzini *et al.* [27], who showed that, while the number of AgNORs were very different in two neuroblastoma cell lines, the rRNA synthesis was the same. In this study, AgNOR quantity was not related to DNA synthesis, the number of NOR carrying chromosomes or the quantity of ribosomal DNA sequences. It was suggested that the increase in AgNOR number following stimulated transcription in other studies was simply related to the entry of cells into mitosis [27]. Thus NORs in rapidly proliferating cells will not have the opportunity to reaggregate after mitosis, therefore resulting in a larger number of stained AgNORs [28]. This concept is supported by numerous studies which have shown a positive correlation between AgNOR numbers and cellular proliferation [16,29–32].

So, while AgNOR number is more clearly a measure of dispersion, alternative means are required to measure AgNOR expression. A possible approach is by the measurement of AgNOR size (see Section 5.2.5). For example, if two or more AgNORs are clumped together this should be reflected in the size of the stained body. This can be assessed simply from photographs by measuring maximum AgNOR diameter [33], or by the measurement of AgNOR area by interactive computer-linked planimetry [34] or automatic image analysis [35,36].

5.1.2 Nuclear DNA ploidy?

Increased numbers of AgNORs in malignant lesions have often been attributed to increased DNA content or aneuploidy leading to a multiplication of acrocentric chromosomes or NOR genes. Suresh *et al.* [37] examined the AgNOR numbers in trophoblastic tissue. Hydropic abortions, complete hydatidiform moles and partial hydatidiform moles show the necessary combinations of ploidy and proliferation disturbances for examining their relationship with AgNOR quantitation. AgNOR counts were found to be higher in partial hydatidiform moles which are known to be triploid but no significant difference was found between complete hydatidiform moles and hydropic abortions which show sharp differences in cell proliferation. In breast carcinoma, AgNOR counts were also found to be significantly related to ploidy [24]. However, in non-Hodgkin's lymphoma, examination showed no correlation between AgNOR number and DNA content, although there was a positive association with the percentage of cells in S phase. This is in agreement with other studies which have shown a relationship between AgNORs and cell proliferation and a lack of association with DNA ploidy [28–30]. It is possible, therefore, that AgNOR numbers reflect ploidy in tissues which are not obscured by cell proliferation [37]. In non-Hodgkin's lymphoma, however, it has been confirmed that the number of AgNORs is not linked to the number of NOR-bearing chromosomes, as seen in metaphase spreads [28].

5.1.3 Differentiation?

Reeves *et al.* [38] measured AgNOR number and size after treating an HL69 leukaemia cell line with dimethyl sulphoxide (DMSO). Induced differentiation by DMSO resulted in a suppression of rDNA transcription and a drop in AgNOR number and size. This response was not observed in control lymphoblastoid cell lines and so the NOR response to differentiation was restricted to malignant cells only. Smetana and Likovsky [39] also describe AgNOR loss in mature stages of erythroid and granulocytic cells compared to earlier stages. Thus increase in AgNOR numbers in malignant tissue might also be attributed to the increased dedifferentiation in neoplastic progression.

5.1.4 Conclusion

It seems that the number and size of AgNORs are not purely reflective of any single feature but are determined by several factors. Cellular proliferation, differentiation, RNA synthesis and ploidy may all be disturbed to some degree in malignancy and all must contribute to the AgNOR picture. The extent to which they affect AgNOR size and number will relate to the particular tumour studied and this in part accounts for the varying reports in the literature. Nevertheless, the quantitation of AgNORs must reflect the degree of disturbance from the normal cycling pattern of the cell. However, these features are also disturbed in benign neoplastic disease and for this reason AgNOR quantitation in some tissues has been of little use in distinguishing benign from malignant conditions.

5.2 TECHNICAL AND QUANTITATIVE ASPECTS OF AgNOR ASSESSMENT

5.2.1 Fixation

The argyrophilic reaction of NOR-associated proteins (NORAPs) is susceptible to methods of fixation. Sulphydryl, disulphide and carboxyl groups on the proteins have been shown to be involved in the binding of silver ions [40] and several fixatives may interact with these sites, preventing uptake. Smith *et al.* [41], in an examination of a series of fixatives, showed that glutaraldehyde and mercuric fixatives as well as additives such as picric acid and potassium dichromate hindered silver binding due to their adverse effects on the sulphydryl and carboxyl groups. Mercuric solutions were unsuitable as mercury and silver compete for the available binding sites. Formaldehyde fixatives gave variable results, although neutral buffered formalin and formol saline were satisfactory. Other studies have shown that formalin-based media gave good AgNOR staining [42]. In the study by Smith *et al.* [41], alcohol-based fixatives gave by far the best results. Fixation time has also been shown to affect AgNOR resolution [43] which is important for accurate AgNOR counting. This is fine for prospective studies but is beyond control in retrospective studies on archival material.

5.2.2 Section thickness

Regarding section thickness, a compromise needs to be met. Thick sections will allow a more accurate estimation of total AgNOR number but increased nuclear overlap will obscure the clarity of the AgNOR structures. Semithin plastic-embedded sections give optimal light microscopic resolution but reduce the visible number of AgNORs per nucleus. This reduces the scale of difference between cells with different AgNOR numbers. Crocker *et al.* [44] suggest that 3 μm sections form a compromise and this has been shown to be satisfactory in a number of studies. An alternative approach in prospective studies is the use of cell imprints [25], the advantages of which are discussed later (see Section 5.3.1).

5.2.3 Staining time

Staining time is crucial to the quantitative assessment of AgNORs, with overstaining resulting in loss of resolution. For this reason it should be standardized for all specimens within a certain study [24,44]. This is contested by Ruschoff *et al.* [35] who in an automatic image analysis study proposed the use of lymphocytes as an internal control to assess if overstaining (AgNOR area $> 0.40\,\mu m^2$) or understaining (AgNOR area $< 0.10\,\mu m^2$) was taking place. While such measuring facilities are not available to every centre, comparable staining procedures and the use of a control tissue with a known AgNOR status should be employed.

5.2.4 AgNOR counting

Counting can be done manually by simply recording the number of AgNORs seen within each nucleus, although even in sections of 3 μm, careful focusing is required to count all the AgNORs in a particular nucleus. An eyepiece graticule can, however, be used to avoid recounting [45]. An alternative approach is to use an interactive computer-linked graphic tablet system (see Chapter 2) so that, as each AgNOR is identified, it is registered digitally on the monitor, thus preventing duplication of counts. A more recent method of enumerating and sizing AgNORs has been to use automatic image segmentation and analysis. While these methods facilitate AgNOR counting, the basic question of what constitutes an AgNOR is a matter of contention and varies from one study to another.

Generally, three AgNOR structures can be identified on histological section (Fig. 5.2) and the central issue is in the assessment of AgNOR clusters. Crocker *et al.* [44] feel that it is important to attempt to enumerate individual AgNORs within clusters. However, Howat *et al.* [46] demonstrated that there was a large degree of interobserver variation in trying to resolve clumped AgNORs, suggesting that these structures should be called AgNUs (silver-stained nucleoli) and counted as single independent events. A comparison of methods has shown that the counting of individual AgNORs within clumps is the only method that allows one to distinguish benign and malignant breast tumours [47], whereas in trophoblastic tissue both methods gave comparable findings [37]. In the author's opinion, the recognition of clustering is crucial in quantitatively assessing the AgNOR status of a cell. If we count a cluster as a single entity then not only is

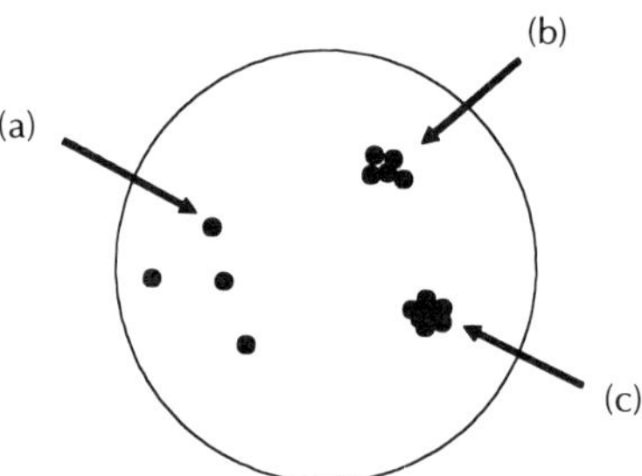

Fig. 5.2 Schematic representation of three principal types of AgNOR structure. (a) Individual AgNOR dots – easy to count; (b) loose AgNOR cluster; (c) AgNORs densely clustered within a nucleolus: sometimes called AgNUs (silver-stained nucleolus).

this fundamentally inaccurate but we lose potentially useful information. If individual AgNORs cannot be accurately defined within clusters then the counting procedure should recognize and take into account the existence of AgNOR clusters or AgNUs. This approach has been adopted in a few studies [48,49]. An alternative solution to this problem might be in the measurement of AgNOR cluster size. Cluster size is strongly correlated with the number of comprising AgNORs [50] and so a calculation of AgNOR content will measure both the extent of AgNOR clumping within an individual nucleus and the number of AgNORs which constitute the clump [35]. In breast cancer cell lines, Ofner *et al.* [51] showed that AgNOR size (area) was the only reliable marker of proliferation.

5.2.5 AgNOR size

In general, the measurement of AgNOR size has been restricted to ultrastructural studies due to the small dimensions seen in light microscopy and some doubt the reliability of measuring AgNOR size using light microscopy [45]. Several workers have measured AgNOR diameter manually from enlarged photographs of stained nuclei. Crocker and Egan [34] did this using interactive image analysis in non-Hodgkin's lymphoma and found an inverse relationship between AgNOR size and number. It must be remembered, however, that the interactive measurement of objects < 15 mm in diameter on a graphic tablet can be subject to excessive variation in the data [52].

A more precise approach to the measurement of AgNOR size on histological preparations is automatic image analysis, i.e., the segmentation and measurement of a digitized image [16,32,34,35,51]. Like Crocker and Egan [34], such studies have shown that an increase in AgNOR number in malignancy is associated with a corresponding decrease in their size. This reaffirms the concept of aggregation and dispersion and stresses the importance of size as a valuable measurement to make. Automatic measurement of a segmented image is not subject to the variation entailed in the tracing of small structures by hand, although thresholding and segmentation of grey-value images can be subjective. The resulting binary image should always be checked against its equivalent histology for accuracy. In addition, automatic image analysis restricts measurements to a single focal plane, thereby reducing the number of countable AgNORs and precluding the absolute counts considered necessary by some workers [44]. However, the examination of a single focal plane is thought to be advantageous by some [35] as it reduces the variations involved in counting by focusing through the nucleus. Still, the choice of an appropriate plane of focus for image analysis may also introduce bias, although this problem might be improved by maximizing the depth of field. An additional advantage of automatic image analysis is that it allows the parallel measurement of number and size and the quotient of these has been used by some as a measure of AgNOR content [35].

Unfortunately, in quantitative AgNOR studies, reproducibility of data is seldom checked. This should be done for measurements of both number and size and it is crucial to assess both intraobserver and interobserver variation.

5.3 EXAMPLES OF HISTOPATHOLOGICAL APPLICATIONS

5.3.1 Non-Hodgkin's lymphoma

In the first paper truly to advocate AgNOR counting in histopathology, Crocker and Nar [20] showed that their number was significantly greater in high-grade (4.4–6.8 AgNORs per nucleus) as opposed to low-grade lymphomas (1.0–1.5 AgNORs per nucleus; Fig. 5.3). These results were confirmed by Boldy *et al.* [25] on cell imprints. The advantages of cell imprints are twofold: (i) the examination of whole cells gives a more realistic picture with regard to the total number of AgNORs per nucleus [26]; and (ii) a greater distinction between low- and high-grade non-Hodgkin's lymphoma can be made. AgNOR size was found to be larger in low-grade ($0.48-1.99\,\mu m^2$) compared to high-grade lymphomas ($0.082-0.19\,\mu m^2$) and a combination of size and number provided a better quantitative separation [34]. This was confirmed in an ultrastructural study by Goodlad *et al.* [53]. This clearcut dicrimination set a baseline for the investigation of AgNORs

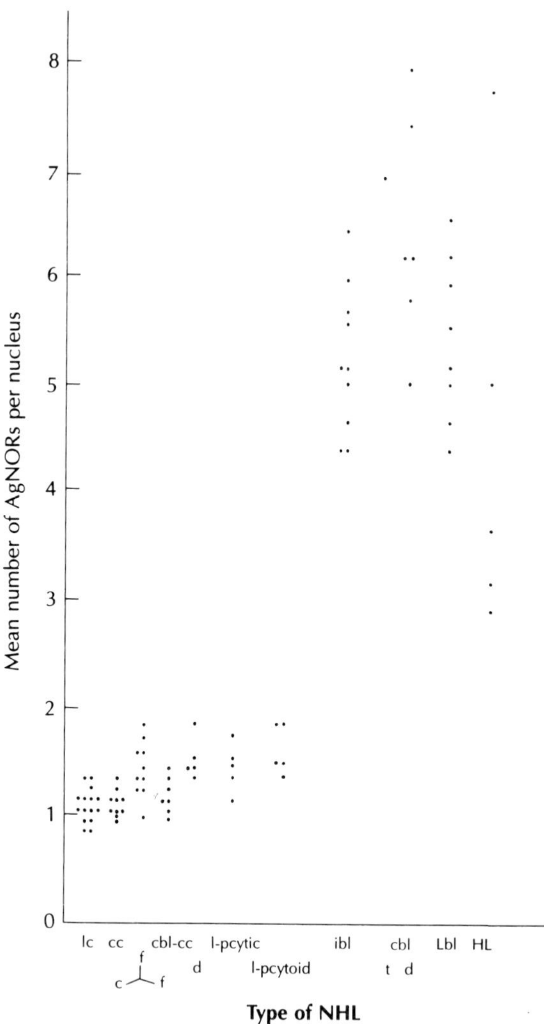

Fig. 5.3 Comparison of AgNOR counts in cases of low-grade lymphomas compared to high-grade lymphomas. lc, lymphocytic; cc, centrocytic, cbl-cc, centroblastic-centrocytic; l-pcytic, lymphoplasmacytic; l-pcytoid, lymphoplasmacytoid; ibl, immunoblastic; cbl, centroblastic; Lbl, lymphoblastic; HL, true histiocytic lymphoma; f, follicular; d, diffuse; c, centre of follicle; i, interfollicular; NHL, non-Hodgkin's lymphoma. From Crocker and Nar [20].

and their association with other cellular features such as nuclear DNA content and cell proliferation [29,30,54,55]. The conclusions reached from these studies indicate that in non-Hodgkin's lymphoma the number of AgNORs is positively associated with the greater proliferation rate encountered in high-grade lesions and may serve as a predictive marker of clinical outcome [55].

These papers on non-Hodgkin's lymphoma also serve to illustrate the variation that exists in the methods used to count AgNORs and in the criteria used to define them. Few reports have assessed the reproducibility of counting [29] and this seems to be a general failure in many studies due to lack of a standardized procedure.

5.3.2 Gastrointestinal neoplasia

Stomach

In the stomach, mean AgNOR numbers showed a steady increase from controls (1.30 per nucleus) through regenerative gastric epithelium (2.10 per nucleus) to early and advanced gastric adenocarcinoma (2.75 per nucleus). While statistical differences were observed, the large overlap between the categories precludes the use of AgNOR counting as an accurate method for distinguishing benign lesions from malignancy, including dysplasia [56]. Higher AgNOR numbers were demonstrated with increasing cellular atypia, as seen in intestinal metaplasia (types I and II), dysplasia and intestinal and diffuse carcinoma [31,57]. This is thought to be correlated with the proliferation or ploidy status of the lesion. An interesting finding was that 'normal' gastric mucosa from carcinoma-bearing stomachs had higher counts (2.10 per nucleus) compared to normal controls (1.54 per nucleus). This advances the concept of a field change but it is not known if this is a secondary change due to the presence of the tumour or a primary premalignant phenomenon.

Colorectum

The number of AgNORs is higher and their size smaller in colonic adenocarcinoma compared to benign hyperplastic polyps, with adenomatous polyps having an intermediate pattern [58]. A clear distinction in counts has been shown between adenocarcinoma (5.53–9.33 per nucleus) and adenomas with severe dysplasia (3.60–5.02 per nucleus) [59]. Kram *et al.* [60] counted AgNORs in 44 cases of colorectal carcinoma and found that they could not be correlated with tumour location, Dukes' classification, differentiation or ploidy status. Similarly, there was no association between AgNOR numbers and survival in rectal adenocarcinoma [43]. Several studies, however, showed that higher counts were associated with decreasing histological differentiation, patients with liver metastases and those who had died within 5 years of follow-up [61–66]. Ofner *et al.* [62] demonstrated that higher numbers (> 4) of scattered AgNORs (i.e., those not occurring as nucleolar clumps) were significantly associated with a poor survival. These results were confirmed by Ruschoff *et al.* [63] who showed that, while there was no significant relationship between AgNOR content and pathological grade or stage, a multivariate survival analysis revealed that it was of independent importance in assessing patient prognosis (Fig. 5.4). These converse findings in colorectal lesions are again most likely due to differing methodologies [64].

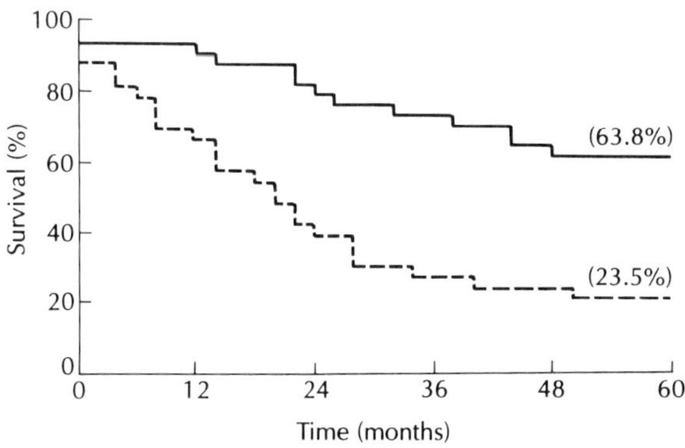

Fig. 5.4 Survival curves for high (---; $n > 7$) versus low (—; $n < 7$) AgNOR counts per tumour cell in patients with colorectal cancer. Survival is significantly ($P < 0.001$) better in the low-count group. From Ruschoff *et al.* [63].

5.3.3 Skin

Several studies have shown an increase in AgNOR numbers in malignant melanoma as compared to benign melanocytic naevi [67–69] (Fig. 5.5). Visual examination of AgNORs was considered sufficient to distinguish benign from malignant lesions [67]. Counts in borderline lesions fell within the range for benign lesions [68,69], aiding their distinction from malignant melanoma. Results from Fallowfield and Cook [48] disagree with this. Using a novel semiquantitative method of assessing AgNOR pattern, they showed that one could not discriminate borderline from malignant lesions in 91% of cases. Other workers have also demonstrated no significant difference in numbers between Spitz naevi and malignant melanoma [70].

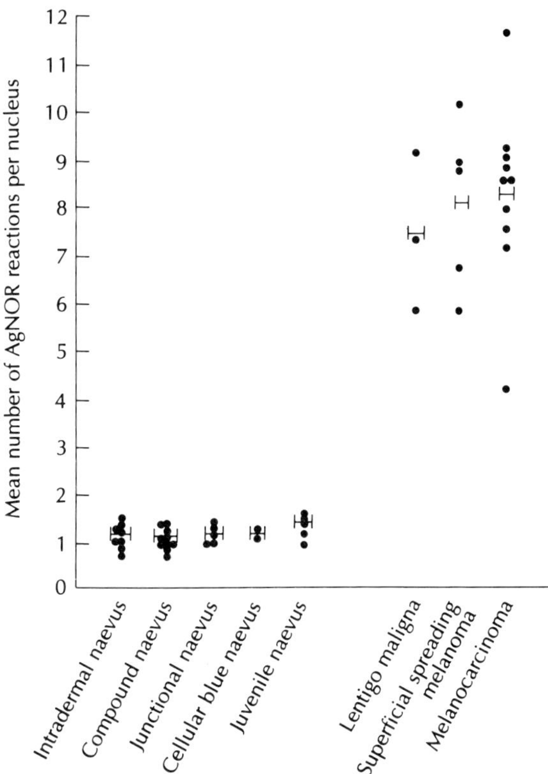

Fig. 5.5 Distribution of mean AgNOR counts per nucleus for benign and malignant skin melanocytic neoplasms. From Crocker and Skilbeck [67].

5.3.4 Gynaecological neoplasia

In an examination of cervical intraepithelial neoplasia (CIN), Rowlands [71] demonstrated overlap in AgNOR counts between CIN I, II and histologically normal specimens. Numbers in CIN III were significantly different from the other categories. These findings were confirmed by Egan *et al.* [33] who also showed a significant difference in AgNOR size between CIN III and the lower grades and it has been proposed that stratified counts within basal, intermediate and parabasal regions are of diagnostic value [72,73]. No significant difference in AgNOR number can be detected between condylomatous lesions and CIN I [73]. A comparison of squamous, adenosquamous and adenocarcinomas showed little difference and no association with proliferation as determined by flow cytometry [74].

Wilkenson *et al.* [75] have shown high AgNOR numbers in both normal proliferative endometrium (8.0 per nucleus) and adenocarcinoma (10.1 per nucleus). Intermediate categories of simple and complex hyperplasia and intraendometrial neoplasia showed comparable mean values of between 6 and 7 AgNORs per nucleus. They propose that a mean AgNOR count >9 in histologically atypical endometrium is highly suggestive of invasive carcinoma. Hansen and Ostergard [76] found the lowest AgNOR count to be in normal proliferative endometrium with an increasing trend, but extensive overlap, through hyperplasia, intraepithelial neoplasia I, II, III and adenocarcinoma. The ratio of AgNOR counts in epithelial cells and stromal cells is similar in hyperplasia with cytological atypia and adenocarcinoma. The difference between these two groups and cystic hyperplasia [77] further supports the idea that atypical hyperplasia is a premalignant lesion.

A study of benign adenomas, borderline lesions and adenocarcinoma in the ovary has illustrated the potential usefulness of AgNOR counting in distinguishing borderline from malignant serous tumours (Fig. 5.6) [78]. In mucinous lesions, borderline tumours fell within the range seen in adenocarcinoma but these were significantly different from benign adenomas. AgNOR counts are of little use in predicting the clinical behaviour of borderline ovarian tumours [79].

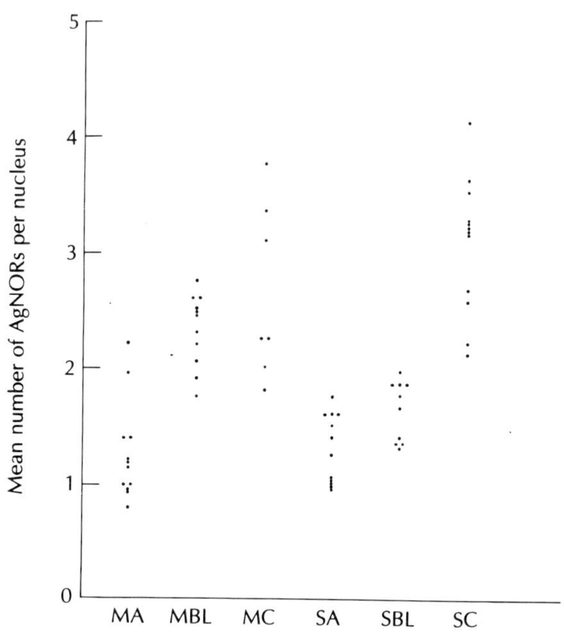

Fig. 5.6 Distribution of mean AgNOR number per nucleus in ovarian tumours, mucinous adenoma (MA), mucinous borderline tumour (MBL), mucinous cystadenocarcinoma (MC), serous adenoma (SA), serous borderline tumour (SBL) and serous cystadenocarcinoma (SC). From Griffiths *et al.* [78].

5.3.5 Breast

AgNOR counts separated benign and malignant breast lesions in almost 100% of cases (Fig. 5.7), although this was only achieved by counting the total number of AgNORs, including those within clusters [80]. In a subsequent analysis [24] which assessed clusters as single events (due to the poor reproducibility found in the method of Smith and Crocker [80]), overlap was seen between benign and malignant cases. This was confirmed by Raymond and Leong [81], and in a cytological study on fine-needle aspiration specimens [82], the conclusion being that AgNOR counting was of limited help in identifying malignancy. These variable results may be attributed to differing counting methods, justifying the need to standardize the procedure between laboratories. While there was no apparent correlation between counts and pathological stage or histological grade, aneuploid tumours tended to have an AgNOR number >3, compared to diploid tumours which were mostly <3 [24]. The flow cytometric assessment of the proliferative cell compartment showed no significant correlation with AgNOR number in breast tumours [24]. A positive association was found with the growth fraction of cells as determined by Ki-67 staining [81] and with hyperploidy in Feulgen-stained samples [83]. In a relatively large study on 230 patients with operable breast cancer, no associ-

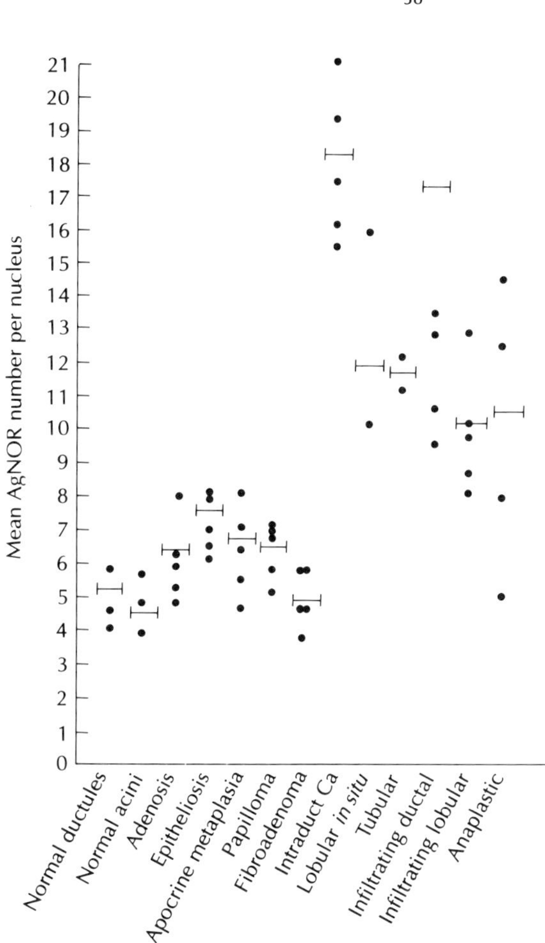

Fig. 5.7 Distribution of mean AgNOR number per nucleus in benign and malignant breast lesions. From Smith and Crocker [80].

ation between AgNOR number and survival was found [84].

5.3.6 Bladder

Examination of AgNOR numbers in bladder tumours showed a stepwise increase from normal through dysplastic to neoplastic lesions [49,85], but these were not statistically significant. Ruschoff *et al.* [86], however, showed that by calculating an AgNOR quotient (dividing AgNOR number by their area), a better discrimination of groups could be obtained, again emphasizing the importance of size as an independent measure of AgNOR status. AgNOR enumeration is reported to have a role in predicting prognosis, but only in superficial transitional cell tumours [87].

5.3.7 Pulmonary neoplasia

Ayres *et al.* [88] illustrated that AgNOR counts could accurately distinguish benign and malignant pleural tissue. AgNOR counts did not discriminate between cases of lung adenocarcinoma, squamous-cell carcinoma, large-cell anaplastic carcinoma, small-cell carcinoma, mesothelioma and carcinoid tumours [89,90]. However, Egan and Crocker [89] point out that AgNOR enumeration might be of use in distinguishing small-cell carcinoma from lymphocyte aggregates in bronchial biopsies but is not useful in its separation from carcinoids (typical or atypical) [91]. As with previous studies on premalignancy, squamous dysplasia of the larynx shows an increase in AgNOR numbers with increasing epithelial atypia [92,93]. AgNORs have no prognostic value in squamous-cell carcinoma of the bronchus [94].

5.3.8 Prostate

Small but statistically significant differences in AgNOR number have been detected between normal (1.76 ± 0.22) and malignant (3.12 ± 0.52) prostate tissues [95]. Benign disease, including granulomatous prostatitis, squamous metaplasia and hyperplasia, can also be distinguished from malignant prostatic tissue by simple assessment of AgNOR number [95–97], although Hansen and Andersen [98] showed that stereological assessment of AgNORs using the disector technique (see Chapter 1) was more sensitive and specific for the detection of malignant cases. In prostatic adenocarcinoma, AgNOR counts are correlated significantly with Gleason grade, with higher numbers in poorly differentiated tumours [95,96,99]. However, AgNORs seem to be poor indicators of prognosis [100].

5.4 CONCLUSION

'Dot-counting' is a laborious procedure and there is

a lack of clarity as to what constitutes an AgNOR. Histopathologists have therefore largely been dubious of the method, regarding it as being too cumbersome for routine practice. A protocol for a standardized approach in the definition and counting of AgNORs should remove ambiguity. New preparatory techniques will further improve their resolution on histological sections. Finally, automatic image analysis provides a means to speed up the process of sizing and counting with minimum effort and increased objectivity. Only if AgNOR quantitation is shown reliably to reflect tumour behaviour or differences in lesions which are otherwise difficult to diagnose differentially, will it become established as an additional special stain of practical use.

References

1 Henderson AA, Warburton D, Atwood KC. Location of ribosomal DNA in the human chromosome complement *Proc Natl Acad Sci USA* 1972; 69: 3394–3398.

2 Evans HJ, Buckland RA, Pardue ML. Location of genes coding for 18S and 28S ribosomal RNA in the human genome. *Chromosoma* 1974; 48: 405–426.

3 Goodpasture C, Bloom SE. Visualization of nucleolar organizer regions in mammalian chromosomes using silver staining. *Chromosoma* 1975; 53: 37–50.

4 Howell WM. Visualization of ribosomal gene activity: silver stains proteins associated with rRNA transcribed from oocyte chromosomes. *Chromosoma* 1977; 62: 361–367.

5 Stocker AJ. Correspondence of silver banding with rRNA hybridisation sites in polytene chromosomes of *Rhynchosciaria hollaenderi*. *Exp Cell Res* 1978; 114: 429–434.

6 Wachtler F, Hopman AHN, Wiegant J, Schwarzacher HG. On the position of nucleolus organizer regions (NORs) in interphase nuclei. *Exp Cell Res* 1986; 167: 227–240.

7 Cheung SW, Sun L, Featherstone T. Visualization of NORs in relation to the precise chromosomal localization of ribosomal RNA genes. *Cytogenet Cell Genet* 1989; 50: 93–97.

8 Miller DA, Breg WR, Warburton D, Dev VG, Miller OJ. Regulation of rRNA gene expression in a human familial 14p+ marker chromosome. *Hum Genet* 1978; 43: 289–297.

9 Scheer U, Raska I. Immunocytochemical localisation of RNA polymerase I in the fibrillar centres of nucleoli. In: Stahl A, Luciani JM, Vagner-Capodana AM (eds) *Chromosomes Today*, vol. 9. London: Allen & Unwin, 1987: 284–300.

10 Spector DL, Ochs RL, Busch H. Silver staining, immunofluorescence, and immunoelectron microscopic localization of nucleolar phosphoproteins B23 and C23. *Chromosoma* 1984; 90: 139–148.

11 Roussel P, Belenguer P, Amalric F, Hernandez-Verdun D. Nucleolin is an AgNOR protein; this property is determined by its amino-terminal domain independently of its phosphorylation state. *Exp Cell Res* 1992; 203: 259–269.

12 Ochs RL, Busch H. Further evidence that phosphoprotein in C_{23} (110 kD/pl 5.1) is the nucleolar silver staining protein. *Exp Cell Res* 1984; 152: 260–265.

13 Pfeifle J, Boller K, Anderer FA. Phosphoprotein pp135 is an essential component of the nucleolus organizer region (NOR). *Exp Cell Res* 1986; 162: 11–22.

14 Escande ML, Gas N, Stevens B. Immunolocalisation of the 100 K nucleolar protein in CHO cells. *Biol Cell* 1985; 53: 99–110.

15 Fakan S, Hernandez-Verdun D. The nucleolus and the nucleolar organizer regions. *Biol Cell* 1986; 56: 189–206.

16 Trere D, Pession A, Derenzini M. The silver-stained proteins of interphasic nucleolar organizer regions as a parameter of cell duplication rate. *Exp Cell Res* 1989; 184: 131–137.

17 Ploton D, Menager M, Heannesson P, Himber G, Pigeon F, Adnet JJ. Improvement in the staining and in the visualization of the argyrophilic proteins of the nucleolar organizer region of the optical level. *Histochem J* 1986; 18: 5–14.

18 Howell WM, Black DA. Controlled silver-staining of nucleolus organizer regions with a protective colloidal developer: a 1-step method. *Experientia* 1980; 36: 1014–1015.

19 Lindener LE. Improvements in the silver staining technique for nucleolar organizer regions (AgNOR). *Histochem Cytochem* 1993; 41: 439–445.

20 Crocker J, Nar P. Nucleolar organizer regions in lymphomas. *J Pathol* 1987; 151: 111–118.

21 de Capoa A, Baldini A, Marlekaj P *et al.* Hormone-modulated rRNA gene activity is visualized by selective staining of the NOs. *Cell Biol Int Rep* 1985; 9: 791–796.

22 Field DH, Fitzgerald PH, Sin FYT. Nucleolar silver-staining patterns related to cell cycle phase and cell generation of PHA-stimulated human lymphocytes. *Cytobios* 1984; 41: 23–33.

23 Goessens G, Thiry M, Lepoint A. Relations between nucleoli and nucleolus-organizing regions during the cell cycle. In: Stahl A, Luciani JM, Vagner-Capodana AM (eds) *Chromosomes Today*, vol. 9. London: Allen & Unwin, 1987: 261–271.

24 Giri DD, Nottingham JF, Lawry J, Dundas SAC, Underwood JCE. Silver-binding nucleolar organizer regions (AgNORs) in benign and malignant breast lesions: correlations with ploidy and growth phase by DNA flow cytometry. *J Pathol* 1989; 157: 307–313.

25 Boldy DAR, Crocker J, Aures JG. Application of the AgNOR method to cell imprints of lymphoid tissue. *J Pathol* 1989; 157: 75–79.
26 Ruschoff J, Plate K, Bittinger A, Thomas C. Nucleolar organizer regions (NORs). Basic concepts and practical application in tumour pathology. *Pathol Res Pract* 1989; 185: 878–885.
27 Derenzini M, Pession A, Farabegoli F, Trere D, Badiali M, Dehan P. Relationship between interpleasic nucleolar organizer regions and growth rate in two neuroblastoma cell lines. *Am J Pathol* 1989; 134: 925–932.
28 Jan-Mohamed RM, Armstrong SJ, Crocker J, Leyland MJ, Hulten MA. The relationship between number of interphase NORs and NOR-bearing chromosomes in non-Hodgkin's lymphoma. *J Pathol* 1989; 158: 3–7.
29 Crocker J, Macartney JC, Smith PJ. Correlation between DNA flow cytometric and nucleolar organizer region data in non-Hodgkin's lymphomas. *J Pathol* 1988; 154: 151–156.
30 Hall PA, Crocker J, Watts A, Stansfeld AG. A comparison of nucleolar organizer region staining and Ki-67 immuno-staining in non-Hogkin's lymphoma. *Histopathology* 1988; 12: 373–381.
31 Rosa J, Mehta A, Filipe MI. Nucleolar organizer regions, proliferative activity and DNA index in gastric carcinoma. *Histopathology*, 1990; 16: 614–616.
32 Derenzini M, Pession A, Trere D. Quantity of nucleolar silver-stained proteins is related to proliferating activity in cancer cells. *Lab Invest* 1990; 63: 137–140.
33 Egan M, Freeth M, Crocker J. Relationship between intraepithelial neoplasia of the cervix and the size and number of nucleolar organizer regions. *Gynecol Oncol* 1990; 36: 30–33.
34 Crocker J, Egan MJ. Correlation between NOR sizes and numbers in non-Hodgkin's lymphomas. *J Pathol* 1988; 156: 233–239.
35 Ruschoff J, Plate KH, Contractor H, Kern S, Zimmermann R, Thomas C. Evaluation of nucleolus organizer regions (NORs) by automatic image analysis: a contribution of standardization. *J Pathol* 1990; 161: 113–118.
36 Ploton D, Visseaux-Coletto B, Canellas JC *et al.* Semi-automatic quantifications of silver-stained nucleolar organizer regions in tissue sections and cellular smears. *Anal Quant Cytol Histol* 1992; 14: 14–23.
37 Suresh UR, Chawner L, Buckley CH, Fox H. Do AgNOR counts reflect cellular ploidy or cellular proliferation? A study of trophoblastic tissue. *J Pathol* 1990; 160: 213–215.
38 Reeves BR, Casey G, Honeycombe JR, Smith S. Correlation of differentiation state and silver staining of nucleolar organizers in the promyelocytic leukaemia cell line HL-60. *Cancer Genet Cytogenet* 1984; 13: 159–166.
39 Smetana K, Likovsky Z. Nucleolar silver-stained granules in maturing erythroid and granulocytic cells. *Cell Tissue Res* 1984; 237: 367–370.
40 Buys CHCM, Osinga J. Selective staining of the same set of nucleolar phosphoproteins by silver and Geimsa. A biochemical and cytochemical study on combined staining of NORs. *Chromosoma* 1984; 89: 387–396.
41 Smith PH, Skilbeck N, Harrison A, Crocker J. The effect of a series of fixatives on the AgNOR technique. *J Pathol* 1988; 155: 109–112.
42 McDermott JG, Kamel HMH, Hamilton P, Carr KE. Variations in the AgNOR expression: technical aspects. *Med Lab Sci* 1989; 46: 510.
43 Griffiths AP, Butler CW, Roberts P, Dixon MF, Quirke P. Silver-stained structures (AgNORs), their dependence on tissue fixation and absence of prognostic relevance in rectal adenocarcinoma. *J Pathol* 1989; 159: 121–127.
44 Crocker J, Boldy DAR, Egan MJ. How should we count AgNORs? Proposals for a standardized approach. *J Pathol* 1989; 158: 185–188.
45 Crocker J. Nucleolar organizer regions. In: Underwood JCE (ed.) *Current Topics of Pathology: Pathology of the Nucleus.* Berlin: Springer Verlag, 1990: 91–149.
46 Howat AJ, Giri DD, Wright AL, Underwood JCE. Silver-stained nucleoli and nucleolar organizer region counts are of no prognostic value in thick cutaneous malignant melanoma. *J Pathol* 1988; 156: 227–232.
47 Smith R, Crocker J. Evaluation of nucleolar organizer region-associated proteins in breast malignancy. *Histopathology* 1988; 12: 113–125.
48 Fallowfield ME, Cook MG. The value of nucleolar organizer region staining in the differential diagnosis of borderline melanocytic lesions. *Histopathology* 1989; 14: 299–304.
49 Ooms EC, Veldhuizon RW. Argyrophilic proteins of the nucleolar organizer region in bladder tumours. *Virchows Arch [A]* 1989; 414: 365–369.
50 Hamilton PW, McDermott J. Is 'AgNOR' size a solution to the problems involved in the quantitative assessment of AgNORs? *J Pathol* 1991; 63: 161A.
51 Ofner D, Hittmair A, Marth C *et al.* Relationship between quantity of silver stained nucleolar organizer regions associated proteins (Ag-NORs) and population doubling time in ten breast cancer cell lines. *Pathol Res Pract* 1992; 188: 742–746.
52 Fleedge JC, Baak JPA, Smeulders AWM. Analysis of measuring system parameters that infuence reproducibility of morphometric assessments with a graphic tablet. *Hum Pathol* 1988; 19: 513–517.
53 Goodlad JR, Crocker J, McCartney JC. Nucleolar ultrastructure in low- and high-grade non-Hodgkin's lymphomas. *J Pathol* 1991; 163: 223–237.
54 Smith FG, Murray PG, Crocker J. Correlation between PCNA and AgNOR scores in non-Hodgkin's lymphomas using sequential staining technique. *J Clin Pathol* 1993; 46: 28–31.
55 Jakic-Razumovic J, Uzarevic B, Petrovecki M, Marusic M, Radman I, Labar B. AgNORs predictive value of prognosis in non-Hodgkin's lymphoma: comparison with flow cytometric cell cycle analysis. *Leuk Lymph*

1992; 7: 165–170.
56 Falck VG, Novelli MR, Wright NA, Alexander N. Gastric dysplasia: inter-observer variation, sulphomucin staining and nucleolar organizer region counting. *Histopathology* 1990; 16: 141–149.
57 Rosa J, Mehta A, Filipe MI. Nucleolar organizer regions in gastric carcinoma and its precursor stages. *Histopathology*, 1990; 16: 265–269.
58 Derenzini M, Romagnoli T, Mingazzini P, Marinozzi V. Interphasic NOR distribution as a diagnostic parameter to differentiate benign from malignant epithelial tumours of human intestine. *Virchows Arch [Cell Pathol]* 1988; 54: 334–340.
59 Yang P, Huang GS, Zhu XS. Role of nucleolar organizer regions in differentiating malignant from benign tumours of the colon. *J Clin Pathol* 1990; 43: 235–238.
60 Kram N, Nessim S, Geller SA. A study of colonic adenocarcinoma, with comparison of histopathology, DNA flow cytometric data and number of nucleolar organizer regions (NORs). *Mod Pathol* 1989; 2: 468–472.
61 Moran K, Cooke T, Forster G *et al.* Prognostic value of nucleolar organizer regions and ploidy values in advanced colorectal cancer. *Br J Surg* 1989; 76: 1152–1155.
62 Ofner D, Totsch M, Sandbichler P *et al.* Silver-stained nucleolar organizer region proteins (Ag-NORs) as a predictor of prognosis in colonic cancer. *J Pathol* 1990; 162: 43–49.
63 Ruschoff J, Bittinger A, Neumann K, Schmitz-Moorman P. Prognostic significance of nucleolar organizing regions (NORs) in carcinomas of the sigmoid colon and rectum. *Pathol Res Pract* 1990; 186: 85–91.
64 Ruschoff J, Plate K, Contractor H, Thomas C. Silver-stained structures (AgNORs), their dependence on tissue fixation and absence of prognostic relevance in rectal adenocarcinoma (letter). *J Pathol* 1990; 161: 89–90.
65 Joyce WP, Fynes M, Moran KT *et al.* The prognostic value of nucleolar organizer regions in colorectal cancer: a 5-year follow-up study. *Ann R Col Surg Engl* 1992; 74: 172–176.
66 Yamaguchi A, Tsukioka Y, Kurosaka Y *et al.* Prognostic value of nucleolar organizer regions in endoscopically biopsied tissues of colorectal cancers. *Oncology* 1993; 50: 121–126.
67 Crocker J, Skilbeck N. Nucleolar organizer region associated proteins in cutaneous melanocytic lesions: a quantitative study. *J Clin Pathol* 1987; 40: 885–889.
68 Leong AS-Y, Gilham P. Silver staining of nucleolar organizer regions in malignant melanoma and melanocytic nevi. *Hum Pathol* 1989; 20: 257–262.
69 Mackie R, White SI, Seywright MM, Young H. An assessment of the value of AgNOR staining in the identification of dysplastic and other borderline melanocytic naevi. *Br J Dermatol* 1989; 120: 511–516.
70 Howat AJ, Giri DD, Cotton DWK, Slater DN. Nucleolar organizer regions in Spitz nevi and malignant melanomas. *Cancer* 1989; 63: 474–478.
71 Rowlands D. Nucleolar organizing regions in cervical intraepithelial neoplasia. *J Clin Pathol* 1988; 14: 1200–1202.
72 Leopardi O, Colavecchio M, Colecchia M, Dede A. Value of AgNOR counts in cervical pathology. *Eur J Gynaecol Oncol* 1992; 13: 539–544.
73 Cardillo MR. Nucleolar organizing regions in human papilloma virus infection and in cervical intraepithelial neoplasia. *Eur J Gynaecol Oncol* 1992; 13: 277–280.
74 Newbold KM, Rollason TP, Luesley DM, Ward K. Nucleolar organizer regions and proliferative index in glandular and squamous carcinomas of the cervix. *J Clin Pathol* 1989; 42: 441–442.
75 Wilkenson N, Buckley CH, Chawner L, Fox H. Nucleolar organizer regions in normal, hyperplastic and neoplastic endometria. *Int J Gynecol Pathol* 1990; 9: 55–59.
76 Hansen AB, Ostergard B. Nucleolar organizer regions in hyperplastic and neoplastic prostatic tissue (letter). *Virchows Arch [A]* 1990; 417: 9–13.
77 Coumbe A, Mills BP, Brown CL. Nucleolar organizer regions in endometrial hyperplasia and neoplasia. *Pathol Res Pract* 1990; 186: 254–259.
78 Griffiths AP, Pickles A, Wells M. AgNORs in diagnosis of serous and mucinous ovarian tumours (letter). *J Clin Pathol* 1989; 42: 1311.
79 Khattech A, Spatz A, Prade M *et al.* Nucleolar organizer regions in ovarian tumours: discrimination between carcinoma and borderline tumours. *Int J Gynaecol Pathol* 1992; 11: 11–14.
80 Smith R, Crocker J. Evaluation of nucleolar organizer region-associated proteins in breast malignancy. *Histopathology* 1988; 12: 113–125.
81 Raymond WA, Leong A S-Y. Nucleolar organizer regions relate to growth fractions in human breast carcinoma. *Hum Pathol* 1989; 20: 741–746.
82 Giri DD, Dundas SAC, Sanderson PR, Howat AJ. Silver-binding nucleoli and nucleolar organizer regions in fine needle aspiration cytology of the breast. *Acta Cytol* 1989; 33: 73–75.
83 Charpin C, Bonnier P, Piana L *et al.* Correlation of nucleolar organizer regions and nuclear morphometry assessed by automatic image analysis in breast cancer with aneuploidy, Ki-67 immunostaining, histopathologic grade and lymph node involvement. *Pathol Res Pract* 1992; 188: 1009–1017.
84 Toikkanen S, Joensuu H. AgNOR counts have no prognostic value in breast cancer. *J Pathol* 1993; 169: 251–254.
85 Cairns P, Suarez V, Newman J, Crocker J. Nucleolar

organizer regions in transitional cell tumours of the bladder. *Arch Pathol Lab Med* 1989; 113: 1250–1252.

86 Ruschoff J, Zimmerman R, Ulshofer B, Thomas C. Silver-stained nucleolar organizer proteins in urothelial bladder lesions. A morphometric study. *Pathol Res Pract* 1992; 188: 593–598.

87 Lipponen PK, Eskelinen MJ, Nordling S. Nucleolar organizer regions (AgNORs) as predictors in transitional cell bladder cancer. *Br J Cancer* 1991; 64: 1139–1144.

88 Ayres JG, Crocker J, Skilbeck NQ. Differentiation of malignant from normal and reactive mesothelial cells using the argyrophil technique for nucleolar organizer region associated proteins. *Thorax* 1988; 43: 366–370.

89 Egan MJ, Crocker J. Evaluation of nucleolar organizer regions in pulmonary pathology. *Thorax* 1990; 45: 225–232.

90 Soomro I, Patel N, Whimster WF. Distribution and estimation of nucleolar organizer regions in various human lung tumours. *Pathol Res Pract* 1991; 187: 68–72.

91 Benbow LW, Cromie CJ. Inability of AgNOR counts to differentiate between bronchial carcinoid tumours and small cell carcinoma of the bronchus. *J Clin Pathol* 1989; 9: 1003–1004.

92 Ashworth MT, Helliwell TR. Nucleolar organizer regions in benign, dysplastic and malignant laryngeal epithelium. *J Pathol* 1988; 154: 35–110.

93 Bryan RL, Allcock PA, Crocker J, Shenoi PH. Nucleolar organiser regions in squamous tumours of the pharynx and larynx. *J Clin Pathol* 1989; 42: 218.

94 Boldy DA, Ayres JG, Crocker J. Waterhouse JA, Gilthorpe M. Interphase nucleolar organizer regions and survival in squamous cell carcinoma of the bronchus: a 10 year follow up study of 138 cases. *Thorax* 1991; 46: 871–877.

95 Kobayashi S, Kuriyama M, Yamamoto N *et al.* Nucleolar organizer regions in prostate cancer. *Adv Exp Med Biol* 1992; 324: 183–188.

96 Ghazizadeh M, Sasaki Y, Oguro T. Aihara K. Silver staining of nucleolar organizer regions in prostatic lesions. *Histopathology* 1991; 19: 369–372.

97 Pavlakis K, Alivizatos G, Mitropoulos D *et al.* Silver-binding nucleolar organizer regions in benign and malignant prostatic lesions. *Urol Int* 1992; 49: 137–140.

98 Hansen AB, Andersen CB. Stereological estimation of nucleolar organizer regions in prostatic tissue with an optical disector. *Acta Pathol Microbiol Immunol Scand* 1992; 100: 135–141.

99 Sakr WA, Sarker FH, Screepatni P, Drozdowicz S, Crissman JD. Measurement of cellular proliferation in human prostate by AgNOR, PCNA, and SPF. *Prostate* 1993; 22: 147–154.

100 Eskelinen M, Lipponen P, Syrjanen K. Nucleolar organizer regions (AgNORs) related to histopathological characteristics and survival in prostatic adenocarcinoma. *Anticancer Res* 1992; 12: 1635–1640.

6

DNA DENSITOMETRY

E.K.W. SCHULTE, D.SEIGNEURIN, F.GIROUD AND G.BRUGAL

With a contribution by P.W. Hamilton

The quantitation of nuclear DNA is increasingly coming into practice in both research and clinical applications. Unfortunately, already existing terms such as ploidy, DNA ploidy, DNA content – defined well before any cytometric approach was possible – have been recycled to designate that which is measured by either flow or image cytometry after appropriate staining. These terms rapidly found their way into the literature before any consensus was established about the biological meaning of the measurements provided by cytometry. This introduction will thus emphasize that DNA ploidy is not ploidy or DNA content.

6.1 DNA PLOIDY IS NOT PLOIDY

Provided that the staining of the nuclear DNA is perfectly stoichiometric, the quantity of dye should represent the quantity of DNA. This quantity may be changed by the operation of three mechanisms: replication, polyploidization and deletion with biological significance and each affecting the size or the number (C) of chromatids and thus the DNA content (c), but not necessarily the number of chromosomes. The number (n) of chromosomes, defined as ploidy according to international nomenclature, is a species feature of all eukaryotic cells. Two species having the same ploidy usually differ in their nuclear DNA content and, two species having the same DNA content do not necessarily have the same number of chromosomes. In normal somatic cells there are two haploid sets of chromosomes of maternal and paternal origin. Such cells are said to be diploid ($2n$) and the chromosomes are comprised of only one chromatid each, therefore $2n = 2C$.

6.1.1 Replication

Cell cycling is the first mechanism by which the number of chromatids (C), and therefore the DNA content (c), changes as a consequence of DNA duplication which occurs during the S phase of the cell division cycle. By the end of S phase each chromosome is comprised of the original chromatid bound to its copy at the centromere level. Then, the number of chromatids ($4C$) is twice the number of chromosomes ($2n$) and the DNA content in G_2 phase ($4c$) is twice the DNA content in G_1 phase, or in non-proliferating cells ($2c$), while the ploidy is identical ($2n$). The M phase following the G_2 phase separates each pair of chromatids, thus generating two cells where $2n = 2C$ again. The cell cycle thus changes the number of chromatids and the DNA content but not the ploidy.

6.1.2 Polyploidization

Polyploidization is the second mechanism changing the number of chromatids. It is frequent in plant cells but also occurs in animal cells after a DNA replication round, which is not followed by a mitosis, thus generating a cell with $4n$ chromosomes and $4C$ chromatids. Such a cell is said to be tetraploid and has a $4c$ DNA content, identical to that of a diploid cell in the G_2 phase of the cycle. Should another DNA replication round occur again, then the cell becomes octoploid (8*n* chromosomes, 8*C* chromatids, 8*c* DNA content), and so on. All cells having a whole-number multiple of both the 2*n* species-characteristic chromosome number and the 2*C* species-specific chromatid number are said to be polyploid. Contrary to the normal cell cycle, polyploidization changes the number of chromatids, and therefore the DNA content accordingly.

6.1.3 Deletion

The third mechanism changes the number of chromatids as the consequence of a change in chromosome number, but not according to an entire multiple of the original 2*n* set and results in a cell said to be aneuploid. This mechanism is not well known but always results from a chromosome loss after abnormal mitosis or endomitosis. This deletion may concern one or several chromosomes, either entirely or only partially, and results in a change in DNA content. Depending on which chromosome, or part of the chromosome, is lost, the cell may remain viable, and in many cases escapes its embryological determination and environmental proliferating regulation to become malignant. Malignant uncontrolled proliferation may again change the ploidy status by further deletions and any other cytogenetic structural abnormalities in the aneuploid cell progeny.

From the above definitions, based on international nomenclature, it is clear that the cell DNA content is not synonymous with ploidy, although one wording is commonly used for the other by the medical community. This confuses any further interpretation of DNA changes (detectable by flow and image cytometry) versus ploidy changes (detectable by karyotyping and *in situ* hybridization techniques) as far as the investigation of malignancy-related chromosome versus DNA damage is concerned. Some other damages to the DNA molecule may contribute to change the DNA content, as measured by cytometry. These are gene amplifications or massive viral infections which can be considered as minor when compared to total or partial chromatid loss detectable by karyotyping.

6.2 DNA PLOIDY IS NOT DNA CONTENT

The measurement of DNA content by either flow or image cytometry is based on the assumptions that the amount of stain represents the amount of DNA and that this amount of stain is correctly measured by the instrument. These assumptions would imply that:

1 the DNA labelling procedure (fluorescent dye, chromogenic reaction or staining) is specific (all DNA is labelled and only DNA), stoichiometric (staining intensity changes proportionally to DNA content) and stable (staining intensity does not change with time or repeated measurements);

2 the instrument used to measure either the light emitted by the fluorescent dye or absorbed by the stain is accurate (giving a result close to the true amount of stain) and reproducible (giving very similar measurements when repeated on the same nucleus), even though not close to the true amount of stain, and linear (giving a result that is perfectly proportional to the amount of stain).

Unfortunately, both the staining procedures and the instrument have well-known limitations such that the final measurement is not representative of the absolute amount of DNA actually present in a nucleus.

6.2.1 Staining limitations

While stoichiometry can easily be verified by routine controls, the specificity is not accessible because there is no alternative method for the cytometric measurement of DNA content at the individual cell level. Specificity is not a concern of cytometrists in routine practice, for example:

1 Very specific fluorescent dyes bind to either G-C (e.g., mithramycin, chromycin A3) or A-T (e.g., Hoechst, DAPI) DNA base pairs and thus detect the DNA only partially and generate measurements that depend on base pair sequence.

2 The chromogenic reactions, like Feulgen, involve an acid hydrolysis that removes some DNA fragments as rapidly as they are released from the decondensed chromatin. These reactions thus detect the DNA only partially and provide measurements

that depend on the euchromatin versus heterochromatin balance.
3 The fixative medium may impair or facilitate further hydrolysis, depending on the way they interact with histones.

6.2.2 Physical limitations

As far as image cytometry of Feulgen-stained nuclei is concerned, the Beer and Lambert laws do not perfectly apply since:
1 the linearity of stain to optical density (OD) is progressively lost as OD runs over 1 unit, which is often the case for heavily stained heterochromatin [1];
2 the distribution of the dye is not spatially homogeneous and thus introduces a distributional error that increases as the pixel size increases over from the resolution power of the optics [2–5];
3 the absorption coefficient of a dye varies with the wavelength of light so that the densitometric calculation only applies for monochromatic light. Since they do not deliver enough intensity for visual observation (unless combined with huge arc lamps), monochromators are not used in routine image cytometry, but filters are used whose centre on the maximum absorption is ± 10 nm, which usually varies from one system to another.

In addition to the above considerations, the preparation and the instrument are optical compromises and are thus responsible for reflection, refraction and diffraction due to the glass slide, mounting medium, lenses and prisms. The light not following the expected geometrical pathways contributes to glare, also called Schwarzchild — Villiger effect, which distorts the ratio between the light beam intensity (I_0) incident to the nucleus and that (I) emerging from the specimen. Therefore, all the pixel ODs calculated as log I_0/I are slightly erroneous. This error increases as the optical field size increases. The use of a high-quality microscope is thus mandatory to decrease this systematic error of densitometric measurements [6,7], which is the most important factor contributing to variations of image cytometry measurements. Glare can be reduced by decreasing the measurement field size. In practice, the field size is slightly larger than the television target size as projected on to the object plane and thus cannot be reduced. Nevertheless, it should be noted that the absorbing nuclei crowding within the microscope field act as a field diaphragm and thus reduce the glare effect, as shown in Fig. 6.1. The measured integrated optical density (IOD) thus increases as the population density increases.

Also, video cameras are sensitive to vibrations and electromagnetic fields, image afterglow and saturation — all factors contributing to the distortion of the signal before digitization. At present, charge-coupled device (CCD) cameras undoubtedly provide the most reproducible results as far as densitometry is concerned [8].

6.2.3 Towards a standardized terminology

The above limitations all contribute to negative errors that have been extensively investigated [5]. It is thus obvious that the true cell DNA content is

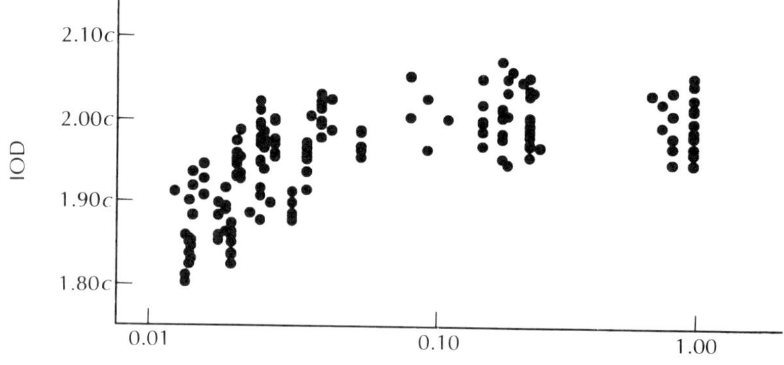

Fig. 6.1 Measurements made on chicken erythrocytes plotted against the fraction of the microscope field occupied by cells surrounding the one currently measured (logarithmic scale). As the proportion of the measuring field occupied by nuclei increases, the negative error due to glare decreases and the measured DNA staining intensities of the erythrocytes thus rise to the expected 2.00c average value. IOD, integrated optical density.

not accessible to cytometric measurements. It is therefore astounding that some commercially available image cytometry systems provide measurements expressed in picograms DNA per nucleus, thus adding to the general confusion and, in addition, deliberately misleading the clinicians using such systems! In this respect, the standardization committees have failed to counter the trend of cytometrists to reuse words which have different definitions that have been well-established for a long time. The most likely reason is that they have not been able to invent a new nomenclature. In spite of the standardization committee's failure, the authors are convinced that terms such as ploidy, DNA ploidy and DNA content to designate the measurements provided by cytometry after specific DNA staining *must be banned* and replaced by specific terms yet to be defined by international nomenclature committees. In what is to follow, this chapter will refer to DNA staining intensity for want of another generally accepted term.

It will be emphasized below that, provided the staining and measuring procedures are correctly performed and controlled, the quantitation of DNA-specific stains can be interpreted in terms of overall proliferative activity and gross cytogenetic aberrations, thus giving a clear indication as to how to proceed further in investigating those tumour characteristics that are of interest for differential diagnosis and prognosis.

6.3 QUANTITATIVE DNA STAINING TECHNIQUES

Various stains and chromogenic reagents for quantitative staining of DNA have been recommended in the literature (Table 6.1), but finally only one of them has gathered worldwide acceptance for DNA cytophotometry, and this is the reaction named after Feulgen and Rossenbeck [9], often simply named Feulgen reaction. Strictly speaking, the Feulgen reaction is not a stain but a chromogenic reaction [10]. Terms like Feulgen stain and Feulgen staining, however, are commonly used. The Feulgen reaction is presently the only staining technique which is stoichiometric for DNA, which means that staining of DNA is both quantitative and specific. All the other methods mentioned in Table 6.1 are quantitative but not specific for DNA. The success of the Feulgen reaction for quantitative DNA staining is certainly based on this uniqueness.

6.3.1 Chemical background of the Feulgen reaction

The Feulgen reaction is a complicated cytohistochemical method which consists of various preparatory steps [11]. Principally, the reaction starts with a procedure called acid hydrolysis: slides with the fixed cytological material are immersed in hydrochloric acid (HCl) which splits off the purine bases adenine and guanine from the DNA molecule, thereby generating aldehyde groups in the purine-free DNA molecule, which is then called apurinic

Table 6.1 Quantitative DNA stains (+, yes; /, no)

Staining procedures	Quantitative	Stoichiometric	References
Feulgen reaction (basic fuchsin)	+	+	[10,12]
Feulgen reaction plus	+	+	[45]
anionic counterstain	+		
Thionin, Feulgen	+	+	[27]
Thionin, Feulgen plus	+	+	[29]
anionic counterstain	+		
Gallocyanin chromalum	+	/	[42]
Methyl green-pyronin Y	+		[10,46]
Thionin alcoholic	+	/	[10,47]
Victoria blue B	+	/	[10,48]

acid (APA). In a second step, the slides are immersed in Schiff's reagent containing a dye which binds covalently to the aldehyde groups. After removal of surplus dye the slides are dehydrated and mounted as usual. In correctly stained material, cell nuclei are stained red-violet, and the cytoplasm and background are unstained. The various steps of the Feulgen reaction become critical when they must be standardized to achieve good reproducibility of staining performance. Therefore, a discussion of the relevant preparatory steps must consider potential sources of error [12–14].

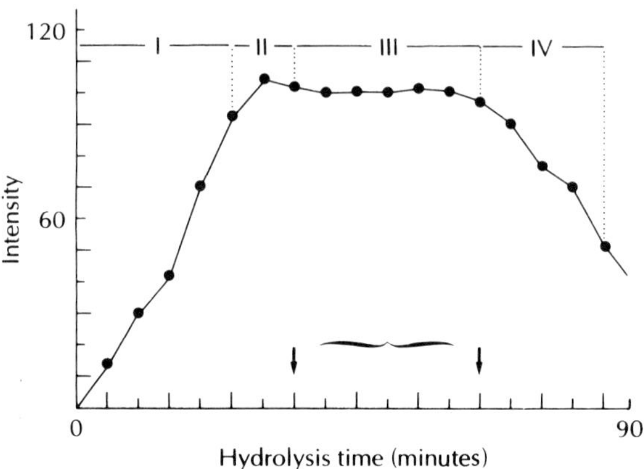

Fig. 6.2 Hydrolysis curve for cytological material after fixation in methanol/formaldehyde acetic acid (MFA) (according to Schulte [13]). Staining intensity (in arbitrary units) was plotted against hydrolysis time. The arrows show the beginning and the end of the plateau phase (III) with the optimum hydrolysis time.

Acid hydrolysis

Routinely, HCl is used, but in principle any acid is suitable. The acid has two effects on the DNA molecule: (i) removal of purine bases, which generates aldehyde groups in the DNA molecule; and (ii) depolymerization of the large APA molecule into smaller fragments. These fragments are partly removed from the cell nuclei by diffusion into the acid solution. Generation of aldehyde groups leads to an increase in nuclear staining intensity, whereas the loss of APA fragments leads to a loss of stainable material from the cell nucleus and thus to a decrease of staining intensity. Thus, we have two countercurrent chemical reactions, each following specific and complicated kinetics; the resulting reaction curve is called the hydrolysis profile or the hydrolysis curve (Fig. 6.2) [13].

This hydrolysis profile can be subdivided into four phases: (I) increase of staining intensity; (II) peak phase with maximum staining intensity; (III) plateau phase with constant staining intensity; and (IV) decrease in staining intensity.

Phase I is characterized by continuous generation of aldehyde groups. The loss of APA fragments is minimal in the beginning, and the amount of stainable material in the cell nucleus increases constantly until phase II is reached — the peak — which can be so short that it is sometimes hardly visible in hydrolysis profiles. During the plateau phase, III, we find a balance between the continuous generation of aldehyde groups and the loss of APA fragments, and consequently, the staining intensity remains constant over a certain period of time. In phase IV, the loss of APA fragments outruns the generation of new aldehyde groups, and the staining intensity decreases. After prolonged hydrolysis we find the generation of the maximum number of aldehyde groups, but all APA fragments have been removed from the cell nucleus, and staining intensity is zero.

In practice, it is important to stop acid hydrolysis during phase III where smaller variations of the hydrolysis time have virtually no influence on staining intensity.

The shape of the hydrolysis curve is influenced by several factors, only some of which can be standardized.

Sensitivity of the DNA molecule

Highly condensed DNA is less sensitive to acid hydrolysis than decondensed DNA: phases I and IV are less steep, and the plateau phase is retarded. DNA compactness, as a biological characteristic of cells, varies between different cell types [15,16] and in the same cell during the cell cycle [17–20]. Cell preparation techniques such as specimen sampling and especially fixation of the material (dry fixation, wet fixation [14–21]) may artificially influence DNA compactness and thus acid sensitivity. The importance of standard fixation techniques for DNA cytometry has been discussed in detail by Giroud and Montmasson [22].

Concentration and temperature of the acid bath

The high temperature of the acid bath shortens all four phases. Phase III may be as short as only a few seconds, and a prominent plateau may not be detectable. If hydrolysis is stopped in the very steep phases I or IV, even minimal variations of processing time lead to considerable variations in staining intensity. Short hydrolysis profiles with an extremely short peak phase are usually found with so-called hot hydrolysis techniques using an acid bath at 60 °C, and frequently it is impossible to stop hydrolysis at the right moment, namely in phase III. More frequently, cold hydrolysis with 4–5 mol/l HCl is performed at about 22 °C [23] where under routine conditions the plateau phase has a length of several minutes. Acid hydrolysis is then stopped by a short rinse of the slide in tap water.

Various additives to the acid bath have been recommended in the literature, these should minimize the loss of APA fragments from the cell nucleus [24]. These additives, however, do not play an important role for practical purposes.

The Schiff reagent

Schiff's reagent is a colourless aqueous reagent which contains a dye mixture called basic fuchsin [13]. Basic fuchsin is normally composed of four cationic triarylmethine dyes [25] — pararosanilin (CI 42 500 [26]) and its methylated homologues rosanilin (CI 42 510 [26]), magenta II (no CI number) and new fuchsin (CI 42 520 [26]). Basic fuchsin of high quality contains a high proportion of pararosanilin. Schiff's reagent is colourless because the relevant dyes are present in their leucoform with sulphite bound to the dye molecules. Coloration of Schiff's reagent (based on basic fuchsin) proves loss of sulphite and deterioration of the solution, which should then be discarded. Various substitutes for basic fuchsin have been recommended, among them the thiazine dye thionin [27,28] (CI 52 000 [26]). The advantage of thionin is that it stains cell nuclei blue (a colour the cytologists and pathologists are used to when they want to check the slide visually), and cytoplasmic counterstaining with eosin Y (CI 45 389 [26]) or Congo red (CI 22 120 [26]) is easily feasible [29]. Schiff's reagent based on thionin is usually not completely colourless.

The rinsing procedure

After staining with the Schiff reagent the material is rinsed in dye-free sulphite water. The sulphite removes surplus dye from the cell nuclei and cytoplasm, and only the covalently bound dye molecules stay fixed to the APA molecule within the cell nucleus. The background of the slide should be completely unstained when the Feulgen reaction has been performed correctly.

6.3.2 Practical considerations to avoid pitfalls

Acid hydrolysis

Acid hydrolysis is the most critical step of the Feulgen reaction [13,30,31]. A correctly performed hydrolysis should be stopped in the plateau phase. It is important to have HCl of suitable molar concentration at the right temperature (5 mol/l HCl at 22 °C or 4.0 mol/l HCl at 27.50 °C [12,32]). Acid of suitable molar strength is commercially available or can easily be prepared from concentrated HCl. Frequently, HCl stored in the refrigerator at 4 °C is used immediately without waiting for the acid to warm up; this leads to retardation of the hydrolytic reaction, which is often stopped before the plateau phase has been reached. The use of temperature-controlled water baths is recommended [33]. Where this is not feasible, scrupulous measurement of the temperature of the acid solution helps to avoid erroneous photometric results.

It is of utmost importance to note that changing the fixative may influence the hydrolysis profile dramatically (by changing chromatin compactness and thus acid sensitivity of the DNA). Changing the fixative means that the hydrolysis curve has to be re-evaluated [22,34,35]. Therefore, it seems a good recommendation to stick to one staining protocol which has been established in the relevant laboratory and was found to give reliable and consistent staining results.

The chromogenic reaction

The staining procedure itself is uncritical. Staining should be carried out for at least 45 min to give the reaction sufficient time to be completed. Schiff reagent of high and consistent quality is commercially available. The reagent should be completely colourless. Two pitfalls must be carefully considered.

1 Two reagents are on the market: one for the detection of aldehydes in chemistry, and one for detection of aldehydes in microscopy. These two reagents differ in dye and sulphite content. Only reagents which are clearly labelled as suitable for microscopy should be used.

2 Schiff's reagent is frequently stored in the refrigerator, and the cold solution (about 4 °C) is often used immediately for staining of the material. At such a low temperature the chromogenic reaction can still be incomplete even after 1 h because the reaction speed decreases remarkably. Give the reagent enough time (about 1 h for a volume of 100 ml) to warm up to room temperature (about 22 °C) in the Coplin jar. Close the Coplin jar carefully to avoid evaporation of sulphur dioxide (SO_2) from the reagent.

The sulphite rinse

Rinsing is uncritical as long as fresh sulphite water is used (not older than 6 h). The solution loses SO_2 on standing, and unspecific background staining can be due to incomplete rinsing with old solutions. Close the Coplin jar carefully to avoid evaporation of SO_2 from the sulphite water. All rinsing procedures, before and after hydrolysis and after the sulphite rinse, can be performed using tap water. Tap water can also be used for the preparation of the sulphite solution. It is, at least for routine purposes, not necessary to use distilled water (which is often recommended). Other reagents for rinsing the slide — partly containing ethanol — are not in common use.

Dehydration, clearing and mounting are not critical as long as normal processing times (several minutes per step) are used. The stained slides should be stored in the dark to avoid bleaching [36,37].

A list of biological and preparatory factors which influence Feulgen stain performance is given in Table 6.2.

Table 6.2 Factors influencing the Feulgen stain performance

Factors	References
Cell type: chromatin compactness	[15–120]
Specimen sampling: (smear, imprint, aspiration biopsy; cytocentrifuged material)	[14,39,40]
Fixation: chemical composition, osmotic pressure, pH of the fixative, wet or dry fixation	[14,21,22,34,39,52]
Acid hydrolysis:	
acid bath: type and molar strength of acid,	[32,34]
temperature of the solution	[14,32,33]
rinsing: type, temperature, chemical composition and pH of the rinsing agent	[53]
Schiff's reagent: dye content and composition	[12,25]
purity and sulphite content	
pH, ionic strength and solvent	
staining time and temperature	
Terminal rinsing procedure: chemical composition and pH	[53,54]
Mounting medium: chemical composition (effect on bleaching of stained material)	[36,37]
Bleaching of slides: conditions of storage	[37,56]
exposure to light	

Standardization of the Feulgen reaction

The application of the Feulgen reaction as a quantitative DNA stain requires a fully standardized staining protocol [12–14,38–40]. Otherwise, widely variable staining results are unavoidable. Table 6.3 gives a list of preparatory steps which must be standardized to guarantee consistent staining. A protocol which proved to be useful in the authors' laboratory for Feulgen staining of cervical smears and breast aspiration biopsies is given in Table 6.4. Table 6.5 gives a corresponding protocol for plastic-embedded liver tissue.

Table 6.3 Preparatory factors which have to be standardized for consistent Feulgen stain performance

Specimen preparation
Use fresh material (fix within 6 h; avoid autolysis)
Use either dry fixed or totally wet fixed material
Avoid unintentional air drying of wet fixed material

Fixation
Regaud fixative (30 min), MFA (60 min) or ethanol (10 min)

Acid hydrolysis
Either 5 mol/l HCl at 22 °C for about 40 min or 4 mol/l HCl at 27.5 °C for about 50 min
If possible, use temperature controlled water bath (variation of temperature ± 0.5 °C)

Rinse
Rinse for about 10 s in tap water to stop hydrolysis

Chromogenic reagent
Use commercial Schiff reagent with a dye content (pararosanilin or basic fuchsin) not less than 0.5% (w/v) in sulphite water
Use Schiff's reagent at 22 °C. Identify solution as 'to be used for microscopy'. If Schiff's reagent is prepared freshly with commercial dyes, use pararosanilin and identify dye batch by CI number

Rinsing procedure
Sulphite water followed by tap water

Mounting
Any commercial mounting medium is suitable

Storage
Store slides in the dark

Table 6.4 Standard Feulgen staining protocol for cervical smears

1 Smear prepared with a cervical brush
2 Immediate wet fixation in ethanol 99% (v/v), 15 min
3 Rinse in ethanol 50% (v/v), 1 min
4 Rinse in tap water, 1 min
5 5 mol/l HCl, 22 °C, 45 min; temperature controlled at ±0.5 °C
6 2 sequential rinses in tap water, 15 s each
7 Schiff's reagent at 22 °C, 60 min (Commercial Schiff reagent 'for microscopy'; if prepared freshly, a standard solution according to Schulte and Wittekind [12] was used)
8 2 rinses in sulphite water [12], 3 min each
9 2 rinses in tap water, 3 min each
10 Ethanol 50%, 70%, 90%, 99% (v/v), 2 min each
11 2 rinses in xylene (toluene), 3 min each
12 Mounting in any commercial resin

Table 6.5 Standard Feulgen staining protocol for plastic embedded liver tissue

1 Freshly cut pieces of liver (not larger than 5 × 5 × 5 mm) is fixed in neutral buffered formaldehyde 3.7% (v/v) for 24 h
2 Rinse for 8 h in running tap water
3 Dehydrate in ethanol 50%, 70%, 80%, 90%, 99% 2 h each
4 Immersion in GMA for 24 h
5 Allow polymerization of GMA for 24 h [57]
6 Cut sections with glass knives, thickness 5 μ [58]
7 Hydrate sections in tap water for 5 min
8 Acid hydrolysis in 5 mol/l HCl at 22 °C for 45 min
9 Rinse in 2 changes of tap water, 30 s each
10 Schiff reagent at 22 °C for 60 min
11 Rinse in two changes of sulphite water, 2 min each
12 Rinse in two changes of tap water, 30 s each
13 Dehydrate in ethanol 50%, 70%, 80%, 90%, 99%, 5 min each
14 Clear in two changes of xylene (toluene), 3 min each
15 Mounting in any commercial resin

GMA, glycolmethacrylate.

6.3.3 Gallocyanin as a quantitative DNA stain

Gallocyanin chromalum (GCA) has been introduced by Einarson [41]. Gallocyanin (CI 51 030 [26]) is a cationic oxazine dye which forms complexes with metals. GCA stains DNA and RNA quantitatively. Thus, it is not specific for DNA. Photometric determination of DNA requires either photometric correction for stained RNA or enzymatic or hydrolytic removal of RNA.

The Einarson GCA staining protocol prescribes staining times of up to 48 h at elevated temperature which makes it impossible to use for routine cytology. Husain and Watts [42] described a modified GCA with staining times of about 15 min. The physicochemical background of the Husain–Watts stain was investigated elsewhere [43]. GCA has been recommended for cytophotometric purposes [44].

As compared with Feulgen, GCA after Husain and Watts has the following advantages: (i) no acid bath; (ii) staining time only 15 min; and (iii) grey-blue cell nuclei (similar to those in the Papanicolaou stain). The disadvantages are: (i) not specific for DNA; (ii) background staining (due to RNA); and

(iii) short shelf-life of the staining solution (about 6 weeks). Specificity of staining can be improved by mild hydrolysis (1 mol/l HCl at 22 °C for 10 min) which removes RNA but not DNA. Anionic counter-staining is possible without loss of GCA from the stained DNA.

GCA stains both wet and dry fixed material. Dry fixed slides are significantly less intensely stained. Ethanol 99% (v/v) for 10 min on wet fixed material or neutral buffered formaldehyde 3.7% (v/v) for dry fixed material are suitable fixatives. If commercial spray fixatives containing polyethylene glycol (PEG) are used, the PEG film on the slide has to be removed prior to staining by washing the slide for 5 min in ethanol 99% (v/v).

Both techniques — the Feulgen reaction and GCA — are equally suitable for cytophotometric determination of DNA. However, they give completely different results when the texture of nuclear chromatin is measured at high optical resolution: acid hydrolysis changes the chromatin structure dramatically, and the chromatin texture of Feulgen-stained cell nuclei is absolutely different from the texture of GCA-stained material.

GCA is all in all less critical than the Feulgen reaction and easier to perform. Nevertheless, the authors prefer the Feulgen reaction due to its substrate specificity and the stability of the staining solution. A careful standardization of the protocol, however, is a prerequisite for consistent staining quality.

6.4 IMAGE CYTOMETRY OF STAINED DNA

6.4.1 Image cytometry system

Until the mid 1970s quantification of DNA was performed using the difficult and time-consuming technique of microspectrometry on Feulgen-stained material. The development of the fluorescence-activated cell sorter led to the application of flow cytometry (FCM) as a method of DNA measurement. This quickly became the 'gold standard' for DNA measurements. It has the one disadvantage that it requires the specimen to be a cell or nuclear suspension. The more recent technique of image cytometry (ICM) is applicable to pathological material prepared by and largely in the same way as for conventional visual analysis.

For most tumours there is a good correlation between DNA indices measured using FCM and ICM [59,60]. However, although FCM is a well-established technique, ICM has many advantages in that it allows a degree of operator interaction and selection of the cells or nuclei to measure or to discard. Direct visualization of the sample using ICM allows subpopulations of cells to be preferentially selected for analysis. This greater specificity of cell selection allows the elimination of confounding populations of inflammatory and stromal cells and permits the identification of small malignant populations that are often missed using FCM. In addition, damaged nuclei and other artefacts can be ignored using ICM, reducing background noise. Simultaneous assessment of morphological criteria and ploidy using ICM provides additional objective information from the one specimen, which is not available if only the FCM technique is used. This extra information may allow ICM to overcome a major drawback of FCM — that it cannot discriminate between normal host cells and tumour cells that have the same DNA staining intensity.

The basic capabilities expected from an ICM system for DNA densitometry are the following.

Speed

The ploidy overview programme should be sufficiently fast to give a representative sample of the specimen at about the usual screening rate of a typical user. In order to be usable in routine, the DNA measurement programme must be fast enough to analyse a few hundred cells in no more than a few minutes.

Log conversion

The signal from the standard television camera is usually approximately linear with light level, and needs to be converted into the logarithmic curve required for true densitometric values. This should be carried out with an accuracy of at least 8 bits to get sufficient accuracy at high-density values.

Image shading

The light level obtained across the field of a microscope is often significantly higher near the centre of the field than near the edges. To allow for this effect, a correction is required with a correction map to give a fixed level across an empty field. This map must be reset whenever the microscope illumination system is changed, or when a new specimen is loaded (because of variations in slide and/or mountant thickness).

Local background correction

In addition to the static variations in brightness across the field, there is often local variation in brightness outside versus inside a nucleus to be measured caused by cytoplasm, bacteria, etc. This effect can be minimized by taking a 'skirt' just around the segmented area, measuring its mean signal level (after shading correction) and then subtracting this local offset from the density values measured in the segmented nucleus.

Segmentation

Segmentation of the nuclei to be measured is one of the major sources of inaccuracy. The most simple method is that based on thresholding with a preset level. This level must be adjustable by the operator, and the segmented portions of the image must be visible for setting and control. In the random-sample programme, this may be sufficiently accurate. In current image analysis systems, the most appropriate segmentation mask may be produced by one or more of the local filtering methods that have been developed (e.g., median filtering high-pass filtering, followed by erosion and dilation and perhaps local smoothing of the outlines produced).

Artefact rejection

In most types of specimens, a substantial proportion of the objects detected by the segmentation algorithm will be cell overlaps, clusters and other non-nuclear artefacts. As these objects will cause errors in the histograms and numerical results if not removed, they must be eliminated by automatic or manual methods. This can be in the form of a simple one-dimensional gate (eliminating objects with abnormally high area or density) or in the form of statistical classifiers (e.g., linear discriminant multiparametric analysis).

6.4.2 Data handling

After having been stained by the Feulgen reaction, the microscopic preparation is scanned by the image cytometry system which measures the OD at each point of the image. The digital values belonging to the nucleus are selected through a segmentation procedure and then summed giving a measurement called the integrated optical density which is closely correlated to the quantity of DNA-specific stain in the nucleus, and less closely to the true DNA content. These raw IODs have to be normalized and corrected before any specimen-to-specimen comparisons can be carried out.

Normalization coefficient

In order to compensate for the variations in staining intensity from one staining bath to another and from one sample to another, the IODs have to be normalized so that the DNA staining intensity of a diploid cell will always be represented by the same numerical figure, say 2.00*c*, whatever the image cytometry system or the staining bath. The IOD_s measured by an image cytometry system are expressed by arbitrary raw numerical figures according to how the calculations are done. Thus, raw IOD_s measured on a given cell by one system may be 61 541 arbitrary units (a.u.) but 158 327 a.u. on another. Such figures must be normalized so that the average DNA staining intensity measured on a reference set of diploid normal cells having a 2*c* DNA content will finally be 2.00*c* (normalized arbitrary units). The normalization coefficient K is calculated so that the reference average IOD of normal non-proliferating cells is IOD $* K = 2.00c$. The normalization coefficient K entirely depends on the measuring instrument used and has to be accurately determined for any given ICM system, even if manufacturers provide this coefficient for the system they distribute.

Correction factors

The reference IOD of normal non-proliferating cells is usually not equal to the IOD measured on specimen cells. This is due to one of the following.

1 The reference normal non-proliferating cells, like most of the differentiated cells, have a chromatin condensation such that a measurement negative error is generated. For example, the DNA staining intensity of a resting lymphocyte is about 15% less than in a stimulated lymphocyte or an epithelial proliferating cell in G_1 phase of the division cycle.

2 For reasons of availability, the reference normal non-proliferating cells are often obtained from non-human material (rat or mouse hepatocytes, chicken or trout blood) and thus differ from human cells in DNA staining intensity because of the difference in DNA content.

Whatever the reference used, the average DNA staining intensity has to be corrected.

If the reference is external, the cells used can be either from the same species (leucocytes, stromal cells, normal epithelial cells) or from another species (trout or chicken erythrocytes, rat hepatocytes) and must be stained in the same bath as the specimens. The reference cells can be put either on the specimen slide or a dedicated one. Measuring such cells provides an average IOD of the external reference (IOD_e) that should differ from the human normal non-proliferating diploid cells of the specimen by a correction factor F_e, whose value has to be determined by separate experiments, to be rerun from time to time. For example, trout erythrocytes have an average DNA staining intensity which is about 60% of human cells (then $F_e = 1.67$). From one staining bath to another, both the IOD_e of the external reference cells and IOD_s of the specimen cells vary but the ratio $IOD_s/IOD_e = F_e$ of cells assumed to be in the same cell-cycle phase is kept constant if the staining of the specimen and reference cells varies to the same extent.

If the reference is internal, it refers to cells of the specimen that can be obviously recognized as normal and are usually lymphocytes, granulocytes or stromal cells. Measuring such cells provides an average IOD of the internal reference (IOD_i) that should differ from the specimen cells of interest by a correction factor F_i, mainly because of differential chromatin condensation, well known to generate a negative error. The F_i value has to be determined by separate experiments to be rerun from time to time. For example, the IOD_i of epithelial cells is about 1.15 times higher than in non-stimulated lymphocytes where the chromatin is more condensed (then $F_i = 1.15$) and thus can be easily identified. From one staining bath to another, both the IOD_i of the internal reference cells and IOD_s of the specimen cells vary but the ratio $IOD_s/IOD_i = F_i$ of cells assumed to be in the same ploidy status is kept constant if the staining of the specimen and reference cells varies to the same extent.

Both the F_e and F_i correction factors depend on the cell types' respective staining specificity and the measuring instrument used. These factors must be accurately determined for any given ICM system, even if manufacturers provide these coefficients for the system they distribute.

External versus internal reference

Among the variety of possible external reference cells, the imprints from liver have the advantage of offering diploid (2*c* DNA content), tetraploid (4*c* DNA content) and octoploid (8*c* DNA content) cell subpopulations whose occurrence rate is age dependent. Measuring these three categories of nuclei makes it possible to check the stoichiometry of the staining and the linearity of the cytometry system used. In spite of this advantage, an internal reference per specimen is always preferred over the external reference for correction purposes, as shown by the following experiment. Mouse hepatocytes and breast fibroadenoma imprints, which are all diploid, were stained in different baths where slightly different acid hydrolysis conditions were applied to the Feulgen reaction in order to obtain staining intensities differing from bath to bath. Measuring mouse hepatocytes as an external reference made it possible to order the baths from A to F according to linearly increasing average staining intensity. Then, as the internal reference, the lymphocytes and stromal cells were measured and their respective average IOD were plotted against bath number after normalization with respect to staining bath A. Figure 6.3 shows that the increase of the DNA staining intensity of both stromal cells and lympho-

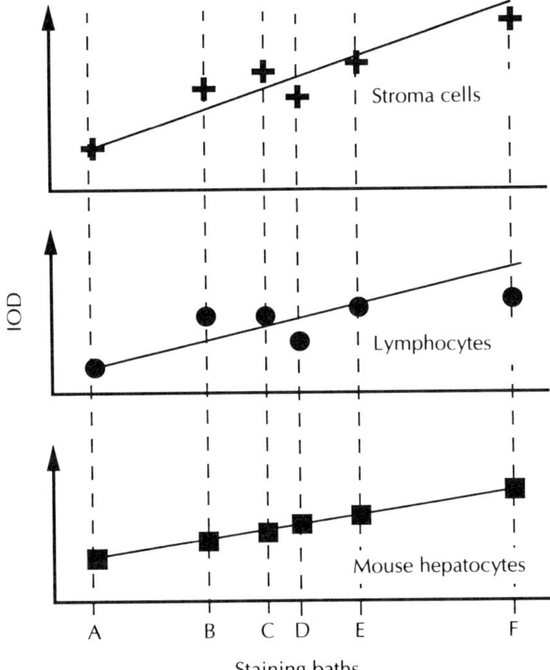

Fig. 6.3 Variation of the Feulgen integrated optical density (IOD) in external reference (mouse hepatocytes), internal reference (lymphocytes) and specimen (stromal) cells as the staining intensity increases from staining baths A to F. Each point represents the average Feulgen IOD (arbitrary units) of 100 cells.

cytes of the human fibroadenoma is not as linear as the increase of the DNA staining intensity of the external reference mouse hepatocytes. The overall ratio between lymphocytes and stromal cells is ± 0.2%, while it is ± 12% between hepatocytes and stromal cells, thus clearly demonstrating that, should the staining intensity vary, the consistency between specimen cells and internal reference lymphocytes is much better than between specimen and hepatocyte external reference. Most likely, mice and humans differ with respect to sensitivity to acid hydrolysis time. It is thus questionable whether one can be used as a reference for the other. However, as a result of the compaction of their chromatin, lymphocytes and granulocytes have a lower measured DNA staining intensity than normal non-proliferating epithelial cells having the same DNA content [61]. Moreover, the rarity of blood cells in a tumour preparation may limit the use of these cells as a DNA reference and thus obliges us to use an external reference from possibly the same species. The importance of the quality of the DNA staining intensity reference and the choice of calibration procedure have been documented in detail by Kiss *et al.* [62].

Standardization

Applying normalization and correction factors is called standardization and involves two of the following three possible sets of raw data:

1 a set of measurements on external reference cells from which an average-value IOD_e and external reference coefficient of variation over the specimen (CV_s) are derived and for which a correction factor F_e has been assessed separately;

2 a set of measurements on internal reference cells from which an average-value IOD_i and internal reference coefficient of variation of the internal reference (CV_i) are derived and for which a correction factor F_i has been assessed separately;

3 a set of measured IOD_s on cells of interest that have to be corrected and normalized.

The objective of standardization is to replace all specimen cell, raw IOD_s, by standard IOD values, then assumed to be independent from the ICM system and from the absolute staining intensities within certain acceptable limits:

1 a stain too pale leads to segmentation difficulties since too many pixels would fall below the detection threshold and would thus be missed by the segmentation mask;

2 a stain too dark would lead to many individual pixel ODs being well over the range of linearity of the Beer and Lambert laws. In both cases a large negative error would be obtained.

The standardization steps are the following.

1 The reference (either external or internal) DNA staining intensity has to be calculated (Fig. 6.4). The location of the reference cell population can be calculated as either:

(a) the peak value of the DNA staining intensity histogram, or

(b) the mean of the DNA staining intensities measured on the reference cells.

If the number of measured reference cells is high, these two values converge, but normally the number

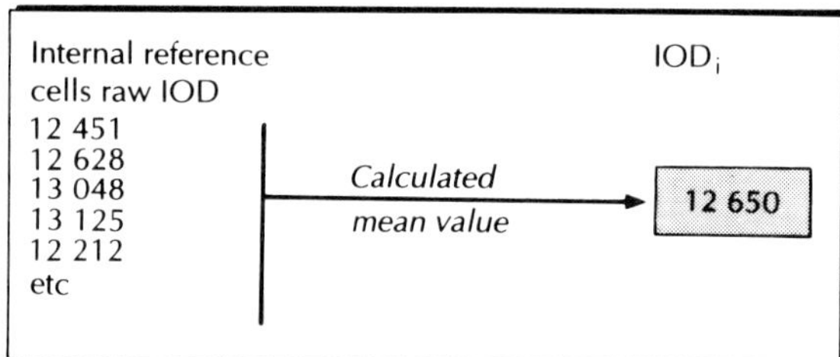

Fig. 6.4 Measuring the integrated optical density (IOD) of internal reference cells.

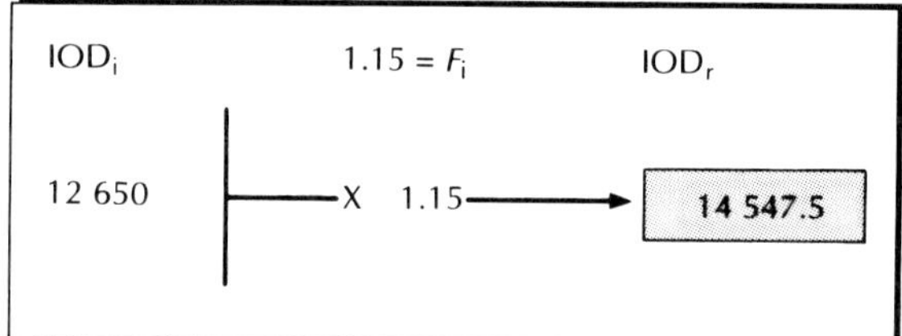

Fig. 6.5 Correction of reference integrated optical density (IOD_r).

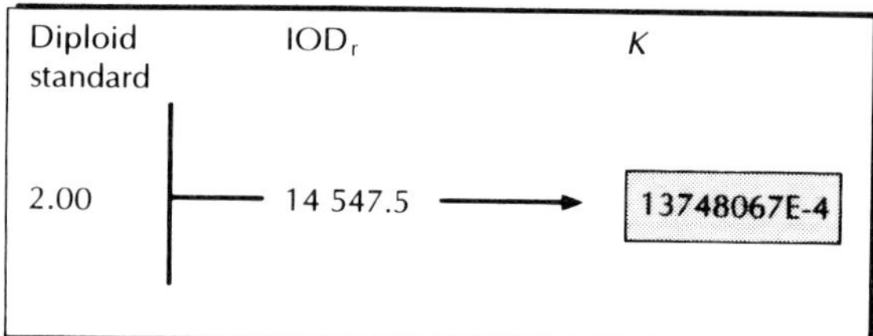

Fig. 6.6 Calculation of normalization coefficient K using the corrected reference integrated optical density (IOD_r).

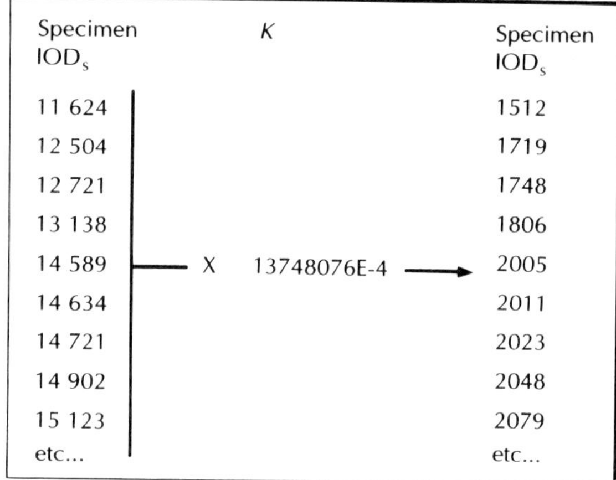

Fig. 6.7 Sample cell integrated optical density (IOD) corrected using the normalization coefficient K.

is low because it is usually time-consuming to select more than 20–50 lymphocytes within a tumour. In that case, using the peak value is better than the mean value because it is less sensitive to any single artefact.

2 The reference (either external or internal) DNA staining intensity has to be corrected by the correction factor to provide the final reference DNA staining intensity (IOD_r), expected to be that of the normal non-proliferating cells of the specimen (Fig. 6.5). The calculation is as follows:

$IOD_r = IOD_e * F_e$ if the external reference is used
$IOD_r = IOD_r * F_i$ if the internal reference is used

3 The final reference DNA staining intensity (Fig. 6.6) can then be used to calculate the normalization coefficient K as follows:

$K = 2.00/IOD_r$

4 Finally, all the IOD_s measured on the specimen cells will be recalculated into IOD_s standard values (Fig. 6.7), using the K coefficient as follows:

$IOD_s = K * IOD_s$

5 The distribution histogram of the standardized DNA staining intensities over the specimen cell population can thus be constructed and displayed for further interpretation (Fig. 6.8).

Coefficient of variation

Given all the limitations mentioned above, a certain variability of the measured DNA staining intensity is expected among cells having identical DNA content because the staining, its measurement and the digitizer (camera and converter) are not perfectly reproducible. The overall variability is estimated by the CV_s. From a set of standardized IOD_s on a specimen comprised of non-proliferating normal cells, the CV_s is calculated as follows:

CV_s = standard deviation of IOD_s/mean IOD_s

This CV_s is comprised of:

1 CV_l due to labelling intensity differences from

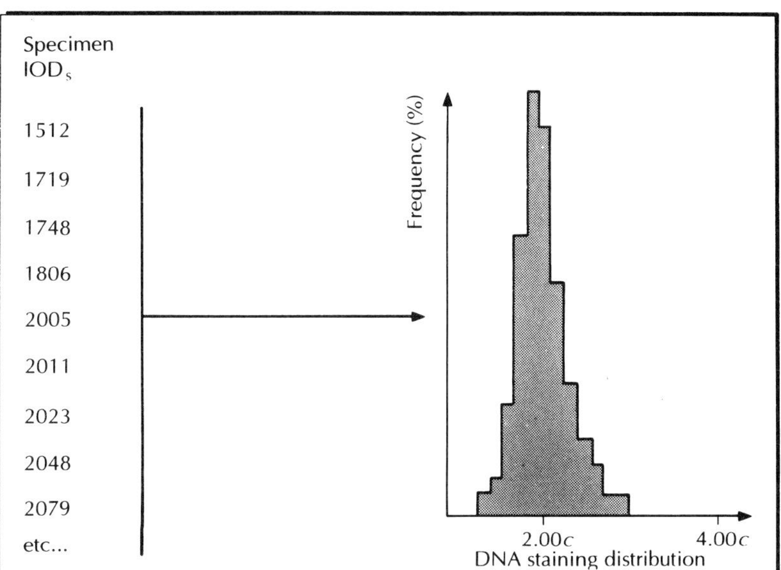

Fig. 6.8 Histogram of specimen cell integrated optical densities (IOD).

cell to cell as a consequence of differential hydrolysis curve and local staining conditions;
2 CV_m due to measurement bias resulting from chromatin pattern and spreading differences from cell to cell, resulting in variation of distributional error, loss of linearity on pixels with high IOD, and cell population density changing the glare effect;
3 CV_n due to non-reproducibility of the instrument digitizer resulting from signal to noise ratio.

The CV_n is very easy to evaluate by repeated measurements on a single cell. It is usually minimized after 30 measurements and stabilizes around 0.5%. Contrarily, the CV_l and CV_m are much more difficult to evaluate individually. All together, they represent the biological variability CV_b, that can be measured by repeated measurements (to keep CV_n to a minimum) on an increasing number of cells of a reference homogeneous population such as a liver imprint. So doing, the CV_b is usually minimized after 50 cells have been repeatedly measured and stabilizes around 2%. Should the same cells be measured only once, the overall CV_s (including CV_n and CV_b) would not behave very differently. Finally, the CV_s which defines the confidence of measurements on individual cells depends on the number of cells having a given DNA staining intensity. Consequently, the DNA histogram class size depends on the CV_s and the number of cells included. Such a DNA histogram, interpretable without statistical restriction on dimensionality, is still to be implemented by manufacturers.

The DNA staining intensity can be measured by ICM but cannot be expected to measure the DNA content of cells, although both features vary accordingly. The various sources of errors due to specimen staining and instrument measurement limitations result in a distribution histogram, the biological meaning of which is difficult to establish. As a matter of fact, the outline of the distribution histogram may be very different depending on the number of classes and/or the class width chosen, as shown in Fig. 6.9. Increasing the number of classes makes an increasing number of peaks appear. Whether these peaks represent cell population subsets with different DNA content is questionable unless each DNA histogram class width is calculated to display similar significance, taking into account the CV and the number of cells in the class. Given a CV, a class has to be wide enough to ascertain a 95% confidence for cells collected in it. Not only does the ascertained difference in DNA staining intensity not convey the true difference in DNA content, but it should also be noted that a 5% difference in DNA staining intensity already represents a difference of two chromosomes of average size in human cells. This remark confirms, if

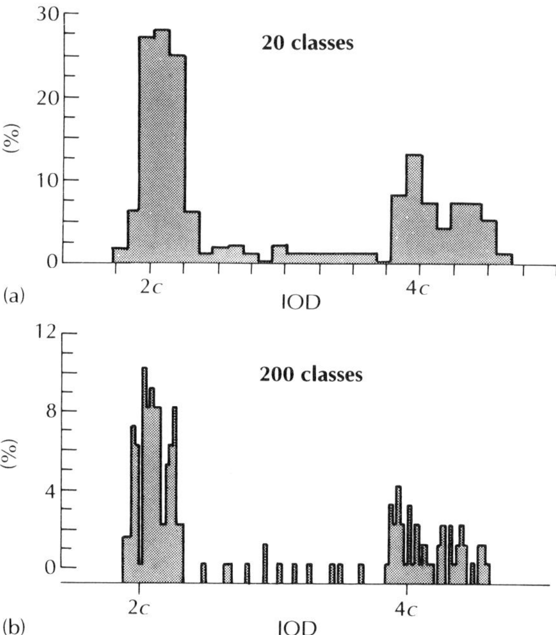

Fig. 6.9 Representation of the histogram distribution of 600 cells according to their DNA staining intensity represented as (a) 20 versus (b) 200 classes. The higher the number of classes, the higher the number of peaks, whose statistical meaning is questionable. IOD, integrated optical density.

necessary, that speaking of ploidy when measuring DNA staining intensity is more than presumptuous.

6.5 INTERPRETATION OF HISTOGRAMS

The distribution of the cell population DNA staining intensities according to a so-called DNA histogram is the commonest way of looking at the results. In addition to this overall assessment of the results, statistical parameters can be calculated to evaluate more objectively the distribution.

6.5.1 Histogram classification

The interpretation of DNA histograms obtained by ICM has been the subject of numerous papers since the first reference classification published by Auer *et al.* [63,64]. In addition to such an overall classification based on the DNA histogram outline, further work has defined a number of DNA distribution-derived parameters. Some depend on the number of histogram classes and tend to be unreliable, while others are more system-independent.

DNA histogram outline

Auer's classification [63–65] was the first attempt to correlate DNA histogram outline to prognosis. It was initially designed for breast cancer but it is now used for other malignancies. Auer's DNA histogram classification defines four types.

Type I has one major DNA peak around the 2*c* DNA content, allowing only a few cells to deviate from this average value.

Type II is characterized by either a peak in the 4*c* region or one peak in 2*c* and one in 4*c*. The few cells in between 2*c* and 4*c* are assumed to be in S phase of the cell division cycle. Only a very small proportion of cells may appear outside the DNA values of a normal cell population, usually in the 8*c* range.

Type III is similar to type II but with a noticeable proportion of cells having a DNA content in between 2*c* and 4*c*. This proportion, lately called S-phase fraction (SPF), is claimed to be an estimate of the proliferative activity of the cell population.

Type IV is characterized by a pronounced and irregular aneuploidy with a DNA content ranging from 2*c* to 6*c* and even higher.

Sperb *et al.* [66] proposed to add a fifth type to the Auer classification to take into account those DNA histograms with a main peak in the 3*c* region. Other authors have emphasized a comparable classification based on the presence of a major 2*c* peak (the tumour is then said to be diploid or near diploid) and a 4*c* peak (the tumour is said to be tetraploid, although a 4*c* peak may result from a lengthening of G_2-M cell-cycle phase duration of diploid cells or a real tetraploidization consequent to endomitosis). The other DNA histograms with non-euploid peaks (2*c*, 4*c*, 8*c*, etc.) are said to be aneuploid. Unfortunately, assigning DNA histogram profiles to these types is highly observer-dependent, especially for heterogeneous tumour-cell populations [67]. Moreover, these classifications based on histogram outline do not make it possible to identify the biological mechanisms responsible for the distribution of cells according to the DNA content actually observed.

Distributional parameters

To obviate the inherent subjectivity of visual classifications of DNA histogram profiles, various order statistics have been proposed to represent the so-called tumour ploidy.

The *DI* (DNA index) is the most popular DNA histogram feature, mainly because it is very simple to derive. It is calculated as the ratio between the DNA staining intensity of a peak of the DNA histogram and the DNA staining intensity of the reference after standardization. Various cell populations are said to be characterized by the following indices: below 1, hypodiploid; 1, diploid or near diploid; 1–2, aneuploid; 2,tetraploid; above 2, hyperploid In case of multiple peaks, each one has a DI and the cell population is said to be heterogeneous with respect to ploidy. Besides the wrong usage of the terms diploid, aneuploid, tetraploid, these preformulated conclusions are misleading for clinicians and just raise additional questions, such as: what is the minimum value of the DI above 1 that ascertains aneuploidy? Which DI should be taken into consideration in cases of heterogeneous populations? How many histogram classes should there be to ascertain the peak value?

The *2.5cER* (2.5*c* exceeding rate) has been formulated to separate non-proliferating and non-aneuploid from proliferating and possibly aneuploid cell populations. It takes into account the proportion of cells having a DNA content higher than 2.5*c*. This feature is not satisfactory since it may increase due to mechanisms as different as increased proliferation rate, occurrence of truly aneuploid or polyploid clones, or increased frequency of cells in S, G_2 or M phase of the cell cycle as a consequence of lengthening of these phases due to genetic disorders.

The *5cER* (5*c* exceeding rate) has been formulated to detect cells whose DNA content is not a consequence of normal diploid cell proliferation, if any [68]. This feature does not apply to tissues which normally contain tetraploid cells (urothelium, liver), where the presence of a few cells having a DNA staining intensity greater than 5*c* is not unusual.

The *2cDI* (2*c* deviation index) is the variance of the DNA staining intensity of the cell population around the normal diploid (2*c*) DNA peak [68,69], expressed as:

$$2cDI = \sqrt{[(1/n)\Sigma(Ci - 2c)2]}$$

where n = number of cells, Ci = DNA staining intensity of individual cells, and $2c$ = reference DNA staining intensity.

The *DE* (distribution entropy) measures the heterogeneity of the DNA staining intensities distribution [70]. Its value is maximum if the measurement values are evenly distributed over all classes and it is nil if all measurements belong to the same class. A division by the logarithm of the number of classes renders the entropy independent from the number of classes.

$$\text{Entropy} = \Sigma pi \times \log 2(pi)/\log 2\ k$$

where pi = probability or frequency of class i and k = number of classes.

Interpretative parameters

The previous distributional parameters, although objective, are not very helpful for further understanding of the biological rationale behind any correlation with tumour prognosis. Other parameters have thus been designed to extract directly biological meaning from the distribution of cells according to their DNA staining intensity.

The DNA-MG (DNA-malignancy grade according to Böcking [71,72]) is a logarithmic transform of the 2cDI, designed to provide a continuous scale [2]:

$$\begin{aligned}\text{DNA-MG} &= 3 * \log(2cDI + 1)/\log 51 \\ &= 1.757 \times \lg(2cDI + 1)\end{aligned}$$

This parameter permits the discrimination of tumours of various tissues with a bad versus good prognosis, using a threshold specific to the tissue considered [71,72]. Unfortunately, the rationale behind the equation are not biological by nature.

The *PB* (ploidy balance) is calculated after the standardized DNA staining intensities are assigned to 10 classes centred on the ploidy values: 2*c*, 2.5*c*, 3*c*, 3.5*c*, 4*c*, 5*c*, 6*c*, 7*c*, 8*c*, >8*c*. Then PB is calculated as the percentage of euploid cells collected in the 2*c*, 4*c* and 8*c* classes minus the percentage of cells collected in the 2.5*c*, 3*c*, 3.5*c*, 5*c*, 6*c*, 7*c*, >8*c*. This parameter varies from +100% (all of the cells are euploid) to −100% (all of the cells are aneuploid) [67]. This parameter is probably close to the real occurrence of cells having an abnormal DNA content.

The *PI* (proliferation index) is calculated after the standardized DNA staining intensities are assigned to 10 classes, as above. The PI is then calculated as the percentage of cells outside the major peak (regardless of its ploidy level) and the related G_2 counterpart (peaks having a whole number multiple of the modal value) [67]. This parameter measures the real occurrence of cells having a DNA content intermediate between G_0–G_1 cells and G_2–M cells, i.e., the S cells of a cycling cell population, whatever their ploidy.

When associated, the PB and PI provide the two main features of neoplasia accessible by DNA staining: the degree of aneuploidy and the proliferation, respectively. Plotting PI and PB data for intralobular breast carcinomas has made it possible to define a triangle of aggression representing tumour samples associated with a bad prognosis (less than 5-year survival) compared to good prognosis (more than 10-year survival) [67].

The *SPF* is the proportion of the cell population in S phase of a cell cycle. Depending on the author, this parameter is calculated in very different ways. Longin *et al.* [73] estimated the S phase as the percentage of tumour cells having a DNAc staining intensity between 2.5*c* and 3.8*c*. Montironi *et al.* [74] used a commercially available programme (Multi-cycle version 2.12, Phenix Flow Systems, San Diego, CA) based on a method proposed by Dean and Jett [75]. A Gaussian distribution fitting algorithm is used to estimate the percentages of cells in G_0–G_1 and G_2. The SPF is then derived from a polynomial curve. The results obtained from image analysis are usually very similar to those obtained from FCM.

The SPF suffers from two main drawbacks. The first concerns the calculation, which makes the improper assumption that only proliferating cells have a DNA staining intensity intermediate between the G_0–G_1 and the G_2 peaks. The second concerns the erroneous interpretation that the higher the SPF, the higher the proliferating activity of the cell population. It has been known for 30 years that an increase in S-phase duration — the cell cycle time and the growth fraction being kept constant — does increase the SPF accordingly. S-phase lengthening subsequent to genetic abnormalities has been reported in all tumours investigated in this respect. As a matter of fact, the literature shows a remarkable correlation between SPF and aneuploidy on an impressive number of tumours whose proliferation kinetic parameters (growth fraction and cell-cycle duration) were unknown, thus demonstrating that increased SPF is obviously correlated to chromosome aberrations.

6.5.2 Histogram reliability

Type of preparation

The sample from which the DNA histogram is obtained can comprise spontaneously exfoliating cells (voided urine or bladder washings), scrapings or brushings material (uterine cervix, bronchiolus), fine-needle aspiration biopsy (breast, prostate) or imprints from the surgical specimen. The cells obtained are smeared, pressed or cytocentrifuged on to a slide, some being isolated and others clumped but kept entire, as opposed to histological sections. Comparative studies on mammary tumours have shown that centrifugation or imprinting does not introduce significant differences in DNA staining measurement [66]. However, it is well-known that cytocentrifugation may alter nuclear shape and size and chromatin pattern, thus providing a potential source of densitometric inconsistency.

Since an increasing number of DNA cytometric studies are being made on histological sections from paraffin-embedded archival material, it must be pointed out that the conditions of applicability, and especially the ratio between nuclear size and section thickness, vary from tumour to tumour and even from clone to clone. Any claim from manufacturers that measuring DNA ploidy on tissue sections is possible is clearly intended to persuade buyers, but is not based on scientific demonstration. Technology has not yet been developed (and may never be!) for this very attractive way of retrospectively investigating the correlation between DNA staining distribution and tumour prognosis. It has been shown that the use of cytological material is definitely preferable to histological sections, takes less time, and can be more selective of malignant material [76], particularly if the new generation of interactive ICM systems like HOME (highly optimized microscope environment) is used [77,78].

Artefact rejection

Ever-increasing sophisticated image analysis techniques improve segmentation and featuring of nuclei stained for DNA, thus increasing the number of nuclei that can be analysed automatically in an acceptable time. One pitfall of fully automatic standalone ICM systems is the processing of cells which are irrelevant, such as non-urothelial cells in bladder washings, stromal cells in fine-needle aspiration biopsy (FNAB) of the breast, etc. The automatic procedure has thus to apply selective processing of those objects within predefined limits of shape and size [79] and reject those that do not. This technique may prove to be either inefficient (if the limits are too tolerant) or troublesome (if the limits are too stringent when compared to unexpected tumour-cell variability). Most of the artefact rejection image-processing capabilities have been exemplified up to a decade ago [80–82] and no significant progress is expected in the near future.

Sampling validity and representativity

Cytometric analysis is most often based on a sample of 200–300 randomly selected cells acquired with no stopping criteria. The question over when to stop the analysis hides two completely different questions about the reliability of the acquired dataset. The first, which refers to validity, is whether the number of analysed cells is sufficient to support the interpretation of the observed distribution DNA histogram *per se*. The second, which refers to representativity, is whether all the possible clones of the tumour are represented in the dataset.

As far as validity is questioned, proper statistics may certainly provide an answer. For example, a Kolmogorov–Smirnof test on every new set of 50 cells would provide a confidence coefficient for the observed distribution which progressively establishes a non-significant difference when a sufficiently large number of cells has been analysed. Surprisingly, such a simple test is not even done in practice. The rule of thumb stating that 300 cells are sufficient may apply for a monomodal cell population, while a heterogeneous population spread from $2c$ to $7c$ may require 3000 cells to ascertain the same significance for the DNA classes. Should the DNA histogram become a medical routine for tumour prognosis, such an arresting criterion based on statistics running during the analysis will have to be used.

As far as representativity is concerned, it is well known that many tumours are heterogeneous and contain several cell clones [83,84] that do not have the same probability of being encountered in a sample. It has been suggested that 10–20% of errors obtained from DNA histogram-based prognosis could be explained by a failure to detect aneuploid clones that are small when compared to the whole tumour-cell population [85]. Improving the detection of such clones may require the selection of cells by a pathologist [79] or an increased number of samples (four for Beerman *et al.* [86] 9–10 for Pennes *et al.* [87]). If the Kolmogorov–Smirnof test is used to test every new set of 50 cells, it may establish a non-significant difference before a new clone, different from those already detected, indicates the opposite. Whether such a clone will be encountered after, say, 10 cells or 10 000 cells is not predictable and not relevant for any statistical test. Should the particular clone be picked up by the sampling method (multiple-direction FNAB, for example), only a pathologist rapidly screening the entire cell population at low resolution would be able cost-efficiently to detect areas of particular interest, record their co-ordinates with a user-friendly marking microscope like HOME [78], and then run the DNA staining quantitation in these selected areas.

6.5.3 Conclusion

FCM, mainly applied during recent years to fundamental biology, is not yet established in clinical routine because it requires tissue disaggregation and destruction of the specimen so that direct control of what is actually measured cannot be implemented. On the other hand, this approach has been quite successful because it is essentially impossible for end-users to build their own system. FCM was thus practised, since the beginning, with a rather limited number of commercially available systems. As a result, communication between users has been facilitated and a consensus rapidly emerged about the possibilities and limitations of the instruments and related methods. A worldwide experience sharing and a rather unified technical jargon emerged. Conversely, the rapid development of computer imaging technology in the last decade enabled practically everybody to plug in a microscope, television camera, image boards and personal computers. Thus each researcher built his or her own ICM system and implemented his or her own ideas on how to analyse images. With as many different systems as users, communication has been incredibly inefficient over the years. The dialogue between deaf people, each one reinventing the wheel, was so noisy that sorting out the specific and real advantages of ICM compared to FCM proved to be impossible. A number of end-users of these quantitative approaches thus held faith in either image or flow according to their scientific and technical environment or just following trends and moods. Nowadays, rationalism seems to be winning! Medical users now want to generate results which are reproducible both within and between different laboratories. They are aware that most commercially established ICM and histometry instruments are respectful of the physical and mathematical requirements progressively defined since the pioneering work of Torbjörn Caspersson, while home-built instruments are not. In addition, user-friendliness and software flexibility have opened a new era during which the quantitative knowledge of cell and tissues will become standardized and will complement the qualitative and subjective but still essential pathologist medical expertise.

6.6 APPLICATIONS OF DNA STATIC CYTOMETRY

P. W. HAMILTON

With the widespread availability of computerized image analysis systems, static DNA cytometry has now been applied to many areas of tumour pathology. However, the variety of techniques used to derive densitometric data and analyse the results makes direct comparisons between different studies extremely difficult. Since many studies have shown the clinical value of this technique it is vital that standardized methodology and consistent terminology are established.

6.6.1 Prostate

DNA cytometry has now been established as a powerful tool in the grading of prostate cancer and this has been supported by a consensus meeting of the World Health Organization [88]. The most convincing evidence comes from a study by Forsslund and Zetterberg [89] where DNA ploidy was measured on a series of patients with a long-term follow-up. Patients who died within 3 years of diagnosis consistently had DNA stemlines at 3*c* and 6*c*, whereas long-term survivors (> 15 years) had stemlines at 2*c* and 4*c* (Fig. 6.10). Multivariate analysis has shown that compared to grade and tumour stage, DNA ploidy is the best predictor of survival [90]. These results are reflected in the additional findings that tumour progression is associated with a higher incidence of DNA aneuploidy [91] and that DNA ploidy and grade are independently important in predicting the presence of metastases [92]. It is likely that centres with the appropriate facilities

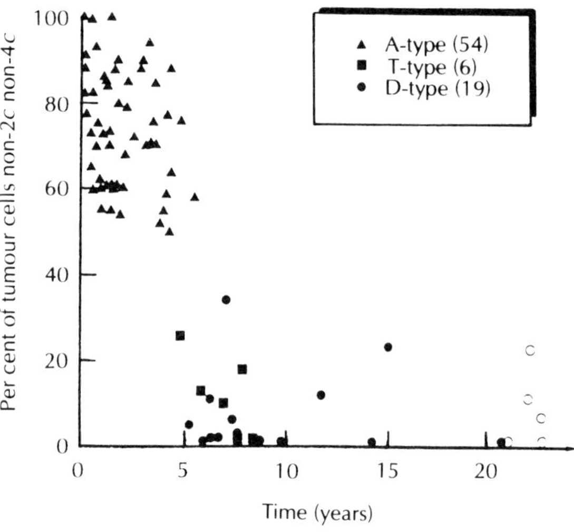

Fig. 6.10 The relationship between the percentage of tumour cells which are non-2*c* or non-4*c* and patient survival. Aneuploid DNA histograms (A-type); tetraploid (T-type); diploid (D-type); (○) diploid tumours; patients still alive at time of study. From Forsslund and Zetterberg [89] with permission.

will adopt this technique routinely in the prognostic assessment of prostate carcinomas.

The characterization and diagnosis of prostatic intraepithelial neoplasia is becoming important in many centres. Montironi *et al.* [93,94] showed a progressive increase in DNA ploidy from nodular hyperplasia, through increasing degrees of prostatic intraepithelial neoplasia to carcinoma.

6.6.2 Breast

The ploidy characteristics of breast cancer have been extensively studied using static cytometry. These studies have shown that increased DNA content is associated with increasing histological grade [95–97], tumour size [98–99], lymph-node invasion [100], oestrogen-receptor status [101,102], c-*erb*-2 oncoprotein and p53 tumour-suppressor gene product overexpression [96] and increased cell proliferation as assessed by Ki-67 labelling indices, and was more commonly found in young women [103]. It is not surprising therefore that several survival studies have proposed that abnormal DNA histograms may be used as an indicator of poor prognosis in breast cancer patients [99,100, 104–106]. Examination of large patient numbers has shown that the DNA profile is an independent variable in assessing prognosis [107] (Fig. 6.11), providing additional information to the other independent features, tumour size and lymph node status [98]. Bocking *et al.* [108] advocate the use of

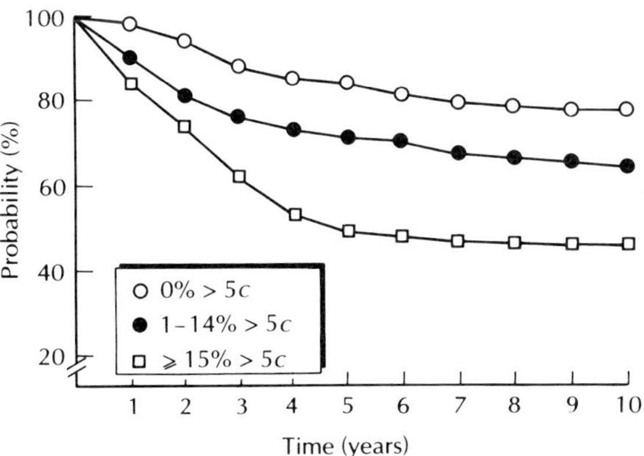

Fig. 6.11 Probability of distant recurrence-free survival in breast cancer patients stratified by the percentage of cells >5*c*. From Fallenius *et al.* [107].

a (malignancy grade DNA-MG), a mathematical formula based on the variance of DNA values around the normal diploid peak (see Section 6.5.1: Interpretative parameters). They have shown this measure to be a reproducible and reliable prognostic indicator in breast cancer. While the evidence from these many studies may seem overwhelming, it is important to be aware that some studies have shown that the association between abnormal DNA ploidy and poor survival disappears when patients are stratified for oestrogen-receptor status [109]. A comparison of DNA modal values between the primary tumour and lymph-node metastases shows good correlation [102,108].

The incidence of DNA aneuploidy is lower in atypical hyperplasia (36%) as compared to ductal carcinoma *in situ* (63%) [110] and is increased further in the comedo variant (91%) [111]. However, the distinction of atypical hyperplasia and well-differentiated intraductal carcinoma could only be made in 69% of cases using DNA cytometry [112]. Lobular and papillary carcinoma *in situ* have a very low incidence of DNA aneuploidy [111].

6.6.3 Colorectum

Patients with DNA aneuploid colorectal tumours, as determined using static cytometry, tend to have shorter survival times than non-aneuploid cases [113,114] and DNA aneuploidy seems to be more frequent in distal tumours [114]. Nevertheless, multivariate studies showed that DNA ploidy was not an independent parameter in the assessment of overall patient survival, particularly when Dukes' stage is included [114,115], but that it may be a good indicator of prognosis in patients who had undergone 'curative' surgical resection [114]. Extensive heterogeneity in DNA patterns exists in colorectal tumours [113,116,117], making the precise assessment of an individual patient difficult unless numerous samples are taken [117].

DNA content is also altered in adenomatous polyps with a continuous increase in ploidy abnormalities from mild dysplasia through to infiltrating carcinoma [118,119]. Alterations in ploidy values are also noted in transitional epithelium adjacent to colorectal tumours, advocating a possible premalignant change in these cells [120].

6.6.4 Bladder

While FCM has been used successfully to screen for bladder cancer and for monitoring treatment (see Section 10.3.3), static ICM is favoured by some. Shabaik *et al.* [121] showed that DNA cytometry of cells from bladder washings had a sensitivity for detecting recurrence of 85% compared to 55% by routine cytology and this has been confirmed by others [122]. However, analysis of cells from washings alone may not be accurate as a discrepancy in DNA profile between washings and tumour imprints has been shown to exist in up to 30% of cases [123]. Again DNA abnormalities have been shown to be associated with histological grade [124,125].

Classification of patients with transitional-cell carcinoma on the basis of their DNA histograms has demonstrated a strong association between ploidy abnormalities and clinical course which is independent of grade and tumour stage [126]. Similarly, Aufferman *et al.* [127] showed that a calculated DNA-MG was strongly related to survival in patients with bladder tumours. This DNA-MG is based on the variance of DNA values around the diploid peak and the importance of this feature in transitional-cell carcinoma prognosis and in predicting progression-free survival is confirmed by Schapers *et al.* [128].

6.6.5 Uterine cervix

Uterine cervical neoplasia was the subject of Caspersson's early studies on DNA content using cytophotometry in which abnormalities were demonstrated in malignant and premalignant lesions [129]. Since then many studies have confirmed that malignant lesions generally show aneuploid DNA distributions [130–133] whilst benign lesions rarely possess cells with a DNA content greater than $5c$ [133–135]. It is for these reasons that the measurement of nuclear OD, either on Papanicolaou or Feulgen-stained smears, may be an important feature in abnormal cell detection for automated cervical screening devices [136–138]. The distance of the aneuploid stemline from the diploid position seems to bear some relevance to the aggressiveness of the tumour and patient survival — patients with high stemline tumours have a worse prognosis [139–143].

The incidence of cells showing DNA aneuploidy increases with increasing grades of cervical dysplasia or cervical intraepithelial neoplasia [130, 144–147] and follow-up of patients with cervical dysplasia has shown that smears demonstrating DNA aneuploidy represent a high-risk group whose lesions are likely to progress to invasive carcinoma (Fig. 6.12) [133,148–150]. However, this view is not shared by Nasiell *et al.* [151], who showed no

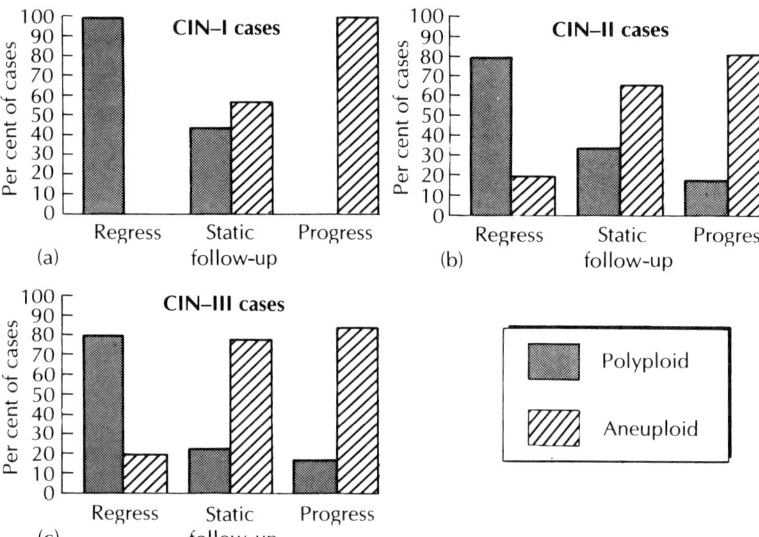

Fig. 6.12 The relative proportions of aneuploid and polyploid DNA profiles in three follow-up groups. Regress, initial abnormal cervical biopsy followed by negative histology or cytology for at least a year. Static, abnormal cervical biopsy with no increase in severity for more than 1 year. Progress, increase in severity of lesion after subsequent biopsy, cervical conization or hysterectomy. From Bibbo *et al.* [149].

difference in the DNA profiles between dysplastic lesions which progressed and those that did not. Dysplasia as a result of human papillomavirus infection (i.e., koilocytosis) often shows polyploidy, i.e., the presence of 2*c*, 4*c*, 6*c* or 8*c* DNA stemlines. Chatelain *et al.* [152] have shown that the detection of aneuploid cells above 9*c* is predictive of the development of invasive cancer.

6.6.6 Thyroid

By classifying DNA ploidy histograms into six types — (I) diploid; (II) triploid; (III) tetraploid; (IV) hyperdiploid; (V) hypertriploid; and (VI) polymorphic — increasing DNA abnormalities were evident with increasing histological grade in thyroid tumours [153]. Overall, malignant tumours show a higher incidence of DNA aneuploidy than benign tumours [153–155] and this was also shown in fine-needle aspiration cytology of the thyroid where the distinction between benign and malignant lesions using DNA quantitation was better than by conventional cytology [156]. The measurement of DNA ploidy may be useful in distinguishing benign and malignant follicular thyroid tumours [157], although in a study by Montironi *et al.* [155] using discriminant analysis, DNA ploidy was not included as one of the quantitative discriminatory variables in the distinction of follicular adenoma and carcinoma. A number of studies have shown a lack of association between DNA ploidy pattern and tumour progression or survival [158,159], although young patients (who generally have a good prognosis) tend to have DNA diploid tumours [158]. However, in medullary thyroid cancer, a multivariate analysis showed that patients with high stage (equal to or greater than stage II) and high variation in DNA ploidy had a shorter disease-free interval [160].

An interesting study by Wallin *et al.* [161] on thyroid tumours of mixed differentiation showed that DNA aneuploidy was present in all of the anaplastic tumour regions but only in one-third of the papillary or follicular differentiated areas. The conclusion made was that anaplastic thyroid carcinoma is not the result of clonal transformation of well-differentiated carcinomas but rather the result of a *de novo* change.

6.6.7 Ovary

As with other malignancies, DNA aneuploidy is commonly found in ovarian carcinoma [162–165]. In serous tumours the specificity of DNA cytometry as a predictor of mortality was higher than conventional histological evaluation (0.92 vs 0.42) and as such may have a role to play in patient prognosis. In borderline serous tumours, Fu *et al.* [163] showed an association between DNA aneuploidy and tumour stage but, in a larger series, de Nictolis *et al.* [165] found no such association. In fact, DNA aneuploidy did not correlate with gross features, the presence or absence of peritoneal implants, the number of mitoses or patient survival [165]. However, patients with implants and a DNA-aneuploid pattern may have a worse prognosis. The role of DNA measurements was further undermined in a study of normal ovarian tissue, borderline mucinous tumours and mucinous carcinomas where DNA content was less useful than morphometric data in the discrimination of the three groups [164]. Conversely, in a number of studies on borderline ovarian tumours, DNA measurements have been shown to be useful in predicting prognosis [166,167].

6.6.8 Lung

Kayser *et al.* [168] showed that the measurement of nuclear DNA content was not associated with tumour size or lymph-node infiltration. In malignant mesothelioma, diploid/polyploid tumours tend to have a good prognosis [169], although because of the wide variation in ploidy values, DNA cytometry is not useful in the distinction between benign and malignant mesothelial lesions [170]. DNA content shows an increasing trend through the sequence from typical carcinoids to atypical carcinoids to small-cell lung carcinomas [171] and may have a role to play in the distinction of premalignant and non-premalignant squamous dysplasias [172].

6.6.9 Skin

DNA aneuploidy is found in basal-cell carcinomas [173] and in malignant melanomas of the skin [174]. There is no association between DNA abnormalities and metastases in primary melanomas [174]. A higher incidence of DNA aneuploidy exists in dysplastic naevi as opposed to compound naevi [175].

6.6.10 Miscellaneous

DNA ploidy analysis by static cytometry has been investigated in numerous other pathological conditions. These include oral tissues [176,177], oesophagus [178], stomach [179–181], pancreas [182–184], liver [185–187], kidney [188,189], larynx [190–193], nervous system [194–199], soft-tissue tumours [200–202] and lymph node/leukaemias [203–208].

References

1 Schulte EK, Wittekind DH. Standardization of the Feulgen reaction: the influence of chromatin condensation of the kinetics of acid hydrolysis. *Anal Cell Pathol* 1990; 2: 149–157.

2 Patau K. Absorption of irregular-shaped objects. *Chromosoma* 1952; 5: 341–362.

3 Mendelsohn ML, Conway TJ, Hungerford DA *et al.* Computer oriented analysis of human chromosomes. I. Photometric estimation of DNA content. *Cytogenetics* 1966; 5: 223–242.

4 Zimmer HG. Microphotometry. In: Neuhoff Y (ed.) *Micromethods in Molecular Biology*. Berlin: Springer 1973: 297–328.

5 Goldstein DJ. Errors in microdensitometry. *Histochem J* 1981; 13: 251–267.

6 Mayall BH, Mendelsohn ML. Deoxyribonucleic acid cytometry of stained human leucocytes. II. The mechanical scanner of CYDAC, the theory of scanning photometry and the magnitude of residual errors. *J Histochem Cytochem* 1970; 18: 383–407.

7 Duijndam WA, van Duijn P, Riddersme SH. Optical errors in scanning stage absorbance cytophotometry. II. Application of correction factors for residual distributional error, glare and diffraction error in practical cytometry. *J Histochem Cytochem* 1980; 28: 395–400.

8 Mac Eachron DL, Gallistel CR, Tretiak OJ. Issues in quantitative imaging. In: Toga AW (ed.) *Three-dimensional Neuro-imaging*. New York: Raven Press, 1990: 39–71.

9 Feulgen R, Rossenbeck H. Mikroskopisch-chemischer Nach-weis einer Nukleinsäure vom Typus der Thymonukleinsäure und die darauf beruhende elektive Färbung von Zellkernen in mikroskopischen Präparaten. *Z Physiol Chem* 1924; 135: 203–249.

10 European Committee for Clinical Laboratory Standards (ECCLS) Subcommittee on reference materials for tissue stains. Parts I and II. *Histochem J* 1992; 24: 217–242.

11 Hardonk MJ, van Duijn P. Studies on the Feulgen reaction with histochemical model systems. *J Histochem Cytochem* 1964; 12: 758–767.

12 Schulte E, Wittekind D. Standardization of the Feulgen–Schiff technique. Staining characteristics of pure fuchsin dyes; a cytophotometric investigation. *Histochemistry* 1989; 91: 321–331.

13 Schulte E. Standardization of the Feulgen reaction for absorption DNA image cytometry: a review. *Anal Cell Pathol* 1991; 3: 167–182.

14 Kiss R, Salmon I, Camby I, Gras S, Pasteels J-L. Characterization of factors in routine laboratory protocols that significantly influence the Feulgen reaction. *J Histochem Cytochem* 1993; 6: 935–945.

15 Mayall BH. Deoxyribonucleic acid cytophotometry of stained human leukocytes. I. Differences among cell types. *J Histochem Cytochem* 1969; 17: 249–257.

16 Mello MLS. Cytochemical properties of euchromatin and heterochromatin. *Histochem J* 1983; 15: 739–751.

17 Fukuda M, Miyoshi N, Hattori T *et al.* Different instability of nuclear DNA at acid hydrolysis in cancerous and noncancerous cells as revealed by fluorescent staining with acridine orange. *Histochemistry* 1986; 84: 556–560.

18 Rasch RW, Rasch EM. Kinetics of hydrolysis during the Feulgen reaction for deoxyribonucleic acid. *J Histochem Cytochem* 1973; 21: 1053–1065.

19 Millett JA, Husain OAN, Bitensky L, Chayen J. Feulgen-hydrolysis profiles in cells exfoliated from the cervix uteri: a potential aid in the diagnosis of malignancy. *J Clin Pathol* 1982; 35: 345–349.

20 Darzynkiewicz Z, Traganos F, Andreeff M, Sharpless T, Melamed MR. Different sensitivity of chromatin to acid denaturation in quiescent and cyclic cells as revealed by flow cytometry. *J Histochem Cytochem* 1979; 27: 478–485.

21 Schulte E. Air-drying as a preparatory factor in cytology: investigation of its influence on dye-uptake and dye binding. *Diagn Cytopathol* 1986; 2: 160–167.

22 Giroud F, Montmasson MP. Reevaluation of optimal Feulgen reaction for automated cytology. Influence of fixatives. *Anal Quant Cytol Histol* 1989; 11: 87–95.

23 Fand SB. Environmental conditions for optimal Feulgen hydrolysis. In: Wied GK, Bahr GF (eds) *Introduction to Quantitative Cytochemistry*. II. New York: Academic Press, 1970: 209–221.

24 Kjellstrand PTT. Control of extraction of deoxyribonucleic acid and apurinic acid by polyethylene glycol in Feulgen hydrolysis. *J Histochem Cytochem* 1977; 25: 371–375.

25 Kasten FH. The chemistry of Schiff's reagent. *Int Rev Cytol* 1960; 10: 1–100.

26 Colour Index (CI) Bradford: *Society of Dyers and*

Colourists and American Association of Textile Chemists and Colorists, 1971.

27 Van Duijn P. A histochemical specific thionin-SO_2 reagent and its use in a bi-color method for deoxyribonucleic acid and periodic acid-Schiff positive substances. *J Histochem Cytochem* 1956; 4: 55–63.

28 Kasten FH. Additional Schiff-type reagents for use in cytochemistry. *Stain Technol* 1958; 33: 39–45.

29 Oud PS, Zahniser DJ, Raaijmakers MCT, Vooijs PG, van de Walle RT. Thionine-Feulgen-Congo red staining of cervical smears for the BioPEPR image-analysis system. *Anal Quant Cytol Histol* 1981; 3: 289–298.

30 Kjellstrand PTT. Mechanisms of the Feulgen acid hydrolysis. *J Microsc* 1980; 119: 391–396.

31 Pöppe C, Pellicciari C, Bachmann K. Computer analysis of Feulgen hydrolysis kinetics. *Histochemistry* 1979; 60: 53–60.

32 Kjellstrand PTT. Temperature and acid concentration in the search for optimum Feulgen hydrolysis conditions. *J Histochem Cytochem* 1977; 25: 129–134.

33 Chatelain R, Willms A, Biesterfeld A, Auffermann W, Böcking A. Automated Feulgen staining with a temperature controlled staining machine. *Anal Quant Cytol Histol* 1989; 11: 211–217.

34 Böhm N. Einfluβ der Fixierung und der Säurekonzentration auf die Feulgen-Hydrolyse bei 28°C. *Histochemie* 1968; 14: 201–211.

35 Kotelnikov VM, Litinskaya LL. Comparative studies of Feulgen hydrolysis for DNA I. Influence of different fixatives and polyethylene glycols. *Histochemistry* 1981; 71: 145–153.

36 Dewse CD, Potter CG. Influence of light and mounting medium on the fading of Feulgen stain. *Stain Technol* 1975; 50: 301–306.

37 Swartz FJ, Nagy ER. Feulgen stain stability in relation to three mounting media and exposure to light. *Stain Technol* 1963; 38: 179–185.

38 Allison DC, Ridolpho PF, Rasch EM, Rasch RW, Johnson TS. Increased accuracy of absorption cytophotometric DNA values by control of stain intensity. *J Histochem Cytochem* 1981; 29: 1219–1228.

39 Mikel UV, Fishbein WN, Bahr GF. Some practical considerations in quantitative absorbance microspectrophotometry: preparation techniques in DNA cytophotometry. *Anal Quant Cytol* 1985; 7: 107–118.

40 Husain OAN, Watts KC. Preparatory methods for DNA hydrolysis, cytochemistry, immunocytochemistry and ploidy analysis. *Anal Quant Cytol Histol* 1987; 9: 218–224.

41 Einarson L. A method for progressive selective staining of Nissl and nuclear substance in nerve cells. *Am J Pathol* 1932; 8: 295–307.

42 Husain OAN, Watts KC. Rapid demonstration of nucleic acids using 'oxidised' gallocyanin and chromic potassium sulphate: methods and applications. *J Clin Pathol* 1984; 37: 99–101.

43 Schulte E, Lyon H, Prento P. Gallocyanin chromalum as a nuclear stain in cytology. I. A cytophotometric comparison of the Husain–Watts gallocyanin chromalum staining protocol with the Feulgen procedure. *Histochem J* 1991; 23: 241–245.

44 Eason PJ, Tucker TH. The preparation of cervical scrape material for automated cytology using gallocyanin chrome-alum stain. *J Histochem Cytochem* 1979; 27: 25–31.

45 Oud P, Henderik J, Huysmans A *et al.* The use of light green and orange II as quantitative protein stains, and their combination with the Feulgen method for the simultaneous determination of protein and DNA. *Histochemistry* 1984; 80: 49–57.

46 Schulte E, Lyon HO, Hoyer PE. Simultaneous quantification of DNA and RNA in tissue sections. A comparative analysis of the methyl green-pyronin technique with the gallocyanin chromalum and Feulgen procedures using image cytometry. *Histochem J* 1992; 24: 305–310.

47 Schulte E, Wittekind D. Standardized thionin–eosin stain in bronchial cytology A substitute for hematoxylin-eosin Y staining. *Anal Quant Cytol Histol* 1989; 11: 131–139.

48 Schulte E, Wittekind D, Kretschmer V. Victoria blue B: a nuclear stain for cytology. A cytophotometric study. *Histochemistry* 1988; 88: 427–433.

49 Boss JMN, Feneley RCL, Mays RGW. Modes of chromatin packing in Feulgen-stained normal and malignant uro-epithelial cell nuclei, and in lymphocytes, in relation to DNA content. *J Microsc* 1976; 108: 291–300.

50 Duijndam WAL, Van Duijn P. The influence of chromatin compactness on the stoichiometry of the Feulgen–Schiff procedure studied in model films. I. Theoretical kinetics and experiments with films containing isolated deoxyribonucleic acid. *J Histochem Cytochem* 1975; 23: 882–890.

51 Schulte E, Wittekind D. Standardization of the Feulgen reaction. The influence of chromatin condensation on the kinetics of acid hydrolysis. *Anal Cell Pathol* 1990; 2: 149–157.

52 Esteban JM, Sheibani K, Owens M *et al.* Effects of various fixatives and fixation conditions on DNA ploidy analysis. A need for strict internal DNA standards. *Am J Clin Pathol* 1991; 95: 460.

53 Larson MLP, Sauaia H. The Feulgen reaction: importance of the wash after hydrolysis. *Acta Histochem* 1980; 67: 6–12.

54 Demalsy P, Callebaut M. Plain water as a rinsing agent preferable to sulfurous acid after the Feulgen nuclear reaction. *Stain Technol* 1967; 42: 133–136.

55 Duijndam WAL, Van Duijn P. The dependence of the absorbance of the final chromophore formed in the Feulgen-Schiff reaction on the pH of the medium. *Histochemie* 1973; 35: 373–375.

56 Kasten FH, Kiefer G, Sandritter W. Bleaching of Feulgen stained nuclei and alteration of absorption

curve after continuous exposure to visible light in a cytophotometer. *Histochemistry* 1962; 10: 547–555.
57 Schulte E. The influence of embedding on the stoichiometry of the pararosaniline–Feulgen stain in histological material. *Acta Histochem* 1990; 38: 255–258.
58 Bennett HS, Wyrick AD, Lee SW, McNeil J. Science and art in preparing tissues embedded in plastics for light microscopy, with special reference to glycol methacrylate, glass knives and simple stain. *Stain Technol* 1976; 51: 71–97.
59 Fausel RE, Burleigh W, Kominsky DB. DNA quantification in colorectal carcinoma using flow and image analysis cytometry. *Anal Quant Cytol Histol* 1990; 12: 21–27.
60 Wilbur DC, Zakowski MF, Kosciol CM, Sojda DF, Pastuszak WT. DNA ploidy in breast lesions. A comparative study using two commercial image analysis systems and flow cytometry. *Anal Quant Cytol Histol* 1990; 12: 28–34.
61 Chatelain R, Willms A, Biesterfield S, Auffermann W, Böcking A. Automated Feulgen staining with a temperature-controlled staining machine. *Anal Quant Cytol Histol* 1989; 11: 211–217.
62 Kiss R, Gasperin P, Verhest A, Pasteels JL. Modification of tumour ploidy level via the choice of tissue taken as diploid reference in the digital image analysis of Feulgen-stained nuclei. *Mod Pathol* 1992; 5: 655–660.
63 Auer GU, Capersson TO, Wallgren AS. DNA content and survival in mammary carcinoma. *Anal Quant Cytol Histol* 1980; 2: 161–165.
64 Auer GU, Eriksson E, Azavedo E *et al.* Prognostic significance of nuclear DNA content in mammary adenocarcinomas in humans. *Cancer Res* 1984; 44: 394–396.
65 Ono J, Auer G. The significance of DNA measurements for the early detection of bronchial cell atypia. *Cytometry* 1983; 3: 340–344.
66 Sperb RA, Arnold W, Bahr GF, Loning T, Gebbers JO. Comparative DNA image cytometry in imprint, cytospin and tissue section preparations of breast carcinoma. *Anal Cell Pathol* 1993; 5: 265–275.
67 Opfermann M, Brugal G, Vassilakos P. Cytometry of breast carcinoma: significance of ploidy balance and proliferation index. *Cytometry* 1987; 8: 217–224.
68 Böcking A, Adler CP, Common HH *et al.* Algorithm for a DNA cytophotometric diagnosis and grading of malignancy. *Anal Quant Cytol Histol* 1984; 6: 1–8.
69 Aufferman W, Böcking A. Early detection of precancerous lesions in dysplasias of the lung by rapid DNA image cytometry. *Anal Quant Cytol Histol* 1987; 7: 218–226.
70 Stenkvist B, Bengtsson E, Eriksson O, Jarkrans T, Nordin B. Image cytometry in malignancy grading of breast cancer. Results in a prospective study with seven years of follow-up. *Anal Quant Cytol Histol* 1986; 8: 293–300.
71 Böcking A, Chatelain R, Biesterfield S *et al.* DNA grading of malignancy in breast cancer. Prognostic validity, reproductibility and comparison with other classifications. *Anal Quant Cytol Histol* 1989; 11: 73–80.
72 Böcking A, Chatelain R, Homge M, Gilissen R, Wohtmann D. Representativity and reproductibility of DNA malignancy. Grading in different carcinomas. *Anal Quant Cytol Histol* 1989; 11: 81–86.
73 Longin A, Fontanière B, Pinzani V *et al.* An image cytometric DNA analysis in breast neoplasms. *Pathol Res Pract* 1992; 188: 466–472.
74 Montironi R, Diamanti L, Santenelli A, Scarpelli M. Computer aided S-phase fraction determination in DNA static cytometric in breast cancer. *Anal Quant Cytol Histol* 1992; 14: 379–385.
75 Dean R, Jett JH. Mathematical analysis of DNA distributions derived from flow microfluorimetry. *J Cell Biol* 1974; 60: 523–527.
76 Uyterlinde AM, Smeulders AWN, Baak JPA. DNA measurement errors with a scanning microdensitometer in cytologic and histologic samples of breast cancers. *Anal Quant Cytol Histol* 1991; 13: 115–122.
77 von Hagen V, Morens A, Krief B. Highly optimized microscopic environment: a new workstation for microscopic analysis in pathology. *Anal Cell Pathol* 1991; 3: 249–256.
78 Brugal G, Dye R, Krief B *et al.* HOME: highly optimized microscope environment. *Cytometry* 1992; 13: 109–116.
79 Mesker WE, Eysackers MJ, Ouwerkerk-van Velsen MCM *et al.* Discrepancies in ploidy determination due to specimen sampling errors. *Anal Quant Cytol Histol* 1989; 1; 87–95.
80 Tucker JH, Eason P, Stark M. Ellipse test for a reduction of false positive signals in automated cytology. *Acta Cytol* 1979; 22: 370–376.
81 Sychra JJ, Bartels PH, Bibbo M, Taylor J, Wied GL. Computer recognition of binucleation with overlapping in epithelial cells. *Acta Cytol* 1979; 22: 22–28.
82 Dytch HE, Bartels PH, Bibbo M, Pishotta F, Wied GL. The rejection of noncellular artifacts in Papanicolaou-stained cells specimens by an automated high-resolution system: identification of important cytometric features. *Anal Quant Cytol Histol* 1983; 5: 241–249.
83 Sasaki K, Hamano K, Kinjo M, Hara S. Intratumoral heterogeneity in DNA ploidy of bladder carcinomas. *Oncology* 1992; 49: 219–222.
84 Carey FA, Lamb D, Bird CC. Intratumoral heterogeneity of DNA content in lung cancer. *Cancer* 1990; 65: 2226–2269.
85 Meyer JS, Wittliff JL. Regional heterogeneity in breast carcinoma: thymidine labelling index, steroid hormone receptors, DNA ploidy. *Int J Cancer* 1991; 47:

213–220.

86 Beerman H, Veldhnizen RW, Blok RAP, Hermans J, Ooms ECM. Cytomorphometry as quality control for fine needle aspiration; a study in 321 breast lesions. *Anal Quant Cytol Histol* 1991; 13: 143–148.

87 Pennes DR, Naylor B, Rebner M. Fine needle aspiration biopsy of the breast. Influence of the number of passes and the sample size on the diagnostic yield. *Acta Oncol* 1990; 34: 673–676.

88 Bocking A, Striepecke E, Auer H, Fuzesi L. Static DNA cytometry. Biological background, technique and diagnostic interpretation. In: Wied GL, Bartels PH, Rosenthal DL, Schenk U (eds) *Compendium on the Computerized Cytology and Histology Laboratory.* Chicago: Tutorials of Cytology, 1994: 107–128.

89 Forsslund G, Zetterberg A. Ploidy level determinations in high grade and low grade malignant variants of prostate carcinoma. *Cancer Res* 1990; 50: 4281–4285.

90 Forsslund G, Esposti PL, Nilsson B, Zetterberg A. The prognostic significance of nuclear DNA content in prostatic carcinoma. *Cancer* 1992; 69: 1432–1439.

91 Peters-Gee JM, Miles BJ, Cerny JC *et al.* Prognostic significance of DNA quantitation in stage D1 prostate carcinoma with the use of image analysis. *Cancer* 1992; 70: 1159–1165.

92 Ross JS, Nazeer T, Church K *et al.* Contribution of HER-2/neu oncogene expression to tumour grade and DNA content analysis in the prediction of prostatic carcinoma. *Cancer* 1993; 72: 3020–3028.

93 Montironi R, Scarpelli M, Galluzzi CM, Diamanti L. Aneuploidy and nuclear features of prostatic intraepithelial neoplasia (PIN). *J Cell Biochem* 1992; 16(suppl): 47–53.

94 Montironi R, Scarpelli M, Sisti S *et al.* Quantitative analysis of prostatic intraepithelial neoplasia on tissue sections. *Anal Quant Cytol Histol* 1990; 12: 366–372.

95 Grigolato P, Valagussa E, Chioda C, Donzelli C. Static cytometry DNA in breast lump with reference to grading. *Eur J Basic Appl Histochem* 1991; 35: 433–440.

96 Siitonen SM, Kallioniemi OP, Helin HJ, Isola JJ. Prognostic value of cells with more than 5c DNA content in node-negative breast cancer as determined by image cytometry from tissue sections. *Hum Pathol* 1993; 24: 1348–1353.

97 Troncone G, Zeppa P, Fulciniti F *et al.* C-*erb*2 expression and DNA ploidy status in breast cancer cells obtained by fine needle aspiration (FAN). *Cytopathology* 1993; 4: 195–205.

98 von Rosen A, Rutqvist LE, Carstensen J *et al.* Prognostic value of nuclear DNA content in breast cancer in relation to tumour size, nodal status and estrogen receptor content. *Breast Cancer Res Treat* 1989; 13: 23–32.

99 Yokoe T, Izuo M, Ishada T, Iino Y, Kawai T. DNA ploidy level and S-phase fraction as prognostic factors in breast cancer. *Jpn J Surg* 1990; 20: 491–497.

100 Charpin C, Andrac L, Lavaut MN *et al.* Image cytomertry of aneuploidy, growth fraction (MoAb Ki-67) and hormone receptors (ER, PR) immunocytochemical assays in breast carcinomas. *Anal Cell Pathol* 1990; 2: 357–371.

101 Larsimont D, Kiss R, d'Olne D *et al.* Correlation between nuclear cytomorphometric parameters and estrogen receptor levels in breast cancer. *Cancer* 1989; 63: 2162–2168.

102 Chang DB, Yang PC, Chang KJ, Luh KT, Kuo SH. Comparison of DNA stemline and cell kinetics between primary breast cancer and its lymph node metastasis. *Anal Quant Cytol Histol* 1993; 15: 32–38.

103 von Rosen A, Fallenius A, Sundelin B, Auer G. Nuclear DNA content in mammary carcinomas in women aged 35 or younger. *Am J Clin Oncol* 1986; 9: 381–386.

104 Mir R, Johnson H, Margolis M, Teplitz S, Wise L. Prognostic significance of DNA measurement determined by image analysis in human breast carcinoma. *J Surg Oncol* 1992; 50: 168–172.

105 Erhardt K, Auer G, Fallenius A *et al.* Prognostic significance of nuclear DNA analysis in histological sections in mammary carcinoma. *Am J Clin Oncol* 1986; 9: 117–125.

106 Theissig F, Dimmer V, Haroske G, Kunze KD, Meyer W. Use of nuclear image cytometry, histopathological grading and DNA cytometry to make breast cancer prognosis more objective. *Anal Cell Pathol* 1991; 3: 351–360.

107 Fallenius AG, Auer GU, Carstensen JM. Prognostic significance of DNA measurements in 409 consecutive breast cancer patients. *Cancer* 1988; 62: 331–341.

108 Bocking A, Chatelain R, Biesterfeld S *et al.* DNA grading of malignancy in breast cancer. Prognostic validity, reproducibility and comparison with other classifications. *Anal Quant Cytol Histol* 1989; 11: 73–80.

109 Gilchrist KW, Gray R, van Driel-Kulker AM *et al.* High DNA content and prognosis in lymph node positive breast cancer. A case control study by the University of Leiden and ECOG. *Breast Cancer Res Treat* 1993; 28: 1–8.

110 Crissman JD, Visscher DW, Kubus J. Image cytophotometric DNA analysis of atypical hyperplasias and intraductal carcinomas of the breast. *Arch Pathol Lab Med* 1990; 114: 1249–1253.

111 Pallis L, Skoog L, Falkmer U *et al.* The DNA profile of breast cancer *in situ*. *Eur J Surg Oncol* 1992; 18: 108–111.

112 Norris HJ, Bahr GF, Mikel UV. A comparative morphometric and cytophotometric study of intraductal hyperplasia and intraductal carcinoma of the breast.

Anal Quant Cytol Histol 1988; 10: 1–9.
113 Koha M, Wikstrom B, Brismar B. Colorectal carcinoma. DNA ploidy pattern and prognosis with reference to tumor DNA heterogeneity. *Anal Quant Cytol Histol* 1992; 14: 367–372.
114 Albe X, Vassilakos P, Helfer-Guarnori K *et al.* Independent prognostic value of ploidy value in colorectal cancer. A prospective study using image cytometry. *Cancer* 1990; 66: 1168–1175.
115 Deans GT, Williamson K, Hamilton PW *et al.* DNA densitometry of colorectal cancer. *Gut* 1993; 34: 1566–1571.
116 Koha M, Brismar B, Wikstrom B. DNA content in primary tumours and lymph node metastases in colorectal adenocarcinoma. *APMIS* 1992; 100: 640–644.
117 Koha M, Caspersson TO, Wikstrom B, Brismar B. Heterogeneity of DNA distribution pattern in colorectal carcinoma. A microspectrophotometric study of fine needle aspirates. *Anal Quant Cytol Histol* 1990; 12: 348–351.
118 Verhest A, Kiss R, d'Olne D *et al.* Characterisation of human colorectal mucosa, polyps, and cancers by means of computerized morphonuclear image analysis. *Cancer* 1990; 65: 2047–2053.
119 Ranaldi R, Bearzi I, Santinelli A, Mannello B, Mariuzzi GM. Quantitative study of the precancerous and malignant lesions in colorectal adenomas. *Pathol Res Pract* 1992; 188: 561–564.
120 Wang Q, Gao H, Chen Y, Wang Y, He J, Jin C. Biopathologic characteristics of DNA content in crypt cells of transitional mucosa adjacent to carcinomas of the rectum and rectosigmoid. *Dis Colon Rectum* 1992; 35: 670–675.
121 Shabaik AS, Pow-Sang JM, Lockhart J, Nicosia SV. Role of DNA image cytometry in the follow-up of patients with urinary tract transitional cell carcinoma. *Anal Quant Cytol Histol* 1993; 15: 115–123.
122 Amberson JB, Laino JP. Image cytometric deoxyribonucleic acid analysis of urine specimens as an adjunct to visual cytology in the detection of urothelial cell carcinoma. *J Urol* 1993; 149: 42–45.
123 Seigneurin D, Rambeud JJ, Bosio C, Louis J. DNA image cytometry of bladder tumours: comparison of washings and tumour imprints from 61 patients. *Anal Cell Pathol* 1993; 5: 39–48.
124 Montironi R, Scarpelli M, Pisani E, Ansuini G, Marinelli F, Mariuzzi G. Noninvasive papillary transitional-cell tumours. Karyometric and DNA content analysis. *Anal Quant Cytol Histol* 1985; 7: 337–342.
125 Montironi R, Scarpelli M, Sisti S, Ansuini G, Pisani E, Mariuzzi G. Prognostic value of computerized DNA analysis in noninvasive papillary carcinomas of the urinary bladder. *Tumori* 1987; 73: 567–574.
126 al-Abadi H, Nagel R. Deoxyribonucleic acid content and survival rates of patients with transitional cell carcinoma of the bladder. *J Urol* 1994; 151: 37–42.
127 Auffermann W, Urquardt M, Rubben H, Wohltmann D, Bocking A. DNA grading of urothelial carcinoma of the bladder. *Anticancer Res* 1986; 6: 27–32.
128 Schapers RF, Ploem-Zaaijer JJ, Pauwels RP *et al.* Image cytometric DNA analysis in transitional cell carcinoma of the bladder. *Cancer* 1993; 72: 182–189.
129 Caspersson T. Quantitative cytochemical studies on normal, premalignant and atypical cell populations from the uterine cervix. *Scand Arch Physiol* 1936; 73: 8–45.
130 Nishaya I, Kikuchi T, Mariya S, Shimotomai K, Sauramura I. Cytophotometric study of premalignant and malignant cells of the cervix in an approach towards automated cytology. *Acta Cytol* 1977; 21: 271–275.
131 Wied GL, Bartels PH, Bibbo M, Sychra JJ. Cytomorphometric markers for uterine cancer in intermediate cells. *Anal Quant Cytol* 1980; 4: 257–263.
132 Wied GL, Bartels PH, Dytch HE *et al.* Diagnostic marker features in dysplastic cells from the uterine cervix. *Acta Cytol* 1982; 26: 475–483.
133 Bocking A, Hilgarth M, Auffermann W *et al.* DNA cytometric diagnosis of prospective malignancy in borderline lesions of the uterine cervix. *Acta Cytol* 1986; 30: 608–615.
134 Winkler B, Crum CP, Fujii T *et al.* Koilocytic lesions of the cervix. The relationship of mitotic abnormalities to the presence of papillomavirus antigens and nuclear DNA content. *Cancer* 1984; 53: 1081–1087.
135 Evans AS, Managhan JM. Nuclear DNA content of normal, neoplastic and 'wart affected' cervical biopsies. *Anal Quant Cytol Histol* 1983; 5: 112–116.
136 Bahr GF, Bartels PH, Dytch HE, Koss LG, Wied GL. Image analysis and its application to cytology. In: Koss LG (ed.) *Diagnostic Cytology and its Histopathological Basis*, 4th edn. Philadelphia: JB Lippincott, 1992; 1572–1612.
137 Bibbo M, Bartels PH, Dytch HE, Wied GL. Cell image analysis. In: Bibbo M (ed.) *Comprehensive Cytopathology*. Philadelphia: WB Saunders, 1991: 965–983.
138 Banda-Gamboe H, Ricketts I, Cairns A *et al.* Automation in cervical cytology: an overview. *Anal Cell Pathol* 1992; 4: 25–48.
139 Atkin NB, Richards BM. Clinical significance of ploidy in carcinoma of the cervix. Its relation to prognosis. *Br Med J* 1962; 2: 1445–1446.
140 Atkin NB. Prognostic significance of ploidy level in human tumours. I. Carcinoma of the uterus. *J Natl Cancer Inst* 1976; 56: 909–910.
141 Fu YS, Reagan JW, Fu AS, Janija KE. Adenocarcinoma and mixed carcinoma of the uterine cervix. II. Prognostic value of nuclear DNA analysis. *Cancer* 1982; 49: 2571–2577.
142 Goppinger A, Freudenberg N, Ross A, Hillemanns H-G, Hilgarth M. The prognostic significance of the DNA distribution in squamous cell carcinomas of

the uterine cervix. *Anal Quant Cytol Histol* 1986; 8: 148–151.

143 Ng ABP, Atkin NB. Histological cell type and DNA values in the prognosis of squamous cell cancer of the uterine cervix. *Br J Cancer* 1979; 28: 322–331.

144 Hrushowetz SB, Lauchlan SC. Comparative DNA content of cells in the intermediate and parabasal layers of cervical intraepithelial neoplasias studied by two-wavelength Feulgen cytophotometry. *Acta Cytol* 1970; 14: 68–77.

145 Pellicer A, Herzog RE. Measurement of nuclear DNA in the management of cervical intraepithelial neoplasia. *Arch Gynecol* 1984; 234: 197–204.

146 Mariuzzi GM, Montironi R, Di Loreto C, Sisti S. Multiparametric quantitation of the progression of uterine cervix preneoplasia towards neoplasia. *Pathol Res Pract* 1989; 185: 606–611.

147 Bibbo M, Bartels PH, Dytch HE, Wied GL. Ploidy patterns in cervical dysplasia. *Anal Quant Cytol Histol* 1985; 7: 213–217.

148 Fu YS, Reagan JW, Richart RM. Definition of precursors. *Gynecol Oncol* 1981; 12: 220–231.

149 Bibbo M, Dytch HE, Alenghat E, Bartels PH, Wied GL. DNA ploidy profiles as prognostic indicators in CIN lesions. *Am J Clin Pathol* 1989; 92: 261–265.

150 Kashyap V, Das DK, Luthra UK. Microphotometric nuclear DNA analysis in cervical dysplasia of the uterine cervix: its relation to the progression to malignancy and regression to normalcy. *Neoplasma* 1990; 37: 497–500.

151 Nasiell K, Auer G, Nasiell M, Zetterberg A. Retrospective DNA analysis in cervical dysplasias as related to neoplastic progression or regression. *Anal Quant Cytol Histol* 1979; 1: 103–106.

152 Chatelain R, Schunk T, Schindler EM, Schindler AE, Bocking A. Diagnosis of prospective malignancy in koilocytic dysplasias of the uterine cervix with DNA cytometry. *J Reprod Med* 1989; 34: 505–510.

153 Salmon I, Gasperin P, Remmelink M *et al.* Ploidy level and proliferative activity measurements in a series of 407 thyroid tumours or other pathologic conditions. *Hum Pathol* 1993; 24: 912–920.

154 Collin F, Salmon I, Rahier I *et al.* Quantitative nuclear cell image analyses of thyroid tumors from archival material. *Hum Pathol* 1991; 22: 191–196.

155 Montironi R, Alberti R, Sisti S *et al.* Discrimination between follicular adenoma and follicular carcinoma of the thyroid: preoperative validity of cytometry on aspiration smears. *Appl Pathol* 1989; 7: 367–374.

156 Liautaud-Roger F, Dufer J, Delisle MJ, Coninx P. Thyroid neoplasms. Can we do any better with quantitative cytology? *Anal Quant Cytol Histol* 1992; 14: 373–378.

157 Salmon I, Gasperin P, Pasteels JL, Heimann R, Kiss R. Relationship between histopathologic typing and morphonuclear assessments of 238 thyroid lesions. Digital cell image analysis performed on Feulgen-stained nuclei from formalin fixed, paraffin embedded materials. *Am J Clin Pathol* 1992; 97: 776–786.

158 Ekman ET, Backdahl M, Lowhagen T, Auer G. Nuclear DNA measurements on thyroid carcinoma in young patients. *Acat Oncol* 1989; 28: 475–479.

159 Soares J, Fonseca I, Limbert E, Falkmer UG, Falkmer S. Prognostic implications of image cytometric assessments of nuclear DNA distribution pattern of neoplastic cells in thyroid medullary carcinoma. A retrospective study using disaggregated, formalin-fixed, paraffin-embedded specimens. *APMIS* 1991; 99: 745–754.

160 Galera-Davidson H, Gonzalex-Campora R, Mora-Marin JA *et al.* Cytophotometric DNA measurements in medullary thyroid carcinoma. *Cancer* 1990; 65: 2255–2260.

161 Wallin G, Backdahl M, Tallroth-Ekman E *et al.* Co-existent anaplastic and well differentiated thyroid carcinomas: a nuclear DNA study. *Eur J Surg Oncol* 1989; 15: 43–48.

162 Erhardt K, Auer G, Bjorkholm E *et al.* Prognostic significance of nuclear DNA content in serous ovarian tumours. *Cancer Res* 1984; 44: 2198–2202.

163 Fu YS, Ro J, Reagan JW, Hall TL, Berek J. Nuclear deoxyribonucleic acid heterogeneity of ovarian borderline malignant serous tumours. *Obstet Gynecol* 1986; 67: 478–482.

164 de Nictolis M, Montironi R, Tommasoni T *et al.* Benign, borderline, and well differentiated malignant intestinal mucinous tumours of the ovary: a clinicopathologic, histochemical, immunohistochemical and nuclear quantitative study of 57 cases. *Int J Gynecol Pathol* 1994; 13: 10–21.

165 de Nictolis M, Montironi R, Tommasoni S *et al.* Serous borderline tumours of the ovary. A clinicopathologic, immunohistochemical and quantitative study of 44 cases. *Cancer* 1992; 70: 152–160.

166 Padberg BC, Arps H, Franke U *et al.* DNA cytophotometry and prognosis in ovarian tumours of borderline malignancy. *Cancer* 1992; 69: 2510–2514.

167 Dietel M, Arps H, Rohlff A, Bodecker R, Niendorf A. Nuclear DNA content of borderline tumours of the ovary correlation with histology and significance for prognosis. *Virchows Arch [A]* 1986; 409: 829–836.

168 Kayser K, Stute H, Tacke M. Minimum spanning tree, integrated optical density and lymph node metastasis in bronchial carcinoma. *Anal Cell Pathol* 1993; 5: 225–234.

169 Dejmek A, Stromberg C, Wikstrom B, Hjerpe A. Prognostic importance of the DNA ploidy pattern in malignant mesothelioma of the pleura. *Anal Quant Cytol Histol* 1992; 14: 217–221.

170 Tierney G, Wilkinson MJ, Jones JS. The malignancy grading method is not a reliable assessment of malignancy in mesothelioma. *J Pathol* 1990; 160: 209–211.

171 Larsimont D, Kiss R, de Launoit Y, Melamed MR.

Characterisation of the morphonuclear features and DNA ploidy of typical and atypical carcinoids and small cell carcinomas of the lung. *Am J Clin Pathol* 1990; 94: 378–383.
172 Auffermann W, Bocking A. Early detection of precancerous lesions in dysplasias of the lung by rapid image cytometry. *Anal Quant Cytol Histol* 1985; 7: 218–226.
173 Bocking A, Schunck K, Auffermann W, Exfoliative-cytologic diagnosis of basal-cell carcinoma, with the use of DNA image cytometry as a diagnostic aid. *Acta Cytol* 1987; 31: 143–149.
174 Rode J, Williams RA, Charlton IG, Dhillon AP, Moss E. Nuclear DNA profiles in primary melanomas and their metastases. *Cancer* 1991; 67: 2333–2336.
175 Fleming MG, Wied GL, Dytch HE. Image analysis cytometry of dysplastic nevi. *J Invest Dermatol* 1990; 95: 287–291.
176 Schulte EK, Joos U, Kasper M, Eckert HM. Cytological detection of epithelial dysplasia in the oral mucosa using Feulgen DNA-image cytometry. *Diag Cytopathol* 1991; 7: 436–441.
177 Chatelain R, Hoffmeister B, Harle F, Bocking A, Mittermayer C. DNA grading of oral squamous carcinomas. A preliminary report. *Int J Oral Maxillo Surg* 1989; 18: 43–46.
178 Munck-Wikland E, Rubiro CA, Auer GU, Kuylenstierna R, Lindham J. Control cells for image analysis of esophageal tissue and the influence of preoperative treatment. *Anal Quant Cytol Histol* 1990; 12: 267–274.
179 Sugihara H, Hattori T, Fujita S, Hirose K, Fukuda M. Regional ploidy variations in signet ring cell carcinomas of the stomach. *Cancer* 1990; 65: 122–129.
180 Bearzi I, Ranaldi R, Santinelli A, Mannello B, Mariuzzi GM. Epithelial dysplasia of the gastric mucosa. A morphometric and ploidy pattern study. *Pathol Res Pract* 1992; 188: 550–555.
181 Böcking A, Biesterfeld S, Liu SQ. DNA distribution in gastric cancer and dysplasia. In: Zahngl, Kawain (eds) *Precancerous Conditions and Lesions of the Stomach*. Heidelberg: Springer Verlag, 1993: 103–120.
182 Weger AR, Glaser KS, Schwab G *et al.* Quantitative nuclear DNA content in fine needle aspirates of pancreatic cancer. *Gut* 1991; 32: 325–328.
183 Rickaert F, Gelin M, van Gansbeke D *et al.* Computerised morphonuclear characteristics and DNA content of adenocarcinoma of the pancreas, chronic pancreas and normal tissues: relationship with histopathologic grading. *Hum Pathol* 1992; 23: 1210–1215.
184 Allison DC, Bose KK, Hruban RH *et al.* Pancreatic cancer cell DNA content correlates with long-term survival after pancreatoduodenectomy. *Ann Surg* 1991; 214: 648–656.
185 Deprez C, Vangansbeke D, Fastrez R *et al.* Nuclear DNA content, proliferation index, and nuclear size determination in normal and cirrhotic liver, and in benign and malignant primary and metastatic hepatic tumours. *Am J Clin Pathol* 1993; 99: 558–565.
186 Zeppa P, Vetrani A, Palombini L *et al.* Evolution of DNA content in small and well-differentiated hepatocarcinoma. *Anal Quant Cytol Histol* 1993; 15: 12–22.
187 Hoso M, Nakanuma Y. Cytophotometric DNA analysis of adenomatous hyperplasia in cirrhotic livers. *Virchows Arch [A]* 1991; 418: 401–404.
188 van den Houte K, Kiss R, de Prez C *et al.* Use of computerized cell image analysis to characterise cell nucleus populations from normal and neoplastic renal tissues. *Eur Urol* 1991; 19: 155–164.
189 Banner BF, Brancazio L, Bahnson RR, Ernstoff MS, Taylor SR. DNA analysis of multiple synchronous renal cell carcinomas. *Cancer* 1990; 66: 2180–2185.
190 Bocking A, Auffermann W, Vogel H, Schlondorff G, Goebbels R. Diagnosis and grading of malignancy in squamous epithelial lesions of the larynx with DNA cytophotometry. *Cancer* 1985; 56: 1600–1604.
191 Franzen G, Olofsson J, Klintenberg C, Brunk U. Prognostic value of malignancy grading and DNA measurements in small glottic carcinomas. *ORL J Otorhinolaryngol Relat Spec* 1987; 49: 73–80.
192 Feichter GE, Maier H, Adler K *et al.* S-phase fractions and DNA ploidy of oropharyngeal squamous epithelium carcinomas compared with histological grade, stage, response to chemotherapy and survival. *Acta Otolaryngol* 1987; 194: 377–384.
193 Munck-Wikland E, Kuylenstierna R, Lindholm J, Auer G. Image cytometry DNA analysis of dysplastic squamous epithelial lesions in the larynx. *Anticancer Res* 1991; 11: 597–600.
194 Salmon I, Kiss R, Dewitte O *et al.* Histopathologic grading and DNA ploidy in relation to survival among 206 adult astrocytic tumour patients. *Cancer* 1992; 70: 538–546.
195 Salmon I, Kiss R, Leviver M *et al.* Characterisation of nuclear DNA content, proliferation index and nuclear size in a series of 181 meningiomas, including benign primary, recurrent and malignant tumours. *Am J Surg Pathol* 1993; 17: 239–247.
196 Salmon I, Kruczynski A, Camby I *et al.* DNA histogram typing in a series of 707 tumours of the central and peripheral nervous system. *Am J Surg Pathol* 1993; 17: 1020–1028.
197 Salmon I, Kiss R. Relationship between proliferative activity and ploidy level in a series of 530 human brain tumours, including astrocytomas, meningiomas, schwannomas and metastases. *Hum Pathol* 1993; 24: 329–335.
198 Gonzalez-Campora R, Diaz Cano S, Lerma-Puertas E *et al.* Paragangliomas. Static cytometric studies of nuclear DNA patterns. *Cancer* 1993; 71: 820–824.
199 Auffermann W, Fohlmeister I, Bocking A. Diagnostic and prognostic value of DNA image cytometry in

myelodysplasia. *J Clin Pathol* 1988; 41: 604–608.

200 Hartnack Federspiel B, Sobin LH, Hellwig EB, Mikel UV, Bahr GF. Morphometry and cytophotometric assessment of DNA in smooth-muscle tumours (leiomyomas and leiomyosarcomas) of the gastrointestinal tract. *Anal Quant Cytol Histol* 1987; 9: 106–114.

201 Sapi Z, Bodo M. DNA cytometry of soft tissue tumours with TV image analysis system. *Pathol Res Pract* 1989; 185: 363–367.

202 Herzberg AJ, Kerns BJ, Honkanen FA *et al.* DNA ploidy and proliferation index of soft tissue sarcomas determined by image cytometry of fresh frozen tissue. *Am J Clin Pathol* 1992; 97(suppl 1): 29–37.

203 Vogt T, Stolz W, Braun-Falco O *et al.* Prognostic significance of DNA cytometry in cutaneous malignant lymphomas. *Cancer* 1991; 68: 1095–1100.

204 Muller CP, Kropff M, Biesterfeld S *et al.* Detection of high risk patients in chronic myelogenous leukemia by DNA-image cytometry. *Anticancer Res* 1991; 11: 617–623.

205 Vuckovic J, Dubravcic M, Matthews JM *et al.* Prognostic value of cytophotometric analysis of DNA in lymph node aspirates from patients with non-Hodgkin's lymphoma. *J Clin Pathol* 1990; 43: 626–629.

206 Bocking A, Chatelain R, Auffermann W *et al.* DNA-grading of malignant lymphomas. II. Correlation with clinical parameters. *Anticancer Res* 1986; 6: 1217–1223.

207 Bocking A, Chatelain R, Auffermann W *et al.* DNA-grading of malignant lymphomas. I. Prognostic significance, reproducibility and comparison with other classifications. *Anticancer Res* 1986; 6: 1205–1216.

208 Auffermann W, Krueger GR, Bocking A. DNA image cytometry in acquired immune deficiency syndrome (AIDS). *Anal Quant Cytol Histol* 1986; 8: 19–24.

7

AUTOMATED IMAGE CYTOMETRY

J. S. PLOEM

7.1 INTRODUCTION

Quantitative microscope analysis in cellular pathology has now been used for several decades, and has resulted in considerable diagnostic and prognostic information [1]. Most applications have been performed with interactive measurement systems since full automation is not always required, desirable or possible [2,3]. Moreover useful diagnostic and prognostic results can often be obtained by interactive methods which are, however, time-consuming and not particularly suited for high-volume routine work. They are also unsuited if the cells to be investigated can be classified as 'rare events' which demand the investigation of large numbers of microscope fields to detect them. Only recently instrumentation research has progressed so far that automated image analysis has become a practical proposition for routine applications [4,5]. This is mainly the result of the availability of powerful personal computers (PCs) and workstations (WSs) which combine easy operation with a reasonable price and which only rarely have technical breakdowns. To arrive at high-speed analysis for the examination of many microscope fields, the current PC or WS still has to be equipped with special image-processing boards. As the power of the PC or WS is expected to increase further due to the development of even faster microprocessors, the need for special image-processing boards will be expected to diminish [6]. The PCs and WSs of today are provided with efficient operating systems and user interfaces which may already be familiar to workers in a clinical routine environment (e.g., MS-DOS/Windows, UNIX/X Windows and Macintosh operating systems with user interface).

Fully automated image analysis requires specially designed microscopes. They have to be equipped with scanning stages, motorized focus control, charge-coupled device (CCD) cameras and automatic slide loading to enable a rapid examination of multiple specimens. As a consequence of the increased use of multiple fluorescence markers in clinical cytology, such microscopes also have to be provided with automated fluorescence epi-illuminators to enable multiwavelength fluorescence microscopy. Furthermore, very sensitive CCD cameras should be incorporated to detect low-intensity fluorescence signals [7,8]. Several microscope systems for automated cytology have been developed during the last decade [9–11]. The automated cytometry system (LEYTAS) in this laboratory is centred around such an automated microscope, the AUTOPLAN (Leica, Wetzlar, Germany). An updated and further advanced version of our system has been developed by Beacton Dickinson (Image Cytometry Systems, Leiden, The Netherlands). Their system is identified as Discovery and shown in Fig. 7.1. The description of the image analysis procedures and applications in this chapter is mainly based on the characteristics and performance of the LEYTAS cytometry system. Although procedures in other systems will show some similarities with the procedures described here, the reader is referred to their specific reports for optimal information [4,12]. A comprehensive overview of automated cytometry systems has been given by Banda-Gamboa *et al.* [3].

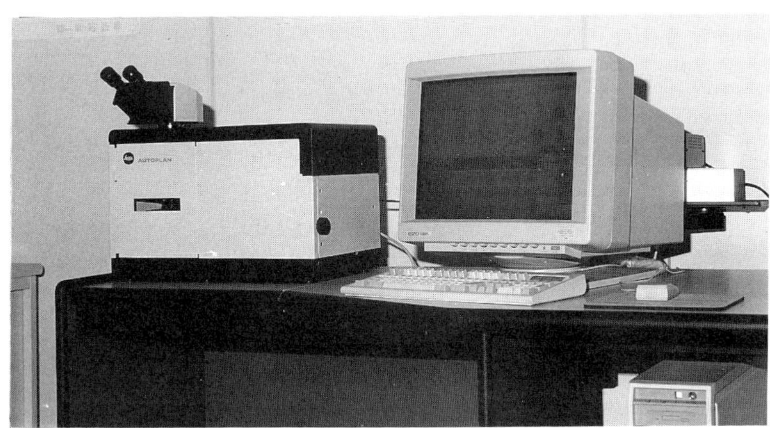

Fig. 7.1 Overview of an automated image cytometry system: automated microscope with one objective allowing two simultaneous magnifications on to two different charge coupled device cameras and a personal computer which contains an extra image cytometry board (Discovery, Becton Dickinson, Image Cytometry Systems, Leiden, The Netherlands). Computer-controlled movement of the objective takes care of rapid focusing. The scanning stage can retrieve microscope specimens from a slide loader (not shown).

7.2 STORING OF CELLULAR IMAGES IN COMPUTER MEMORY

7.2.1 Image acquisition

To obtain an image of a cell or a nucleus, a microscope objective and possibly a projective lens or an eyepiece are needed. When high resolution is used, it should be realized that high-power objectives with a high numerical aperture (NA) only have a very small part of the object in sharp focus. A 60× objective with an NA of 1.40 combined with 10× eyepieces for instance has a focal depth of merely 0.6 µm. This means that the images obtained by the cytometer are very dependent on the focal plane selected by the autofocus system of the cytometer. When larger microscope fields are analysed, the non-flatness of high NA objectives constitutes additional problems. Large fields are, however, necessary when speed is required in the analysis of specimens, such as in the screening of entire microscope slides. The rationale is that the electronic cycle time of an image cytometer only covers the analysis of one microscope field. After movement of the stage to the next field, the inevitable mechanical vibrations of the stage have to decrease before starting the next cycle and this causes a delay in the analysis procedure. The larger the microscope field using the same speed of stage movement the faster the progress in the examination of an entire microscope slide.

Special microscope objectives have been constructed for cytometry. An example is the 40× NA 1.30 from Leica. The lens system of this objective is corrected for non-flatness, allowing the analysis of 512 × 512 µm fields, whereas the depth of focus is moderately larger than that of 100× objectives. This facilitates autofocusing.

In many modern image cytometers an image of the objective can be directly projected on the camera surface without the use of a projective lens or eyepieces. This has become possible by the manufacturing of objective lenses, in which all corrections for optical errors, like insufficient flatness, chromatic abberations, coma, etc., are incorporated in the objective itself. In most earlier microscope designs, this correction was partly carried out in the eyepieces. Sometimes a combination of an objective with an adjacent negative tube lens is chosen for demagnification of the image to increase the image brightness. Since the intensity of a fluorescence image increases with a square-power function when the magnification is decreased, it is important to keep the magnification low. Modern CCD cameras have such fine sensitive elements (0.7 µm) that images of lower magnification can still be effectively analysed. In this way low magnification objectives with maximum NA can provide very bright fluorescent images on a CCD surface with acceptable resolution.

7.2.2 Object and image plane scanners

A scanning stepping stage enabling the measurement of multiple fine (0.5 μm) spots was used in the early measurement systems. The light signal from each scanned spot was recorded with a photomultiplier. In flying spot scanners a small illuminated spot is moved over the specimen by vibrating mirrors. Here also a photomultiplier is used to record the light. Flying spot scanning is used in most laser scanning microscopes. Both scanning stage and flying spot scanners have the advantage that only one small spot (0.5–1 μm) in the microscope specimen is illuminated per time unit. This prevents scattered light from reaching the photomultiplier. Thus the level of glare will be sufficiently low to allow correct absorption measurements of even the darker smaller objects in the specimen. This is of considerable advantage, since glare can substantially disturb correct measurement of absorption signals in heterogeneous cell populations [13].

If television or CCD cameras with a large number of detecting elements are placed at the level of the image projected by the microscope objective, the system is defined as an image plane scanner, in contrast to the stage and flying spot scanners which are known as object plane scanners. Image plane scanners have the disadvantage that the whole microscope field is illuminated simultaneously, causing scattered light from the entire field to reach the camera, and an amount of glare that has to be corrected for.

7.2.3 Digitization of the image

In a cytometer, the signal from the photomultiplier or television or CCD camera is digitized by an analog to digital converter and stored in computer memory as a grey value. If the digitization is performed in 256 steps, the value 0 of the grey-value scale equals no light or total darkness, whereas the value 255 stands for maximum light, meaning that no absorbing structure is situated in the light path.

Storage of grey values in the modern, more powerful image cytometers is done in 512×512 or 1024×1024 picture elements or pixels. This means that the image of a cell is stored in rows and columns. In connection with the statistical requirements for the analysis of cell populations [14], enough computer memory should be available to store a minimum of 400 measured cell images, composed of about $128 \times 128 = 16\,384$ pixels each.

7.3 IMAGE OPERATIONS FOR THE DETECTION OF CELLS

Thresholding or segmentation is an important pixel operation and is used in the discrimination between the object and the background (Fig. 7.2). Thresholding can transpose a grey-value image into a binary one, showing on the computer display the areas occupied by cells as 1s and the background as 0s. Thresholding has to be performed as precisely as possible since weakly stained thin cytoplasm of a cell can slope very gradually into the background. This scene can be compared to a rather flat beach where the rise of a few centimetres of water can cover a lot of beach. Cell sizes are therefore very dependent on accurate thresholding procedures.

Several types of pixel operations can be applied to the grey values. The grey values in the image can be transformed into grey values of maximal contrast (grey-value stretching). It is also possible to inverse the image from a positive into a negative-like image. A fluorescent image which is white on a black background will then be inverted to a dark image on a white background. This can have certain advantages for computational purposes.

7.3.1 Mathematical morphology operations

These types of operations have been described by Serra [15]. *Erosion* is an example of a basic operation of mathematical morphology. Erosion can remove one pixel from the entire outer rim of a nucleus. If this operation is repeated a few times, all the pixels representing the binary image of a nucleus can be removed. Of course the smaller nuclei will be eroded first. After a few erosion steps only parts of the abnormally large nuclei will remain in the image. This can be used in certain applications to detect large nuclei with strongly increased DNA content, which often are polyploid or aneuploid tumour cells. Furthermore, erosions can be used to separate

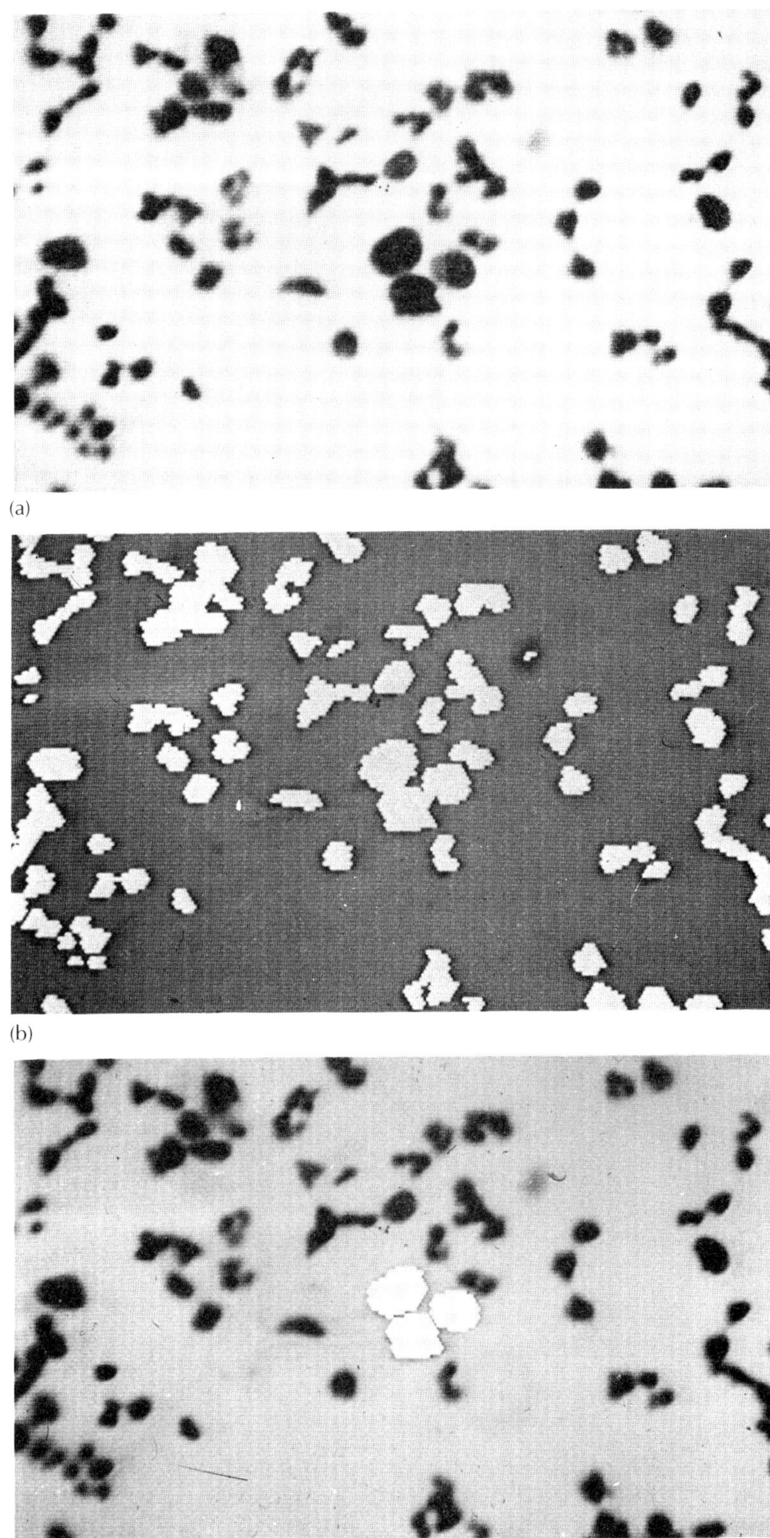

Fig. 7.2 (a) Cervical cells as seen in the analog image. (b) The thresholded image. Note that the three nuclei in the centre are connected. Using more extensive image analysis algorithms, it is possible to separate these nuclei (c).

nuclei which are just touching each other. The importance of separating touching nuclei is shown in Figs 7.2b and c. By thresholding only, the three nuclei in the centre of Fig. 7.2b are connected, whereas image operations have separated the three nuclei in Fig. 7.2c.

Another important operation is *dilation*. With this algorithm a pixel is added to the entire border of a cell or nuclear image. Small holes in cell or nuclear images hampering image recognition can be filled with one or more dilation steps. *Skeletonization* shrinks an object by repeated erosions; it stops when only one line skeleton of a cellular shape remains. This procedure can detect overlapping cells or nuclei since the skeletonization of such structures leads to typical forms of skeletons which can be recognized by the computer program (Fig. 7.3). An *opening* is an erosion followed by a dilation. It separates two objects connected by a small bridge. First the bridge is eroded away, with the consequence that also the outer zone of the objects disappears. Subsequently the objects are restored to their original shape by performing the same number of dilation steps as the number of erosions. The small bridge, however, will not be reconstituted with this opening algorithm since the bridge was completely eroded away. For cytology these operations have been proven to be extremely effective in the recognition of certain cell types, the removal of artefacts such as overlapping cells and the separation of touching cells. These mathematical morphology type of procedures can be carried out on entire microscope images by pipelined processing and require often less than 100 ms per microscope field of $512 \times 512\,\mu m$ [16,17].

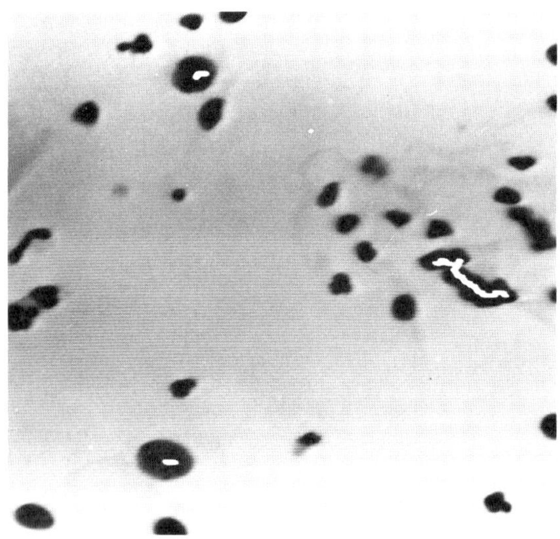

Fig. 7.3 Cervical cells which have been subjected to a skeleton procedure to reject detected artefacts. In two objects (single cells) the result of the skeletonization is a short line; in the third object (overlapping cells = artefact), it is a long line with side branches. The latter shape fulfils the criteria of an artefact, and the object will be rejected.

7.4 CELL PREPARATION AND STAINING FOR AUTOMATED IMAGE CYTOMETRY

Not all slides with cells are suitable for the image analysis routines and instrumentation available at this moment. Cell preparations with numerous overlapping cells and dirt are difficult to analyse automatically. Interactive image cytometry also needs well-isolated cells, although the preparation requirements are less stringent than for automated cytometry as the operator selects the cells to be measured. Many investigators in automated cytometry have therefore used special cell preparation methods to achieve better cell isolation and removal of dirt [18–22].

An efficient procedure to remove debris is to collect the cells in preservation fluid and to wash the cell suspension by centrifugation. Syringing with thin needles (e.g., 21-gauge) is often included to break up cell clumps. Automated syringe pumps facilitate this step and moreover increase its reproducibility. Excessively high cellularity should also be avoided in cytometry, which can be achieved by measuring the cell concentration before slide preparation. Different methods can be used such as a Coulter counter or the measurement of the 90° scatter from a light source directed at the cell suspension.

In automated cytometry the cells should be in a monolayer on the glass slide. This can be adequately achieved by cytocentrifugation. Based on a method by Leif *et al.* [23], a cytocentrifugation bucket was developed at the laboratory of the author [20] to deposit already fixed cells on the slide. High **g** forces need to be used to adhere the cells to the slide, which should be precoated with a substance such as polylysine with a high molecular weight [24]. The cells of the resultant monolayers are approximately in one focal plane and have a well-preserved morphology. Oud *et al.* [25] have developed an automated system to produce monolayers from cell suspensions. The system collects cells on a filter tape by filtration and transfers it to glass slides by means of pressure fixation. These preparation procedures can be applied to fresh, unfixed cells as well as cells isolated from paraffin-embedded tissue. The preparation of single cells from paraffin-embedded tissue was first described by Hedley *et al.* [26] for flow cytometry, and later adapted for image cytometry by van Driel-Kulker *et al.* [21]. Both procedures involve the cutting of thick sections (30–50 μm) which are rehydrated and enzyme-treated.

An improved automated cell selection of crowded cell smears can often also be obtained by not staining DNA and cytoplasm simultaneously, or by choosing a method with two absorbent or fluorescent dyes which can be visualized sequentially. When only the nuclei are stained, cell overlap is less of a problem in cell selection than with staining of the total cell. Several sequential staining methods for image cytometry have been described [27,28]. Their use often requires more complex image cytometry instrumentation with automated filter rotors and several cameras (colour, black and white) looking at the same cell observed at a different wavelength.

In interactive image cytometry it is possible either to avoid measurement of cells which appear to be stained unsatisfactorily, or to adapt the segmentation threshold. In fully automated image cytometry inadequately stained cells are not selected and measured, since very lightly stained cells can often not be separated from the background. If the threshold for image segmentation is lowered, areas in the background in another part of the image may also be detected. In general this means that staining procedures must be chosen such that the staining contrast is high. Staining procedures that lead to relatively high local extinctions do not, however, always provide linear relations between the concentration of the stained macromolecules and the measured integrated optical density; they suffer from non-linearity in the stoichiometry of the measured cytochemical staining result. This becomes clearly evident in the measurements of DNA-stained rat liver cells. These cells are polyploid and should have measurement values of 2, 4 and 8 U. If the staining is non-linear, this relationship cannot be reproduced. In routine practice a compromise between automatic detectability and accurate measurement must sometimes be accepted. This does not need to lead to false conclusions. Since automated image cytometry can also detect rarely occurring cells with very abnormal DNA content, it means that aneuploid cells with, for example, 6*C* DNA content can still be detected with sufficient accuracy as proof of the existence of a 3*C* stemline. Whether this nucleus is measured as 5.8 or 6.2*C* does not hamper the diagnosis of aneuploidy. In both cases the nucleus is definitely aneuploid. In this context it should be realized that flow cytometry may have difficulties in detecting a small number of aneuploid cells of more than twice the normal DNA content, since doublet-cell nuclei will yield the same measured value. In image cytometry such doublets are recognized as artefacts. In automated cytometry this is for the larger part done by the programme; remaining artefacts can be recognized via the stored images which are displayed on a screen. The above arguments should not of course detract from trying to obtain staining procedures which have a high contrast and are stoichiometric. It only illustrates that fully automated cell selection requires an image that is optimal for image segmentation.

7.5 MULTIPARAMETER WIDE-FIELD MICROSCOPE

An important problem in image cytometry instrumentation is the necessity to analyse cells at different microscope magnifications. Like the visual inspection procedure by a cytopathologist, a low microscope magnification is also preferred in image cytometry for rapid screening of the entire specimen in search of interesting or suspect cells. After selection of such cells, a closer inspection of their morphology is often needed at high microscope magnification. The low- and high-magnification

(LM and HM) possibilities can be obtained by sequentially employing LM and HM objectives. With a motor-driven revolver for objectives this can be performed under computer control. An even more efficient solution is a microscope which produces two magnifications of the same cells simultaneously on to two different television cameras, like the AUTOPLAN. The instrument incorporates a 40× NA 1.30 wide-field immersion objective. The light after passing this objective is split into two synchronously usable light channels for LM (20×) and HM (80×). The 20× magnification in the LM channel is achieved by using the 40× objective in combination with a 2× demagnifying tube lens. In both channels a television or CCD camera is used to capture the image. To achieve a similar illumination for both cameras, the light is divided by a beam-splitter with interference coating in a ratio of 1:16, which is in proportion to the magnification ratio of 1:4 for the LM and HM channel, respectively. The LM of 20× in combination with an oil immersion objective of an NA of 1.30 has been especially chosen to capture 512 × 512 μm microscope fields and for obtaining very bright images to facilitate analysis of fluorescent images.

7.5.1 Automatic focusing

Rapid screening of cytological specimens demands the analysis of many microscope fields. Here rapid autofocusing methods are of paramount importance, since most microscope slides are wedge-shaped if the thickness is evaluated in the order of microns. This requires focusing for almost every microscope field to be examined. In addition, all cells selected at LM will be measured at HM, requiring renewed focusing. For optimal performance of an image cytometer in the autofocusing process, the objective should be moved rather than the heavier scanning stage [10]. A computer-driven motor attached to a small gearbox moves the objective in subunits of microns required for exact focusing. Information for movement of the motor is obtained from the image analysis part of the cytometer. Even when using the relatively light objective for autofocusing, the total time needed for this process is a major contributor in the total screening time of a whole slide. Economy in the time needed for focusing is therefore important to obtain reasonable screening times in routine clinical cytology.

7.5.2 Multiparameter analysis

With regard to the basic principles for multiparameter analysis of pathological samples, the Leica AUTOPLAN image cytometer microscope was designed similarly to the approach used in multiparameter flow cytometry. By using multiple antibodies marked by cytochemical stains with differently coloured end-products, several types of macromolecules can be analysed simultaneously. For this purpose the image cytometer is provided with computer-operated filterwheels in the illumination light path, a computer-operated fluorescence epi-illuminator and combinations of different types of cameras, like black and white and colour CCD cameras. Since the measured values from the different colour signals are all stored in the list mode of the computer memory, many combinations of cellular parameters can be made in the final analysis of the stored data. In contrast to flow cytometry, where similar data handling based on list mode data is used, image cytometry offers the advantage that multiparameter data can be directly combined with the images of the selected cells stored in the computer memory. This link of biochemical topology with cell morphology opens new areas of investigation for the pathologist.

7.6 ARTEFACT REJECTION IN AUTOMATED CYTOMETRY

In interactive cytometry the human observer selects the cells to be measured, and avoids overlapping cells, badly stained cells or cells covered with dirt. Automated cytometry, however, requires automated and efficient artefact rejection procedures. If a significant percentage of the selected and measured objects were artefacts, it would be very difficult to interpret the data. Major efforts must therefore be devoted to avoid artefacts. In Section 7.4 we have already discussed methods of cell preparation and staining to diminish dirt, overlapping cells, etc. In our image analysis system artefact rejection can be performed at two levels [29]. The first level is at LM when typical or suspect cells are selected for further measurement at higher magnification. Mathematical morphology operations are very well suited for fast artefact rejection algorithms. A few erosion steps can remove most of the small dirt particles and, by adding an opening, the original size of the cells will be restored after the removal of the small dirt particles from the binary image. In automated cytology, overlapping cells constitute the main artefact problem. Skeletonization algorithms in combination with the detection of triple points (see Fig. 7.3) are very effective in removing such artefacts [16,17]. Leucocytes and groups of leucocytes can be removed from the image by other mathematical morphology algorithms [16].

Objects surviving artefact rejection at LM will be measured at HM, whereafter these are subjected to a second group of artefact recognition procedures, like thresholds in size or bending energy. The latter procedure will eliminate oddly shaped objects [30]. The combination of adequate cell preparation, staining and image algorithms at both LM and HM can lead to satisfactory results (Table 7.1). As a last artefact rejection procedure, the images of the stored cells (Fig. 7.4) are inspected by the operator of the cytometer. If one or two objects of the stored images depicted on the screen are still recognizable as an artefact, the observer can remove these by typing in the identification number. Thus the measurement data will be composed of single cells only. Such data merely need the presence of a few aneuploid cells to permit the diagnosis of aneuploidy for the entire specimen. In contrast, flow cytometry would require a well-separated significant peak of the histogram, since these data are often contaminated with doublets, triplets and nuclei with dirt. If the objects measured in flow cytometry are not sorted on to a slide, the ratio of single cells cannot be verified. In many practical applications this is not

Table 7.1 Objects (alarms) detected during cervical screening. Visual evaluation of the stored images (see Fig. 7.4) shows that the number of artefacts is relatively low. Note also the large difference between average numbers of single cells in the positive and the negative specimens

Reference diagnosis	Average numbers of alarms per slide			
	Alarms	Nuclei	Overlap	Dirt
Negative ($n = 1223$)	12.0	5.8	3.9	2.3
Dysplasia ($n = 160$)	87.7	70.9	13.3	3.5
Positive ($n = 117$)	189.0	151.1	31.6	6.3

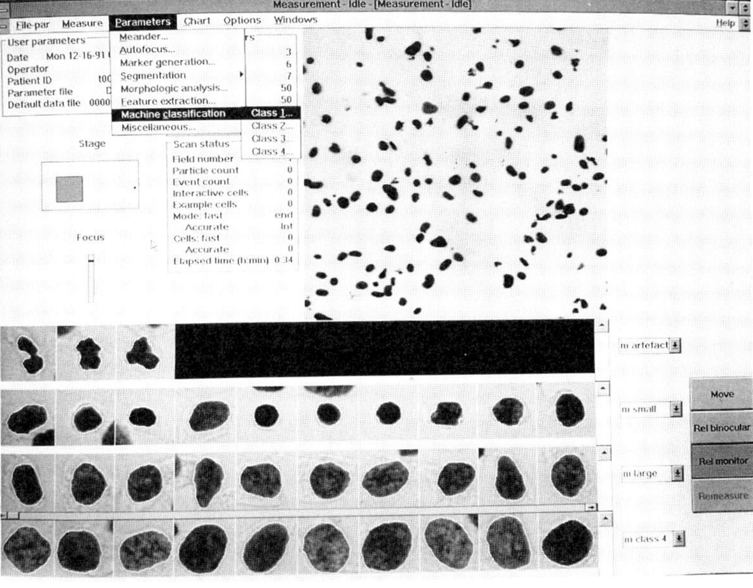

Fig. 7.4 Cells automatically selected by the Discovery from a microscope slide of an ovarian carcinoma. By activating the pull-down options of the Window menu, the part of the screen for display of the selected cells can be varied.

considered an important problem, provided one does not search for rare events. Of course, rare event detection suffers more from artefact contamination than the analysis of dominant stemlines containing many single nuclei. In image cytometry it is also possible to verify that objects with extreme values are indeed single cells. Due to data storage in list mode, all data of one object can be combined and this option allows display of a specific cell on the screen or even in the microscope. If it can be demonstrated with a high degree of certainty that objects with extreme values are indeed single cells, important conclusions can sometimes be made. One example consists of the demonstration of heterogeneity in a tumour sample containing, as well as a typical stemline, rare aneuploid cells which may have consequences for diagnosis and prognosis [31].

7.7 DATA ACQUISITION PROGRAMS AND DATA PROCESSING

It should be realized that the analysis of a cellular specimen on a microscope slide requires an adequate statistical strategy [14,32]. Usually 50 000–100 000 cells are present on a slide prepared by cytocentrifugation techniques. It is not possible to measure all these cells in a reasonable time with image cytometry. It is, however, feasible to select representative samples of cell populations from such a slide. If a cytometer were able to measure and store the images of about 500 nuclei at HM in about 15 min, we would have to select these 500 nuclei at LM in such a way that statistically significant information is obtained about the major cell populations present on the slide.

7.7.1 DNA heterogeneity in tumours

In the case of DNA measurements in a tumour-cell specimen, we would first like to get information about the normal cells. Since such nuclei are often present in larger numbers it might be sufficient to select about 200 nuclei in the 2*C* DNA range in 10–20 microscope fields at LM. Since the cell selection process operates by selecting cells above certain thresholds, cell selection in the 2*C* range means in fact the selection of cells with 2*C* DNA content and more. With the rapid mathematical morphology algorithms such a selection is possible on the basis of size and density of the nuclei while analysing total microscope fields (512 × 512 μm). The image cytometer should have a datafield programmed in a user-friendly interface like Windows (Fig. 7.5) where the number of nuclei to be measured in

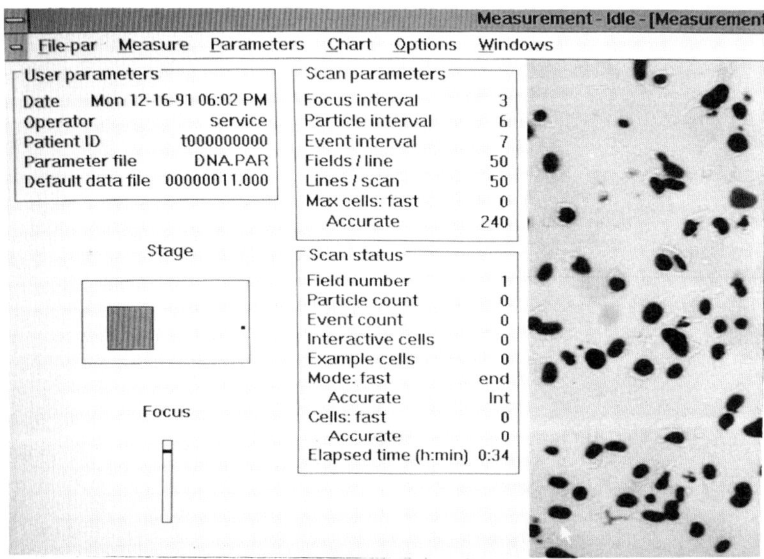

Fig. 7.5 Display of the Discovery analysis status. The system keeps track of various counting processes (scan status) and shows the used parameters on request (scan parameters).

certain DNA ranges can be entered. In the 100–200 ms needed for the selection of these cells no accurate measurements are performed. The selected nuclei are placed in the centre of the microscopic field and measured accurately via the HM channel of the image cytometer. Histogram analysis of these 200 nuclei will give information on the normal cells and possibly about the peak position of an aneuploid tumour. A diploid tumour cannot be distinguished from normal cells on the basis of its DNA content of the main cell population. Next we should search nuclei in another DNA range (e.g., 3–4*C* DNA). Nuclei below about 2.4*C* are no longer selected by entering this next range for mathematical morphology nuclear selection algorithms in the Windows datafield for cell selection. Depending on the frequency of this type of cell, another 20–40 microscope fields are examined. Finally, selection of all nuclei above 4 C is entered in the cell selection datafield. Smaller nuclei are no longer selected and, since the frequency of these high-DNA-content nuclei in the specimen is often quite low, fewer nuclei are selected in each microscopic field and also fewer nuclei have to be measured at HM. Less time is now needed per field. This procedure provides an excellent possibility to investigate heterogeneous tumours with small centres of abnormal cells which will appear only infrequently in the total cell sample [2]. Yet the mere presence of such abnormalities may strongly influence diagnosis and prognosis. Recent *in situ* hybridization studies using chromosome-specific DNA probes for the investigation of interphase nuclei have often demonstrated unsuspected marked heterogeneity of human tumours based on the observation of multiple copies of the same chromosome in some nuclei [33].

7.7.2 Statistical considerations

To be able to judge the statistical significance of the above cell selection procedure, the investigator must demonstrate that the cell selection procedures of the image cytometer occur in a randomized way and will not be biased by artefact rejection algorithms. In other words, artefact rejection should not also remove certain cell types, and care should be taken to tune the settings of the artefact rejection to the application on hand. Furthermore, slightly hypodiploid or hyperdiploid stemlines are difficult to demonstrate in image cytometry. This is due to the contribution of variation in cell preparation, staining and instrument performance. Under equilibrium staining conditions in flow cytometry this variance is less. In image cytometry it is advisable to concentrate on the doubling of DNA values in dividing cell populations. These nuclei occur less frequently, but are easily detectable in image cytometry since they can be well-distinguished from artefacts like doublet nuclei. For the same reason, nuclei with DNA values higher than 5*C* can be well-detected, even if their frequency is very low. The presence of such nuclei can often be well-correlated to prognosis [31,34]. In some cases, such as in cervical lesions, care should be taken to exclude polyploidization (2, 4 and 8*C*) of nuclei caused by viral infections when the significance of 5*C* exceeding cells is investigated.

7.7.3 The advantage of list mode in the storage of cellular data

Much progress has been achieved in flow cytometry by storing all measured cellular parameters in list mode in the computer memory. This has the advantage that the investigator does not need to know which cellular parameters will be combined before the experiment is started. The most significant combination can thus be assessed after the measurement process, if necessary, even in a different computer. The more cellular parameters that are measured, the more fruitful the study of parameter combinations will be. In image cytometry a similar approach can be chosen. The data can be displayed in histograms (Fig. 7.6) and scatter plots (Fig. 7.7). Ample operator interaction with this data display is feasible. Four histograms or scatter plots can be evaluated simultaneously (Fig. 7.8). Through the mouse option, modern data-handling programs of an image cytometry system may allow the operator to point out certain cells or populations directly in a histogram or scatter plot. Of these selected populations, statistical calculations can be automatically performed (Fig. 7.9). Selected populations can also be transported to another histogram or a scatter plot (Fig. 7.10). For example, the transport option allows

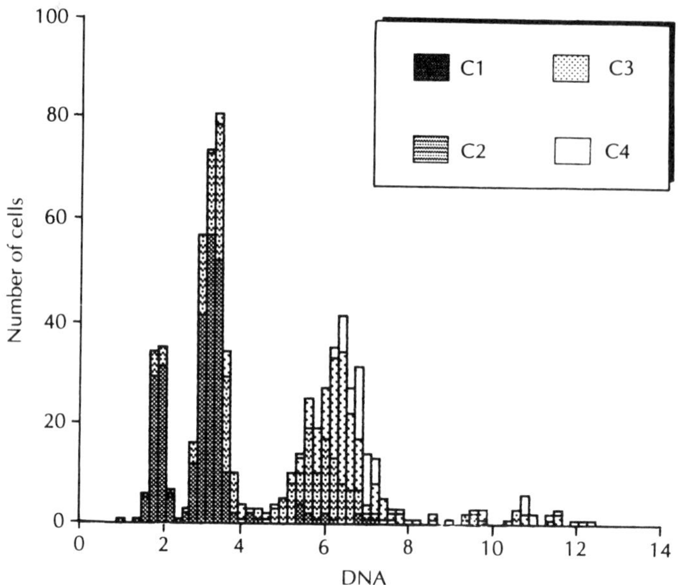

Fig. 7.6 DNA histogram from an ovarian tumour. The nuclei have been automatically selected by means of criteria with increasing demands for density and size, which are depicted in different shadings. The lower criteria (criterion c1 in the picture) have darkest shading.

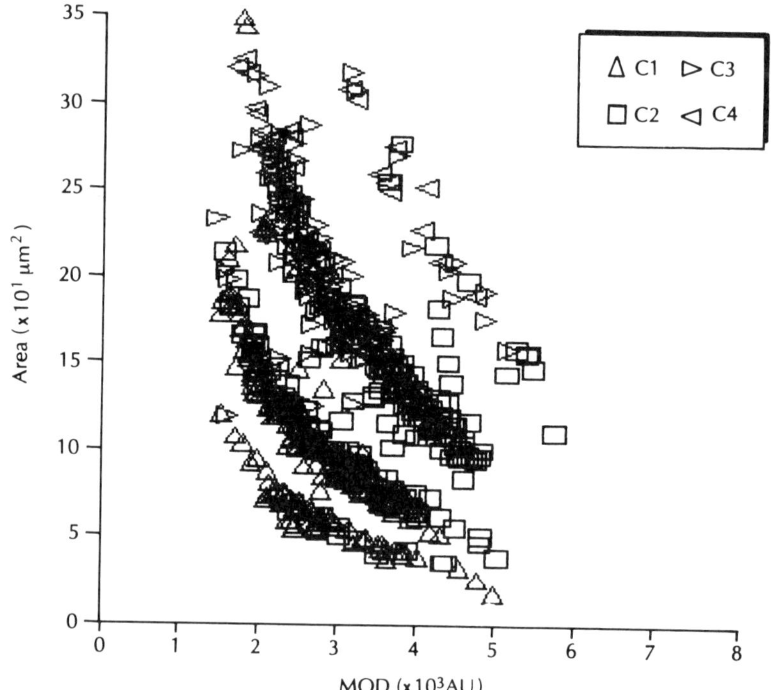

Fig. 7.7 Scatter plot of the DNA histogram of Fig. 7.6. The cells are now displayed according to their area (*x*-axis) and mean optical density (MOD) (*y*-axis). AU, arbitrary units.

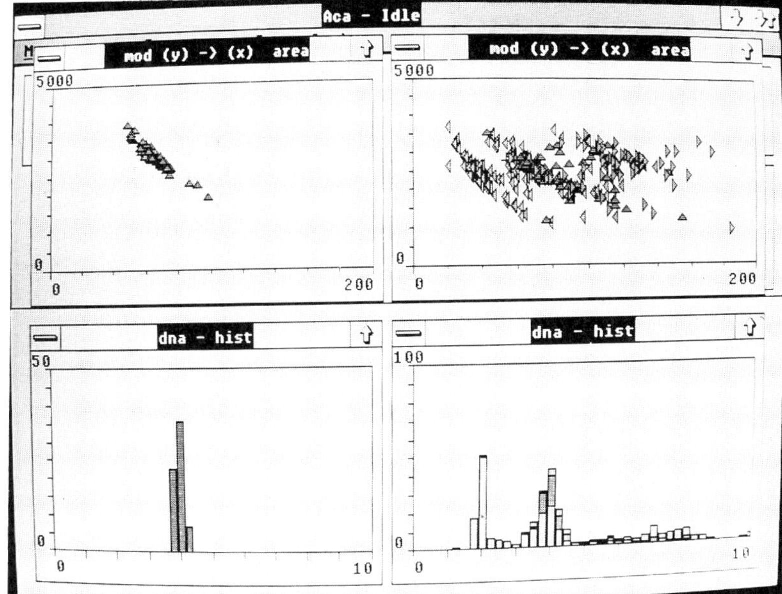

Fig. 7.8 The programme incorporates the display of four histograms or scatter plots simultaneously. The left side shows 4*C* liver cells in a scatter plot and histogram. The right shows the scatter plot and histogram of a tumour.

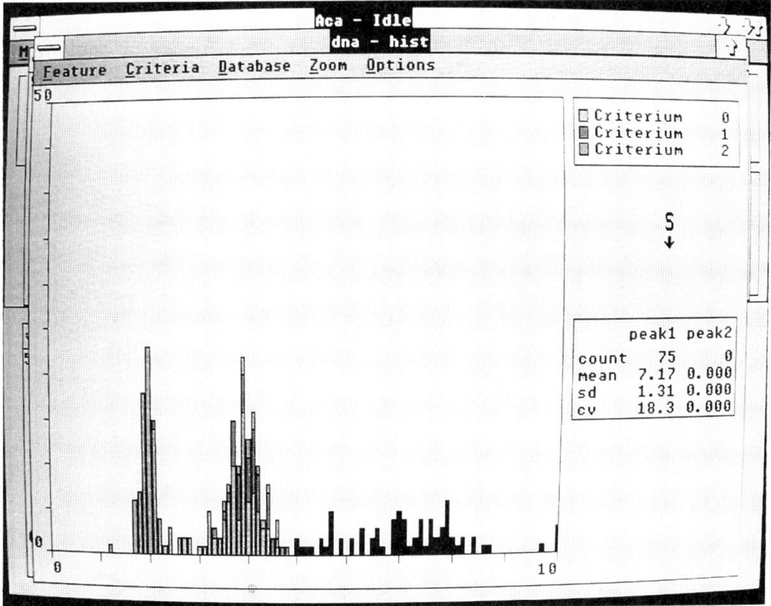

Fig. 7.9 In this DNA histogram the cells with more than 5*C* DNA content have been marked. The program will then calculate population data, which can be seen on the right.

the evaluation of variation in the area and mean optical density of cells with a certain DNA content (Fig. 7.11). Furthermore, images of selected cells or cell populations can be searched for in the file of the computer memory and displayed on the monitor for visual inspection. This enables verification that a certain high value really corresponds to a single, very abnormal cell. For instance, in a specimen containing 100 000 cells, a few truly aneuploid nuclei can then allow one to decide that there is aneuploidy, even when more than 99% of the nuclei are diploid.

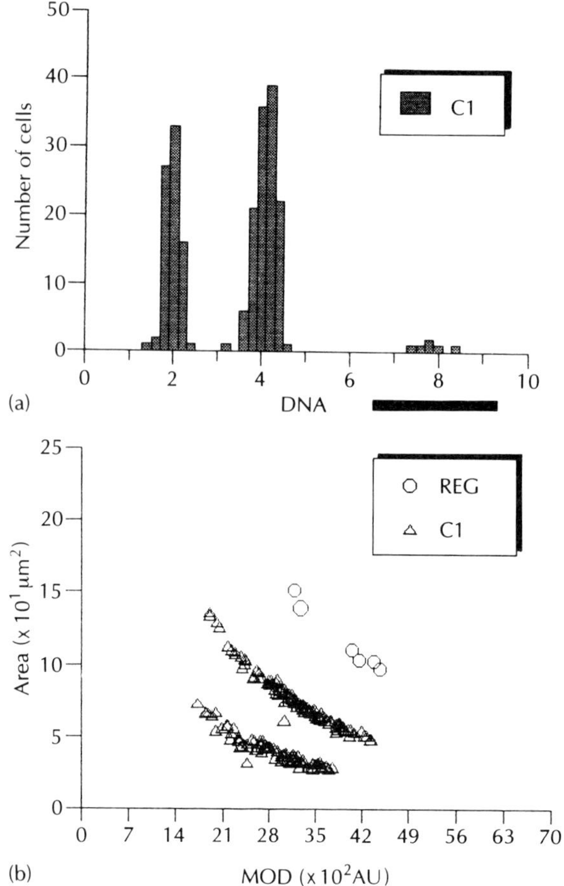

Fig. 7.10 Demonstration of selection of certain cell populations in a histogram and of transportation of this selection into a scatter plot via the list mode data. AU, arbitrary units; MOD, mean optical density.

7.8 EXAMPLES OF CLINICAL APPLICATIONS

An automated cytometry system should allow the analysis of several types of cellular material. Most important are the settings for the cell selection, but also artefact rejection should be adapted according to cell type. Furthermore, it should be possible to adjust the settings for the overall cell segmentation and for the range of the autofocus steps if preparations with a different contrast are analysed. Using LEYTAS, the settings for the algorithms can be optimized in a separate step-by-step procedure where the result of each algorithm can be evaluated individually. Thereafter the settings can be fixed for analysis of the whole slide.

The applications carried out with LEYTAS can be divided into two main groups. The first type is aimed at detecting cells of low frequency and covers cervical screening, detection of early virus infections, of metastatic cells in bone marrow and of very rare mutant cells in the peripheral blood. The second type of application aims at analysis of tumour samples to gain prognostic information.

7.8.1 The detection of rare events in pathology

The detection of rare events such as very abnormal cancer cells requires a special strategy in cytometry. In flow cytometry all cells in the sample are measured at high speed. In practice a small number of artefacts like doublet or triplet nuclei will always be measured. This can of course be limited by using precise time-of-flight analysis, slit scanning or multiple antibodies. For example, if a clinical cytological sample contains only a very small percentage of high-DNA-content cells, the number of artefacts may even exceed the number of detected high-DNA-content nuclei. This would require cell sorting on to microscope slides to verify visually which objects are a single nucleus with high DNA content and which objects are artefacts.

In image cytometry a different strategy can be followed. The procedure is to select cell nuclei over a certain threshold, defined by the operator. Since the DNA by such rapid selection operations is not actually measured but estimated on the basis of features such as the nuclear size, the threshold is rather inaccurate. For the purpose of rapidly screening a large cytological sample, however, this procedure is quite effective. Following cell selection at LM, each selected object is measured at HM (e.g., 0.25 μm pixel separation).

Like flow cytometry, image cytometry cell selection also results in the detection of artefacts. Due to very effective artefact rejection algorithms at LM as well as HM the number of detected artefacts in image cytometry can be kept low. Moreover, visual inspection of the stored images of the detected cells or cell nuclei allows visual removal of remaining artefacts. If any doubt remains about the interpret-

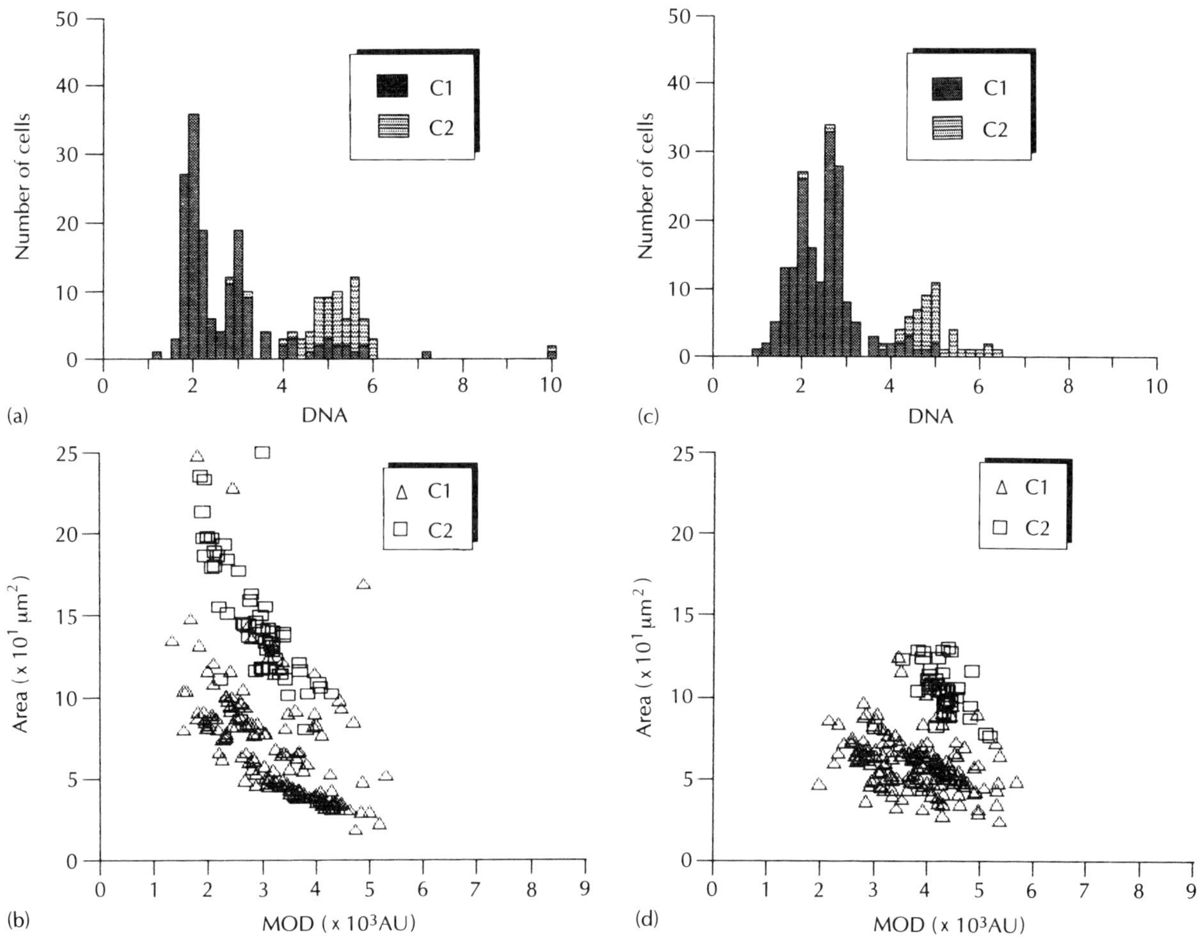

Fig. 7.11 DNA histograms (a and c) and mean optical density (MOD)/area scatter plots (b and d) of two cases of breast carcinoma stage 1. In the region to the right of the 4*C* (4*C* exceeding region) the two DNA histograms do not differ greatly. In the corresponding scatter plots, however, a difference in the distribution of cells exceeding 4*C* is seen. The areas of the cell nuclei depicted in (b) show a much larger variation than the case depicted in (d). AU, arbitrary units.

ation of a recorded image, the cells can be automatically relocated in the microscope for visual inspection of the actual microscope image. As a result, rare events can be detected in image cytometry with a high degree of certainty, which is of considerable interest in the early diagnosis of disease.

Cervical screening

Since the development of the cervical smear method directed at early cancer diagnosis, the screening load has been steadily increasing. This has stimulated research for methods which could automate the screening process. In more recent decades it also became apparent that the conventional (visual) screening process led to considerable numbers of false-negative screening results [35]. Therefore, present research in automation is not only directed at decreasing the screening workload, but also and most importantly at obtaining a very low false-negative rate.

We followed this approach in the development of a method for the automated screening of cervical smears using LEYTAS. Recently this system has been tested in a semiroutine setting in a clinical laboratory, where 1500 cervical smears were automatically analysed [36,37]. The smears were prepared from cervical cell suspensions which were centrifuged on glass slides and stained with a Feulgen procedure (acriflavine). All smears were first visually classified by four different cytologists to obtain a reference diagnosis for the machine result.

The smears were then analysed with LEYTAS, which consisted of automatic cell counting and the search for abnormal cells by means of specific cell detection criteria which had been optimized in earlier experiments [17]. The whole set of 1500 slides was screened with identical criteria for cell detection as well as for artefact rejection and the total screening process was carried out without any operator interaction. After termination of the screening, each slide was characterized by a number of detected cell-like objects (alarms) and its ratio in relation to a total cell count. Thresholds in the number and ratio of alarms led to a false-negative error of zero in the group of smears diagnosed as cervical intraepithelial neoplasia (CIN) III or carcinoma ($n = 117$). The false-positive machine rate was 16.5% in 1223 morphologically negative specimens. For the CIN I and CIN II group the false-negative ratios were 12.6 and 3.1% (Table 7.2). The advantage of a system such as LEYTAS is that images of the alarms are stored and displayed on a television monitor (see Fig. 7.4). This allows a fast visual evaluation of the alarms. True alarms such as single cells can thus be distinguished from falsely selected objects such as overlaps. Also a morphological diagnosis of the selected cells can be given, which was demonstrated in the test of the 1500 cervical smears. All positive specimens and 97.5% of the negatives were correctly classified using the images of the selected cells.

Table 7.2 Results of completely automated screening of cervical smears. The classification into machine-positive or −negative is based on a threshold in the number and ratio of alarms

Reference diagnosis	Machine classification			
	Negative	Positive	FNR (%)	FPR (%)
Negative ($n = 1223$)	1021	202	–	16.5
Dysplasia 31 ($n = 95$)	12	83	12.6	–
Dysplasia 32 ($n = 65$)	2	63	3.1	–
Positive ($n = 117$)	0	117	0	–

FNR, false-negative rate; FPR, false-positive rate.

Early detection of virus-infected white blood cells

An early diagnosis of virus infections, e.g., infection with human cytomegalovirus (CMV) is now feasible by means of a direct antigen method using monoclonal antibodies against an early protein (pp65) of CMV. Antigen-positive (CMV-pp65) leucocytes appear in the circulation in frequencies from one in 1000 000 to one in 100 cells, and manual counting indicated that changes in frequency have prognostic value. Automated search and counting of these low-frequency CMV-positive cells were performed using immunoenzymatically stained blood smears which were counterstained with haematoxylin to allow autofocusing of the image cytometer. Furthermore, endogenous peroxidase was inactivated with glucose oxidase. The density of the labelled cells was about five times higher than the non-labelled cells using this staining procedure. The analysis resulted in a count of the non-labelled cells and, after visual evaluation of the stored images of the detected objects, in a count of the CMV-positive cells. The sensitivity of the system proved to be higher than one per 100 000 but less than one per 1000 000 white blood cells. The procedure was used in the evaluation of patients with a kidney transplant, who are prone to CMV infection [38]. The screening time, however, is still too long for routine use (60 min for 1 million cells).

Metastatic cancer cells

Marrow aspirates taken at the time of surgery for primary breast cancer often show cancer cells. These can be detected by immunocytochemical staining of bone-marrow smears. However, these cells appear rarely (< 1 in 10 000) and visual screening is time-consuming. Using LEYTAS and reproducible preparation with counterstaining of non-labelled cells it was possible to automate the screening. The selected objects resembling a positive cell were relocated in the microscope to verify this diagnosis. The preparations investigated with LEYTAS showed a good correlation with the visual counts [39].

Mutant research

Environmental carcinogenic factors such as radiation and chemicals may cause point mutations in human cells. Some point mutations occur in erythrocytes and can be visualized by immunological detection of abnormal haemoglobin (HbS). Strong polyclonal antibodies against HbS result in high fluorochrome isothiocyanate (FITC) fluorescence intensities in red cells containing HbS and low fluorescence readings of normal (HbA-containing) red cells. The contrast in the microscope image was quite sufficient for automated image cytometry with LEYTAS, which for this application was equipped with a multichannel microscope to allow absorption analysis of the unlabelled red blood cells and fluorescence analysis of the FITC-marked cells. Since the frequency of these mutants can be as low as one in 10 million cells, artefact rejection needed to be quite rigorous. The procedure was first to focus and count all erythrocytes along one row of microscope fields, by using dia-illumination with violet light (415 nm). After one 8 cm scan line, illumination was changed under computer control from dia-illumination to epi-illumination. All the fields of the scan line were re-examined following a fitted curve through the previously defined focus positions to permit detection of the fluorescing objects. From each detected object both the fluorescence and the absorption image were stored and displayed. Verification of detected objects suspected of being an HbS-containing cell was done in the microscope. Although automated screening of this large number of cells is still very time-consuming, it could be established that exposure to carcinogenic substances led to a higher mutant frequency than is present in control persons [40].

7.8.2 Tumour analysis

Both fresh and archival material can be analysed by automated cytometry. However, most LEYTAS studies have been performed with monolayer smears from paraffin-embedded tissue. The advantage of using archival material is that the outcome of the disease is already known, which allows a direct evaluation of the prognostic significance of the measured parameters. Another advantage of paraffin-embedded tissue is that a diagnostic 5 μm section of the same tissue block can be used to control visually the cells to be analysed. The ratio of tumour versus normal cells can be estimated. If the ratio is very low, a special procedure is used to isolate the tumour cells from the block. To that purpose the whole block is fluorescently stained and mounted on the stage of a fluorescence microscope equipped with incident illumination. Aided by the diagnosis of the 5 μm section, the fluorescent structures can be interpreted to locate the tumour cells. Subsequently the objective is turned away and a hollow bore mounted in an objective holder is positioned over the tumour area. By using the microscope microscrew, the bore is pressed into the tissue (Fig. 7.12). This procedure allows separate preparation

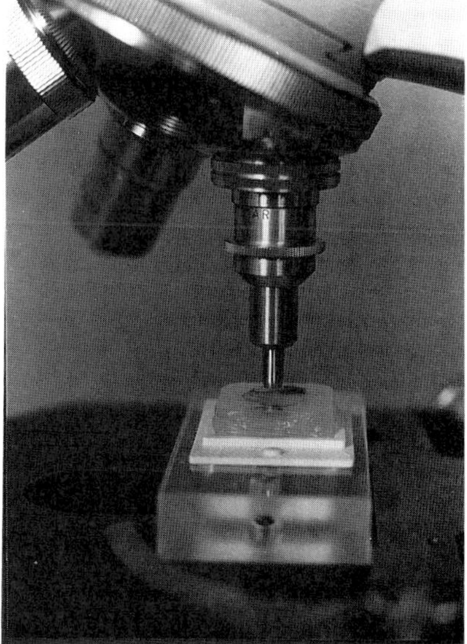

Fig. 7.12 Photograph of the hollow bore fitted into the objective holder to cut specific areas from the tissue block.

of the bored tissue and leaves the rest of the block intact [41].

The LEYTAS procedure to analyse tumour cells is described in Section 7.7. Using this strategy, prognostic archival studies have been performed on ovarian, breast and bladder cancer, soft-tissue sarcomas and thymomas.

Ovarian carcinoma

In 45 patients with advanced ovarian cancer, a significant difference in survival between diploid and non-diploid cases could be demonstrated. The combined results of ploidy and the number of cells exceeding $5C$ resulted in three groups of patients. Patients with a diploid tumour had a median survival of more than 60 months. Patients with a non-diploid malignancy and less than 100 cells exceeding $5C$ were an intermediate group with a median survival of 42 months, whereas the remaining patients with a non-diploid tumour and more than 100 cells exceeding $5C$ showed a median survival of 15 months. Comparison with clinical parameters in a multivariate analysis showed that ploidy and cells exceeding $5C$ had the highest impact on survival [31].

Bladder carcinoma

The impact of ploidy in combination with cells having more than $5C$ DNA content was shown in a study by Stoeckle *et al.* [34] and in a more recent analysis of 140 bladder carcinomas (stage Ta, T1 and T2). In the latter study the DNA histograms were divided into four classes (diploid, two borderline groups and aneuploid) on the basis of rates exceeding 2 and $5C$. Comparison to survival showed a similar behaviour for the diploid and the first borderline group, whereas the second borderline group corresponded to the aneuploid category. An important difference between the two borderline groups was the rate exceeding $5C$. This rate alone was highly correlated with survival ($P = 0.0001$).

Breast carcinoma

Based on the work by Auer *et al.* [42], who found that short survival was correlated to aneuploidy, we performed cytometry studies of early as well as more advanced stages of breast carcinoma. The majority of cases proved to be aneuploid, including the stage I tumours. In this category 10 patients died; nine of these had an aneuploid histogram. However, in the group of patients with an aneuploid histogram no difference could be observed between long- and short-term survivors. In breast cancer more parameters are needed to predict the disease course.

Soft-tissue sarcoma and thymoma

These investigations demanded adaption of the artefact rejection algorithms to avoid the rejection of the elongated nuclei (sarcoma) and of the small lymphocytes (thymoma). The ploidy classification correlated significantly with grading of the sarcomas. In most cases ploidy characteristics of recurrences or metastases were similar to the primary tumour [43]. In the thymoma study the measured area and mean optical density were used to quantify the different cell populations in this tumour. Higher stages were more frequently associated with non-diploid histograms and with a higher ratio of cells exceeding a certain size threshold.

7.9 CONCLUSION

Progress is being made in automated cytometry through advances in microscope and camera design leading to better image acquisition; imaging operations, preparative and staining techniques also give greater cell separation and contrast. This is allied to advances in computer hardware and software which are capable of storing vast numbers of microscopic images, processing large amounts of data and allowing selected images to be recalled on demand for expert operator assessment and verification. The speed of automated image cytometry procedures is improving. Its merits lie in the detection of rare events in pathology and possible applications include cervical smear screening and the assessment of tumour tissue where abnormal cells occur at low frequency.

References

1 Baak JPA. *Manual of Quantitative Pathology in Cancer Diagnosis and Prognosis.* Berlin: Springer Verlag, 1991.

2 Ploem JS, van Driel-Kulker AMJ, Ploem-Zaaijer JJ. Automated cell analysis for DNA studies of large cell populations using the LEYTAS image cytometry system. *Pathol Res Pract* 1989; 185: 671–675.

3 Banda-Gamboa H, Ricketts I, Cairns A, Hussein K, Tucker JH, Husain N. Automation in cervical cytology: an overview. *Anal Cell Pathol* 1992; 4: 25–48.

4 Brugal G. Pattern recognition, image processing, related data analysis and expert systems integrated in medical microscopy In: *Ninth International Conference on Pattern Recognition.* Washington: IEEE Comput. Soc. Press, 1988: 286–293.

5 Husain OAN, Watts KC, Lorriman F *et al.* Semi-automated cervical smear pre-screening systems: an evaluation of the CYTOSCAN-110. *First Conference of the European Society for Analytical Cellular Pathology. Anal Cell Pathol* 1989; 1: 266 (abstract).

6 van Vliet LJ, Young IT, ten Kate TK, Mayall BH, Groen FCA, Roos R. Athena: a Macintosh-based interactive karyotyping system. In Lundsteen C, Piper J (eds) *Automation of Cytogenetics.* Berlin: Springer-Verlag, 1989: 47–66.

7 Vrolijk J, Verwoerd NP, Bonnet J, Beverloo HB, Tanke HJ. A system for time-resolved fluorescence microscopy and quantitation of *in situ* hybridisation products (abstract). *Cytometry* 1990; 4(suppl): 83.

8 Nederlof PM, van der Flier S, Raap AK, Tanke HJ. Quantification of inter- and intra-nuclear variation of fluorescence *in situ* hybridization signals. *Cytometry* 1992; 13: 831–838.

9 Young IT, Balasurbamanian DL, Dunbar R, Peverini L, Bishop RP. SSAM: solid-state automated microscope. *IEEE Trans Biomed Eng* 1982; 29: 70–82.

10 Wasmund HF, Ploem JS. Ein computergesteuertes Mikroskop als Baustein eines automatisierten Prescreening Systems. *Microsc Acta* 1983; 6(suppl): 135–144.

11 Jaggi B, Poon SSS, Pontifex B, Fengler JJP, Palcic B. Evaluation of a quantitative microscope for image cytometry (abstract). *Cytometry* 1990; 4(suppl): 18–19.

12 Tucker JH, Shippey GF. Basic performance tests on the CERVIFIP linear array prescreener. *Anal Quant Cytol* 1983; 5: 129–137.

13 Duijndam WAL, Smeulders AWM, van Duijn P, Verweij AC. Optical errors in scanning stage absorbance cytophotometry I. Procedures for correcting apparent integrated absorbance values for distributional glare and diffraction errors. *J Histochem Cytochem* 1980; 28: 388–394.

14 Bartels PH, Weber JE, Bibbo M. Ploidy pattern analysis: statistical considerations. *Anal Quant Cytol* 1985; 7: 126–130.

15 Serra J. *Image Analysis and Mathematical Morphology.* London: Academic Press, 1982.

16 Meyer F. Iterative image transformations for automatic screening of cervical smears. *J Histochem Cytochem* 1979; 27: 128–135.

17 van Driel-Kulker AMJ. Automated image analysis applied to the diagnosis of cervical cancer. Thesis. University of Grenoble, France, 1986.

18 Bahr GF, Bibbo M, Oehme M, Puls JH, Reale FR, Wied GL. An automated device for the production of cell preparations suitable for automatic assessment. *Acta Cytol* 1978; 22: 243–249.

19 Rosenthal DL, Stern E, McLatchie *et al.* A simple method of producing a monolayer of cervical cells for digital image prccessing. *Anal Quant Cytol* 1979; 1: 84–88.

20 van Driel-Kulker AMJ, Ploem-Zaaijer JJ, van der Zwan M, Tanke HJ. A preparation technique for exfoliated and aspirated cells allowing different staining procedures. *Anal Quant Cytol* 1980; 2: 243–246.

21 van Driel-Kulker AMJ, Mesker WE, van Velzen I, Tanke HJ, Feichtinger J, Ploem JS. Preparation of monolayer smears from paraffin-embedded tissue for image cytometry. *Cytometry* 1985; 6: 268–272.

22 Tanaka N, Ikeda H, Ueno T, Okamoto Y, Hosoi S. CYBEST-CDMS Automated cell dispersion and monolayer smearing device for CYBEST. *Anal Quant Cytol* 1981; 3: 96–102.

23 Leif RC, Gall S, Dunlap LA, Ratley C, Zucker RM, Leif SB. Centrifugation cytology: IV The preparation of fixed stained dispersions of gynecologic cells. *Acta Cytol* 1975; 19: 159–168.

24 Tucker JH, Husain OAN. Trials with the cerviscan experimental prescreening device on polylysine-prepared slides. *Anal Quant Cytol* 1981; 3: 117–120.

25 Oud PS, Haag DJ, Zahniser DJ *et al.* Cytopress: automated slide preparation of cytologic material from suspension. *Cytometry* 1986; 7: 8–17.

26 Hedley DW, Friedlander ML, Taylor IW, Rugg CA, Musgrove EA. Method for analysis of cellular DNA content of paraffin-embedded pathological material using flow cytometry. *J Histochem Cytochem* 1983; 31: 1333–1335.

27 Cornelisse CJ, Ploem JS. A new type of two-color fluorescence staining for cytology specimens. *J Histochem Cytochem* 1976; 24: 72–81.

28 Oud PS, Zahniser DJ, Raaijmakers MCT, Vooijs PG, Van de Walle RT. Thionine–Feulgen–Congo red staining of cervical smears for the BioPEPR image analysis system. *Anal Quant Cytol* 1981; 3: 289–294.

29 van Driel-Kulker AMJ, Ploem-Zaaijer JJ. Image cytometry in automated cervical screening. *Anal Cell Pathol* 1989; 1: 63–77.

30 Young IT, Walker EJ, Bowie JE. An analysis technique for biological shape. *Inform Contr* 1974; 25: 357–370.

31 Rodenburg CJ, Ploem-Zaaijer JJ, Cornelisse CJ *et al.* Use of DNA image cytometry in addition to flow cytometry for the study of patients with advanced ovarian cancer. *Cancer Res* 1987; 47: 3938–3941.
32 Weber JE, Bartels PH, Bartels HG, Bibbo M. Discrimination of DNA ploidy patterns by order statistics. *Anal Quant Cytol* 1987; 9: 60–68.
33 Hopman AHN, Moesker O, Smeets AWGB, Pauwels RPE, Vooys GP, Ramaekers FCS. Numerical chromosome 1, 7, 9 and 11 aberrations in bladder cancer detected by *in situ* hybridization. *Cancer Res* 1991; 51: 644–651.
34 Stoeckle M, Tanke HJ, Mesker WE, Ploem JS, Jonas U, Hohenfellner R. Automated DNA-image cytometry: a prognostic tool in infiltrating bladder carcinoma. *World J Urol* 1987; 5: 127–132.
35 Bogdanitch W. The Pap test misses much cervical cancer through lab's errors. *Wall Street J* 1987; Nov 27th.
36 van Driel-Kulker AMJ, Strohmeier R, Naujoks H, Ploem JS. System evaluation of LEYTAS in cervical cancer screening (abstract). *Anal Cell Pathol* 1989; 1: 266.
37 Naujoks H, Strohmeier R, Bicker T, van Driel-Kulker AMJ, Knepfle CFHM, Ploem JS. Interobserver variability in the cytological diagnosis of 1500 Papanicolaou stained cervical monolayer specimens. *Pathol Res Pract* 1990; 186: 150–153.
38 Jiwa NM. Early detection of human cytomegalovirus infections in transplant recipients. Thesis, University of Leiden, The Netherlands 1989.
39 Mansi JL, Mesker WE, McDonnell T, van Driel-Kulker AMJ, Ploem JS, Coombes RC. Automated screening for micrometastases in bone marrow smears. *J Immunol Methods* 1988; 112: 105–111.
40 Tates AD, Bernini LF, Natarajan AT *et al.* Detection of somatic mutants in man: HPRT mutations in lymphocytes and hemoglobin mutations in erythrocytes. *Mutation Res* 1989; 213: 73–82.
41 van Driel-Kulker AMJ, Eysackers MJ, Dessing MTM, Ploem JS. A simple method to select specific tumor areas in paraffin blocks for cytometry using incident fluorescence microscopy. *Cytometry* 1986; 7: 601–604.
42 Auer G, Eriksson E, Azavedo E, Caspersson T, Wallgren AS. Prognostic significance of nuclear DNA content in mammary adenocarcinomas in humans. *Cancer Res* 1984; 44: 394–396.
43 Pape H, Poettgen C, Ploem JS, van Driel-Kulker AMJ, Wurm R, Schmitt G. The prognostic value of DNA content measured by image cytometry in soft tissue sarcoma. *Ann Oncol* 1992; 3(suppl 2): 89–92.

PART 2
FLOW CYTOMETRY

8

THE FLOW CYTOMETER

P. W. HAMILTON AND A. D. CROCKARD

Flow cytometry is an extremely powerful tool for the analytical and quantitative characterization of cells. A flow cytometer is essentially a complex measuring device which can detect small intensities of light either scattered or emitted from a cell. If the intensities are proportional to the cellular components causing them, then light measurement (photometry) will allow these features to be quantified.

Prior to this chapter, quantitative cellular analysis has been largely concerned with measurements made from tissue sections. Sections allow a clear visualization of the tissue morphology within which the measured cells lie, but restrict the automated measurement of cellular features due to image complexity. True automated image quantitation is made easier by the examination of free-lying cells in the form of cytological preparations. Flow cytometry utilizes an extension of this rule as it requires a *suspension* of dispersed single cells for analysis. While most body fluids (e.g., blood) form a natural cell suspension, certain methods have been developed to disaggregate solid tissue for flow cytometry (see Chapter 9).

As with image analysis, the ability sequentially to analyse free-lying cells imparts speed and precision to the measurement process. The disadvantage of a cell suspension, as with a cytological smear, is that tissue morphology is lost and the resulting sample comprises a mixture of components derived from the tissue under study. This may cause problems when analysis of a specific cell type is desired. Various methods can be used to enrich cell populations and reduce contamination.

Flow cytometry has now become an extremely useful technique in many areas of disease research and this is reflected in the volume of literature which has appeared over the past number of years. Advantages lie in its speed and versatility and it is possible to analyse up to 1000 cells per second with high precision. The simultaneous development of a variety of fluorescent markers and monoclonal antibodies has allowed the flow cytometric measurement of various cellular features, including nuclear DNA content, cell surface and intracellular antigens, cell proliferation markers and intracellular pH. The retention of the cell as a whole unit allows an *in vivo* analysis of these characteristics, giving flow cytometry advantages over quantitative biochemical methods. However, flow cytometry may also be used to examine individual cellular components, e.g., nuclei, chromosomes, mitochondria, etc., if they can be extracted and suspended in a suitable medium. For this reason, most of the following text will refer to the objects being analysed from suspension as particles.

8.1 BRIEF OVERVIEW OF THE FLOW CYTOMETRY TECHNIQUE

The speed and precision of flow cytometry are due to a unique combination of electronic, optical and biochemical technology. The common design of a laser-based flow cytometer is shown in Fig. 8.1. The particles (cells, nuclei, chromosomes, bacteria) for analysis are dispersed in suspension (a). This sample suspension is fed into a flow chamber (b) in which the particles are hydrodynamically focused

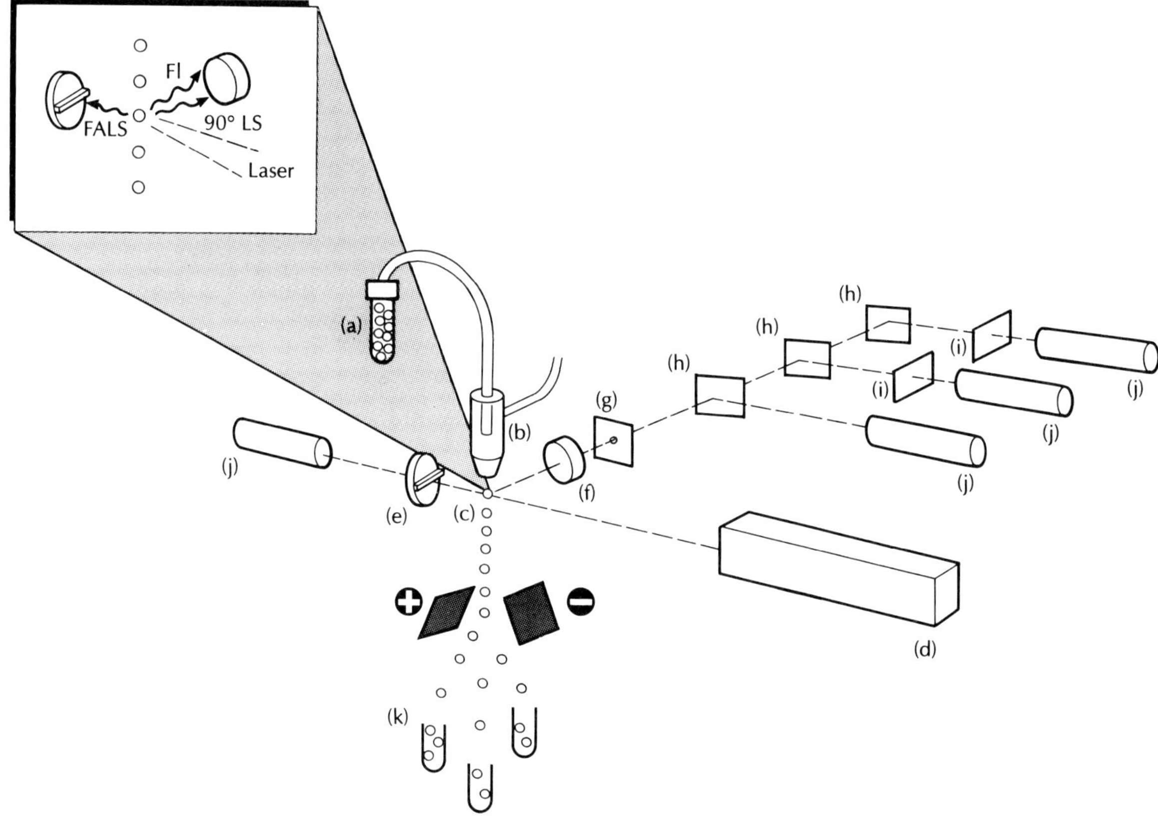

Fig. 8.1 Typical laser-based flow cytometer with orthogonal design. (a) Cell suspension; (b) flow chamber; (c) single cell stream; (d) laser; (e) forward-angle optical lens with obscuration bar; (f) 90° or orthogonal optical lens; (g) pinhole aperture; (h) dichroic mirrors; (i) absorption filters; (j) photodetectors; (k) cell-sorting region. (Inset) Close-up of detection region. The laser striking the cell results in light scatter and fluorescence in all directions. Forward-angle light scatter (FALS) is detected at low angles to the direction of the laser beam. Light scatter (90° LS) and fluorescence (Fl) are detected by a lens at right angles to the laser beam.

into a central stream in single file (c). A very-high-intensity light source (laser or arc lamp) (d) is focused on this stream and as each particle physically passes through the laser beam, light is scattered in all directions. Optical channels collect forward-angle light scatter (FALS) (e) and light scattered at an angle of 90° (90° LS) to the direction of the laser (f). If the cells have been specifically stained with a fluorochrome, excitation by the light source will cause the fluorochrome molecules to fluoresce. Fluorescence is also collected in the 90° light channel (see Fig. 8.1, inset) and a pinhole aperture (g) excludes extraneous light. Specific wavebands of light can be selected for measurement using dichroic mirrors (h) and absorptive filters (i). Photodetectors (j) measure the intensity of scattered and fluorescent light, the electrical output signal of which is directly proportional to the quantity of incident light. Analogue-to-digital conversion of this signal allows the quantitative data to be stored in the computer memory and retrieved for analysis. As the cells leave the point of analysis they can be partitioned into droplets of fluid. Cells which possess defined light characteristics can be given an electrical charge and deflected from the main stream (k). This function can be used to separate specific populations physically and is called cell sorting.

The geometry of the design shown in Fig. 8.1 is

termed *orthogonal* because of the perpendicular arrangement of the laser, stream and light collection axes.

Light scatter and fluorescence are the major characteristics which are quantified using flow cytometry. Before a more detailed examination of the flow cytometric technique, a brief description of these light phenomena is given.

8.2 LIGHT SCATTER

Light scatter is the result of reflection and refraction (Fig. 8.2) from a particle and has been shown to provide information specific to its characteristics. The physics of light scatter are complex and have been given elsewhere [1].

FALS has been shown to increase with the size of a particle. However, limitations of this measurement are fourfold.

1 Scatter is only proportional to size when the particle is near-spherical.

2 FALS is strongly affected by the wavelength of light and its absorption by the particle.

3 The refractive index of the particle surface, the internal components of the particle and the suspending medium will all alter the FALS intensity.

4 Minor changes in optical alignment of the flow cytometer will affect the reproducibility of this measurement [2].

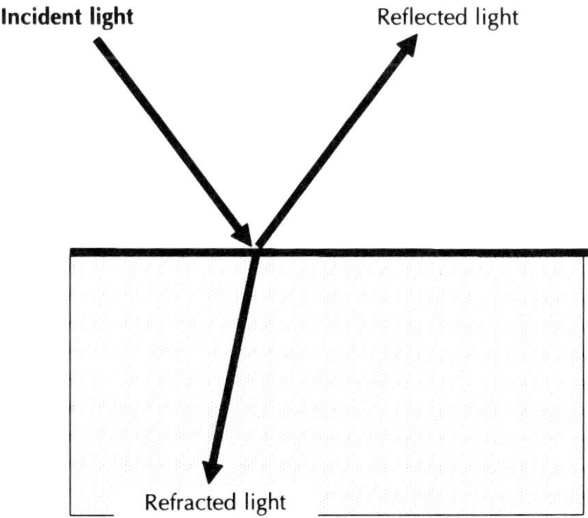

Fig. 8.2 Reflected and refracted light scatter.

Nevertheless, FALS is and will continue to be used as a rough guide to particle size and as a method to distinguish particle populations.

Light scattered at right angles (90 °LS) is determined by the reflective and refractive characteristics of the particle surface and its internal components. In cells this measurement can give a good index of cytoplasmic granularity and so, in combination with FALS, it has been used to discriminate haemopoietic cells and, in particular, blood lymphocytes, monocytes and granulocytes [3].

8.3 FLUORESCENCE

Certain molecules, when stimulated by light photons of a specific wavelength, are raised to a higher energy state. In the process of returning to their basic state the molecules emit light which has a higher wavelength and lower energy than that used to excite them. This emission is called fluorescence. It is distinguished from phosphorescence by the speed at which the molecule returns to its ground state after excitation: fluorescence rapidly disappears when the excitation light is removed, whereas phosphorescence continues for variable times.

Many different compounds have fluorescent properties and these are collectively termed fluorophores. The *extinction coefficient* of a fluorophore is the power of the molecule to absorb light. This varies depending on the wavelength of the excitation light (*excitation range*) and the *absorption maximum* is that wavelength which invites the maximum extinction coefficient. The *quantum efficiency* is the number of photons emitted for every photon absorbed. The *emission range* is the wavelengths of light that are emitted from the fluorophore after excitation.

The intensity of excitation light determines the degree of fluorescence. However, overexposure to extreme light intensities will result in damage to the fluorophore and bleaching of the fluorescence.

The advantage of certain fluorophores (fluorochromes) is that they can be made to bind to certain cellular components, rendering them fluorescent. The basis of quantitative fluorescence analysis is that the binding of a fluorochrome to a specific cellular component is *stoichiometric*, i.e., proportional to the quantity of the component. The intensity of emitted fluorescence should then be in direct proportion to this. The specificity of the fluorochrome/target reaction will, in part, determine the *accuracy* of the measurements. For example, non-specific binding of the fluorochrome to components other than the target will give an overestimation of the quantity and numbers of the feature or cells being studied.

The wavelength and intensity of excitation light and emitted fluorescence are important in the choice of fluorochrome for flow cytometric quantitation. The spectral properties for a series of commonly used fluorochromes are given by Waggoner [4].

A variety of techniques can be used to label components with fluorescent compounds. Certain fluorochromes directly attach themselves to cellular compounds, e.g., propidium iodide intercalates with double-stranded DNA (see Chapter 10); fluorochrome isothiocyanate (FITC) covalently binds to protein. Alternatively, fluorochromes can be attached to primary or secondary antibodies for the detection of specific antigens within the cell or on the cell surface, e.g., FITC-conjugated antibody detection of 5-bromodeoxyuridine for quantitative cell proliferation analysis (see Chapter 11) or the detection of cell-surface antigens in cell phenotyping (see Chapter 12). Finally, other probes are sensitive to their microenvironment and display varying fluorescence characteristics under different conditions, e.g., carboxyfluorescein diacetate in the measurement of intracellular pH; Indo-1 for the study of intracellular free calcium [Ca^{2+}].

Certain cellular constituents are naturally fluorescent. This intrinsic *autofluorescence* results in a background of 'noise' which can interfere with the fluorescent signal produced by the feature of interest. This is particularly true when labelled features emit low intensities of light which are not much higher than the background fluorescence, i.e., the signal/noise ratio is low. The subtraction of background fluorescence from the detected labelled fluorescence is an index of the *sensitivity* of the measuring system. Various techniques have been devised to improve the signal/noise ratio, including modified immunological methods to enhance fluorescence and optic/electronic adjustments to improve the collection of fluorescent light.

8.4 THE FLOW CYTOMETER IN MORE DETAIL

8.4.1 The flow chamber

In flow cytometry the particles must be made to flow one by one through a narrow stream so that each passes individually through the point of interrogation (the light source). This is accomplished in the flow chamber and is governed by the laws of hydrodynamics.

The velocity profile of a fluid passing through a narrow tube is parabolic (Fig. 8.3). This means that the velocity of the stream is greater towards the centre of the tube than at its periphery, where contact with the walls slows the fluid down. This is called *laminar flow*. Pressure decreases as velocity increases, and particles entered into the flow are drawn into the central axis of the stream, a process known as hydrodynamic focusing.

The basic design of a flow chamber is shown in Fig. 8.4. An inlet allows isotonic fluid to pass through the chamber and exit through a narrow orifice or channel, creating the hydrodynamic characteristics described above. The sample particle suspension is fed into the centre of this chamber by a tube and each particle is singly focused in the centre of the flowing stream, leaving the flow chamber one by one and enclosed in fluid (hence the name sheath fluid).

The rate of sample throughput can be controlled by altering the differential pressure between the sample and the sheath fluid. Alternatively, the

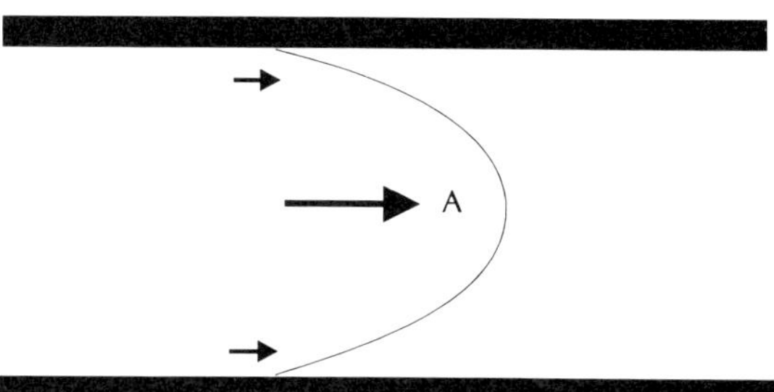

Fig. 8.3 Laminar flow of a fluid through a narrow tube. Particles are dragged to the point labelled A on the parabolic profile, which has the highest velocity and lowest pressure.

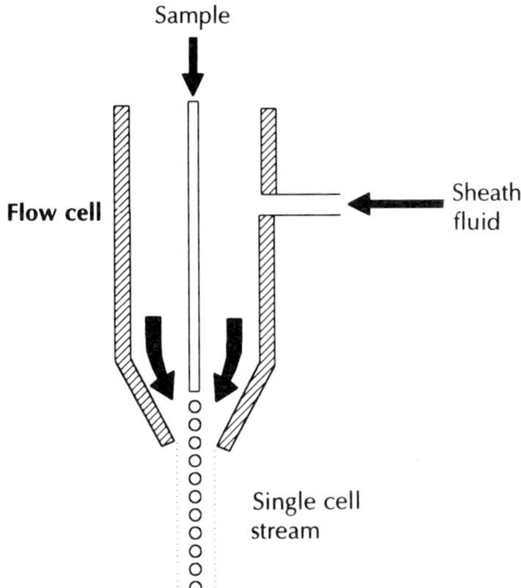

Fig. 8.4 The flow chamber. Sheath fluid provides a constant flow through the chamber orifice. Cells fed into the centre of the chamber are hydrodynamically focused, leaving the orifice one at a time.

sample can be injected into the flow chamber at varying rates by a syringe under accurate motor control.

Flow chambers can be broadly categorized into opened and closed systems.

Open chambers

In laser-based instruments the laminar stream flows through the orifice at the conical end of the chamber. Analysis of stream particles by the light source takes place immediately after the stream leaves the chamber. This can be as low as 5 µm below the exit point of the flow chamber and is named stream-in-air analysis. An alternative form of open chamber exits for cytometers with an arc lamp source [4].

Closed chambers

In closed systems light source intersection with the particles takes place inside a rectangular tube which is an extension of the conical chamber nozzle. The flat sides of the flow channel allow the use of oil immersion optics in some closed systems to improve light collection and sensitivity. However, contamination of the channel and its effect on light measurement may present problems [5].

Both types of chamber can be used to initiate droplet formation for cell sorting (see Section 8.5).

8.4.2 Light sources

A strong light source is required to excite sufficient fluorescence and light scatter needed for quantitative analysis. Two suitable light sources have been exploited in flow cytometry – the arc lamp and the laser.

Arc lamps

Arc lamp illumination in flow cytometry is usually provided by a 100 W high-pressure mercury (Hg) lamp or alternatively 75 W xenon (Xe) lamp. A process of epi-illumination is generally used, where the excitation and emitted light share the same optical channel. This reduces the intensity of detected background light scatter which occurs in the optical design of laser-based systems. Emission lines produced by an Hg arc lamp are limited. Unfortunately, lack of an emission line at 488 nm reduces the sensitivity of arc lamps in the measurement of FITC fluorescence – an important fluorescent conjugate in many antibody studies. Selection of the required wavelength is achieved using optical filters. While arc lamps are cheap in comparison to lasers, they do have a lower light output. This requires oil immersion optics to focus as much light on the sample as possible and collect the lower amounts of fluorescence obtained. Arc lamps also have a short lifetime and decay of the lamp electrodes causes intensity flicker, which is detrimental to accurate cytometry.

Lasers

The incorporation of the laser (*l*ight *a*mplification by *s*timulated *e*mission of *r*adiation) as a light source in flow cytometry has bestowed several advantages over the arc lamp. These include a higher light intensity of monochromatic light and a wider range of emission lines, including ultraviolet. The argon (Ag) ion laser is a common choice for flow cytometric analysis. It is generally run at 488 nm, permitting the excitation and analysis of various fluorochromes, including propidium iodide, FITC, acridine orange and phycoerythrin. Other types of lasers include krypton (Kr) ion lasers, helium–neon (He–Ne) atomic lasers, helium–cadmium (He–Cd) molecular lasers and diode lasers.

8.4.3 Optical system

The quantitative analysis of cells by light in flow cytometry requires the light source, stream and optical collection lenses to be accurately aligned.

Optical lenses

In laser-based systems optical lenses are positioned to collect: (i) light scattered in the forward direction; (ii) light scattered at right angles (orthogonal) to the laser beam; and (iii) fluorescence which is also collected through the orthogonal lens (Fig. 8.1).

As the orthogonal lens is responsible for collecting low intensities of fluorescent light, it is desirable to maximize this by using a lens with a large numerical aperture (NA). Increasing the NA of a lens also increases its working distance, so that within the confined space of the sensing region the NA is physically restricted. The use of closed chambers and immersion optics allows the NA to be increased and a greater amount of light to be collected. A pinhole aperture is aligned in the optical channel to eliminate stray light from sources other than the particle under analysis.

As right-angle-scattered light and fluorescence are collected by the same lens and follow the same optical path, they must be separated before measurement. This is achieved using dichroic filters, as described later.

The forward angle lens is responsible for collecting FALS (0–20°). An obscuration bar (see Fig. 8.1) is positioned to protect this lens from the directly oncoming laser beam. Whilst this reduces the amount of FALS that is collected, it prevents direct laser light from entering the optical detection channel and reduces the FALS signal/background noise ratio.

Optical filters

The choice of suitable filters is essential in flow cytometry, as in any form of fluorescence microscopy. Filters are designed to transmit portions of the wavelength spectrum and so confine the spectral range of both excitation and emission light. The optical filtering of *excitation* light is common in arc lamp-based instruments which give a wide range of emission peaks, whereas laser light is monochromatic. The filtering of *emitted* light is, however, crucial to both types of system, first to distinguish scattered light from fluorescent light and second, to select the specific wavelength of fluorescence that is emitted by the labelled feature.

A large range of filters have become available for the separation and detection of specific wavelengths of light. *High-pass* filters transmit light above a certain wavelength (Fig. 8.5a), *low-pass* filters transmit light below a specific wavelength (Fig. 8.5b) and *band-pass* filters transmit light over a narrow wavelength band (Fig. 8.5c).

Filtering is achieved either by *reflection* or *absorption* of the unwanted wavelengths, whilst the desired spectral components continue through the filter to the detector. Those which reflect light are called interference filters and can be used to split a beam into two spectral components. Dichroic mirrors are generally high-pass interference filters which reflect light below a certain wavelength, yet allow light above that wavelength to pass through (see Fig. 8.6). In this way fluorescence can be separated from light scatter in the orthogonal light channel. A dichroic mirror intersects the emitted light at a 45° angle (see Fig. 8.6). Fluorescence, which is at a higher wavelength than the scattered light, passes through the mirror while scattered light (which is the same wavelength as the excitation light) is reflected into a different optical channel for separate detection. Dichroic mirrors are used in a similar fashion to separate two different wavelengths of fluorescent light for individual detection and measurement (see Fig. 8.6).

Absorptive filters are also used in flow cytometry systems and have a much sharper transmission threshold than interference filters. Absorptive filters do, however, themselves exhibit a small degree of fluorescence at certain wavelengths and this may

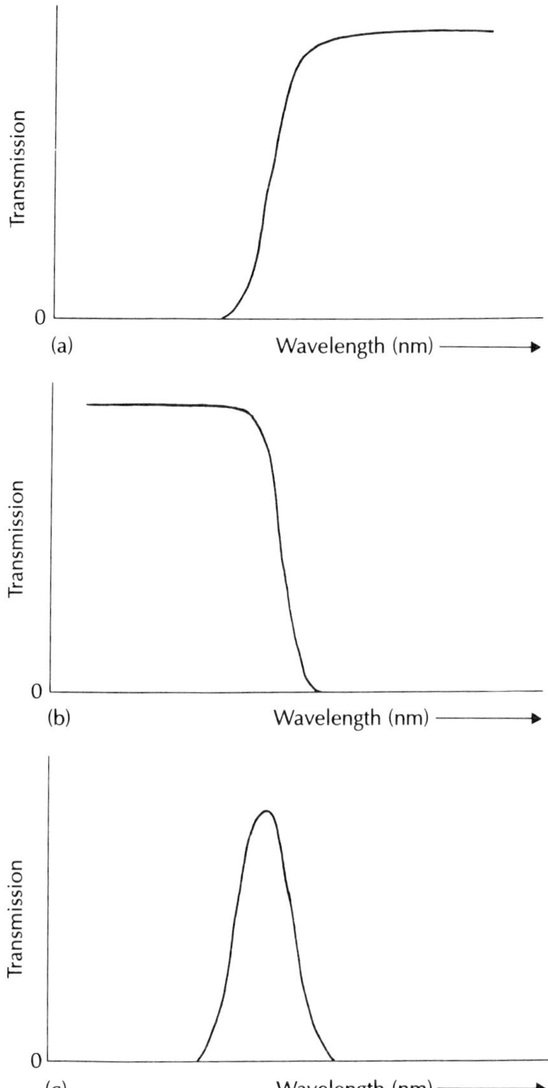

Fig. 8.5 Transmission spectra of (a) high-pass filter; (b) low-pass filter; (c) band-pass filter.

reach the detector. Additionally, the absorptive layers of the lens are susceptible to degradation and loss of transmission characteristics and this needs to be checked regularly (see Section 8.6).

8.4.4 Light detectors, pulse processing and analogue-to-digital converters (ADCs)

Detection of 90° LS and fluorescence is carried out by photomultiplier tubes (PMTs). A PMT is an instrument which releases electrons in response to light. Contact of these electrons with a series of electron-emissive electrodes results in massive exponential amplification of the initial signal. In flow cytometry, a PMT should be highly sensitive to photon particles over a wide spectral range.

As FALS is of a much higher intensity than fluorescence, a more robust solid-state detector is required. As stated previously, the obscuration bar prevents the laser from reaching the detector, so reducing noise from sources other than particle scatter.

The output of both types of detector, after conversion by a preamplifier, is a voltage pulse of between 0 and 10 V. This voltage is read by a pulse amplifier which can be manually adjusted to control amplification of the signal. Amplification can generally be linear or logarithmic, the latter permitting the simultaneous analysis of pulses with widely differing strengths. The pulse amplifier may also be set to filter out signals below a certain voltage, so reducing background 'noise' from unwanted detections. The geometric characteristics of the final amplified pulse are then converted into numerical format by an ADC, allowing the data to be read by a computer. As the speed at which particles travel through the detection region is often greater than that at which conversion to digital format takes place, the voltage pulse is often held in capacitor 'memory' until the ADC is ready.

The pulse height (peak), width and integral area are generally measured to characterize the signal from a single particle (see Fig. 8.7). The *peak* measurement provides information on the fluorescence density of the particle, i.e., how bright it is. One must bear in mind, however, that brightness is a function of particle size, as well as the number of fluorescent molecules contained within it. Shapiro [6] gives a good descriptive example of this phenomenon. To measure the total amount of fluorescent material within a particle the *integral* area of the pulse must be measured. This is the common choice of measurement to assess total cellular fluorescence. The *width* of the pulse represents the duration that the particle remains within the laser beam. If the width of the laser beam at the point of interrogation is smaller than the diameter of the

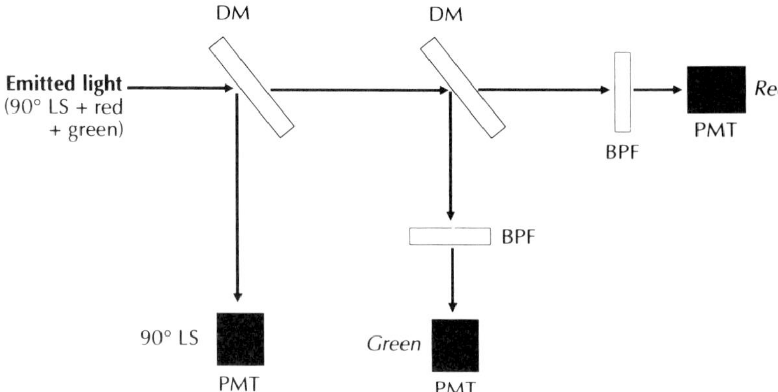

Fig. 8.6 A typical filter arrangement for the separation of 90° light scatter (LS), red fluorescence and green fluorescence. The spectral components are split by dichroic mirrors (DM) and detected by photomultiplyer tubes (PMT). Band-pass filters (BPF) ensure that only light within the desired spectral range is detected by the PMT.

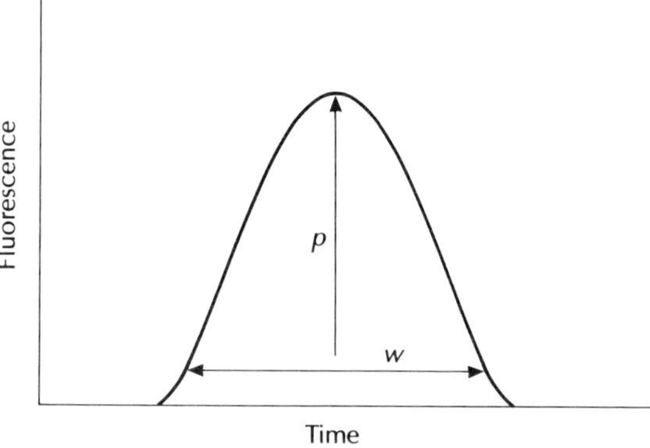

Fig. 8.7 The measurements made from the voltage pulse which characterize the light scatter/fluorescence from a particle. *p*, peak height; *w*, width; integral area = area under the curve.

particle, then the pulse width can give useful information about particle size. This principle has been exploited in slit scan flow cytometry.

A separate ADC is responsible for converting each pulse dimension into digital (numerical) format. The conversion process allocates each measurement into one of a limited number of intervals (channels) depending on the size of the analogue signal. The number of channels which can be used depends on the bit size memory location of the ADC. For example, an 8-bit ADC will allow a scale of 0–255 to be used, i.e., 256 channel locations. Increasing the bit resolution of the ADC and the number of channels will improve the resolution of the measurements (e.g., to 1024 channels).

As each particle is analysed, the results can be displayed in the form of a frequency histogram – number of particles falling into each channel number (see Chapter 10; Fig. 10.1). Alternatively, if two measurements are being made simultaneously by two ADCs, then this data can be presented in the form of bivariate dotplot (see Chapter 12; Fig. 12.5) or bivariate frequency histogram. Most flow cytometers, therefore, have an on-board computer which can store and display the data for interpretation and statistical analysis.

8.4.5 Data analysis

The software allows individual samples to be given an identification name or number under which they can be stored in the computer memory and later retrieved. The data may be stored in the form of a histogram, which later allows analysis of histogram characteristics only. Alternatively, it can be collected in *list mode* which stores each data point to memory and so allows manipulation and reanalysis of the original flow cytometric measurements. Collection of data in list mode is expensive in terms of computer memory.

Prior to running a sample through the flow cytometer, certain specifications can be made within the software to control the data which are collected for final display and analysis. For example, the number of particles that one wishes to analyse can be entered (e.g., 10 000). When this number is reached the computer will stop collecting data from the ADCs and display final results even though cells are continuing to flow through the system.

Included within these 10 000 events will be particles which are of no relevance to or are detrimental to the analysis, e.g., debris. So, within a histogram, gates can be positioned to exclude unwanted populations of particles. On a subsequent run only particles falling within, and meeting the characteristics set by, the gates will comprise the 10 000 events collected for analysis.

Most system software also permits various analyses to be performed on the histogram data. For example, percentages of cells falling within defined gates can be calculated, relative fluorescence intensities measured, statistical measures of data variation (e.g., coefficient of variation; CV) made on univariate distributions, and complex algorithms can be used in specific applications such as the identification of cell cycle stages in the analysis of nuclear DNA content.

The various flow cytometers which are currently on the market have different types of computer hardware which run a variety of operating systems and data analysis software. This presents enormous problems when one wishes to compare and analyse data from various centres as part of a research programme, a multicentre clinical trial or quality-control exercise. It is now possible, however, to convert flow cytometric data from a variety of systems into data file formats which can be read by different computer systems (e.g., RISK-based processors, PCs, Apple Macs) and analysed using various software packages. This allows the transmission of data to other database, spreadsheet, statistics or graphics programmes. Apart from promoting the interchange of cytometric data between centres, the ability to transfer and analyse data on another computer release the flow cytometer processor for data collection functions.

A recent initiative has been to establish a flow cytometry data file standard for international use. This has been commissioned by the Society for Analytical Cytology [7]. The data file recommendation [8], which is based on an earlier proposal [9], is designed to include all information relevant to a flow cytometric measurement, including the type of flow cytometer, the sample analysed, the data obtained and the results of the analysis. These data are written in a format which can be read by any computer system and the adoption of such a standard by all centres should encourage better data communication between groups worldwide.

8.5 CELL SORTING

Whilst the vast majority of applications of flow cytometry are of an analytical nature, an additional important function that can be performed is that of physical separation or sorting of distinct cell populations. The design characteristics of purely analytical flow cytometers and those capable of cell sorting are different and this is reflected in the higher cost for cell-sorting systems.

The ability to sort cells is based on the fact that the stream of fluid emerging from the flow chamber nozzle will break into distinct droplets at a distance from the nozzle. Application of a constant vibration to the stream allows droplet formation to be stabilized. In most flow cytometers this is achieved by a vibrating piezoelectric crystal in contact with the flow chamber, resulting in the formation of precisely uniform droplets (Fig. 8.8). If the flow rate is a fraction of the frequency of the piezoelectric transducer then each droplet should contain an individual cell.

Droplet formation occurs immediately after the cells have passed through the laser beam, where their scatter and fluorescence characteristics have been recorded. From these analytical data, cells with particular quantitative characteristics can be defined and sort criteria preprogrammed by the operator into the computer memory. If, on intersection with the laser, a cell meets these specific criteria then the droplet, which contains that cell, is given a static charge (Fig. 8.8). High-voltage deflector plates are positioned so that, as the charged droplet passes between them, it is deflected into a suitable collection vessel. In this way particles of interest, with specific light scatter or fluorescence characteristics, can be collected. Purity of a sorted population may be determined by reanalysis of the sample, ensuring that a majority of the cells fall within the thresholds defined by the operator.

An alternative method for cell sorting has recently been developed and implimented in the FACS sort instrument from Beckton Dickinson. A small mechanical arm sweeps in and out of the stream under control from the sorting logic and catches cells

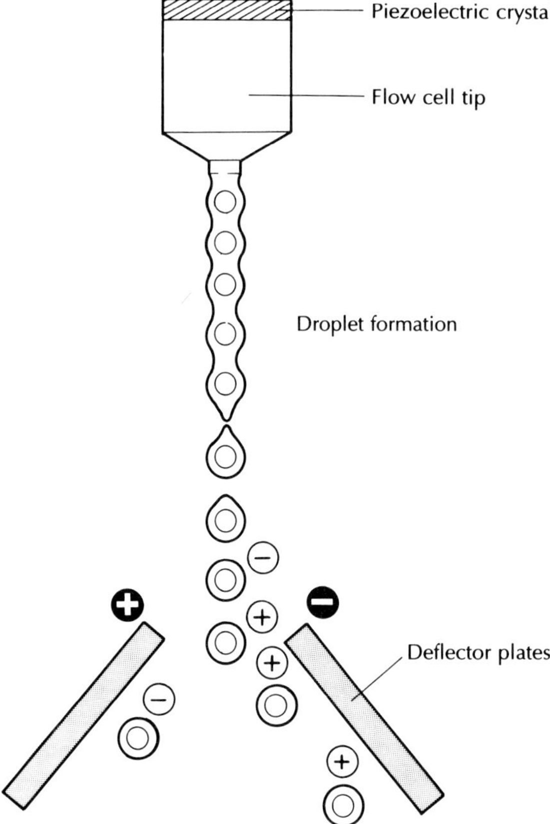

Fig. 8.8 Droplet formation and deflection in the process of cell sorting.

having specific fluorescent and light-scattering properties. This has been demonstrated to provide comparable results with the droplet-based approach in terms of both purity and yield.

Two issues which may affect the choice of methods for cell sorting are first, the required purity of the cells, and second the required yield. Both are limited by the number of starting cells, the sort time available and the quality of the label used for identification of the cells of interest. To achieve satisfactory levels of purity, particularly for infrequent cells, some preselection steps may be necessary, e.g., density centrifugation, sedimentation, immunomagnetic separations. Alternatively, high speed sorts, in which the instrument ignores coincident cells, may result in sufficient enrichment to allow a second conventional sort to achieve the desired purity. As sorting is a compromise, it is inevitable that in the pursuit of purity, cell loss (up to 50%) will occur. This must be allowed for in experimental design.

8.6 QUALITY ASSURANCE

To ensure instrument reliability and precision, quality control schemes, which incorporate the use of reference standards, are employed. Examples of reference standards commonly used in flow cytometry are:

1 uniform monodisperse synthetic microspheres (beads) of known light scatter and fluorescence intensity;

2 glutaraldehyde-fixed chicken erythrocytes;

3 fixed bovine thymocyte nuclei.

With all reference preparations it is important that the particles are uniform and remain stable over a period of time. In addition, the nature and intensity of the fluorochromes used in reference materials should be similar to those pertaining in the experimental situation. A routine instrument quality control programme should incorporate the following.

1 Optical alignment with calibration beads or fixed erythrocytes. The precision of measurements, made from particles which should give identical results such as beads, can be assessed by the coefficient of variation (CV) of the distribution. In DNA flow cytometry (see Chapter 10) the CV of the main DNA peak is often used as a measure of precision: in studies using propidium iodide as the DNA stain, cases having CV $>$ 10% are often excluded from the analysis (see Section 10.2).

2 Calibration of fluorescence intensity with particle mixtures of varying fluorescent intensities.

3 Setting of compensation parameters for overlapping emission spectra of differing fluorochromes.

Monitoring and recording of these day-to-day performance indicators will ensure optimal instrument performance and allow initiation of troubleshooting procedures when the limits of acceptability of the results are exceeded.

8.7 CONCLUSION

The flow cytometer represents a unique combination

of optics, mechanics and fluidics. It is a complex instrument and instruction is usually necessary to maintain optical/stream alignment which is crucial for successful particle analysis and cell sorting. If the instrument is properly aligned, data collection is relatively straightforward and can be carried out with minimal knowledge of the instrument. Cell sorting is a more difficult procedure, requires experience and is considerably more time-consuming. In commercial instruments currently available, most operations can be software controlled from a single computer monitor. This makes operation and data collection a relatively easy process. There is no doubt that for a routine pathology department a flow cytometer would be an expensive research tool but for the academic department with interests in the biological characteristics of diseased cells it is an instrument with tremendous potential.

References

1 Salzman GC, Singham SB, Johnston RG, Bohren CF. Light scattering and cytometry. In: Melamed MR, Lindmo T, Mendelsohn ML (eds) *Flow Cytometry and Sorting*, 2nd edn. New York: Wiley-Liss, 1990: 81–107.

2 Salzman GC, Wilder ME, Jett JH. Light scattering with stream-in-air flow systems. *J Histochem Cytochem* 1979; 27: 264–267.

3 Salzman GC, Crowell JM, Martin JC *et al.* Cell classification by laser light scattering: identification and separation of unstained leukocytes. *Acta Cytol* 1975; 19: 374–377.

4 Waggoner AS. Fluorescent probes for flow cytometry. In: Melamed MR, Lindmo T, Mendelsohn ML (eds) *Flow Cytometry and Sorting*, 2nd edn. New York: Wiley-Liss, 1990: 209–225.

5 Steen HB. Characteristics of flow cytometers. In: Melamed MR, Lindmo T, Mendelsohn ML (eds) *Flow Cytometry and Sorting*, 2nd edn. New York: Wiley-Liss, 1990: 81–107.

6 Shapiro HM. *Practical Flow Cytometry*, 2nd edn. New York: Alan R. Liss, 1988.

7 Dean PN, Bagwell CB, Lindmo T, Murphy RF, Slazman GC. Introduction to flow cytometry data file standard. *Cytometry* 1990; 11: 321–322.

8 Datafile Standards Committee of the Society for Analytical Cytology. Datafile standard for flow cytometry. *Cytometry* 1990; 11: 323–332.

9 Murphy RF, Chused TM. A proposal for a flow cytometric data file standard. *Cytometry* 1984; 5: 553–555.

9

DISAGGREGATION OF SOLID TUMOURS

K. E. WILLIAMSON

Tissue dissociation is a prerequisite for the flow cytometric analysis of solid tumour samples and for *in vitro* assay [1,2]. Flow cytometry can be used to assess DNA content, to measure intracellular components and to identify and purify subpopulations of cells for subsequent cytokinetic studies [3]. Cell suspensions allow uniform incorporation of labels and random counting of cells [4], which are not possible in tissue fragments. The inward movement of molecules into isolated slices of tissue is not a matter of simple diffusion because the labels are consumed as they diffuse into tissues.

Animal tissues contain a mixture of proteins, glycoproteins, lipids, glycolipids and mucopolysaccharides. The aim of tissue dissociation is to break down successfully this complex matrix with minimal alteration to the cell surfaces or intercellular structures. The method of dissociation is dependent on the source, nature and age of the tissue. Epithelial tissues are tightly bound by adhering junctions (e.g., tight junctions) and communicating junctions (e.g., gap junctions). Current methods involve the use of enzymes, chelating agents, mechanical force or a combination of these to produce suspensions of either whole cells or bare nuclei. In certain cases it may be possible to disaggregate cells simply by altering the pH or osmolality. Cells from parenchymal tissues, e.g., liver, are easier to obtain than those from epithelial tissues which are tightly bound by desmosomes. There is no universal procedure for tissue dissociation and it is often necessary to develop a method which is tailored to a specific analysis.

9.1 EVALUATION OF CELL SUSPENSIONS

The resultant cell or nuclear suspensions must be assessed to determine how representative they are of the original solid tumour. The notorious heterogeneity present in some solid tumours can mean that, although a suspension is representative of a single tumour sample, it does not necessarily represent the whole tumour. Unfortunately this evaluation is often overlooked in the pursuit of other data [5]. Certain studies require an assessment of viability, other cell functions, structure and morphology, and some antigenicity or DNA profiles.

Any tissue disaggregation procedure will cause cell/nuclear damage and it is necessary to be aware of the type and extent of these alterations so that results can be correctly interpreted [6]. It is important to assess both surface and internal cell damage. Gross morphological assessment will detect some of the more obvious sublethal damage, such as swollen cells, but more subtle changes may only be identified with more detailed investigations, e.g., immunohistochemistry, protein determinations or cell-function analysis. There is evidence that damaged cell-surface structures are rapidly regenerated following enzymatic treatment and that morphologically discernible changes are also repaired. Some studies advocate the removal of damaged cells using density gradient centrifugation, Ficoll–Paque or cell elutriation techniques. All studies should provide information about representivity, cell/nuclear yields per gram of tissue and cell/nuclear damage.

9.2 ENUCLEATION TECHNIQUES

The loss of plasma membranes, cytoplasmic features and viability does not preclude the analysis of DNA content or nuclear configurations using flow cytometry. Therefore the difficulty in producing intact cells for flow cytometric analysis has lead to the development and use of enucleation techniques which are relatively straightforward and can be applicable to many different tissue types. Suspensions of nuclei have been prepared successfully using detergents such as nonidet P-40 and Triton X-100 [7,8]. Both Hedley's method [9] and subsequent modifications [10] have been extensively used in retrospective studies to extract nuclei from formalin-fixed paraffin-embedded tissue. The damage that results from the disruption of the desmosomes or when the cytoplasm is stripped from the nucleus is largely unknown. One group have demonstrated that in certain enucleation techniques 80–90% of the nuclear membranes are destroyed [2]. It is difficult to determine the representivity of the nuclear suspension to the original tumour. Crude cytokinetic analysis is feasible because the percentages of cells in different stages of the cell cycle should remain constant when DNA profiles from the resultant nuclear suspensions are compared with the DNA profiles obtained using other reliable methods, e.g., fine-needle aspiration (FNA) [11]. The disadvantages of enucleation techniques are that morphological assessment is difficult, no cytoplasmic markers can be evaluated and no calculation of selective cell loss is made.

9.3 ENZYMATIC DISAGGREGATION

In procedures using enzymatic disaggregation, washing is necessary to remove the red blood cells, debris and dead cells from the tissue. The tissue is then minced into small pieces so that the largest surface area is exposed to the enzymatic action. This can be aided with the use of a mechanical tissue chopper which uniformly slices the tissue using a blade. Such instruments can produce millimetre cubes of tissue in under 30 s.

Despite the fact that the optimal activity of enzymes rarely occurs at a neutral pH, at 37 °C, most disaggregation methods are attempted under physiological conditions for a minimal period to limit cell damage and prevent postdisaggregation lysis. The degree of purity of single enzymes is always of concern – particularly collagenase for which no pure enzyme preparation exists. Crude collagenase preparations from *Clostridium histolyticum* contain not only several collagenases but also a protease, clostripain and an aminopeptidase. Trypsin can contain chymotrypsin, elastase, ribonuclease, deoxynuclease and amylase. However, crude preparations of enzymes have been found to be more effective in tissue disaggregation than their purified counterparts; this is attributable to the activities of these contaminants [2]. Heterogeneity of the enzyme preparation can mean that optimized methods are no longer effective when new batches of enzyme preparations are used.

Cocktails of enzymes containing trypsin and/or pronase in combination with collagenase and DNase have been successfully used to disaggregate solid tumours [2,12]. In the analysis of colorectal tissue optimal results have been achieved by serially disaggregating colorectal tumour tissue in a solution containing 0.02% collagenase, 0.02% DNase and 0.05% pronase [13].

The enzymes collagenase, pronase, pepsin, trypsin and chymotrypsin will release cells from most tissues. However, elastase is required to digest the fibrous connective tissue glycoprotein elastin found in arteries, heart and liver [14]. Collagen is the major component of animal extracellular connective tissue and collagenase is an enzyme capable of digesting tendon and muscle. Collagenases are unstable in phosphate buffers and require calcium ions for optimal activity. The proteases, trypsin and pronase, are used to disrupt intercellular junctions. Trypsin, which is a serine protease, hydrolyses ester and peptide bonds involving carbonyl groups. Trypsin can be rather harsh and it has been demonstrated that it destroys membrane-bound immunoglobulins [15]. Despite this it has been used successfully for the dissociation of solid tumours. Its action is inhibited by the presence of serum. Pronase has a broad substrate specificity and results in higher yields of viable cells than either collagenase or trypsin. Hyaluronidase degrades hyaluronic acid, which is a constituent of the extracellular matrix. DNase has also been used in many enzyme cocktails to clear the viscous DNA released from damaged cells which can cause clumping problems. Aggregation of nuclei and cells is a major problem associated with the preparation of samples for flow cytometric analysis. Possible remedies include minimal centrifugation, low cell or nuclei density, the slow addition of diluents to the pellets while they are being vortexed and the addition of 10% serum to the suspensions.

During disaggregation it is advisable to expose the cells to the enzyme for the shortest possible period of time. This can be achieved using serial disaggregation which employs multiple but short incubations in the harmful enzyme solutions. After each disaggregation period the released cells are withdrawn from the enzyme solution and fresh enzyme solution is added to the remaining tissue. As previously, this not only maximizes overall cell yield but also minimizes subpopulation-specific selection and cell damage [5].

9.4 MECHANICAL DISAGGREGATION

Mechanical procedures involve the passage of homogenized or ground tissue through sieves or meshes, triturating with fine- or wide-bore pipettes or needles to tease cells from fragments of tissue or releasing cells from the cut surface of tumour samples with a glass slide held at an angle of 45°. These procedures are most successful on tissues without well-developed desmosomes, e.g., bladder, breast and colon [16].

9.4.1 FNA

FNA has been successfully used to obtain cells from lymphomas and solid tumours [17]. One of the advantages of FNA is that aggregates of tumour cells as well as glandular and other epithelial structures are more friable than supporting stroma and are therefore selectively sampled during FNA procedures. Additionally, FNA allows immediate access to viable tumour cells in suspension and reduces the effects of heterogeneity because of the ability to sample multiple areas.

9.4.2 Chelating agents

The divalent ions Ca^{2+} and Mg^{2+} are involved in cellular adhesion and help to maintain the integrity of cell surfaces. Therefore tissue dissociation can be enhanced either by the complexing of these ions using chelating agents, e.g., ethylenediaminetetraacetic acid (EDTA) and citrate or by omitting these ions from the media. Unfortunately, because most of the cellular calcium and magnesium ions are located in the mitochondria, prolonged exposure to chelating agents will affect metabolism.

9.5 CONCLUSION

Few authors include data on the evaluation of the cell/nuclear suspensions which form the basis of their investigations, although the importance of tissue disaggregation is well-documented [14,16]. Scientific advances in the fields of tissue culture and flow cytometry cannot be fully realized unless there is renewed interest and development in the art of tissue disaggregation.

References

1 Bashor MM. Dispersion and disruption of tissues. In: Jakoby WB, Pasten IH (eds) *Methods in Enzymology*, vol. 58. New York: Academic, 1979: 119–129.

2 Ensley JF, Maciorowski Z, Pietraszkieicz H *et al.* Solid tumour preparation for flow cytometry using a standard murine model. *Cytometry* 1987; 8: 479–487.

3 Vindelov LL. Christensen IJ. Review of techniques and results obtained in one laboratory by an integrated system of methods designed for routine clinical flow cytometric DNA analysis. *Cytometry* 1990; 11: 753–770.

4 Ota DM, Drewinko B. Growth kinetics of human colorectal carcinoma. *Cancer Res* 1985; 45: 2128–2131.

5 Pallavicini MG. Solid tissue dispersal for cytokinetic analysis. In: Gray JW, Darzynkiewicz Z (eds). *Techniques for Analysis of Cell Proliferation.* New Jersey: Humana Press, 1986; 139–162.

6 Waymouth C. To disaggregate or not to disaggregate. Injury and cell disaggregation, transient or permanent? *In Vitro* 1974; 10: 97–111.

7 Thornthwaite JT, Sugarbaker EV, Temple WJ. Preparation of tissues for DNA flow cytometric analysis. *Cytometry* 1980; 1: 229–237.

8 Vindelov LL, Christensen IJ, Nissen NI. A detergent-trypsin method for the preparation of nuclei for flow cytometric DNA analysis. *Cytometry* 1983; 3: 323–327.

9 Hedley DW, Friedlander ML, Taylor IW, Rugg CA, Musgrove EA. Method for analysis of cellular DNA content of paraffin-embedded pathological material using flow cytometry. *J Histochem Cytochem* 1983; 31: 1333–1335.

10 Schutte B, Reynders MMJ, Bosman FT, Blijham GH. Flow cytometric determination of DNA ploidy level in nuclei isolated from paraffin-embedded tissue. *Cytometry* 1985; 6: 26–30.

11 Engelholm, SA, Spang-Thomsen M, Brunner N, Nohr I, Vindelov LL. Disaggregation of human solid tumours by combined mechanical and enzymatic methods. *Br J Cancer* 1985; 51: 93–98.

12 Hood DL, Petras RE, Edinger M, Fazio V, Tubbs RR. Deoxyribonucleic acid ploidy and cell cycle analysis of colorectal carcinoma by flow cytometry. A prospective study of 137 cases using fresh whole cell suspensions. *Am J Clin Pathol* 1990; 93: 615–620.

13 Williamson K, Halliday I, Hamilton P *et al. In vitro* BrdUrd incorporation of colorectal tumour tissue, *Cell Prolif* 1993; 26: 115–124.

14 Waymouth C. Methods for obtaining cells in suspension from animal tissues. In: Pretlow TG II, Pretlow TP (eds) *Cell Separation: Methods and Applications*, vol. 6. New York: Academic Press, 1982: 1–30.

15 Russell SW, Doe WF, Hoskins RG, Cochrane CG. Inflammatory cells in solid murine neoplasms. I. Tumour disaggregation and identification of constituent inflammatory cells. *Int J Cancer* 1976; 18: 322–330.

16 Brattain M. Tissue disaggregation. In: Melamed MR, Mullaney P, Mendelsohn ML (eds) *Flow Cytometry and Sorting*. New York: Wiley, 1979: 193–203.

17 Vindelov L. Flow cytometric analysis of nuclear DNA in cells from solid tumors and cell suspensions. *Virchows Arch B Cell Pathol* 1977; 24: 227–242.

10

DNA PLOIDY ANALYSIS BY FLOW CYTOMETRY

J. C. MACARTNEY AND R. S. CAMPLEJOHN

10.1 INTRODUCTION

During the last 10 years there has been an explosive increase in the number of studies of human cancer using the technique of DNA flow cytometry (DNA FCM). This has been due in large measure to Hedley's discovery that pathological material processed for histological examination can also be used for FCM [1]. Prior to this, workers relied on fresh tissue which limited the rate of acquisition of new cases, and many of these series consist of mixtures of solid tumours, lymphomas and leukaemias [2]. Nevertheless, they quickly validated the results obtained using static cytophotometry (see Chapter 6). Although a number of important early publications deal with the DNA FCM of a single tumour type, Hedley's method opened the way to examination of large series of tumours which, hopefully, were well-characterized clinically and pathologically.

DNA FCM measures the DNA ploidy of tissues. This is the amount of DNA in cells which are in the G_1/G_0 phase of the cell cycle. Normal cells usually have a diploid DNA content but may rarely be polyploid (i.e., have direct multiples of the normal diploid DNA content, as in adult liver). Cells which contain irregular amounts of DNA are said to be aneuploid. Cells with less than the DNA diploid content are termed hypodiploid, which is generally a relatively infrequent finding in tumours. Conversely, hyperdiploid cells contain more than the diploid DNA content and the degree of abnormality can be specified as a DNA index (DI) relative to the normal DI of 1.0 in diploid cells, e.g., triploid cells have a DI of 1.5, tetraploid cells have a DI of 2.0. DNA FCM can also be used to estimate the proportion of cells synthesizing DNA, the S-phase fraction or SPF, which is often used as a measure of proliferative activity. Light scatter and volume can be measured and the method can be combined with immunofluorescent detection of antigens in multiparameter studies. Figures 10.1 and 10.2 show examples of single-parameter DNA plots of the type to be expected from a normal population of cells with a diploid DNA content (Fig. 10.1) and a mixed population of cells with both diploid and aneuploid DNA contents (Fig. 10.2).

Most studies using DNA FCM have one or more of the following three aims: (i) to assess whether DNA aneuploidy is diagnostic of malignancy; (ii) to relate DNA abnormalities and SPF to histopathological findings such as tumour type and grade; and (iii) to determine the prognostic effect of ploidy and SPF. In a minority of studies DNA FCM findings are used to test the hypothesis that DNA aneuploidy causes tumour progression as opposed to being merely a result of progression. There have been a number of useful recent reviews on these and other aspects of DNA FCM, such as the technical and theoretical background [3–10]. In this chapter we concentrate on the relationship between tumour pathology and prognosis and the results of DNA FCM. In order to avoid needless repetition we use the terms aneuploidy, diploidy, FCM, etc., interchangeably with the preferred terminology – DNA aneuploidy, DNA diploidy, DNA FCM [11].

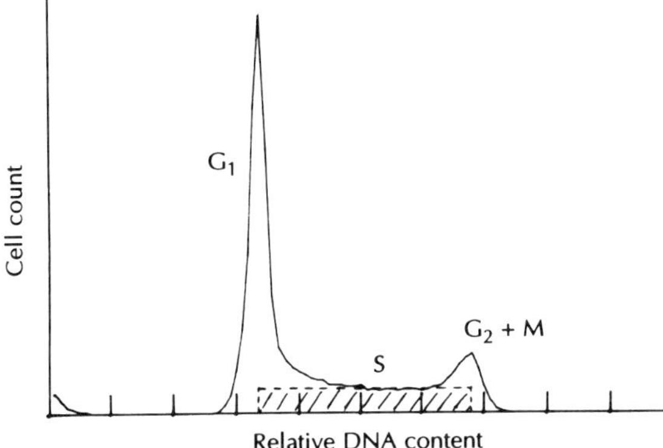

Fig. 10.1 A DNA flow cytometry tracing for a population of cells with a normal diploid DNA content. The shaded area represents the proportion of cells in the S phase of the cell cycle. The G_1 peak corresponds to cells in the G_0/G_1 phase of the cell cycle and the $G_2 + M$ peak corresponds to cells in the G_2 and mitotic phases of the cell cycle. The size of the peaks is proportional to the number of cells in each phase of the cycle.

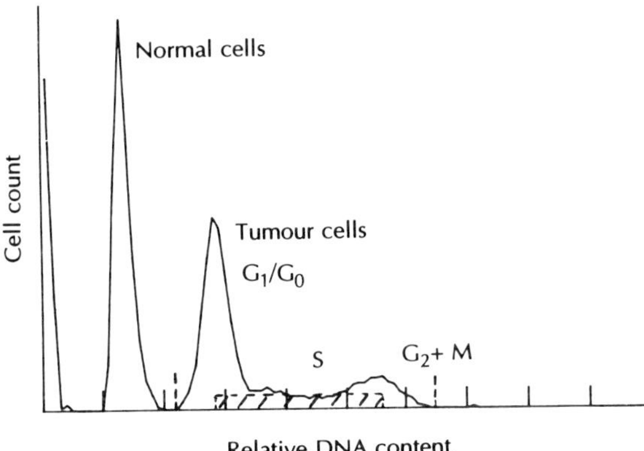

Fig. 10.2 A DNA flow cytometry profile from a mixed population of normal and tumour cells. The G_1/G_0 peak for the tumour cells is shifted to the right, i.e., it is hyperdiploid with respect to normal cells in G_1/G_0. The shaded area corresponds to the proportion of tumour cells in the S phase of the cell cycle.

10.2 TECHNICAL ASPECTS

Detailed technical aspects are considered in Chapters 9 and 10 and in a number of recent reviews [3,4,6]. However, certain facts need to be emphasized as they affect the interpretation of individual flow cytometric analyses and the conclusions drawn from clinical series. First, criteria used to identify aneuploidy are not uniform. A particular problem is the identification of an aneuploid peak close to the normal diploid DNA peak. In part this represents a limitation of FCM. If the peaks are very close they may merge to give a broader peak with a high coefficient of variation. For this reason many workers interpret wide G_1/G_0 peaks as representing aneuploidy. This has been confirmed using image cytometry, which is more sensitive to minimal abnormalities [12]. However, readers should be aware that it is also possible to obtain wide G_1/G_0 peaks for a number of other reasons, including poor technique and inadequate staining of cells with the fluorescent DNA-binding dye. In a situation where the true result is unknown without confirmation by an independent technique, we do not feel that it is possible to make a confident diagnosis of aneuploidy from the existence of a wide G_1 peak [5].

There are also some problems associated with measurement and interpretation of SPF values. Authors vary as to whether they measure the SPF or $S + G_2/M$ fraction. The latter give higher values. Moreover, there is conflict as to the correct approach to measuring SPF in aneuploid tumours. It is quite clear from the literature that, even though workers claim to be using a standard technique to measure SPF, in fact their results may differ markedly, suggesting that there are unidentified biasing factors at work. This can be clearly seen in certain published lymphoma series where there is no clear evidence that case selection is the confounding variable. Finally, it should be recognized that the SPF is a static index rather like the mitotic index. Although a high SPF is usually associated with high proliferative activity, it must be recognized that it is only a crude guide and gives no detailed information on flux rate of cells around the cell cycle [13]. Indeed it should not be assumed that tumours are necessarily more 'proliferative' than normal tissues [14].

10.3 DNA FCM OF TUMOURS

10.3.1 Gastrointestinal tract

Gastric cancer

In advanced gastric cancer aneuploidy is present in at least one-half to three-quarters of cases [15–21]. In some series it is more frequently associated with intestinal-type differentiation in tumours [15,18] and there is frequently marked heterogeneity of ploidy [22]. Values for SPF are generally reported to be higher in the DNA aneuploid cases. This has been most convincingly demonstrated in a multiparameter study where bromodeoxyuridine uptake in aneuploid cells has been quantified by FCM [21]. In early gastric cancer and dysplasia of the gastric mucosa the proportion of aneuploid cases is lower [17,18,23] and a progressive increase in the SPF has been reported in the transition between normal gastric mucosa, gastritis, early gastric cancer and advanced gastric cancer [23].

There are relatively few studies on the prognostic significance of aneuploidy in gastric cancer. In some series it had no effect on survival [16,20]. In others aneuploidy and a high SPF were adverse prognostic factors [21], although this effect may be much weaker than conventional prognostic variables such as stage and resection margin involvement [18,19]. Currently, therefore, there is some evidence that ploidy status has a weak effect on the prognosis of advanced gastric cancer.

Colorectal carcinoma and adenomas

A thorough overview of the results of DNA FCM in colorectal cancer [24] includes many of the older published series. DNA aneuploidy occurs in approximately two-thirds of colorectal cancers; multiple aneuploid cell lines were found in around one-third of cases. The occurrence of aneuploidy has been reported to be associated with poor histological differentiation and with vascular invasion (reviewed in [24–29]). In general, aneuploid tumours have higher SPF values [29].

The relationship between Dukes' stage and ploidy status has been a vexed question. An early series claimed that aneuploidy was a more frequent finding in Dukes' stage C carcinomas compared with Dukes' A cases [30] and this has been observed in several more recent series [24], although it is not a universal finding [31]. Crissman *et al.* [24] conclude that aneuploidy occurs in 30–60% of Dukes' stage A and B cases polled from published series, as compared with 70–75% of Dukes' stage C. The variation depends in part on whether prospective or retrospective surveys are used.

There is also evidence that the frequency and degree of aneuploidy increase in the transition from mild dysplasia to invasive colorectal cancer [32]. In unselected series of colorectal adenomas the incidence of aneuploidy is around 12%, although there is considerable variation in different series [33–36] and there is a positive correlation between the finding of aneuploidy and the diameter and degree of dysplasia of the polyp. An increased incidence of aneuploidy has also been demonstrated in adenomas from patients with a strong family history of carcinomas, implying that it is a marker of increased risk [37]. However, the series is small and biased by the inclusion of polyps which show invasive tumour. Moreover, none of this evidence proves that aneuploidy *causes* tumour progression, as implied by some authors. There are also inconsistencies in the evidence. In familial polyposis where the risk of cancer rises with age, the incidence of aneuploidy did not rise, as might be predicted [38]. Furthermore, there is stability of ploidy between primary and metastatic colorectal cancer [39] and, where they differ, this is probably the result of inadequate sampling of the primary [40].

The existence of ploidy heterogeneity within tumours is of considerable importance when assessing the relationship between aneuploidy stage, tumour progression and prognosis. In one early study the heterogeneity of colorectal cancer was emphasized [41]. However, in a study designed to assess the problem of ploidy heterogeneity [42], 63% of colorectal carcinomas were homogeneous with respect to DNA ploidy and only minimal heterogeneity was found in a further 23%. If a full-thickness slice across the tumour was analysed, 79% of tumours showed no evidence of heterogeneity. Jass *et al.* [40] examined the stability of ploidy between primary site and metastases and concluded that in the 25% of cases where there were differences, this was due to inadequate sampling of the primary. Taken together, these findings suggest that it would be wise to sample two sites in the primary tumour but it is probably unnecessary to examine more than this number.

Dukes' stage of colorectal cancer and the presence of vascular invasion are important prognostic factors [43]. In view of the positive correlation between these factors and the occurrence of aneuploidy, it is hardly surprising that patients with aneuploid carcinomas have a worse overall survival than those with diploid tumours. However, in some series this does not achieve significance [44] and in nearly all series where multivariate analysis is used to compare the relative prognostic importance of aneuploidy with other factors, it is less important than stage [25,45–48]. A high SPF has also been claimed to be an adverse prognostic factor but confirmatory studies are required [49].

The major problems associated with assessing claims of a prognostic role for DNA FCM were clearly delineated by Crissman *et al.* in their review [24]. Particular difficulties were caused by biased survival curves and biased distributions of tumour stage and location in the FCM studies as compared with large clinicopathological series. To this list can be added other confounding factors such as small case numbers with inadequate or absent follow-up, inadequate sampling to account for tumour heterogeneity, and confusion between the curability and operability of colorectal cancer. Currently, there does not appear to be a convincing case that DNA FCM provides more significant prognostic data than conventional clinicopathological assessment.

Premalignancy in ulcerative colitis

The incidence of colorectal carcinoma is increased in long-standing ulcerative colitis and is often associated with the development of colorectal mucosal dysplasia. There are a number of reports based on retrospective series where DNA FCM has been used as an adjunct to the histological detection of dysplasia in order to identify patients at risk [50–54]. Aneuploidy is found in 10–12% of mucosal samples and may be associated with high-grade dysplasia. However, there are problems in making use of this finding. First, the frequency of aneuploidy is low and there is therefore a high false-negative rate. Second, in all the series, DNA aneuploidy is encountered in non-dysplastic mucosa in patients without evidence of carcinoma. The explanation of this finding is uncertain but it may be linked with reports of aneuploidy in histologically normal colorectal mucosa from sites peripheral to coincident colorectal cancer [55]. The claim that FCM is useful for the screen detection of cancer in ulcerative colitis should be viewed with caution in the light of the high incidence of false-positives and false-negatives and the absence of prospective studies. Indeed, the cost-effectiveness of cancer screening in this condition has been questioned [56].

Other gastrointestinal disease

Aneuploidy has been reported in the dysplasia associated with Crohn's colitis [57], Barrett's oesophagus [58], oesophageal carcinoma [59], gastric lymphomas [60], carcinoid tumours [61], gastrointestinal smooth-muscle and related tumours [62] and hepatocellular carcinoma [63]. In some of these series it is also claimed to be an adverse prognostic factor but further work is required to verify these findings.

10.3.2 Breast cancer

A large number of the earlier flow cytometric studies of breast cancer were restricted to looking at DNA ploidy, and many only investigated the association between flow cytometric parameters and other pretreatment variables, not survival. These studies are considered very briefly, mainly by reference to a comprehensive review article by Merkel and McGuire [64]. Most space in this section will be given to studies in which DNA ploidy and SPF are related to long-term survival.

DNA aneuploidy has been found in most studies to be more common in high-grade tumours. The correlation of ploidy with other clinicopathological variables is less certain. Some groups report an association between the frequency of DNA aneuploidy and tumour size, while other groups did not find this and a similar story is to be found with nodal status and DNA ploidy [64]. The relationship between steroid receptor status and DNA ploidy is also uncertain. Merkel and McGuire [64] found 11 studies involving 2553 patients in which DNA aneuploidy occurred more commonly in oestrogen receptor-negative tumours and six studies involving 752 patients in which no relationship or a non-significant trend was found. Our studies [65] would fit into this second group. The impression from reviewing the literature is that many of these parameters may be inter-related but that the correlations are weak.

As regards SPF, there is little evidence that it correlates with tumour size or nodal involvement but many studies find a correlation with steroid receptor status. SPF does correlate — usually strongly — with tumour grade in all studies in which this association was investigated. Interestingly, a recent study [66] found that in breast cancer patients who had taken oral contraceptives from an early age (< 20 years), a higher incidence of aneuploid and high SPF tumours was seen.

There is some disagreement in the literature as to whether DNA ploidy is predictive for survival and whether any prognostic power is independent of other clinicopathological factors. Many of the earlier studies are reviewed by Merkel and McGuire [64]. In node-negative disease a number of recent reports illustrate the disagreement. Four studies failed to find any significant association between ploidy and survival in node-negative patients [67–70]. Whereas Toikkanen *et al.* [71] found an association between patients with DI > or < 1.2 and survival on univariate analysis, this predictive ability was lost on multivariate analysis. In contrast, Clark *et al.* [72] found that DNA ploidy was predictive for relapse-free survival even in a multivariate analysis, although tumour grade was not a factor included in this analysis. A similar lack of agreement exists concerning the relationship between DNA ploidy and survival in node-positive disease, with some studies finding no association, others an association on univariate analysis only and some a statistically independent relationship [64,65,67,73]. In summary, it would seem that many studies find, at least on univariate analysis, an association between DNA ploidy and survival but that if a multivariate analysis, which includes tumour grade, is performed this predictive power is in most cases lost.

In the past 5 years more studies have looked at SPF as well as DNA ploidy. In both node-negative and node-positive patients, tumour SPF was found in virtually all published studies to correlate — usually strongly — with survival [64–66,70–76]. There are, however, disagreements as to whether SPF has independent prognostic significance, particularly if tumour grade is included in the multivariate analysis. At least one study has found SPF to be of independent value in a multivariate analysis, including grade [73]. A number of other studies have reported it to be of independent prognostic value when other clinicopathological parameters such as steroid receptor status, tumour size, age, etc., were included but not tumour grade [65,68,70,72,74,75]. In general, it seems that SPF is a stronger prognostic indicator than DNA ploidy in breast cancer. Further, SPF may be of real value in patient management. For example, in node-negative disease the consistent finding of a strong correlation of SPF with subsequent recurrence [68,70,73] suggests that this parameter may be of value in selecting which patients are suitable for adjuvant chemotherapy. This would help identify high-risk patients for whom adjuvant chemotherapy would be appropriate, and equally importantly, would avoid low-risk patients being given unnecessary toxic therapy. An example of how risk might be assessed is given in Fig. 10.3; in this case (data from O'Reilly *et al.* [68]) a combination of SPF and tumour size was found to give the best discrimination of prognostic groups.

The value of flow cytometric measurements in breast cancer may be improved by including other parameters. In many recent studies investigators have measured light scatter or volume to improve discrimination in the analysis of DNA results [6]. However, the addition of further parameters may yield still more information. Staining of tumour samples with antibodies to cytokeratins can help avoid contamination of histograms with both debris and non-epithelial cells [77]. Many other potentially useful parameters may be measured flow cytometrically at the same time as DNA, for example steroid receptors [78].

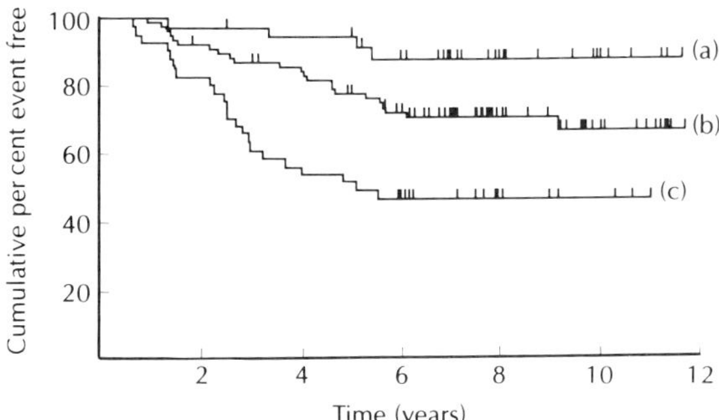

Fig. 10.3 Relapse-free survival for node-negative breast cancer patients: (a) tumours < 1.0 cm; (b) tumours > 1.0 cm + low S-phase fraction (SPF); (c) tumours > 1.0 cm + high SPF. Data from O'Reilly *et al.* [68].

10.3.3 Male genital and urinary systems

The natural history of prostatic carcinoma is strongly dependent on the stage and histological grade of the tumour [79]. Nevertheless, particularly in the moderately differentiated group of tumours, the behaviour of individual tumours is unpredictable. DNA FCM has, therefore, been used with the aim of identifying tumours which have a more aggressive potential and might be treated more vigorously. Well-differentiated prostatic cancers tend to be DNA diploid, whereas poorly differentiated cancers tend to be aneuploid and tumours of intermediate grade show variable ploidy status, although this distinction has become blurred in some more recent series [80–83]. Tetraploidy is relatively frequent in prostatic cancer and may be linked with an intrinsic tendency to tetraploidy in non-neoplastic prostatic tissue [80]. Despite the strong correlation between grade and ploidy status, the use of DNA FCM as an alternative to histological grading is not justified because of the high incidence of false-negatives [84,85].

There are a number of series where a significant survival advantage for diploid prostatic cancers has been demonstrated [86–88], although some series may be biased as they fail to find that histological grade is a prognostic factor [87]. However, before accepting that DNA FCM has a role in the management of prostatic cancer, it should be noted that there are major contrasts in the treatment of prostatic cancer in different centres which might account for discrepant results. In a series from the UK, Ritchie *et al.* [89] failed to find that ploidy was a significant factor in prognosis using multivariate analysis. In contrast, in a series of publications from the Mayo Clinic on uniformly staged and treated patients, aneuploidy was an important prognostic factor [90–92].

There have been relatively few DNA FCM studies of testicular cancers. They show a high incidence of DNA aneuploidy and high SPF, and the DI of teratomas is higher than seminomas [93,94]. SPF values are reported to correlate with prognosis in advanced germ-cell tumours [95] but paradoxically high SPF values are found in good-prognosis spermatocytic seminomas [96]. DNA FCM has not only been used to detect aneuploidy in aspirates from the contralateral testis in association with carcinoma *in situ* and following a previous orchidectomy for cancer [97], but also in the undescended testis in the absence of tumour [98].

Transitional-cell carcinoma of the bladder is a common tumour for which a large number of clinical and pathological prognostic factors have been identified [99]. The natural history of this tumour depends crucially on whether it is invasive or superficial and also on histological differentiation. DNA FCM shows that the incidence of DNA aneuploidy is higher in invasive carcinomas of stage T_3 and T_4 and in poorly differentiated tumours [100,101]. Because of these associations, patients with DNA aneuploid tumours have a worse prognosis in terms of survival [102] or response to intravesical therapy [103]. Early claims may have been overstated as there is also evidence that the prognostic effect only operates in superficial bladder cancer [104] or in more advanced tumours showing tetraploidy [105] and a recent series showed no difference in the survival of aneuploid and diploid groups of tumour [106] although SPF is higher in aneuploid and high-grade tumours [107]. FCM has also been used with considerable success in the screen detection of urinary bladder cancer [108,109] and for monitoring treatment [103].

Small series of squamous and adenocarcinomas of the bladder have been published. Primary renal carcinoma exhibited heterogeneous ploidy patterns with no reported link with stage or effect on prognosis [110,111].

10.3.4 Female genital tract

Common ovarian cancers show a wide range of appearance and behaviour from relatively benign to highly aggressive carcinomas. Important prognostic factors include the International Federation of Obstetricians and Gynaecologists (FIGO) stage of the tumour and histopathological borderline malignancy. Early DNA flow cytometric studies showed that there is a clear relationship between the ploidy status of ovarian carcinomas and their clinical stage [112], and this has been confirmed in more recent series [113–119]. More advanced ovarian carcinomas show a higher incidence of aneuploidy, which is associated with reduced survival and higher histological grade. Borderline tumours are more likely to be diploid and their inclusion in flow cytometric series may therefore contribute significantly to the improved survival associated with diploid ovarian cancer.

In stage I and II ovarian cancer, well-differentiated tumours are more likely to be diploid and survival is better in this group [120] and it has been shown that a combination of ploidy status, mitotic index and morphometric estimates of tumour epithelial volume percentage is highly predictive of outcome [121]. In stages III and IV ovarian cancer a similar prognostic role for ploidy has been claimed [113–119,122]. However, small numbers of borderline tumours are included in some of these series, which may in theory have biased results [122]. Moreover if only stage IV tumours or advanced abdominal tumours are analysed, ploidy ceases to have a prognostic effect [122,123] and the role of ploidy appears to be less important than morphometric assessment in these very advanced tumours [124].

Small flow cytometric series of less common ovarian tumours have been published. Granulosa tumours have an unpredictable prognosis in a minority of cases but there are conflicting results on the usefulness of ploidy for predicting behaviour [125,126]. This may represent the effects of misdiagnosis, with the inclusion of high-grade undifferentiated tumours [127].

There have been repeated attempts to use FCM as an automated approach to screening cervical cytology specimens for evidence of premalignant changes. Despite the use of multiparameter cytometric approaches, these have not succeeded because of the high incidence of false-positive and false-negatives [128,129] and it is unlikely that FCM will find a role in cervical cytology screening because of technical limitations. Although early reports showed a positive association between the presence of aneuploidy and higher grades of cervical intraepithelial neoplasia (CIN), more recent studies have shown a high incidence in CIN I and the changes associated with human papillomavirus infection [130–132].

There is conflict between the results of flow cytometric studies of invasive squamous carcinoma of the cervix. Older studies showed that there was a link between the degree of DNA aneuploidy and overall survival and between SPF and tumour recurrence [133,134]. However, no effect of ploidy on survival was reported in more recent retrospective and prospective series [135,136]. This may reflect the effects of treatment and differences in the age structure of patients in various series since aneuploidy and SPF increase with age and after the menopause [137,138].

Endometrial carcinoma shows a much lower incidence of aneuploidy than other human solid tumours and there is agreement that the results of DNA FCM have prognostic value. Aneuploidy and a high SPF are associated with more poorly differentiated carcinoma, increasing age and postmenopausal hormone status [139–142]. They also carry a worse prognosis and there is evidence that inclusion of information on hormone receptor status improves the prognostic precision [143,144].

Apart from isolated series of cervical adenocarcinoma, uterine leiomyomas and sarcomas, and stromal tumours, probably the other most significant area of application for DNA FCM is in the investigation and diagnosis of molar pregnancies. FCM can be used to identify triploidy, which is found in a high percentage of partial moles and is associated with a benign clinical course [145,146]. However it is questionable whether triploidy should be equated with a diagnosis of partial mole since the incidence of triploidy is known to be high in early spontaneous abortions. More questionably, cytometric analysis has also been used to predict malignant transformation in hydatidiform moles [147].

10.3.5 Carcinoma of the lung and head and neck region

There have been several studies documenting a prognostic advantage for diploid carcinomas of the lung in series excluding small-cell carcinoma [148–151]. For individual histological subtypes there are similar findings with squamous-cell carcinoma [151], but results for adenocarcinoma are conflicting [148,152,153]. In small-cell carcinoma of the lung there is pronounced regional variation of ploidy status within tumours and there is no clear indication that ploidy has any effect on the natural history of these tumours. Similarly, DNA FCM does not appear to be useful in the assessment of potentially aggressive carcinoid tumours [154]. There are several reports that the finding of DNA aneuploidy is an adverse prognostic factor in head and neck cancer, which is associated with poorly differentiated squamous carcinoma [155,156].

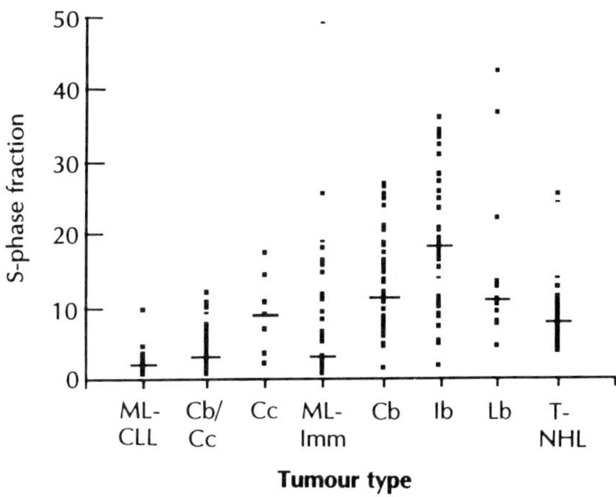

Fig. 10.4 S-phase fractions for 358 non-Hodgkin's lymphomas which have been classified using the Kiel classification. ML-CLL, malignant lymphoma lymphocytic; Cb/Cc, centroblastic/centrocytic, follicular; Cc, centrocytic; ML-lmm, lymphoplasmacytoid; Cb, centroblastic; Ib; immunoblastic; Lb, lymphoblastic; T-NHL, T-cell lymphoma.

10.3.6 Lymphomas

We have recently reviewed the results of DNA FCM of lymphomas in detail and only a résumé is given here [157,158]. DNA aneuploidy is more frequent and SPF values are higher in high-grade non-Hodgkin's lymphoma (NHL) compared with low-grade NHL. Because of the relatively frequent finding of DNA diploidy using single-parameter DNA FCM and the wide scatter of SPF (Fig. 10.4), NHL cannot be discriminated from reactive lymphoid tissue with certainty. With the exception of mycosis fungoides, B-cell NHL show a higher incidence of aneuploidy (30%) than T-cell NHL (13%). However, if multiparameter FCM is used, the frequency of aneuploidy in B-cell NHL rises to 80% [159], suggesting that the incidence of aneuploidy is underestimated in single-parameter studies. In Hodgkin's disease, single-parameter DNA FCM detects aneuploidy in a minority of cases (10%), but this figure is probably a considerable underestimate because of the lack of sensitivity in detecting relatively sparse numbers of Sternberg–Reed cells.

There is good evidence from four retrospective studies that SPF is a significant prognostic factor in low-grade follicle-centre cell NHL [160,161] whereas ploidy status is unimportant. Figure 10.5 shows the effect of SPF on the survival of follicular NHL. Results for high-grade NHL are more difficult to reconcile because of differences in treatment, type of NHL included in clinical series and data analysis [162–168] and there are contradictions between

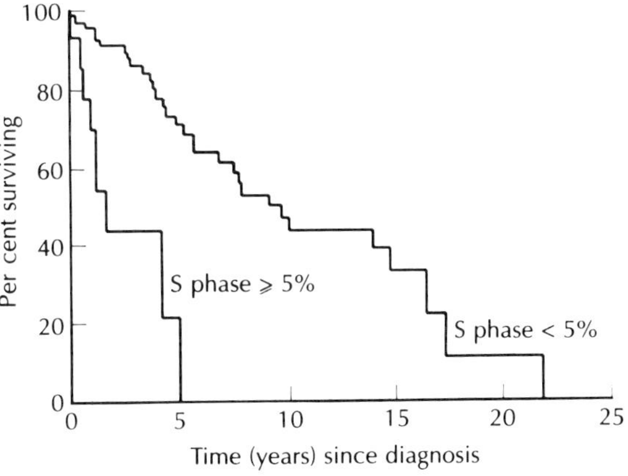

Fig. 10.5 Cumulative survival curves for follicular non-Hodgkin's lymphoma with S-phase fractions (SPF) below ($n = 67$) and above ($n = 16$) 5%. The survival of patients with tumours of higher SPF is significantly worse ($P < 0.01$).

the findings of some of these series. Although the overall impression is that a high SPF affects prognosis adversely in high-grade NHL, this cannot be regarded as proven.

10.3.7 Miscellaneous neoplasms

There are a huge number of DNA FCM studies of other types of tumour. Recently there has been a considerable number of small series of rather rare neoplasms published. In malignant melanoma both aneuploidy and high SPF have been claimed to be adverse prognostic findings [169], but there are more recent results disputing this claim [170]. Aneuploidy has also been reported in both benign and malignant melanocytic lesions [171]. In thyroid cancers aneuploidy is least common in papillary carcinoma and most frequent in undifferentiated carcinoma and has been correlated with aggressive behaviour [172–174]. However, DNA aneuploidy cannot be used to distinguish follicular adenomas from follicular carcinomas since aneuploidy occurs in both [175]. Similarly, it is doubtful whether DNA FCM can be used to discriminate parathyroid carcinoma from adenomas and hyperplasia, as has been claimed [176], since in other series aneuploidy was encountered in the benign conditions [177].

Aggressive behaviour has been correlated with the presence of aneuploidy and high SPF in gliomas, although non-aggressive meningiomas may also be aneuploid [178,179]. In soft-tissue tumours aneuploidy is associated with high-grade histology [180] and has been claimed to be of diagnostic and prognostic usefulness in bone tumours [181,182]. However, it does not predict aggressive behaviour in giant-cell tumours of bone [183]. Conflicting results of DNA FCM analysis have been reported in thymomas, which probably reflect different histological criteria for diagnosing thymic carcinoma [184,185]. No role for DNA FCM has been demonstrated in the clinical assessment of paragangliomas [186].

10.4 CONCLUSION

A characteristic finding of many of the DNA FCM studies reviewed above is the increasing frequency of DNA aneuploidy as tumours progress from premalignancy to widely invasive tumour. A number of authors imply that this progression is due directly to tumour-cell DNA aneuploidy. Although the facts are consistent with this hypothesis, many of the arguments are circular. These arguments also depend on the sensitivity of single-parameter DNA FCM to the presence of small numbers of DNA aneuploid cells which may show only minimal deviation from diploidy. It is well-known that under these conditions DNA FCM is not a very sensitive technique for detecting aneuploidy. DNA aneuploidy *can* be detected in these early neoplastic lesions if looked for more critically using a more sensitive technique and for this reason it would be unwise to assume that aneuploidy is causally linked with tumour progression.

DNA aneuploidy is sometimes also equated with a diagnosis of malignancy but the evidence does not support this conclusion, e.g., meningiomas, benign melanocytic lesions, ulcerative colitis, etc. The existence of substantial numbers of DNA diploid solid tumours is bound to cause a high false-negative rate if aneuploidy is used as the criterion for diagnosis of a tumour. For these reasons the use of single-parameter DNA FCM as a diagnostic procedure without independent histological confirmation is doomed to failure.

Many earlier DNA FCM reports enthusiastically claimed an important prognostic role for the technique in evaluating tumour behaviour. In general DNA aneuploid tumours and tumours with a high SPF show poorer survival than diploid, low-SPF tumours. Unfortunately much of the published work is of doubtful significance because of a failure to take account of other important prognostic factors. When this is done, in many cases, aneuploidy appears to be a bad prognostic indicator only because it is linked with other indicators of poor prognosis. In contrast, in childhood neuroblastoma and medulloblastoma, the presence of aneuploidy confers a survival advantage [187,188]. Despite this serious criticism of much of the published work, there is good evidence that DNA FCM has an important role in the assessment of breast cancer, ovarian and endometrial cancer and NHL; and a more questionable role in bladder and prostatic cancer. With increased understanding of the effects of other prognostic factors, treatment protocols and tissue-sampling strategies, and a better understanding of the limitations of cytometry, there is no reason why DNA FCM cannot continue to give valuable insights into the biological behaviour of cancers. In our opinion the speed and consistency of DNA FCM will outweigh its disadvantages and there is now a need to re-examine cytometric findings in the more common human solid tumours.

Acknowledgement

We are extremely grateful to Annette Shaw for the help she has given in preparing and typing this chapter.

References

1 Hedley DW, Friedlander ML, Taylor IW, Rugg CA, Musgrove EA. Method for analysis of cellular DNA content of paraffin-embedded pathological material using flow cytometry. *J Histochem Cytochem* 1983; 31: 1333–1335.

2 Barlogie B, Drewinko B, Schumann J *et al.* Cellular DNA content as a marker of neoplasia in man. *Am J Med* 1980, 69: 195–203.

3 Melamed MR, Lindmo T, Mendelsohn ML (eds) *Flow Cytometry and Sorting*, 2nd edn. New York: Wiley–Liss, 1990.

4 Ormerod MG. *Flow Cytometry. A Practical Approach.* Oxford: IRL Press, 1990.

5 Camplejohn RS, Macartney JC. Flow cytometry. In: Hall PA, Levison DA, Wright NA. *Assessment of Cell Proliferation in Clinical Diagnosis.* Springer Verlag, 1991: 95–111.

6 Camplejohn RS. Flow cytometry in clinical pathology. In: Herrington CS, McGee JOD (eds) *Diagnostic Molecular Pathology.* Oxford: IRL Press, 1992.

7 Frankfurt OS, Slocum HK, Rustum YM *et al.* Flow cytometric analysis of DNA aneuploidy in primary and metastatic human solid tumors. *Cytometry* 1984; 5: 71–80.

8 Friedlander ML, Hedley DW, Taylor IW. Clinical and biological significance of aneuploidy in human tumours. *J Clin Pathol* 1984; 37: 961–974.

9 Merkel DE, Dressler LG, McGuire WL. Flow cytometry, cellular DNA content, and prognosis in human malignancy. *J Clin Oncol* 1987; 5: 1690–1703.

10 Hedley DW. Flow cytometry using paraffin-embedded tissue: five years on. *Cytometry* 1989; 10: 229–241.

11 Hiddeman W, Schumann J, Andreeff M *et al.* Convention on nomenclature for DNA cytometry. *Cytometry* 1984; 5: 445–446.

12 McFadden PW, Clowry LJ, Daehnert K, Hause LL, Koehe SM. Image analysis confirmation of DNA aneuploidy in flow cytometric DNA distributions having a wide coefficient of variation of the G_0/G_1 peak. *Am J Clin Pathol* 1990; 93: 637–642.

13 Wright N, Alison M (eds) Chapter 3. In: *The Biology of Epithelial Cell Population'*, vol. 1. Oxford: Clarendon Press, 1984: 97–282.

14 Steel GG. *Growth Kinetics of Tumours.* Oxford: Clarendon Press, 1977.

15 Macartney JC, Camplejohn RS, Powell G. DNA flow cytometry of histological material from human gastric cancer. *J Pathol* 1986; 148: 273–277.

16 Ballantyne KC, James PD, Robins RA, Baldwin RW, Hardcastle JD. Flow cytometric analysis of the DNA content of gastric cancer. *Br J Cancer* 1987; 56: 52–54.

17 Sowa M, Yoshino H, Kato Y, Nishimura M, Kamino K, Umeyama K. An analysis of the DNA ploidy patterns of gastric cancer. *Cancer* 1988; 62: 1325–1330.

18 Tosi P, Leoncini L, Cintorino M *et al.* Flow cytometric analysis of DNA ploidy patterns from deparaffinised formalin-fixed gastric cancer tissue. *Int J Cancer* 1988; 42: 868–871.

19 Wyatt JI, Quirke P, Ward DC *et al.* Comparison of histopathological and flow cytometric parameters in prediction of prognosis in gastric cancer. *J Pathol* 1989; 158: 195–210.

20 Kimura H, Yonemura Y. Flow cytometric analysis of nuclear DNA content in advanced gastric cancer and its relationship with prognosis. *Cancer* 1989; 67: 2588–2593.

21 Ohyama S, Yonemura Y, Miyazaki I. Flow cytometric cell cycle analysis using a monoclonal antibody to bromodeoxuridine on gastric cancers. *J Jpn Surg Soc* 1989; 90: 1848–1854.

22 de Aretxabala X, Yonemura Y, Sugiyama K *et al.* Gastric cancer heterogeneity. *Cancer* 1989; 63: 791–798.

23 Macartney JC, Camplejohn RS. DNA flow cytometry of histological material from dysplastic lesions of human gastric mucosa. *J Pathol* 1986; 150: 113–118.

24 Crissman JD, Zarbo RJ, Chan KM, Visscher DW. Histopathologic parameters and DNA analysis in colorectal adenocarcinoma. *Pathol Annu* 1989; 24 (part 2): 103–147.

25 Giaretti W, Danova M, Geido E *et al.* Flow cytometric DNA index in the prognosis of colorectal cancer. *Cancer* 1991; 67: 1921–1927.

26 Kouri M, Pyrhonen S, Mecklin JP *et al.* The prognostic value of DNA ploidy in colorectal carcinoma: a prospective study. *Br J Cancer* 1991; 62: 976–981.

27 Emdin SO, Stenling R, Roos G. Prognostic value of DNA content in colorectal carcinoma. A flow cytometic study with some methodologic aspects. *Cancer* 1987; 60: 1282–1287.

28 Scivetti P, Danova M, Riccardi A, Fiocca R, Dionigi

P, Mazzini G. Prognostic significance of DNA content in large bowel carcinoma: a retrospective flow cytometric study. *Cancer Lett* 1989; 46: 213–219.
29 Hood DL, Petras RE, Edinger M, Fazio V, Tubbs RR. Deoxyribonucleic acid ploidy and cell cycle analysis of colorectal carcinomas. A prospective study of 137 cases using fresh whole cell suspensions. *Am J Clin Pathol* 1990; 93: 615–620.
30 Wolley RC, Schreiber K, Koss LG, Karas LG, Sherman A. DNA distribution in human colon carcinomas and its relationship to clinical behaviour. *J Nat Cancer Inst* 1982; 69: 15–22.
31 Melamed MR, Enker WE, Banner P, Janov AJ, Kessler G, Darzynkiewicz Z. Flow cytometry of colorectal carcinoma with 3 year follow-up. *Dis Colon Rectum* 1986; 29: 184–186.
32 Giaretti W, Santi L. Tumor progression by FDN flow cytometry in human colorectal cancer. *Int J Cancer* 1990; 45: 597–603.
33 Goh HS, Jass JR. DNA content and the adenoma–carcinoma sequence in the colorectum. *J Clin Pathol* 1986; 39: 387–392.
34 Quirke P, Fozard JB, Dixon ME, Dyson JE, Giles GR, Bird CC. DNA aneuploidy in colorectal adenomas. *Br J Cancer* 1986; 53: 477–481.
35 Giaretti W, Sciallero S, Bruno S, Geido E, Aste H, Di Vinci A. DNA flow cytometry of endoscopically examined colorectal adenomas and adenocarcinomas. *Cytometry* 1988; 9: 238–244.
36 Scott NA, Weiland LH, Dozois RR, Beart RW, Lieber MM. DNA aneuploidy in solitary colonic adenomas and the future risk of colorectal cancer. *Dis Colon Rectum* 1988; 31: 423–425.
37 Sciallero S, Bruno S, Di Vinci A, Geido E, Aste H, Giarette W. Flow cytometric DNA ploidy in colorectal adenoma and family history of colorectal cancer. *Cancer* 1988; 61: 114–120.
38 Quirke P, Dixon MF, Day DW, Fozard JB, Talbot I, Bird CC. DNA aneuploidy and cell proliferation in familial adenomatous polyposis. *Gut* 1988; 29: 602–607.
39 Tsushima K, Nagorney DM, Rainwater LM *et al.* Prognostic significance of nuclear deoxyribonucleic acid ploidy patterns in resected hepatic metastases from colorectal cancer. *Surgery* 1987; 102: 635–643.
40 Jass JR, Mukawa K, Richman PI, Hall PA. Do aggressive subclones with primary colorectal cancer give rise to liver metastases? *Int J Colorectal Dis* 1989; 4: 109–117.
41 Quirke P, Dyson JE, Dixon MF, Bird CC, Joslin CA. Heterogeneity of colorectal adenocarcinomas evaluated by flow cytometry and histopathology. *Br J Cancer* 1985; 51: 99–106.
42 Scott NA, Grande JP, Weiland LH, Pemberton JH, Beart RW, Liber MM. Flow cytometric DNA patterns from colorectal cancers — how reproducible are they? *Mayo Clin Proc* 1987; 62: 331–337.
43 Jass JR, Love SB, Northover JMA. A new prognostic classification of rectal cancer. *Lancet* 1987; 1: 1303–1306.
44 Rognum TO, Thorud E, Ludn E. Survival of large bowel carcinoma patients with different DNA ploidy. *Br J Cancer* 1987; 56: 633–636.
45 Goh HS, Jass JR, Atkin WS, Cuzick J, Northover JM. Value of flow cytometric determination of ploidy as a guide to prognosis in operable rectal cancer: a multivariate analysis. *Int J Colorectal Dis* 1987; 2: 17–21.
46 Jones DJ, Moore M, Schofield PF. Prognostic significance of DNA ploidy in colorectal cancer: a prospective flow cytometric study. *Br J Surg* 1988; 75: 28–33.
47 Wiggers T, Arends JW, Schutte B, Volvics L, Bosman FT. A multivariate analysis of pathologic prognosticators in large bowel cancer. *Cancer* 1988; 61: 386–395.
48 Halvorsen TB, Johannesen E. DNA ploidy: tumour site and prognosis in colorectal cancer. A flow cytometric study of paraffin-embedded tissue. *Scand J Gastroenterol* 1990; 25: 141–148.
49 Harlow SP, Eriksen BL, Poggensee L *et al.* Prognostic implications of proliferative activity and DNA aneuploidy in Astler–Coller Dukes' stage C colonic adenocarcinoma. *Cancer Res* 1991; 51: 2403–2409.
50 Hammarberg C, Slezak P, Trigukait B. Early detection of malignancy in ulcerative colitis. A flow cytometric DNA study. *Cancer* 1984; 53: 291–295.
51 Brje B, Hstmark J, Skagen DW, Schrumpf E, Laerum OD. Flow cytometry specimens from ulcerative colitis, colorectal adenomas and carcinomas. *Scand J Gastroenterol* 1987; 22: 1231–1237.
52 Fozard JBJ, Quirke P, Dixon MF, Giles GR, Bird CC. DNA aneuploidy in ulcerative colitis. *Gut* 1987; 28: 1414–1418.
53 Melville DM, Jass JR, Shepherd NA *et al.* Dysplasia and deoxyribonucleic acid aneuploidy in the assessment of precancerous changes in chronic ulcerative colitis. Observer variation and correlations. *Gastroenterology* 1988; 95: 668–675.
54 Lofberg R. Studies in longstanding ulcerative colitis with special reference to malignant transformation of the colorectal mucosa. *Acta Chir Scand Suppl* 1989; 552: 1–45.
55 Wersto RP, Greenebaum E, Deitch D, Kersbergen K, Koss LG. Deoxyribonucleic acid ploidy and cell cycle events in benign colonic epithelium peripheral to carcinoma. *Lab Invest* 1988; 58: 218–225.
56 Gyde S. Screening for colorectal cancer in ulcerative colitis: dubious benefits and high costs. *Gut* 1990; 31: 1089–1092.
57 McKinley MJ, Budman DR, Kahn E. High grade dysplasia in Crohn's colitis characterized by flow cytometry. *J Clin Gastroenterol* 1987; 9: 452–455.
58 McKinley MJ, Budman DR, Gruenberg D, Bronzo RL, Weissman GS, Kahn E. DNA content in Barrett's esophagus and esophageal malignancy. *Am J Gastro-*

enterol 1987; 82: 1012–1015.
59 Kaketoni K, Saito T, Kobayashi M. Flow cytometric analysis of nuclear DNA content in esophageal cancer. Aneuploidy as an index for highly malignant potential. *Cancer* 1989; 64: 887–891.
60 Joensuu H, Soderstrom KO, Klem PJ, Eerola E. Nuclear DNA content and its prognostic value in lymphoma of the stomach. *Cancer* 1987; 60: 3042–3048.
61 Kuyari H, Joensuu H, Klemi P, Asola R. A flow cytometric analysis of 23 carcinoid tumours. *Cancer* 1988; 61: 2517–2520.
62 el-Naggar AK, Ro JY, McLemore D, Garnsey L, Ordonez N, MacKay B. Gastrointestinal stromal tumours: DNA flow cytometric study of 58 patients with at least 5 years of follow-up. *Mod Pathol* 1989; 2: 511–515.
63 Fujimoto J, Okamoto E, Yamanaka N, Toyosaka A, Mitsonabu M. Flow cytometric DNA analysis of hepatocellular carcinoma. *Cancer* 1991; 67: 939–944.
64 Merkel DE, McGuire WL. Ploidy, proliferative activity and prognosis. DNA flow cytometry of solid tumours. *Cancer* 1990; 65: 1194–1205.
65 O'Reilly SM, Camplejohn RS, Barnes DM, Millis RP, Rubens RD, Richards MA. DNA index, S phase fraction, histological grade and prognosis in breast cancer. *Br J Cancer* 1989; 61: 671–674.
66 Olsson H, Ranstam J, Baldetorp B *et al.* Proliferation and DNA ploidy in malignant breast tumors in relation to early oral contraceptive use and early abortions. *Cancer* 1991; 67: 1285–1290.
67 Beerman H, Kuin PM, Hermans J, van de Velde CJH, Cornelisse CJ. Prognostic significance of DNA ploidy in a series of 690 primary breast cancer patients. *Int J Cancer* 1990; 45: 34–39.
68 O'Reilly SM, Camplejohn RS, Barnes DM, Millis RR, Rubens RD, Richards MA. Node negative breast cancer: prognostic subgroups defined by tumour size and flow cytometry. *J Clin Oncol* 1990; 8: 2040–2046.
69 Keyhani-Rofagha S, O'Toole RV, Farrar WB, Sickle-Santanello B, De Cenzo J, Young D. Is DNA ploidy an independent prognostic indicator in infiltrative node-negative breast adenocarcinoma? *Cancer* 1990; 65: 1577–1582.
70 Sigurdsson H, Baldtorp B, Borg A *et al.* Indicators of prognosis in node-negative breast cancer. *N Engl J Med* 1990; 322: 1045–1053.
71 Toikkanen S, Joensuu H, Klemi P. Nuclear DNA content as a prognostic factor in T_1-T_2 breast cancer. *Am J Clin Pathol* 1990; 93: 471–479.
72 Clark GM, Dressler LG, Owens MA, Pounds G, Oldtker T, McGuire WL. Prediction of relapse or survival in patients with node-negative breast cancer by DNA flow cytometry. *N Engl J Med* 1989; 320: 627–633.
73 Toikkanen S, Joensuu H, Klemi P. The prognostic significance of nuclear DNA content in invasive breast cancer — a study with long-term follow-up. *Br J Cancer* 1989; 60: 693–700.
74 Kallioniemi O-P, Blanco G, Alavaikko M *et al.* Improving the prognostic value of DNA flow cytometry in breast cancer by combining DNA index and S-phase fraction. *Cancer* 1988; 62: 2183–2190.
75 Muss HB, Kute TE, Case LD *et al.* The relation of flow cytometry to clinical and biologic characteristics in women with node negative primary breast cancer. *Cancer* 1989; 64: 1894–1900.
76 Uyterlinde AM, Baak JPA, Schipper NW, Peterse H, Matze E, Meijer CL. Further evaluation of the prognostic value of morphometric and flow cytometric parameters in breast cancer patients with long term follow up. *Int J Cancer* 1990; 45: 1–7.
77 Ferroro M, Spyratos F, Le Doussal V, Desplaces A, Rouesse J. Flow cytometric analysis of DNA content and keratins by using CK7, CK8, CK18, CK19 and KL1 monoclonal antibodies in benign and malignant human breast tumors. *Cytometry* 1990; 11: 716–724.
78 Remvikos Y, Vuttai M, Laine-Bidron C, Jollivet A, Magdelenat H. Progesterone receptor detection and quantification in breast tumors by bivariate immunofluorescence/DNA flow cytometry. *Cytometry* 1991; 12: 157–166.
79 Gitte RF. Carcinoma of the prostate. *N Eng J Med* 1991; 324: 236–245.
80 Tribukait B, Ronstrom L, Eposti PL. Quantitative and qualitative aspects of flow DNA measurements related to the cytologic grade in prostatic cancer. *Anal Quant Cytol* 1983; 5: 107–111.
81 Lundberg S, Carstensen J, Rundquist I. DNA flow cytometry and histopathological grading of paraffin-embedded prostate biopsy specimens in a survival study. *Cancer Res* 1987; 47: 1973–1977.
82 Willumsen H, Thorup J, Nrgaard J, Hansen OH. Nuclear DNA content in prostatic carcinoma measured by flow cytometry: a retrospective study on paraffin-embedded tissue. *Acta Pathol Microbiol Scand Suppl* 1988; 4: 120–125.
83 Neill WA, Norval M, Habib FK. Nuclear DNA analysis of prostate tissue: correlation with stage and grade tumour. *Urol Int* 1989; 44: 141–146.
84 Seppelt U, Sprenger E, Hedderich J. Investigation of automated DNA diagnosis and grading of prostatic cancer. *Anal Quant Cytol* 1986; 8: 152–157.
85 Klein FA, Ratliff JE, White FK. DNA distribution patterns of prostatic tissue obtained at time of transurethral resection. *Urology* 1988; 31: 260–265.
86 Fordham MV, Burge AH, Matthews J, Williams G, Cooke T. Prostatic carcinoma cell DNA content measured by flow cytometry and its relation to clinical outcome. *Br J Surg* 1986; 73: 400–403.
87 Stephenson RA, James BC, Gay H, Fair WR, Whitmore WF, Melamed MR. Flow cytometry of prostatic cancer: relationship of DNA content to survival. *Cancer Res* 1987; 47: 2504–2507.
88 Lee SE, Currin SM, Paulson DF, Walther PJ. Flow

cytometric determination of ploidy in prostatic adenocarcinoma: a comparison with seminal vesicle involvement and histopathological grading as a predictor of clinical recurrence. *J Urol* 1988; 140: 769–774.

89 Ritchie AW, Dorey F, Layfield LJ, Hannah J, Lovrekovich H, de Kernion JB. Relationship of DNA content to conventional prognostic factors in clinically localised carcinoma of the prostate. *Br J Urol* 1988; 62: 245–260.

90 Winkler HZ, Rainwater LM, Myers RP *et al.* Stage D1 prostatic adenocarcinoma: significance of nuclear DNA ploidy patterns studied by flow cytometry. *Mayo Clin Proc* 1988; 63: 103–112.

91 Nativ O, Winkler HZ, Raz Y *et al.* Stage C prostatic adenocarcinoma: flow cytometric nuclear DNA ploidy analysis. *Mayo Clin Proc* 1989; 64: 911–919.

92 Montgomery BT, Nativ O, Blute ML *et al.* Stage B prostate adenocarcinoma. Flow cytometric DNA ploidy analysis. *Arch Surg* 1990; 125: 327–331.

93 Kleinhaus G, Hacker-Klom U, Gohde W, Korner F, Schumann J. Studies of the cell kinetics of human malignant testicular tumors. *Urologie* 1986; 25: 294–297.

94 Oosterhuis JW, Castedo SM, de Jong B *et al.* Ploidy of primary germ cell tumours of the testis. Pathogenetic and clinical relevance. *Lab Invest* 1989; 60: 14–21.

95 Sledge GW, Eble JN, Roth BJ, Wuhrman BP, Fineberg N, Einhorn LH. Relation of proliferative activity to survival in patients with advanced germ cell cancer. *Cancer Res* 1988; 48: 3864–3868.

96 Kysala B, Matoska J. Flow cytometry analysis of ploidy and proliferation activity in classical and spermatocytic seminoma. *Neoplasm* 1991; 38: 3–11.

97 Nagler HM, Kaufman D, O'Toole KM, Sawczuk IS. Carcinoma *in situ* of the testis: diagnosis by aspiration flow cytometry. *J Urol* 1990; 143: 359–361.

98 Clausen OP, Giwercman A, Jorgensen N, Bruun N, Frimodt-Muller C, Shakkeback NE. DNA distributions in maldescended testis; hyperdiploidy without evidence of germ cell neoplasia. *Cytometry* 1991; 12: 77–81.

99 Raghavan D, Shipley WU, Garnick MB, Russell PJ, Ritchie JP. Biology and management of bladder cancer. *N Eng J Med* 1990; 322: 1129–1138.

100 Gustafson H, Tribukait B. Characterization of bladder carcinoma by DNA flow analysis. *Eur Urol* 1985; 11: 410–417.

101 Malmstrom PU, Vasko J, Wester K, Norlen BJ, Busch C. Flow cytometric analysis of deparaffinized nuclei in urinary bladder carcinoma. Comparison of different isolation methods and relation to histological grade and state. *Acta Pathol Microbiol Scand* 1989; 97: 811–819.

102 Blomjous CE, Schipper NW, Vos W, Baak JP, et Voogt HJ, Meijer CL. Comparison of quantitative and classical prognosticators in urinary bladder carcinoma. A multivariate analysis of DNA flow cytometric, nuclear morphometric and clinicopathological features. *Virchows Arch A Pathol Anat Histopathol* 1989; 415: 421–428.

103 Bretton PR, Herr HW, Fair WR, Whitmore WF, Melamed MR. Flow cytometry as a predictor of response and progression in patients with superficial bladder cancer treated with bacillus Calmette–Guerin. *J Urol* 1989; 141: 1332–1336.

104 Blomjous EC, Schipper NW, Baak JP, Vos W, De Voogt HJ, Meijer CL. The value of morphometry and DNA flow cytometry in addition to classic prognosticators in superficial urinary bladder carcinoma. *Am J Clin Pathol* 1989; 91: 243–248.

105 Jacobsen AB, Lunde S, Ous S *et al.* T_2/T_3 bladder carcinoma treated with definitive radiotherapy with emphasis on flow cytometric DNA ploidy values. *Int J Radiat Oncol Biol Phys* 1989; 17: 923–924.

106 Lipponen PK, Eskelinen MJ, Collan Y *et al.* DNA ploidy and S phase fraction in human bladder cancer. Relation to survival and histological grade (WHO). *Urol Int* 1990; 17: 923–924.

107 de Vita R, Forte D, Maggi F, Eleuteri P, Di Silverio F. Cellular DNA content and proliferative activity evaluated by flow cytometry versus histopathological and staging classifications in bladder tumors. *Eur Urol* 1990; 19: 65–73.

108 Badalament RA, Fair WR, Whitmore WF, Melamed MR. The relative value of cytometry and cytology in the management of bladder cancer: the Memorial Sloan-Kettering Group Cancer Center experience. *Semin Urol* 1988; 6: 22–30.

109 Klein FA, White FK. Flow cytometry deoxyribonucleic acid determinations and cytology of bladder washings: a practical experience. *J Urol* 1988; 139: 275–278.

110 Ljungberg B, Stenling RI, Roos G. DNA content in renal carcinoma with reference to tumor heterogeneity. *Cancer* 1985; 56: 503–508.

111 Ljungberg B, Forsslund G, Stenling R. Prognostic significance of the DNA content in renal cell carcinoma. *J Urol* 1986; 135: 422–426.

112 Friedlander ML, Taylor IW, Russell P, Musgrove EA, Hedley DW, Tattersall MHW. Ploidy as a prognostic factor in ovarian cancer. *Int J Gynecol Pathol* 1983; 2: 55–63.

113 Iversen OE, Skaarland E. Ploidy assessment of benign and malignant ovarian tumors by flow cytometry. A clinicopathologic study. *Cancer* 1987; 60: 82–87.

114 Blumenfeld D, Braby PS, Ben-Ezra J, Klevecz RR. Tumor DNA content as a prognostic feature in advanced epithelial ovarian carcinoma. *Gynecol Oncol* 1987; 27: 389–402.

115 Kallioniemi OP, Punnonen R, Mattila J, Lehtinen M, Koivula T. Prognostic significance of DNA index, multiploidy and S phase fraction in ovarian cancer. *Cancer* 1988; 61: 334–339.

116 Rodenberg CJ, Cornelisse CJ, Hermans J, Fleuren GJ. DNA flow cytometry and morphometry as prognostic

indicators in advanced ovarian cancer: a step forward in predicting clinical outcome. *Gynecol Oncol* 1988; 29: 176–187.
117 Kuhn W, Kaufman M, Feichter GE, Rummel HH, Schmid H, Heberling D. DNA flow cytometry, clinical and morphological parameters as prognostic factors for advanced malignant and borderline ovarian tumors. *Gynecol Oncol* 1989; 33: 360–367.
118 Iemi PJ, Joensuu H, Maenpaa J, Kiilholma P. Influence of cellular DNA content on survival in ovarian carcinoma. *Obstet Gynecol* 1989; 74: 200–204.
119 Brescia RJ, Barakat RA, Beller U *et al.* The prognostic significance of nuclear DNA content in malignant epithelial tumours of the ovary. *Cancer* 1990; 65: 141–147.
120 Punnonen R, Kallioniemi OPI, Mattila J, Joivula I. Prognostic assessment in stage I ovarian cancer using a discriminant analysis with clinicopathological and DNA flow cytometric data. *Gynecol Obstet Invest* 1989; 27: 213–216.
121 Baak JP, Wisse-Brekelmans EC, Uyterlinde AM, Schipper NW. Evaluation of the prognostic value of morphometric features and cellular DNA content in FIGO 1 ovarian cancer patients. *Anal Quant Cytol Histol* 1987; 9: 287–290.
122 Friedlander ML, Hedley DW, Swanson C, Russell P. Prediction of long term survival by flow cytometric analysis of cellular DNA content in patients with advanced ovarian cancer. *J Clin Oncol* 1988; 6: 282–290.
123 Sahni K, Tribukait B, Einhorn N. Flow cytometric measurement of ploidy and proliferation in effusions of ovarian carcinoma and their possible prognostic significance. *Gynecol Oncol* 1989; 35: 240–245.
124 Baak JP, Schipper NW, Wisse-Brekelmans EC *et al.* The prognostic value of morphometrical features and cellular DNA content in *cis*-platin treated late ovarian cancer patients. *Br J Cancer* 1988; 57: 503–508.
125 Hitchcock CL, Norris HJ, Khalifa MA, Wargotz ES. Flow cytometric analysis of granulosa cell tumor. *Cancer* 1989; 64: 2127–2132.
126 Klemi PJ, Joensuu H, Salmi T. Prognostic value of flow cytometric DNA content analysis in granulosa cell tumor of the ovary. *Cancer* 1990; 65: 1189–1193.
127 Chadha S, Cornelisse CJ, Schaberg A. Flow cytometric DNA ploidy analysis of ovarian granulosa cell tumors. *Gynecol Oncol* 1990; 36: 240–245.
128 Sprenger E, Sandritter W, Naiyoks H, Hilgarth M, Wagner D, Vogt-Schaden M. Routine use of flow-through photometric prescreening in the detection of cervical carcinoma. *Acta Cytol* 1977; 21: 435–438.
129 Linden WA, Ochlich K, Baisch H *et al.* Flow cytometric prescreening of cervical smears. *J Histochem Cytochem* 1979; 27: 529–535.
130 Perticarari S, Presani G, Michelutti A, Facca MC, Alberico S, Mandruzzato GP. Flow cytometric analysis of DNA content in cervical lesions. *Pathol Res Pract* 1989; 185: 686–688.
131 Watts KC, Campion MJ, Butler EB, Jenkins D, Singer A, Hussain OA. Quantitative deoxyribonucleic acid analysis of patients with mild cervical atypia: a potentially malignant lesion? *Obstet Gynecol* 1987; 70: 205–207.
132 Hughes RG, Neill WA, Norval M. Nuclear DNA analysis of koilocytic and premalignant lesions of the uterine cervix. *Br Med J* 1987; 294: 267–269.
133 Jakobsen A. Prognostic impact of ploidy level in carcinoma of the cervix. *Am J Clin Oncol* 1984; 7: 475–480.
134 Strang P, Eklund G, Stendahl U, Frenkendal B. S-phase rate as a predictor of early recurrence of carcinoma of the uterine cervix. *Anticancer Res* 1987; 7: 807–810.
135 Dyson JE, Joslin CA, Rothwell RI, Quirke P, Khoury GG, Bird CC. Flow cytofluorimetric evidence for the differential radioresponsiveness of aneuploid and diploid cervix tumours. *Radiother Oncol* 1987; 8: 263–272.
136 Davis JR, Aristizabal S, Way DL, Weiner SA, Hicks MJ, Hagaman RM. DNA ploidy, grade and stage in prognosis of uterine cervical cancer. *Gynecol Oncol* 1989; 32: 4–7.
137 Strang P. Cytogenetic and cytometric analysis in squamous cell carcinoma of the uterine cervix. *Int J Gynecol Pathol* 1989; 8: 54–63.
138 Strang P, Stendahl U, Frankendal B, Lindgren A. Flow cytometric DNA patterns in cervical carcinoma. *Acta Radiol* 1986; 25: 249–254.
139 Quillamor RM, Furlong JW, Hoschner JA, Wynn RM. Relative prognostic significance of DNA flow cytometry and histologic grading in endometrial carcinoma. *Gynecol Obstet Invest* 1988; 26: 332–337.
140 Britton LC, Wilson TO, Gaffey TA, Lieber M, Wieand HS, Podratz KC. Flow cytometric analysis of stage I endometrial carcinoma. *Gynecol Oncol* 1989; 35: 317–322.
141 Rosenberg P, Wingren S, Simonsen E, Stal O, Risberg B, Nordenskjold B. Flow cytometric measurements of DNA index and S phase on paraffin-embedded early stage endometrial cancer: an important prognostic indicator. *Gynecol Oncol* 1989; 35: 50–54.
142 Strang P, Stendahl U, Trbukait B, Wagenius G, Boman K. Age, menopausal status and DNA-content in endometrial cancer. *Anticancer Res* 1989; 9: 1079–1082.
143 Iversen OE, Utaaker E, Skaarland E. DNA ploidy and steroid receptors as predictors of disease course in patients with endometrial carcinoma. *Acta Obstet Gynecol Scand* 1988; 67: 531–537.
144 Lindahl B, Alm P, Ferno M *et al.* Prognostic value of steroid receptor concentration and flow cytometrical DNA measurements in stage I–II endometrial carcinoma. *Acta Oncol* 1989; 28: 595–599.
145 Hemming JD, Quirke P, Womack C, Wells M, Elston CW, Bird CC. Diagnosis of molar pregnancy and persistent trophoblastic disease by flow cytometry. *J Clin Pathol* 1987; 40: 615–620.

146 Laye JM, Driscoll SG, Yavner DL, Olivier AP, Mark SD, Weinberg DS. Hydatidiform moles. Application of flow cytometry in diagnosis. *Am J Clin Pathol* 1988; 89: 596–600.
147 Martin DA, Sutton GP, Ulbright TM, Sledte GW, Stehman FB, Ehrilich CE. DNA content as a prognostic index in gestational trophoblastic neoplasia. *Gynecol Oncol* 1989; 34: 383–388.
148 Isobe H, Miyamoto H, Shimizu T *et al.* Prognostic and therapeutic significance of the flow cytometric nuclear DNA content in non-small cell lung cancer. *Cancer* 1990; 65: 1391–1395.
149 Volm M, Hahn EW, Mattern J, Muller T, Vogt-Moykopf I, Weber E. Five year follow-up of independent clinical and flow cytometric prognostic factors for the survival of patients with non-small cell lung carcinoma. *Cancer Res* 1988; 48: 2923–2928.
150 Zimmerman PV, Hawson GA, Bint MH, Parson PG. Ploidy as a prognostic determinant in surgically treated lung cancer. *Lancet* 1987; 2: 530–533.
151 Sahin AA, Ro JY, et-Naggar AK *et al.* Flow cytometric analysis of the DNA content of non-small cell lung cancer. *Cancer* 1990; 65: 530–537.
152 Asamura H, Nakajima T, Mukai T, Shimosato Y. Nuclear DNA content by cytofluorometry of stage 1 adenocarcinoma of the lung in relation to postoperative recurrence. *Chest* 1989; 96: 312–318.
153 Cibas ES, Melamed MR, Zaman MB, Kimmel M. The effect of tumour size and tumour cell DNA content on the survival of patients with stage I adenocarcinoma of the lung. *Cancer* 1989; 63: 1552–1556.
154 Jones DJ, Hasleton PW, Moore M. DNA ploidy in bronchopulmonary carcinoid tumours. *Thorax* 1988; 43: 195–199.
155 Kokal WA, Gardine RL, Sheibani K *et al.* Tumour DNA content as a prognostic indicator in squamous cell carcinoma of the head and neck regions. *Am J Surg* 1988; 156: 267–280.
156 Sakr W, Hussan M, Zarbo RJ, Ensley J, Crissman JD. DNA quantitation and histologic characteristics of squamous cell carcinoma of the upper aerodigestive tract. *Arch Pathol Lab Med* 1989; 113: 1009–1014.
157 Macartney JC, Camplejohn RS. DNA flow cytometry of no-Hodgkin's lymphomas. *Eur J Cancer* 1990; 26: 635–637.
158 Macartney JC, Camplejohn RS. DNA flow cytometry. In: Crocker J (ed.) *Cell Proliferation in Lymphomas.* Oxford: Blackwell Scientific Publications, 1992: 99–114.
159 Braylan RC, Benson NA, Nourse VA. Cellular DNA of human neoplastic B cells measured by flow cytometry. *Cancer Res* 1984; 44: 5010–5016.
160 Griffin NR, Howard MR, Quirke P. Prognostic indicators in centroblastic-centrocytic lymphoma. *J Clin Pathol* 1988; 41: 866–870.
161 Macartney JC, Camplejohn RS, Morris R, Hollowood K, Clarke D, Timothy A. DNA flow cytometry of follicular non-Hodgkin's lymphoma. *J Clin Pathol* 1991; 44: 215–218.
162 Bauer KD, Merkel DE, Winter JN *et al.* Prognostic implications of ploidy and proliferative activity in diffuse large cell lymphomas. *Cancer Res* 1986; 46: 3173–3178.
163 Young GAR, Hedley DW, Rugg CA, Iland HJ. The prognostic significance of proliferative activity in poor histology non-Hodgkin's lymphoma: a flow cytometry study using archival material. *Eur J Cancer Clin Oncol* 1987; 23: 1497–1504.
164 McLaughlin P, Osborne BM, Johnston D *et al.* Nucleic acid flow cytometry in large cell lymphoma. *Cancer Res* 1988; 48: 6614–6619.
165 Wooldrige TN, Grierson HL, Weisenburger DD *et al.* Association of DNA content and proliferative activity with clinical outcome in patients with diffuse mixed cell and large cell non-Hodgkin's lymphoma. *Cancer Res* 1988; 46: 6608–6613.
166 Cowan RA, Harris M, Jones M, Crowther D. DNA content in high and intermediate grade non-Hodgkin's lymphoma — prognostic significance and clinicopathological correlations. *Br J Cancer* 1989; 60: 904–910.
167 Lehtinen T, Aine R, Lehtinen M *et al.* Flow cytometric DNA analysis of 199 histologically favourable of unfavourable non-Hodgkin's lymphomas. *J Pathol* 1989; 157: 27–36.
168 Aine R, Lehtinen T, Lehtinen M *et al.* Flow cytometric analysis of DNA ploidy in large cleaved cell lymphomas. *Hematol Oncol* 1990; 8: 339–346.
169 Kheir SM, Bines SD, Vonroenn JH, Soong SJ, Urist MM, Coon SJ. Prognostic significance of DNA aneuploidy in state I cutaneous melanoma. *Ann Surg* 1988; 207: 455–461.
170 Soreson FB, Kristensen IB, Grymer F, Jakobsen A. DNA level, tumor thickness, and stereological estimates of nuclear volume in stage I cutaneous malignant melanoma. A comparative study with analysis of prognostic impact. *Am J Dermatopathol* 1991; 13: 11–19.
171 Newton JA, Camplejohn RS, McGibbon DH. The flow cytometry of melanocytic skin lesions. *Br J Cancer* 1988; 58: 606–609.
172 Schelfhout LJ, Cornelisse CJ, Goslings BM *et al.* Frequency and degree of aneuploidy in benign and malignant thyroid neoplasms. *Int J Cancer* 1990; 45: 16–20.
173 Klemi PS, Joensuu H, Eerola E. DNA aneuploidy in anaplastic carcinoma of the thyroid. *Am J Clin Pathol* 1988; 89: 154–159.
174 Hrafnkelsson J, Stal O, Enestrom S *et al.* Cellular DNA pattern S phase frequency and survival in papillary thyroid cancer. *Acta Oncol* 1988; 27: 329–333.
175 Cusick EL, Ewen SW, Krukowski ZH, Matheson NA. DNA aneuploidy in follicular thyroid neoplasia. *Br J Surg* 1991; 78: 94–96.
176 Obara T, Fujimoto Y, Hirayama *et al.* Flow cytometric DNA analysis of parathyroid tumours with special

reference to its diagnostic and prognostic value in parathyroid carcinoma. *Cancer* 1990; 65: 1789–1793.

177 Obara T, Fujimoto Y, Kanaji Y *et al.* Flow cytometric DNA analysis of parathyroid tumors. Implication of aneuploidy for pathologic and biologic classification. *Cancer* 1990; 66: 1555–1562.

178 Coons SW, David JR, Way DL. Correlation of DNA content and histology in prognosis of astrocytomas. *Am J Clin Pathol* 1988; 90: 289–293.

179 Nishizaki T, Orita T, Furutani Y, Ikeyama Y, Aoki H, Sasaki K. Flow cytometric DNA analysis and immunohistochemical measurement of Ki-67 and BUdR labelling indices in human brain tumors. *J Neurosurg* 1989; 70: 379–384.

180 Kroese MC, Rutgers DH, Wils IS, Van Unnick JA, Roholl PJ. The relevance of the DNA index and proliferation rate in the grading of benign and malignant soft tissue tumors. *Cancer* 1990; 65: 1782–1788.

181 Bauer HCF. Kreibergs A, Silversward C, Tribukait B. DNA analysis in the differential diagnosis of osteosarcoma. *Cancer* 1988; 61: 2532–2540.

182 Look AT, Douglas EC, Meyer WH. Clinical importance of near diploid tumor stem lines in patients with osteosarcoma of an extremity. *N Engl J Med* 1988; 318: 1567–1572.

183 Ladanyi M, Traganos F, Havos AG. Benign metastasizing giant cell tumors of bone. A DNA flow cytometric study. *Cancer* 1989; 64: 1521–1526.

184 Asamura H, Nakajima T, Mukai K, Noguchi M, Shimosato Y. Degree of malignancy of thymic epithelial tumors in terms of nuclear DNA content and nuclear area. An analysis of 39 cases. *Am J Pathol* 1988; 133: 615–622.

185 Davies SE, Macartney JC, Camplejohn RS, Morris RW, Ring NP, Corrin B. DNA flow cytometry of thymomas. *Histopathology* 1989; 15: 77–83.

186 Van der Mey AG, Cornelisse CJ, Hermans T, Gerpstra JL, Schmidt PH, Fleuren GJ. DNA flow cytometry of hereditary and sporadic paragangliomas (glomus tumours). *Br J Cancer* 1991; 63: 298–302.

187 Brenner DW, Barranco SC, Winslow BH, Shaeffer J. Flow cytometric analysis of DNA content in children with neuroblastoma. *J Pediatr Surg* 1989; 24: 204–207.

188 Yasue M, Tomita T, Engelhard H, Gonzales-Crussi F, McLone DG, Bauer KD. Prognostic importance of DNA ploidy in medulloblastoma of childhood. *J Neurosurg* 1989; 70: 385–391.

11

CELL KINETIC STUDIES USING FLOW CYTOMETRY

G. D. WILSON

Flow cytometry (FCM) is essentially the art of bringing suspended cells one by one to an excitation source and detection system by the means of a flow channel. Having achieved this, the attributes which make the technology unique are its sharpness or fidelity of measurement, speed, sensitivity, ability to make several measurements simultaneously and its quantitative power [1]. FCM is a new methodology, with most advances occurring over the past 15 years, and is still under intense development, improvement and continuing change. Many of the proposed analytical applications have not been extensively tested on different cell types and other methods are not yet routine. Methods which have been published earlier are often subject to ongoing modification or improvement and new probes are frequently introduced.

FCM has already made a significant impact on research in various fields of cell and molecular biology and medicine. One of the areas which has greatly benefited from new FCM procedures has been cell kinetic research. Since the first description of the cell cycle by Howard and Pelc [2], studies on DNA synthesis, cell cycle traverse and cell proliferation were significantly advanced through the use of the radiolabelled DNA precursor, tritiated thymidine (^{3}HTdR) [3]. Much of the knowledge concerning growth and differentiation in hierarchical normal tissues and in experimental and human tumours has been gained through the meticulous application of the per cent labelled mitosis (plm) technique first reported by Quastler and Sherman [4]. The field of tumour cell kinetics was comprehensively summarized in *Growth Kinetics of Tumours* by Steel [5]. This book remains an important reference for those who wish to understand the basic theory of growing populations, how to measure and analyse cell kinetic data and results obtained using the plm technique in experimental and human tumours.

The most disappointing aspect of cell kinetics has been its failure to influence profoundly the treatment of human cancer. There can be no doubt, in most clinicians' and biologists' minds, that cellular proliferation must be one of the most important factors influencing treatment response and outcome. Many studies in the 1960s and 1970s sought to utilize parameters such as the labelling index (LI) as a prognostic indicator, and many of the early studies on chemotherapy and cell synchronization *in vivo* were based on cell kinetic studies. Yet cell kinetic information has been relegated to the background by many oncologists. The lack of confidence in cell kinetic concepts in predicting treatment response, or use in treatment planning, arises from both the awareness that proliferation was only one of the factors involved in the tumour response and that the available cell kinetic techniques were not readily applicable to the clinical situation. The use of autoradiography to quantitate the incorporation of ^{3}HTdR meant that the technique was slow (requiring weeks of exposure of tissue sections to photographic emulsion), laborious (quantitation was by counting labelled nuclei or mitoses) and required multiple biopsies if cell cycle traverse rates were to be measured. These characteristics, in addition to the ethical constraints of administering a radioactive precursor of DNA to patients, restricted most studies to *in vitro* incorporation of tumour explants or cell suspensions.

The advent of FCM has introduced renewed interest in cell kinetic research. The technique of measuring S-phase fractions (SPFs) from FCM-derived DNA profiles is analogous to LI measurements, but requires no DNA precursor. The technique is rapid, quantitative and universally applicable. However, both LI and SPF are cytostatic measurements giving only information on the number of cells in a particular phase of the cell cycle at the time of the measurement.

The real advance in cell kinetic FCM technology has been the development of methods to measure cytodynamic information, cell cycle-related proteins and manipulate staining techniques to dissect and exploit the stainability of DNA. This chapter will be dealing with the use of monoclonal antibodies to recognize incorporation of 5-bromo, 2-deoxyuridine (BrdUrd), administered *in vivo*, into DNA of human solid tumours and the use of FCM to measure cell kinetic parameters, which is our own area of expertise [6]. However, in addition to this technique, there are several methods which will be described which can be used to produce cytodynamic information with FCM. These include the technique of quenching of Hoechst 33258 fluorescence by incorporated BrdUrd developed by Latt [7]. An alternative to this technique was developed by Crissman and Steinkamp [8], in which two non-intercalating DNA-specific fluorochromes, the AT-binding Hoechst 33342 and the GC-binding mithramycin (MI) were used in BrdUrd-labelled cells.

Static information on cell proliferation parameters can be obtained using multivariate cell analysis by combining DNA measurements with protein [9] or RNA [10] or by exploiting the denaturability of DNA *in situ* [11]. From these approaches, the basic cell cycle distribution can be dissected further to identify quiescent cells in G_0, G_1, S and G_2, and also mitotic cells.

Several nuclear and surface proteins are expressed in varying amounts in different phases of the cell cycle. Some proteins are oncogene products and may have a direct regulatory function in cell proliferation; other proteins, such as proliferating cell nuclear antigen (PCNA), Ki-67, and DNA polymerase are not coded by oncogenes and their expression may be secondary to proliferative changes in the population. Studying these proteins, using relatively simple immunochemical techniques, may facilitate a better understanding of the mechanisms regulating proliferation and differentiation as well as describing kinetic parameters of the cell cycle.

11.1 CYTODYNAMIC MEASUREMENTS

11.1.1 BrdUrd incorporation *in vivo*

The techniques which I shall be describing in this section were made possible by the development of monoclonal antibodies recognizing the halogenated pyrimidines incorporated into DNA [12]. Subsequently, flow cytometric methods were devised to measure simultaneously the uptake of BrdUrd and total DNA content [13]. The combination of using monoclonal antibodies and FCM for detection of BrdUrd meant that the DNA precursor did not have to be radiolabelled, as was the case for ^{3}HTdR and autoradiography. This reopened the possibility of *in vivo* administration to exploit techniques, developed at the Gray Laboratory, to measure both LI and duration of S phase (T_S), and from these to calculate the potential doubling time (T_{pot}) of the tumour from a single biopsy taken several hours after the administration of BrdUrd [14]. The speed and quantitative power of FCM meant that results could be obtained within 24 h and, potentially, could be used as a diagnostic as well as a prognostic parameter. This represents the only method to obtain a time parameter technique in human tumours (the T_S) using current FCM methods. With this in mind, more detail will be given to this method than the others cited in this section.

11.1.2 BrdUrd administration and surgical procedures

The majority of patients have received 200 mg of BrdUrd administered from a single push in 20 ml of 0.9% saline. Several sources of BrdUrd have been used in our studies. Initially, a preparation suitable for human use was obtained from the National

Cancer Institute Investigational Drugs Branch (Bethesda, Maryland). This is probably the most common source for BrdUrd or iododeoxyuridine (IdUrd). Second, a commercial preparation was obtained from Takeda Chemical Industries (Osaka, Japan). More recently, BrdUrd has been prepared at the Department of Pharmacy, University of Strathclyde, Glasgow.

The biopsy or surgical resection was usually performed between 4 and 8 h after the injection of BrdUrd, to allow sufficient time for the BrdUrd-labelled cells to redistribute through their cell cycle. The half-life of BrdUrd is short (10–15 min), such that it is only incorporated into S-phase cells at the time of injection.

No toxicity has been observed to be clinically associated with the injection of BrdUrd or IdUrd at the doses given for cell kinetic studies. Informed consent was obtained from all patients.

A portion of each biopsy or resection was fixed in 70% ethanol for FCM and an adjacent portion fixed in formal saline for histopathological examination and immunohistochemistry.

11.1.3 Tissue processing and BrdUrd staining

The procedures involved in the processing of tumour tissue into nuclei and staining for BrdUrd uptake and DNA content have been described in detail elsewhere [15]. The staining procedure has evolved over the years from one which initially produced a cell suspension using various enzyme cocktails, to its present form which produces nuclei using pepsin. There are advantages and disadvantages to any dissociation procedure. The major disadvantage of pepsin digestion is that it prevents simultaneous staining of BrdUrd with a cytoskeletal or cell-surface marker which may help to identify different cell types, particularly in diploid human tumours. However, the advantages of the pepsin procedure are manifold. First, the procedures required at the hospital or operating theatre are minimal. The piece of tissue is simply fixed in 70% ethanol and stored at 4 °C. There is no need for prompt collection and processing of tissue. This also means that there does not have to be FCM on site, as the tissue can be posted to a centre which has a facility; this has opened up the possibility for multicentre studies. Second, the yield of nuclei per gram of tissue is greatly increased in comparison to mechanical or enzymatic methods to produce cell suspensions. This feature has made it possible to analyse small amounts of tissue (20–100 mg) and also means that the dissociation procedure is the same for each tumour type. The final advantage of pepsin digestion is that the quality of both BrdUrd detection and DNA staining has been improved by the removal of cytoplasm. This step abolishes much of the non-specific antibody staining and improves the resolution of the DNA distributions.

As regards the staining procedure, the partial denaturation of double-stranded DNA using 2 mol/l hydrochloric acid (HCl) is a critical step. This is necessary, as most monoclonals, recognizing the halogenated pyrimidines, cannot access their epitope in double-stranded DNA. However, this step is a balance between unmasking sufficient antibodybinding sites and not disrupting the stoichiometry of propidium iodide (PI) intercalation into doublestranded DNA. It is likely that various tumours and tissue will denature differently. However, it is not often possible to optimize the denaturation procedure for each tumour, due to the limitation of the material provided. Through experience, we have arrived at 12 min in HCl as a time period which provides acceptable staining profiles in most tumours studied.

It is usually advisable to use indirect fluorescence labelling, as there may not be sufficient detection of a directly labelled monoclonal antibody. It is also important not to have too many nuclei, as this may saturate the labelling reagents; our staining procedure is designed for a maximum of 4×10^6 nuclei.

11.1.4 Data acquisition

The data presented in this chapter have been collected on either an Ortho Cytofluorograph Systems 50-H or a Becton Dickinson FACScan. However, all commercial machines are capable of analysing data of this type, with one proviso. It is important, with any study involving DNA, to have the capability of pulse processing such that doublets, triplets, etc., can be excluded. This is particularly important for double-staining studies of DNA and BrdUrd, as cell doublets may well have BrdUrd labelling and could interfere with the analysis of cell progression through the cycle. Routinely, laser excitation is at 488 nm at a power of 200 mW in the Ortho set-up, but only 15 mW in the FACScan. In the Ortho FCM, the exciting wavelength is deflected using a 510 nm long-pass dichroic filter. Green fluorescence is collected with a 530 nm band-pass (510–550 nm) and red fluorescence with a 620 nm long-pass filter, after deflection with a 590 nm short-pass dichroic. The FACScan is prealigned and set up to detect fluorochrome isothiocyanate (FITC; FL1, green fluorescence), phycoerythrin (PE) and duochrome (FL3). The DNA signal (red fluorescence) can be collected in FL2 or FL3. Compensation will be required to subtract spectral overlap of FL1 and FL2. Typically, 5–15% is necessary, depending on the intensity of the FITC signal. No compensation is required if FL3 is used.

Under normal conditions, 10 000 events are collected in list mode (more may be required if there are few proliferating cells), and the green fluorescence signals can be collected on log or linear scales; the red (PI) must be on linear.

11.1.5 Data analysis

The potential doubling time

The parameter of interest in this section is T_{pot}. Many clinical studies have demonstrated, particularly in radiotherapy, that tumours may undergo rapid (compensatory) proliferation during treatment [16,17]. A predictive test which could identify patients whose tumours may be capable of rapid repopulation may be of clinical benefit to select more appropriate treatment schedules. Fowler [18] and others have identified the T_{pot} to be the best available predictor of the effective doubling time of clonogenic cells.

The T_{pot} represents the time taken for a cell population to double its number, taking into account the presence of dividing and non-dividing cells, but in the absence of cell loss [5]. The potential doubling time is given by the formula:

$$T_{pot} = \lambda \frac{T_S}{LI}$$

where LI is the fraction of cells synthesizing DNA, T_S is the duration of S phase of the proliferating cells and λ is a correction factor for the age distribution of the cell population and varies typically between 0.693 and 1.0 in mammalian cells. A value of 0.8 has been assigned to this parameter based on calculations in experimental tumours.

The relative movement method

The first procedure to calculate T_{pot} from a single observation was devised at the Gray Laboratory by Begg *et al.* [14]. The procedure depends upon several critical assumptions. Figure 11.1a depicts a schematic representation of the cell cycle showing the progression of a pulse-chased cohort of BrdUrd-labelled cells.

At time 0, immediately after labelling, only cells in S phase show evidence of BrdUrd incorporation. The first assumption made by the Begg method is that the distribution of labelled cells is uniform throughout S phase. Figure 11.1b shows results obtained from V79 cells, labelled *in vitro* for 20 min with 20 μM BrdUrd. If the assumption of uniform distribution were true, then a computer region, set around all cells showing BrdUrd uptake, should give a mean DNA content (on the *x*-axis) equal to that of mid-S. To quantitate this function, the term relative movement (RM) was described. The mean DNA content of the BrdUrd-labelled cohort is expressed as a function of the difference in DNA content between the G_1 and G_2 populations:

$$RM = \frac{FL_{BrdUrd} - FL_{G1}}{FL_{G_2+M} - FL_{G1}}$$

where FL_{BrdUrd} is the mean DNA content of the BrdUrd-labelled cohort, progressing through S phase, and FL_{G1} and FL_{G_2+M} are the mean DNA contents of the G_1 and $G_2 + M$ populations respectively. Thus, immediately after labelling with BrdUrd, the RM should be 0.5.

The next critical assumption is that the progression of the BrdUrd-labelled cells through S phase is linear. Figure 11.1a (centre panel) shows that, at some time after BrdUrd incorporation, the labelled cohort has progressed some way through S phase; some cells now reside in G_2, whilst others (the late S-phase cells at the time of labelling) have

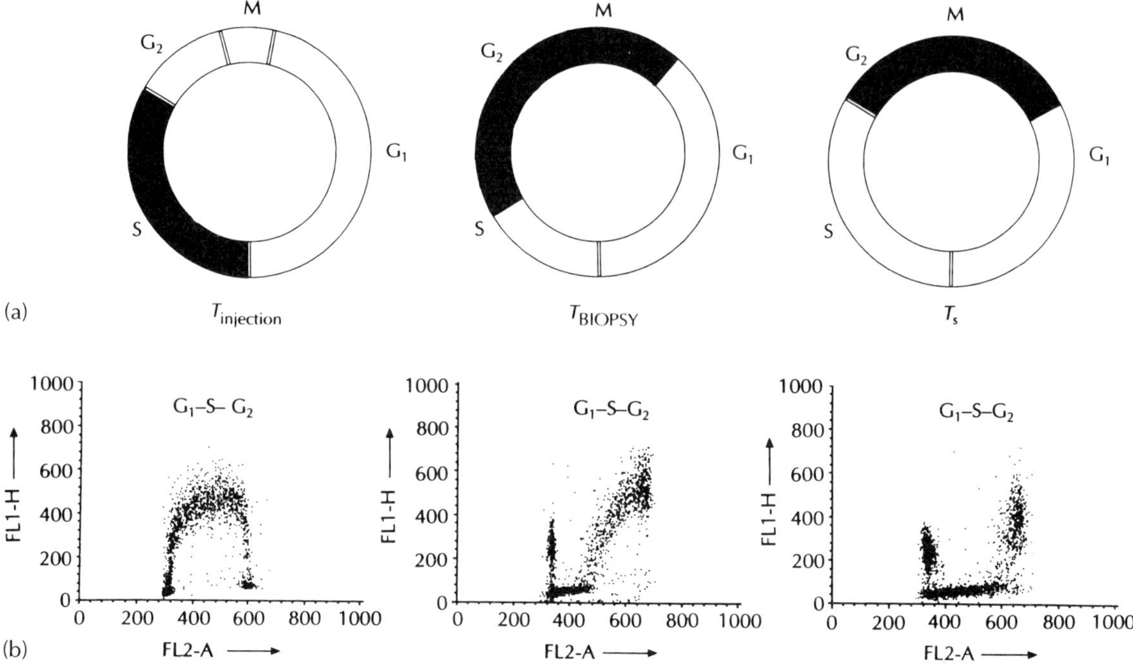

Fig. 11.1 Progression of a 5-bromo, 2-deoxyuridine (BrdUrd) labelled cohort of cells through the cell cycle. (a) A schematic representation of the cell cycle and the position of a cohort of BrdUrd-labelled cells (shaded area) at time T injection, immediately after pulse labelling; at time T_{BIOPSY}, several hours after labelling and at time T_S, where all BrdUrd-labelled cells have either divided or reside in $G_2 + M$. (b) Actual data obtained from V79 cells *in vitro*. The profiles were obtained immediately after labelling and at 3 and 6 hours (which is the T_S). The bivariate cytograms represent DNA content (FL2-A) against BrdUrd uptake (FL1-H).

divided and entered G_1. In Fig. 11.1b it is evident that the BrdUrd-labelled cells form two distinct populations on the basis of their DNA content, one population still progressing through S phase and G_2, whilst the other represents cells which have divided and now reside in G_1. It is the former population that is used to measure RM; this population will show an increase in mean DNA content and the RM will increase.

If the assumption of linear progression through S phase is made, then the BrdUrd-labelled cohort will move through this phase, synchronized according to their DNA content. Thus, as shown in the right-hand panels of Fig. 11.1a and b, at the time T_S the only cells which are BrdUrd-labelled, and have not yet divided, will reside in G_2 and these cells would have been the cells in early S phase at the time of BrdUrd incorporation. By definition, the RM at time T_S will equal 1.0.

With these assumptions, a single observation, made some hours after an injection of BrdUrd (as in the middle panels of Fig. 11.1), allows the computation of T_S from:

$$T_S = \frac{1.0 - 0.5}{RM - 0.5} \times T_{BIOPSY}$$

where T_{BIOPSY} is the time interval between injection and biopsy. The timing of the observation is important. It must be long enough to see sufficient redistribution of the BrdUrd-labelled cells such that the divided cells can be discriminated from those still moving through S phase. It is important that evidence of BrdUrd-labelled cells in G_1 is observed, otherwise the estimation of T_S may not be reliable, possibly due to a long $G_2 + M$ period which will weight the RM towards 1.0 and tend to underestimate T_S [19]. However, it is also not advisable that the period between injection and biopsy be too long, otherwise the measurement of RM will be performed on too few cells as the majority will have divided. It is our experience that a period of between 4 and 8 h between injection and biopsy yields suitable profiles for T_S estimation.

In profiles, obtained some time after the injection of BrdUrd, the LI calculated as the percentage of cells which have incorporated BrdUrd will not be the true LI due to cell division. An approximation to the original LI can be made by measuring the number of BrdUrd-labelled cells which have divided ($BrdUrd_{(G1)}$), the total BrdUrd-labelled cells ($BrdURD_{(tot)}$) and the total cell number (Total). The corrected LI will equal:

$$LI = \frac{\left(BrdUrd_{(tot)} - \dfrac{BrdUrd_{(G1)}}{2}\right)}{\left(Total - \dfrac{BrdUrd_{(G1)}}{2}\right)} \times 100$$

Several alternative methods have been proposed to calculate T_S and T_{pot} from a single observation. The most recent procedure has been proposed by White *et al.* [20] and is termed the v function. This procedure attempts to overcome some of the assumptions made in the Begg method using more rigorous mathematical modelling. The term is a function of the fraction of labelled-divided cells at the time of observation and the labelled undivided cells which relates T_S to T_{pot}.

11.1.6 Examples of human tumour profiles

Figure 11.2a shows the DNA profile and Fig. 11.2b the bivariate cytogram of DNA versus BrdUrd obtained from a biopsy of a diploid squamous-cell tumour from the retromolar area removed 5.6 h after the injection of BrdUrd. The DNA profile shows the presence of one DNA stemline and the BrdUrd/DNA profile clearly shows the redistribution of BrdUrd-labelled cells. One population has divided and resides in G_1 at channel 30, whilst the BrdUrd-labelled cells, still progressing through S phase, have increased their DNA content and are skewed towards the G_2 DNA value. The T_S, calculated from this latter population, was estimated to be 8.6 h and the corrected LI was 7.5%. The computed T_{pot} for this tumour was 3.8 days.

The situation is often more complex in solid tumours due to the presence of abnormal DNA stemlines. Fig. 11.2c and d show the DNA profile and bivariate distribution of a squamous-cell tumour from the tonsil subject to biopsy 6 h after injection with BrdUrd; the DNA index was 1.85. The BrdUrd profile shows that the majority of the proliferation is associated with the aneuploid cells, although some proliferating cells were present in the diploid population, indicated by the BrdUrd-labelled cells which have divided at channel 16. In the aneuploid population, the redistribution of BrdUrd-labelled cells around the cell cycle is again clear. Those cells which have divided reside in G_1 at channel 33, whilst those cells still progressing through S phase had increased their DNA content and the resultant distribution is again skewed towards $G_2 + M$. The LI, in this specimen, was 8.4% for the total cell population, but was 11.8% for the aneuploid cells alone. The T_S was calculated for the aneuploid cells and was estimated to be 9.9 h. These two parameters give a T_{pot} for the aneuploid population of only 2.8 days.

11.1.7 Proliferation parameters of human solid tumours

The common thread in all studies of proliferation in human tumours, irrespective of the technique of measurement, has been the heterogeneity of proliferative characteristics both within a single group of tumours and between tumours from different sites of origin [21]. The application of the BrdUrd technique to study proliferation has proven no exception. Indeed, Fig. 11.3 shows that not only is the LI an important variable amongst different tumours, but that the T_S, which was once thought to be relatively constant, also shows considerable heterogeneity. In Fig. 11.3, the median values of T_S vary from less than 10 h in tumours from the head and neck to almost 16 h in the cervix. There is some suggestion that the T_S tends to increase along the aerodigestive tract. It is also evident that tumour groups which have short median T_S values tend to have lower median LIs and vice versa. This general observation tends to suggest, as one might expect, that the length of a cell-cycle phase will determine the probability of seeing a cell in that particular

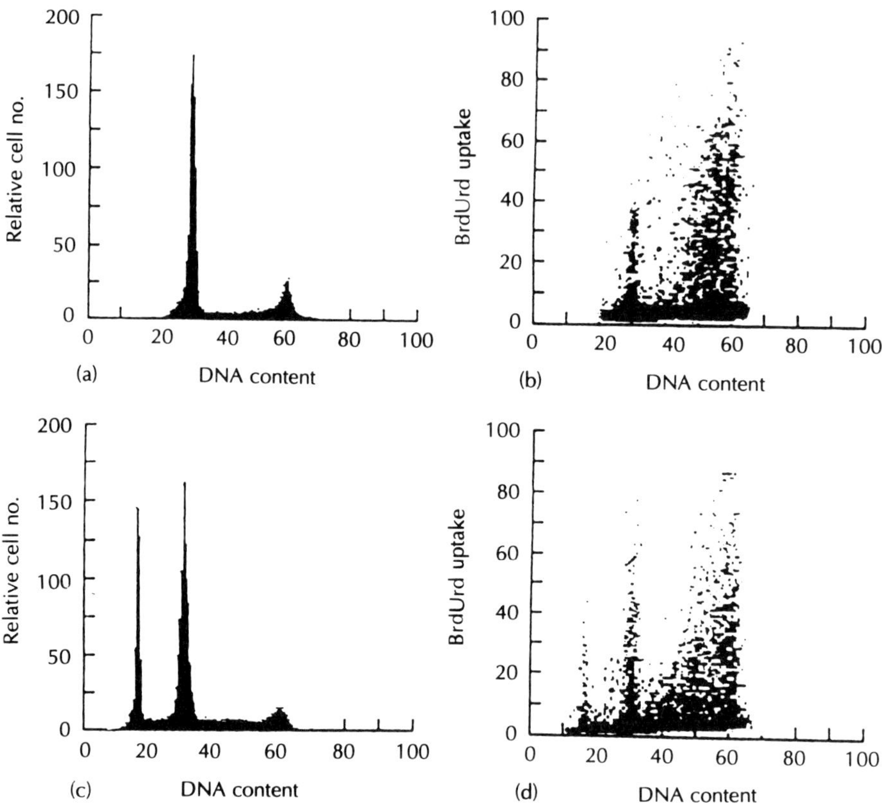

Fig. 11.2 Examples of staining profiles obtained from human solid tumours. (a) The DNA profile; (b) the bivariate distribution of DNA content (*x*-axis) versus 5-bromo, 2-deoxyuridine (BrdUrd) uptake (*y*-axis) of a squamous-cell tumour from the retromolar area biopsied 5.6 h after an injection of BrdUrd. (c) and (d) The DNA profile and bivariate distribution of DNA content and BrdUrd uptake of an aneuploid squamous-cell tumour from the tonsil, biopsied 6 h after injection of BrdUrd.

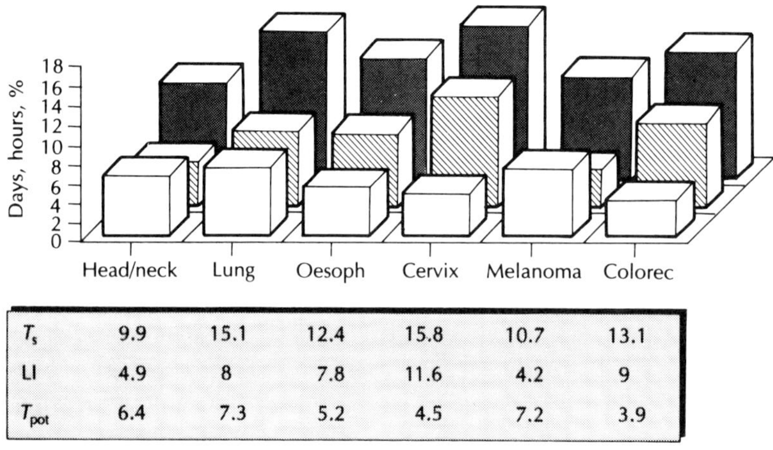

	Head/neck	Lung	Oesoph	Cervix	Melanoma	Colorec
T_s	9.9	15.1	12.4	15.8	10.7	13.1
LI	4.9	8	7.8	11.6	4.2	9
T_{pot}	6.4	7.3	5.2	4.5	7.2	3.9

Fig. 11.3 Comparison of median labelling index (LI; □), duration of S-phase (T_S; ▨) and potential doubling time (T_{pot}; ■) for different groups of human tumours. The bars represent median values for each proliferation parameter in the six major groups of tumours studied. The *y*-axis is interchangeable for LI (%), T_S (h) and T_{pot} (days). The data in each bar represent at least 30 to over 100 tumours studied for each group of tumours.

phase. This again highlights the importance of knowing the cytodynamic data. A single piece of information, such as LI, may be misleading and ambiguous when considered alone. This latter point is important, as a tumour with a high LI but relatively long T_S could give the same T_{pot} as a tumour with a low LI but relatively short T_S. This would appear to be the case, as the median T_{pots} do not vary greatly between the different groups, even though the LI does.

11.1.8 Heterogeneity of proliferation

Median values give an indication that, for instance, colorectal tumours are proliferating more rapidly than lung. However, within each group of tumours there is considerable variation in each of the parameters of proliferation, emphasizing the need to know information on an individual tumour basis. The results obtained in 164 tumours from the head and neck region are summarized as frequency distributions for each cell kinetic parameter in Fig. 11.4. This pattern of variation in each cell kinetic parameter is repeated for each group of tumours. It is clear from Fig. 11.4 that there is tremendous variation in all parameters. The degree of interspecimen heterogeneity is important, as any method which has to rely on a single measurement from biopsy material is open to criticism that the biopsy may not be representative of the tumour as a whole. If the heterogeneity within a specimen approaches or exceeds the heterogeneity between specimens, then it is unlikely that any pretreatment measurement of proliferation will be a good predictor of treatment outcome.

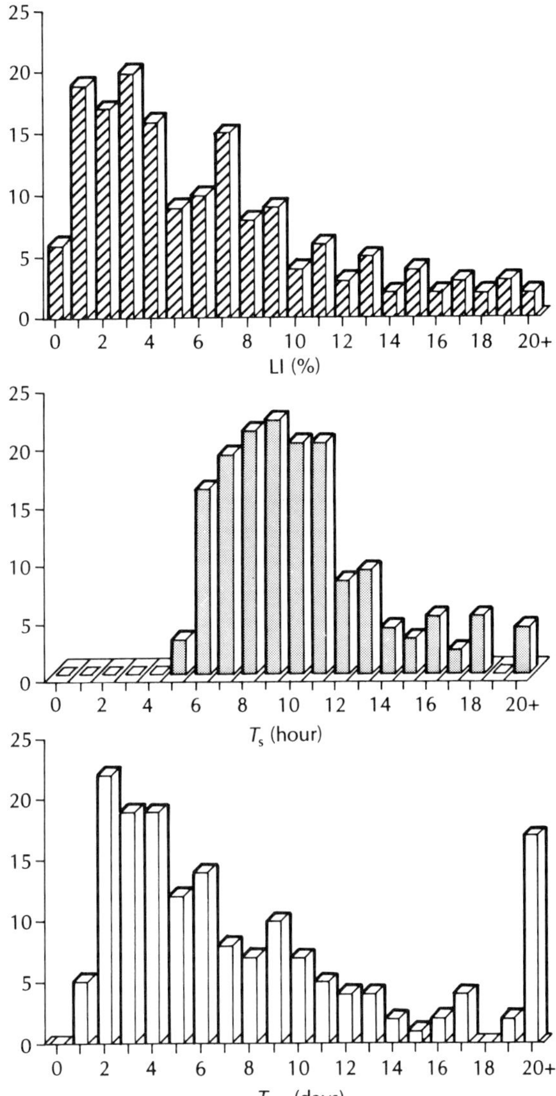

Fig. 11.4 Heterogeneity of proliferation parameters, showing the frequency distribution of labelling index (LI), duration of S-phase (T_S;) and potential doubling time (T_{pot}) for head and neck tumours, showing the variation in each parameter.

We have addressed heterogeneity in a collaborative study on colorectal tumours [22]. In 58 of 100 patients with carcinoma of the colorectum, studied by BrdUrd incorporation, multiple samples (two to six) were taken from each tumour. In these specimens, each parameter showed coefficients of variation (CVs) ranging from 30 to 50%,which does approach the CVs seen in the group as a whole (68%). However, in many ways, this study was the worst possible scenario to relate to biopsy material, as specimens were deliberately chosen from peripheral quadrants and the core of the tumour, which may have been necrotic. In a subset of patients in this study, biopsy-like samples were removed at random from areas of viable, peripheral tumour. In this group of patients, the CVs for each parameter were, in the majority of cases, reduced to a level close to 20%. This level is close to the methodological variation within the assay of about 15%, which has been assessed by processing replicates of single tumours which have been minced randomly.

It is our experience that intertumour heterogeneity has been much more significant than intratumour heterogeneity and that tumours from different sites show different degrees of variability. It is important, in all studies using FCM, that tissue adjacent to the area removed for FCM is studied by histology to assess histopathological features. In addition, we use immunohistochemistry routinely to assess the tissue spatial distribution of proliferation as this information is lost in FCM due to the prerequisite for a single cell suspension. Immunohistochemical localization of BrdUrd furnishes information on the microscopic heterogeneity of the biopsy material as well as the opportunity to calculate LIs based on histopathological discrimination of tumour cells; it is now an integral part of our proliferative classification of tumours.

11.1.9 Proliferation and histopathological features

If proliferation is to be an important prognostic and possibly diagnostic parameter, it must show significant independence from existing clinical parameters. Cellular differentiation has long been identified as an important feature relating natural history to response of tumours. As a general rule, poorly differentiated tumours have been thought to have a shorter history and grow faster than differentiated tumours and, although they may respond more quickly to treatment, they tend to recur locally more rapidly and show distant metastasis sooner. It would not be unreasonable to assume that this was consistent with differences in proliferative characteristics. However, this does not appear to be the case in our studies of squamous-cell cancer of the head and neck [23] or adenocarcinomas of the colorectum [22].

Figure 11.5 shows the distribution of individual proliferation parameters and DNA index as a function of histological grade in squamous-cell cancer of the head and neck. It is apparent that there is overlapping spread of each parameter throughout the four grades defined by Broders [24], such that a highly differentiated tumour may be proliferating as rapidly or slowly as a poorly differentiated, anaplastic, invading tumour. The only relationship that is apparent is that grade 1 tumours tend to be diploid (75%), whilst there was a preponderance of aneuploidy in grade 2 (37%), 3 (40%) and 4 (35%) tumours.

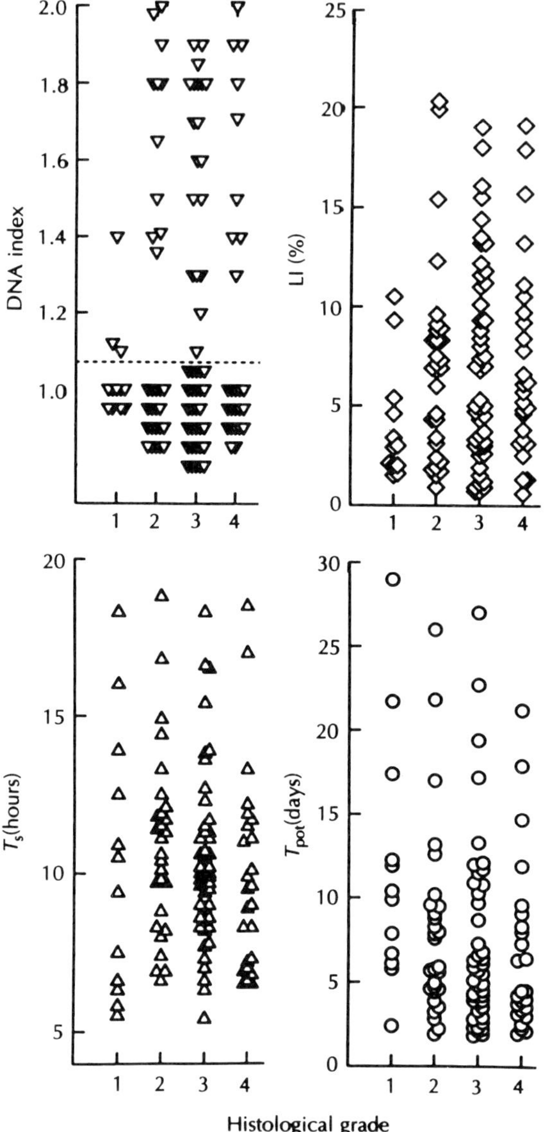

Fig. 11.5 Relationship between proliferation and histological grading in squamous-cell cancer of the head and neck. Data from individual tumours were plotted according to histological grade. The dotted line in the DNA index data represents the discrimination of diploid from aneuploid tumours.

This pattern was repeated in our studies of colorectal adenocarcinomas [22] in which there was no relationship between T_{pot} and either histopathological differentiation or Dukes' classification. In both studies, there was also no apparent relationship with age or sex.

Although T_{pot} shows little relationship with other clinical features in studies outlined above, this may not be the case for other tumour groups. It is well-established that proliferation is associated with stage and nodal status in breast cancer [25].

11.1.10 T_{pot} and clinical outcome

The acid test of T_{pot} measurements will be their ability to predict clinical outcome and whether they are important enough to be used to determine treatment modalities or schedules on an individual patient basis. As stated earlier, there is evidence that suggests that proliferation is important in determining clinical outcome [26] but measurements have yet to influence treatment.

Studies involving T_{pot} measurements are, by definition, prospective and it is too early to assess their clinical utility. However, measurements of T_{pot} are currently incorporated into two major, multicentre, randomized trials. Both of these trials are investigating the therapeutic benefit gained by accelerating radiotherapy compared to conventional fractionation schedules. At Mount Vernon Hospital, Saunders and Dische [27] have pioneered the use of three fractions of 1.5 Gy/day, given over a continuous 12-day period in a schedule known as CHART (continuous, hyperfractionated, accelerated radiotherapy). In a pilot study, this schedule proved to be of substantial benefit when compared to age-matched conventionally treated patients. We have made an initial evaluation of patients treated in this study who also received an injection of BrdUrd. In the CHART-treated patients, there was no significant influence of any of the proliferation parameters on local tumour or survival. This result was as predicted, as the schedule is designed to prevent repopulation during treatment. It is in the conventional, 6- or 7-week treatment regime that rapidly proliferating tumours would be expected to do badly. This latter prediction is now being tested in a multicentre trial, throughout the UK and Europe, of CHART versus conventional treatment.

Preliminary data on the significance of T_{pot} measurements are available from an EORTC trial of accelerated (5 weeks) versus conventional (7 weeks) radiotherapy [28]. Early results show that 'slowly' proliferating tumours ($T_{pot} > 4.2$ days) have a high probability of maintaining local tumour control and survival regardless of the treatment arm, whereas 'fast' proliferating tumours ($T_{pot} < 4.2$ days) showed a significant decrease in local tumour control and survival in the conventional treatment arm but not in the accelerated treatment group.

It will be some time before the significance of T_{pot} measurements is fully established. However, it is encouraging that clinicians are already incorporating them into the clinical trial scenario; this represents a major advance over previous cell kinetic techniques.

11.2 FLUOROCHROME QUENCHING TECHNIQUES

11.2.1 Hoechst/BrdUrd quenching

When BrdUrd is incubated with cells in sufficient concentration to compete with thymidine for incorporation into newly synthesized DNA, the fluorescence of thymidine-specific dyes such as Hoechst 33258 (H33258) or 33342 (H33342) is partly suppressed and no longer proportional to DNA content [7]. At a certain level of BrdUrd incorporation, combined with a certain dye concentration, this fluorescence suppression (quenching) is such that the fluorescence of an S-phase cell stays exactly the same despite an increase in DNA during transit through the cell-cycle phase. Upon mitosis, the fluorescence is halved. By staining cells simultaneously with H33342 and ethidium bromide (EB), whose binding is not compromised by BrdUrd substitution of thymidine, cell-cycle division can be followed for up to three mitotic cycles by the shift in the ratio of H33342/EB binding [29].

A representation of the type of data obtained by this technique is shown in Fig. 11.6. A number of kinetic parameters can be derived by analysing temporarily spaced samples of a growing cell culture. The technique does not have a widespread application in solid tumour research because it is necessary continually to expose cells to 65–100 μM BrdUrd under controlled conditions. However, a

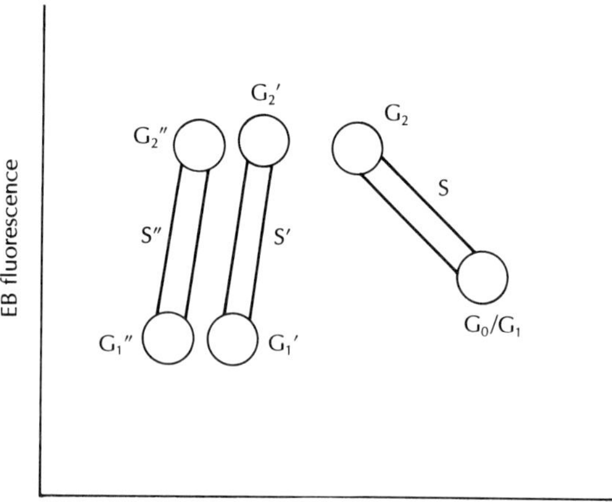

Fig. 11.6 Schematic cytogram of Hoechst 33342 (H33342) 5-bromo, 2-deoxyuridine (BrdUrd) quenching technique. Three successive cell cycles are shown from a population of cells cultured continuously in the presence of BrdUrd. Note that the ratio of DNA of G_2 compared to a G_1 cell, in the first cell cycle (no prime), is 2 on the ethidium bromide (EB) axis but considerably less than 2 on the H33342 axis due to quenching. At the first division, both the H33342 and EB fluorescence is halved, forming the $G_{1'}$ population. No increase in H33342 fluorescence is seen during the second cycle. A third cell cycle can be recognized (G_1'', S′, G_2''), but further cell cycles merge into each other as the effect of H33342 fluorescence halving at division diminishes.

number of highly specific cell-cycle lesions are being defined in human genetic disorders whose common denominator is a disturbance of cellular proliferation. Fanconi's anaemia consists of accumulations of cells in the G_2 compartments of the first and second cell cycles after activation [30]. Elevated G_2 phase accumulations are also displayed by ataxia telangiectasia cells in response to irradiation. The BrdUrd/H33342 technique has proved useful as a clinical test quantitatively to assess cell blocking in the G_2 compartment of these disorders [31].

11.2.2 Differential analysis of Hoechst/BrdUrd quenching

An alternative to the Hoechst quenching technique is to exploit differential fluorescence analysis of DNA fluorochromes detecting BrdUrd-labelled cells [8]. This technique uses pulse-labelled cells (30 min), unlike the quenching method, and two DNA intercalating fluorochromes, H33342 (A-T binding) and mithramycin (MI) (G-C binding). Using dual-wavelength excitation (ultraviolet and 458 nm), blue (H33342) and green-yellow (MI) fluorescence emissions are measured, and a differential amplifier subtracts the blue fluorescence from the green-yellow signal on a cell-by-cell basis; the resulting difference signal must then be amplified. The cells which are in S phase exhibit a significant BrdUrd-H33342 quenching and this results in a greater differential fluorescence signal compared with that of the cells in G_1 and $G_2 + M$ phases.

Although this technique uses much more complicated FCM, it is simple and rapid and requires only one-step staining. It can produce profiles similar to those obtained by the anti-BrdUrd monoclonal antibody method, but it does not require any denaturation steps and therefore minimizes cell loss and, more importantly, can be combined with important cellular markers for DNA, RNA and protein, including cellular antigens.

11.3 DETECTION OF CYCLING AND QUIESCENT CELLS

11.3.1 Multivariate DNA analysis

Nuclear protein

Simultaneous analysis of several cellular components combined with DNA allow the direct assessment of cell growth at various phases of the cell cycle. There is a close coupling of the metabolic patterns of protein content with RNA and DNA content in the maintenance of the state of balanced growth. However, in response to drugs, etc., the cell division patterns can be grossly perturbed, leading to an uncoupling of transcriptional and translational activity. The importance of individual cell-cycle-related proteins will be discussed in the next section. However, combining DNA with a total nuclear protein measurement can provide information on subpopulations with the cell cycle [9]. This is usually achieved by staining RNAse-treated isolated nuclei with FITC (protein) and PI (DNA). The combination can subdivide the basic cell cycle into seven components by recognizing both early and late G_1, S and G_2 compartments, as well as mitotic cells, due to the variation in nuclear protein content with cell-cycle position. It has also been found that nuclei accumulate excess amounts of proteins in response to stress [32] (heat or osmotic shock). The technique is useful to study the redistribution of a population of cells following perturbation with drugs or ionizing radiation, and may be useful to predict the response of a cell population to hyperthermia. The technique has been applied to solid tumours [33].

RNA

Biochemical measurements have indicated that non-cycling cells have lower RNA content than cycling cells. The simultaneous detection of RNA and DNA has been studied extensively by Darzynkiewicz and colleagues [10] using the metachromatic fluorochrome acridine orange (AO). An alternative approach has been to use a combination of H33342 (DNA) and pyronin y (RNA) [34]. In a variety of mammalian cell lines, studied during growth and quiescence, these FCM techniques have shown none or minimal overlap in RNA values of the quiescent cells compared to cycling cells, the quiescent cells having significantly lower levels.

The studies with AO exploit the differential staining of double-stranded versus single-stranded nucleic acids. The dye intercalates with double-stranded DNA and fluoresces green (530 nm maximum emission) when excited with blue (488 mm) light, whilst condensation of the fluorochrome results from the interaction with RNA. The luminescence of these condensed products emits at red wavelengths (640 nm).

The technique requires stringent staining protocols. First, it is necessary to denature selectively any double-stranded RNA to ensure that all cellular RNA is single-stranded but that DNA remains in its double helical conformation. This is usually achieved with chelating agents (ethylene diaminetetraacetic acid; EDTA, citrate) in the presence of AO. Alternatively, permeabilization by detergent (Triton X-100) in the presence of 0.08 N HCl followed by AO and chelating agents can improve then differential stainability of RNA versus DNA [35]. AO has two functions in this reaction: it selectively denatures double-stranded RNA and then differentially stains RNA. It is the higher affinity of AO to single-stranded RNA than to single-stranded DNA that is responsible for the specificity of the denaturing reaction. However, this can only be achieved over a narrow concentration range of free dye. If the concentration is too high, DNA can be denatured; if too low, there may be incomplete denaturation of RNA.

The methods can be applied to a variety of cell types. However, cells of the lymphocyte or monocyte lineage stain particularly well. Correlated measurements of RNA and DNA have distinguished several distinct compartments of the cell cycle in addition to the traditional four main phases of the cycle; Darzynkiewicz and colleagues were able to classify 12 different compartments [36]. RNA measurements have been introduced into the clinic for the characterization of leukaemias, lymphomas, myelomas and other proliferative diseases (see Darzynkiewicz [37] for review). RNA has been shown to be a strong prognostic parameter in the malignancies so far studied.

11.3.2 DNA denaturation and accessibility *in situ*

DNA, in chromatin, is stabilized by interactions with histones and other nuclear proteins. Studies on the stability of DNA *in situ* may prove an insight into chromosome structure. There are two main methods to probe these interactions: (i) measurement of DNA sensitivity to denaturation, under acid conditions, using AO [11]; and (ii) studies of DNA accessibility to several DNA-binding fluorochromes after HCl extraction of histones [38].

DNA sensitivity to denaturation

This technique has shown that DNA sensitivity to denaturation is closely correlated with the degree of chromatin condensation. Studies have shown great differences in DNA stability between various cell types, cells in different phases of the cell cycle, differentiated versus non-differentiated cells and even within individual chromosomes. Again this technique, as with the differential DNA versus

RNA staining, depends on the shift in wavelength emission of AO when binding to double-stranded or single-stranded nucleic acids. In this case, RNA is removed by RNAse treatment and partial denaturation of DNA achieved by acid or heat. The application of this technique to cell kinetics is that cell-cycle subcompartments can be identified. Mitotic cells are very sensitive to denaturation, quiescent cells have condensed chromatin and late G_1 and early S-phase cells are most resistant to the denaturing conditions. A potential problem with AO, which has restricted its use in solid tumours, is that its specificity for nucleic acids is not absolute; the dye can stain other polyanions as well (glycosaminoglycans or proteoglycans). Tissues which contain normal fibroblasts, mast cells, chrondrocytes and keratinocytes may have unacceptably high fluorescence.

DNA accessibility

DNA accessibility to different fluorochromes is restricted by chromosomal proteins. The extent of DNA available for binding depends not only on the size of the probe but also chromatin structure in differentiated or quiescent cells [38]. The smaller intercalating probes (AO, EB) demonstrate a change in binding during differentiation, whilst the larger probes (actinomycin D), with bulky chains protruding into the grooves of DNA, show lowered fluorescence in quiescent and mitotic cells.

11.4 CELL PROLIFERATION-ASSOCIATED PROTEINS

A number of monoclonal antibody probes are now available which recognize cellular proteins associated with proliferation and which can be measured by FCM. Using the quantitative power of FCM and simultaneous staining of total DNA content, the cell-cycle expression of these proteins can be elucidated in experimental cell systems and tumours. Some of these proteins may be expressed in response to changes in the proliferative activity of the population, whilst others are oncogene products probably having a direct regulatory function in cell proliferation, differentiation and transformation. The study of these proteins may provide a better understanding of the mechanisms regulating cell growth but, on a more practical level, they can provide intrinsic cell kinetic parameters which may have prognostic value.

Figure 11.7 summarizes the cell-cycle distribution of a number of proliferation-associated proteins which have been studied using FCM [39]. All of these proteins have been studied in experimental systems and some have found their way into clinical studies. They represent a diverse collection of proteins of cell membrane, cytoplasmic and nuclear localization and function as receptors, DNA synthesis-involved enzymes and proteins, oncogene products as well as epitopes of unknown origin. This list is by no means exhaustive, but represents the most commonly studied proteins.

11.4.1 Transferrin receptor

Transferrin is the major serum iron-binding protein and is required by proliferating cells to transport

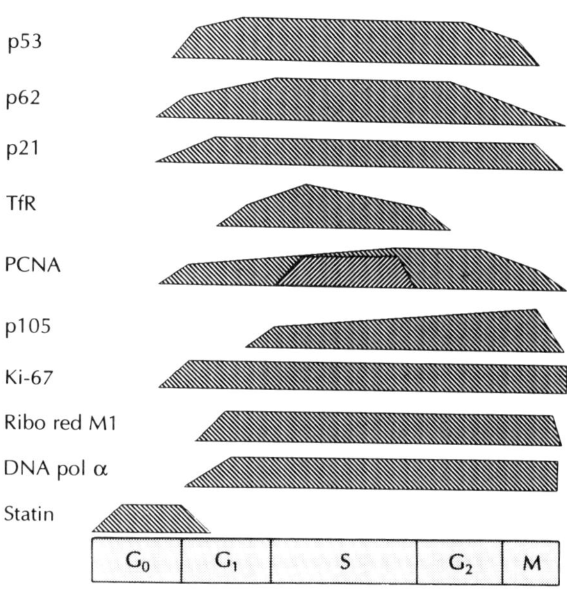

Fig. 11.7 Schematic representation of cell-cycle distribution of proliferation-associated proteins. The shape of each distribution is an approximation of results obtained from flow cytometry studies. Two distributions appear for proliferating cell nuclear antigen, which can show differential staining depending on fixation and processing. Adapted from Danova *et al.* [39].

iron into the cell [40]. The transferrin receptor (TfR) is a 180 kDa dimeric glycoprotein located in the cell membrane responsible for the endocytosis of iron. Evidence suggests that TfR is coupled to the initiation of DNA synthesis and is strongly correlated with SPF in a variety of leukaemias and solid tumours [41].

11.4.2 Ribonucleotide reductase M_1 subunit

Ribonucleotide reductase catalyses the first unique, rate-limiting step in DNA synthesis, the conversion of ribonucleotides to deoxyribonucleotides [42], and is composed of two subunits. Levels of the M_1 subunit are sustained throughout the proliferating cell cycle and it is absent or low in quiescent cells [43]. The M_1 subunit is induced by mitogen stimulation of G_0 cells and has been shown to have a half-life of 24 h. Most work has been restricted to *in vitro* studies as the protein is localized in the cytoplasm and detection is highly dependent upon fixation and processing procedures.

11.4.3 DNA polymerase α

Several antibodies have been raised against DNA polymerase α [44], which is thought to be the polymerase responsible for the synthesis of the first nascent strands of DNA at the origin of replication and is then subsequently responsible for lagging strand synthesis [45]. It would appear that the distribution of this enyme is intranuclear in proliferating cells and correlates with growth fraction. In resting cells, diffuse staining is seen throughout the cytoplasm. The detection of DNA polymerase α is fixation- and processing-dependent, requiring fixation in 4% paraformaldehyde.

11.4.4 Ki-67

The monoclonal antibody, Ki-67 [46], recognizing a proliferation-associated nuclear antigen, is probably the most widely used of the proliferation probes. Yet the epitope recognized by the antibody has not been fully characterized, although it is thought to be a non-histone protein which is highly susceptible to protease treatment. However, even though the fixation and permeabilization procedures are critical for artefact-free detection of the antigen, there is good correlation between Ki-67 reactivity and proliferation through the cell cycle [47,48]. Ki-67 staining can be used for a wide variety of studies in cell cultures, stimulated lymphocytes and solid tumours. Much of the work with Ki-67 has utilized immunohistochemical procedures, where it offers a convenient estimation of proliferation capacity and has shown clinical relevance in a variety of tumours, including breast cancer and non-Hodgkin's lymphoma [49]. FCM studies with Ki-67 suffer from the lability of the antigen and care must be taken in the preparation of cells or nuclei from solid tumours and the fixation and staining conditions. Potentially, FCM could provide a rapid and quantitative technique to study Ki-67 and has the advantage that it could be combined with other markers of proliferation, such as PCNA, to give even more detailed information [50].

11.4.5 PCNA

PCNA is a 36 kDa nuclear polypeptide essential for the correct functioning of DNA polymerase δ, the polymerase involved in leading strand DNA synthesis [45]. PCNA appears to inhibit the action of poly (adenosine diphosphate-ribose) polymerase, an elongation inhibitor.

Synthesis of PCNA occurs in late G_1 and throughout S phase, although the protein is detectable throughout the proliferating cell cycle due to its long half-life (20 h) [51]. It persists in growth-arrested cells but is absent in long-term quiescent cells [52]. It exists in at least two forms, one which is tightly bound to chromatin and associated with S-phase cells, and a second which shows diffuse staining throughout the nucleoplasm [52]. The existence of two forms can be exploited using different fixation and permeabilization conditions to detect total PCNA, which correlates to an index similar to growth fraction or to detect tightly bound PCNA, which is highly S-phase specific [53]. Figure 11.8 shows results from our own laboratory in which V79 Chinese hamster fibroblasts were stained with the monoclonal antibody PC10 [54] as intact methonal fixed cells or as Non-Idet P-40 extracted nuclei with postfixation in methanol. Virtually all

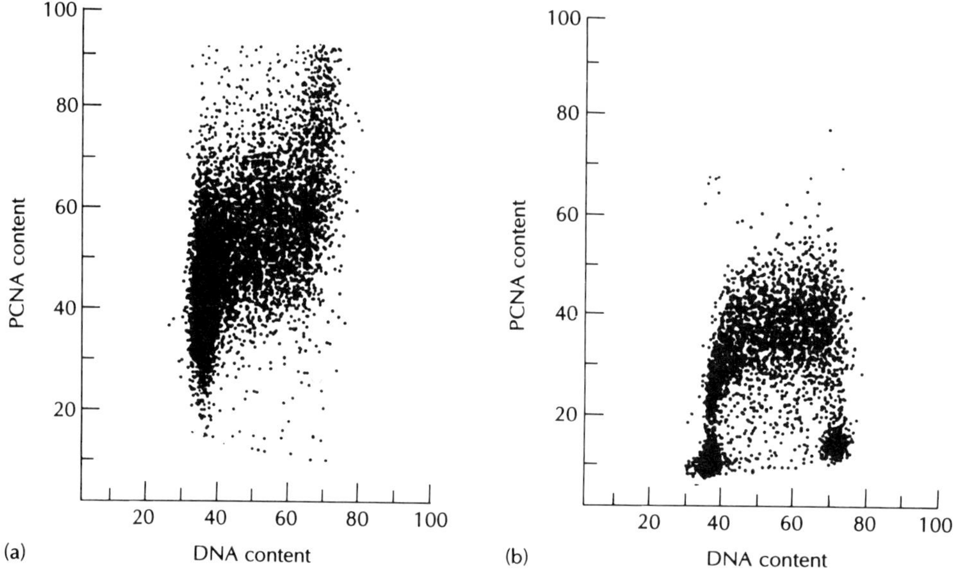

Fig. 11.8 Differential detection of total proliferating cell nuclear antigen (PCNA) and chromatin-associated PCNA in V79 cells using the monoclonal antibody PC10. Bivariate cytograms of DNA content (x-axis) versus PC10 content (y-axis) for intact methanol-fixed cells (a) and Non-Idet P-40 extracted nuclei postfixed in methanol (b). All intact cells stain with PCNA, whilst positivity is restricted to S-phase cells in the extracted nuclei. It should be noted that these profiles were obtained at different photomultiplier settings, such that the fluorescence intensity of the S-phase nuclei is 15% of that obtained in S-phase intact cells.

intact cells show positivity to PC10, which increases through the cell cycle. This is similar to the type of profile which would be obtained with many of the proteins described in this section. However, detergent extraction and postfixation produce profiles almost identical to a BrdUrd pulse-labelling and are highly S-phase specific, with G_1 and G_2 cells being essentially negative.

There is some confusion in this area at present as the monoclonal antibodies which have been raised appear to recognize different epitopes to the autoantibodies which were originally described in patients with systemic lupus erythematosus, and unexpected staining distributions have been described in tissue sections of some human tumours [55]. However, with proper characterization in experimental systems using FCM, PCNA detection offers a versatile approach to the study of proliferation.

11.4.6 p105

p105 is a component of interchromatin granules and has been studied by FCM [56]. Expression of p105 varies widely in different phases of the cell cycle. It has been shown that expression increases as cells progress from early to late G_1 and from G_2 to mitosis.

p105 detection has been studied in a variety of human tumours both prospectively and retrospectively from paraffin-embedded material. In colonic cancer, p105 measurements have been used to complement histological grading and are currently being related to histology and clinical outcome [57].

11.4.7 Statin

Unlike the other proteins cited in this section, statin is characteristically found in non-proliferating cells and its expression disappears upon cell activation [58]. A monoclonal antibody (S-30) was produced by immunization of a mouse with the detergent-insoluble extract of senescent human fibroblasts. The antibody was shown to recognize a 57 kDa nuclear protein which has been termed statin. Statin appears to be a component of the nuclear envelope in senescent and quiescent cells. The expression of statin during the cell cycle is inversely correlated to PCNA and evidence suggests that statin may also exist in two forms, detergent-soluble and -insoluble [59]. The expression of this protein could be used as a marker for quiescent cells in solid tumours.

11.4.8 p62 c-*myc* oncoprotein

The c-*myc* gene codes for a 62 kDa DNA-binding protein. Monoclonal and polyclonal antibodies have been used to study the expression of p62 in a wide variety of neoplasms, including cervix, testis, colonic, ovarian, uterine cervix and breast cancer, using both fresh and archival material [60–63]. The results obtained with c-*myc* detection are complex as it has been shown to correlate with differentiation, proliferation and malignant transformation in different systems. In normal testicular tissue, the p62 level was low and was elevated in teratoma and seminoma [60]. On the contrary, p62 levels were much higher in normal cervical mucosa compared to uterine carcinomas, in which there were decreasing p62 levels as tumours progressed from stage I to stage III [63]. Recently, we have failed to demonstrate any relationship between p62 expression and T_{pot} in colorectal cancer [64].

11.4.9 p21 *ras* oncoprotein

The expression of the c-*ras* protein, p21, is not strictly related to cell-cycle phases. It is a 21 kDa protein localized on the inner surface of the cell membrane and binds with high affinity to guanosine triphosphate or diphosphate, functioning as a signal transducer linking extracellular growth factors to second messenger systems, resulting in the initiation of DNA synthesis. This function is impaired in tumour cells in which p21 has undergone transformation; this can result in inappropriate proliferation [65]. The overexpression of p21 in a variety of human tumours has been related to the malignant phenotype. However, in terms of proliferation, it has been demonstrated that injection of cells with anti-p21 antibodies prevents their entry into S phase [66], whilst injection of the oncogene form of H-*ras* results in rapid proliferation of quiescent cells [67].

11.4.10 p53

This 375 amino acidic nuclear phosphoprotein was first detected because it formed a tight complex with SV40 large-T antigen [68]. Early studies suggested the p53 was a dominant transforming oncogene able to immortalize primary cells and bring about full transformation in combination with an activated *ras* gene [69]. It is now apparent that transforming p53 genes are all mutant and that the wild-type gene can suppress the activity of transforming genes in transfection assays. It has also been demonstrated that growth suppression induced by wild-type p53 protein selectively down-regulated PCNA expression. Abnormalities on p53 expression have been reported in a number of tumour types [70,71] and it would appear that p53 is one of the most common proto-oncogenes to undergo mutation. The relevance of p53 to proliferation characteristics of solid tumours has yet to be established but is the subject of much current investigation.

11.5 CONCLUSION

FCM can now offer a myriad of approaches to study proliferation in tumour cells, ranging from overt cell kinetic measurements to the more subtle investigation of individual proliferation-associated proteins. Many of these measurements should be regarded as proliferation indices and should not have a descriptive cell kinetic term, such as growth fraction, ascribed to them. This is particularly relevant to the proliferation proteins whose expression correlates with the progression from a quiescent to a proliferating state *in vitro*, but whose expression in cells going into quiescence is not known in human tumours. FCM has many attributes, but it must always be remembered that cell morphological information is lost and interpretation of diploid tumours must be viewed with caution. It is important to combine FCM with immunohistochemical studies if a complete understanding of individual tumour proliferation is to be gained.

Acknowledgements

This work is supported by the Cancer Research Campaign. I would like to acknowledge the contribution made to this work by my late colleague and friend Nic McNally and by Christine Martindale at the Gray Laboratory. These studies would not be possible without the enthusiasm of our clinical colleagues, Professor Stanley Dische and Dr Michele Saunders, at the Marie Curie Research Wing, Mr Hamish Laing in the Department of Plastic Surgery, Mount Vernon Hospital, Northwood, and Mr David Rew at Southampton General Hospital. I would like to thank Mrs Dorothy Brown for preparation of the manuscript.

References

1 Mendelsohn ML. The attributes and applications of flow cytometry. In: Laerum OD, Lindmo T, Thorud E (eds) *Flow Cytometry*, vol. IV. Oslo: Universitetsforlaget, 1980: 15–27.
2 Howard A, Pelc SR. Nuclear incorporation of ^{32}P as demonstrated by autoradiographs. *Exp Cell Res* 1951; 2: 178–187.
3 Taylor JH, Woods PS, Hughes WL. The organisation and duplication of chromosomes using tritiated thymidine. *Proc Soc Natl Acad Sci USA* 1957; 43: 122–128.
4 Quastler H, Sherman FG. Cell population kinetics in the intestinal epithelium of the mouse. *Exp Cell Res* 1959; 17: 420–428.
5 Steel GG. *Growth Kinetics of Tumours*. Oxford: Clarendon Press, 1977.
6 Wilson GD, McNally NJ, Dische S *et al.* Measurement of cell kinetics in human tumours *in vivo* using bromodeoxyuridine incorporation and flow cytometry. *Br J Cancer* 1988; 58: 423–431.
7 Latt SA. Microfluorometric detection of deoxyribonucleic acid replication in human metaphase chromosomes. *Proc Soc Natl Acad Sci USA* 1973; 70: 3395–3402.
8 Crissman HA, Steinkamp JA. A new method for rapid and sensitive detection of bromodeoxyuridine in DNA-replicating cells. *Exp Cell Res* 1987; 173: 256–261.
9 Roti Roti JL, Higashikubo R, Blair OC, Uygur N. Cell-cycle position and nuclear protein content. *Cytometry* 1982; 3: 91–96.
10 Traganos F, Darzynkiewicz Z, Sharpless T, Melamed MR. Simultaneous staining of ribonucleic and deoxyribonucleic acids in unfixed cells using acridine organise in a flow cytofluorometric system. *J Histochem Cytochem* 1977; 25: 45–46.
11 Darzynkiewicz Z, Traganos F, Sharpless T, Melamed MR. Cell cycle-related changes in nuclear chromatin of stimulated lymphocytes as measured by flow cytometry. *Cancer Res* 1977; 37: 4635–4640.
12 Gratzner HG. Monoclonal antibody to 5-bromo and 5-iododeoxyuridine: a new reagent for detection of DNA replication. *Science* 1982; 218: 474–475.
13 Dolbeare F, Gratzner HG, Pallavicini M, Gray JW. Flow cytometric measurement of total DNA content and incorporated bromodeoxyuridine. *Proc Soc Natl Acad Sci* 1983; 80, 5573–5577.
14 Begg AC, McNally NJ, Shrieve DC, Karcher H. A method to measure the duration of DNA synthesis and the potential doubling time from a single sample. *Cytometry* 1985; 6: 620–626.
15 Wilson GD, McNally NJ, Dische S *et al.* Measurement of cell kinetics in human tumours *in vivo* using bromodeoxyuridine incorporation and flow cytometry. *Br J Cancer* 1988; 58: 423–431.
16 Withers HR, Taylor JMG, Maciejewski B. The hazard of accelerated tumour clonogen repopulation during radiotherapy. *Acta Oncol* 1988; 27: 131–146.
17 Taylor JMG, Withers HR, Mendenhall WM. Dose–time considerations of head and neck squamous cell carcinomas treated with irradiation. *Radiother Oncol* 1990; 17: 95–102.
18 Fowler JF. Potential for increasing the differential response between tumours and normal tissues: can proliferation rate be used? *Int J Radiat Oncol Biol Phys* 1986; 12: 641–645.
19 Begg AC. Derivation of cell kinetic parameters from human tumours after labelling with bromodeoxyuridine or iododeoxyuridine. In: Denekamp J, Hirst DG (eds) *The Scientific Basis of Modern Radiotherapy*. London: British Institute of Radiology Report 1989; 19: 113–119.
20 White RA, Terry NHA, Meistrich ML, Calkins DP. Improved method of computing potential doubling time from flow cytometric data. *Cytometry* 1990; 11: 314–317.
21 Meyer JS. Cell kinetic measurements of human tumours. *Hum Pathol* 1982; 13: 874–877.
22 Rew DA, Wilson GD, Taylor I, Weaver PC. Proliferation characteristics of human colorectal carcinomas measured *in vivo*. *Br J Surg* 1991; 78: 60–66.
23 Dische S, Saunders MI, Bennett MH, Wilson GD, McNally NJ. Cell proliferation in squamous cancer. *Radiother Oncol* 1989; 15: 19–23.
24 Broders AC. The microscopic grading of cancer. In: Pack GT, Livington EM (eds) *The Treatment of Cancer and Allied Diseases*, vol. 1. New York: Paul B. Hoeber, 1940: 19–41.
25 Mcguire WL, Dressler LG. Emerging impact of flow cytometry in predicting recurrence and survival in breast cancer patients. *J Nat Cancer Inst* 1985; 75: 405–410.
26 Tubiana M, Courdi A. Cell proliferation kinetics in human solid tumours; relation to probability of meta-

static dissemination and long term survival. *Radiother Oncol* 1989; 15: 1–18.
27 Saunders MI, Dische S. Radiotherapy employing three fractions each day over a continuous period of 12 days. *Br J Radiol* 1986; 59: 523–525.
28 Begg AC, Hofland I, Moonen L. *et al.* The predictive value of cell kinetic measurements in a European trial of accelerated fractionation in advanced head and neck tumours: an interim report. *Int J Radiat Oncol Biol Phys* 1990; 19: 1449–1453.
29 Rabinovitch PS, Kubbies M, Chem YC, Schindler D, Hoehn H, BrdU-Hoechst flow cytometry: a unique tool for quantitative cell cycle analysis. *Exp Cell Res* 1988; 174: 309–318.
30 Kubbies M, Schindler D, Hoehn H, Rabinovitch PS. Cell cycle kinetics by BrdU-Hoechst flow cytometry: an alternative to the differential metaphase labelling technique. *Cell Tissue Kinet* 1985; 18: 551–559.
31 Schindler D, Kubbies M, Hoehn H, Schinzel A, Rabinovitch PS. Presymptomatic diagnosis of Fanconi's anaemia. *Lancet* 1985; ii: 947–949.
32 Roti Roti JL, Winward RT. The effects of hyperthermia on the protein-to-DNA ratio of isolated HeLa cell chromatin. *Radiat Res* 1978; 74: 159–169.
33 Pollack A, Moulis H, Bloxck NK, Irwin GL. Quantitation of cell kinetic responses using simultaneous flow cytometry measurements of DNA and nuclear protein. *Cytometry* 1984; 5: 473–481.
34 Shapiro HM. Flow cytometric estimation of DNA and RNA content in intact cells stained with Hoechst 33342 and pyronin Y. *Cytometry* 1982; 2: 143–150.
35 Darzynkiewicz Z, Traganos F, Sharpless T, Melamed MR. Lymphocyte stimulation: a rapid multiparameter analysis. *Proc Natl Acad Sci USA* 1976; 73: 2881–2886.
36 Darzynkiewicz Z, Traganos F, Kapuscinski J, Staiano-Coico L, Melamed MR. New cell cycle compartments identified by flow cytometry. *Cytometry* 1980; 1: 98–108.
37 Darzynkiewicz Z. Cellular RNA content a feature correlated with cell kinetics and tumor prognosis. *Leukemia* 1988; 2: 777–787.
38 Darzynkiewicz Z, Traganos F, Kapuscinski J, Staiano-Coico L, Melamed MR. Accessibility of DNA *in situ* to various fluorochromes: relationship to chromatin changes during erythroid differentiation of Friend leukaemia cells. *Cytometry* 1984; 5: 355–363.
39 Danova M, Riccardi A, Mazzini G. Cell cycle-related proteins and flow cytometry. *Haematologica* 1990; 75: 252–264.
40 Aisen P, Brown EB. Structure and function of transferrin. *Prog Hematol* 1989; 9: 25–56.
41 Sutherland R, Delia D, Schneider C *et al.* Ubiquitous cell-surface glycoprotein on tumor cells is proliferation-associated receptor specific for transferrin. *Proc Natl Acad Sci USA* 1981; 78: 4515–4519.
42 Thelander L, Reichard P. Reduction of ribonucleotides. *Annu Rev Biochem* 1979; 48: 133–158.
43 Mann GJ, Musgrove EA, Fox RM, Thelander L. Ribonucleotide reductase M1 subunit in cellular proliferation quiescence and differentiation. *Cancer Res* 1988; 48: 5151–5156.
44 Alama A, Nicolin A, Conte PF, Drewinko B. Evaluation of growth fractions with monoclonal antibodies to human alpha-DNA polymerase. *Cancer Res* 1987; 47: 1892–1896.
45 Tsurimoto T, Stillman B. Multiple replication factors augment DNA synthesis by the two eukaryotic DNA polymerases alpha and delta. *Embo J* 1989; 8: 3883–3889.
46 Gerdes J, Lemke H, Baisch H, Wacker HH, Schwab U, Stein H. Cell cycle analysis of a cell proliferation associated with human nuclear antigen defined by the monoclonal antibody Ki-67. *J Immunol* 1984; 133: 1710–1715.
47 Baisch H, Gerdes J. Simultaneous staining of exponentially growing versus plateau phase cells with the proliferation-associated antibdy Ki-67 and propidium iodide: analysis by flow cytometry. *Cell Tissue Kinet* 1987; 20: 387–391.
48 Sasaki K, Murakami T, Kawasaki M, Takahashi M. The cell cycle associated change of the Ki-67 reactive nuclear antigen expression. *J Cell Physiol* 1987; 133: 578–584.
49 Hall PA, Levison DA. Assessment of cell proliferation in histological material. *J Clin Pathol* 1990; 43: 184–192.
50 Landberg G, Tan EM, Roos G. Flow cytometric multiparameter analysis of proliferating cell nuclear antigen/cyclin and Ki-67 antigen. A new view of the cell cycle. *Exp Cell Res* 1990; 187: 111–118.
51 Bravo R, MacDonald-Bravo H. Change in the nuclear distribution of cyclin (PCNA) but not its synthesis depend on DNA replication. *Embo J* 1985; 4: 655–661.
52 Bravo R, MacDonald-Bravo H. Existence of two populations of cyclin/proliferating cell nuclear antigen during the cell cycle: association with DNA replication sites. *J Cell Biol* 1987; 105: 1549–1554.
53 Kurki P, Ogata K, Tan EM. Monoclonal antibodies to proliferating cell nuclear antigen (PCNA)/cyclin as probes for proliferating cells by immunofluorescence microscopy and flow cytometry. *J Immunol Methods* 1988; 109: 49–59.
54 Waseem NH, Lane DP. Monoclonal antibody analysis of PCNA structural conservation and detection of nucleolar form. *J Cell Sci* 1990; 96: 121–129.
55 Hall P, Levison DA, Woods AL *et al.* Proliferating cell nuclear antigen (PCNA) immunolocalisation in paraffin sections: an index of cell proliferation with evidence of deregulated expression in some neoplasms. *J Pathol* 1990; 164: 285–294.
56 Clevenger CV, Epstein AL, Bauer KD. Quantitative analysis of a nuclear antigen in interphase and mitotic cells. *Cytometry* 1987; 8: 280–286.
57 Bauer KD, Clevenger CV, Endow RK, Murad T, Epstein

AL, Scarpelli DG. Simultaneous nuclear antigen and DNA content quantitation using paraffin embedded colonic tissue and multiparameter flow cytometry. *Cancer Res* 1986; 46: 2428–2434.

58 Wang E, Krueger JG. Application of a unique monoclonal antibody as a marker for nonproliferating subpopulations of cells of some tissue. *J Histochem Cytochem* 1985; 33: 587–594.

59 Ching G, Wang E. Characterisation of two populations of statin and the relationship of their synthesis to the steady state of cell proliferation. *J Cell Biol* 1990; 110: 255–259.

60 Sikora K, Evan GI, Steward K, Watson JV. Detection of the c-*myc* oncogene product in testicular cancer. *Br J Cancer* 1985; 52: 171–174.

61 Watson JV, Sikora K, Evan GI. A simultaneous flow cytometric assay for c-*myc* oncoprotein and DNA in nuclei from paraffin embedded material. *J Immunol Methods* 1985; 83: 179–192.

62 Locker AP, Dowle CS, Ellis IO *et al.* C-*myc* oncogene product expression and prognosis in operable breast cancer. *Br J Cancer* 1989; 60: 669–672.

63 Hendy-Ibbs P, Cox H, Evan GI, Watson JV. Flow cytometric quantitation of DNA and c-*myc* oncoprotein in archival biopsies of uterine cervix neoplasia. *Br J Cancer* 1987; 55: 275–282.

64 Rew DA, Taylor I, Cox H, Watson JV, Wilson GD. The c-*myc* protein is a marker of DNA synthesis but not of malignancy in human gastrointestinal tissues and tumors. *Br J Surg* 1991; 78: 1080–1083.

65 Willingham MC, Paston I, Shih TY, Scolonick EM. Localisation of the *src* gene product of the Harvey strain of murine sarcoma virus to the plasma membrane of transformed cells by electron microscopic immunocytochemistry. *Cell* 1980; 19: 1005–1014.

66 Mulcahy LS, Smith MR, Stacey DW. Requirement for *ras* proto-oncogene function during serum-stimulated growth of NIH 3T3 cells. *Nature* 1985; 313: 241–244.

67 Feramisco JR, Gross M, Kamata T, Rosenberg M, Sweet RW. Microinjection of the oncogene form of the human H-*ras* (T-24) protein results in rapid proliferation of quiescent cells. *Cell* 1984; 38: 109–112.

68 Lane DP, Crawford LV. T antigen is bound to a host protein in SV40-transformed cells. *Nature (Lond)* 1979; 278: 261–263.

69 Parada LF, Land H, Weinberg RA, Wolf D, Rotter V. Co-operation between gene encoding p53 tumour antigen and *ras* in cellular transformation. *Nature (Lond)* 1984; 312: 649–651.

70 Baker SJ, Fearon ER, Nigro JM *et al.* Chromosome 17 deletions and p53 gene mutations in colorectal carcinomas. *Science* 1989; 244: 217–221.

71 Iggo R, Gatter K, Bartek J, Lane D, Harris AL. Increased expression of mutant forms of p53 oncogene in primary lung cancer. *Lancet* 1990; 335: 675–679.

12

IMMUNOLOGICAL APPLICATIONS OF FLOW CYTOMETRY

A. D. CROCKARD AND C. S. SCOTT

Flow cytometry was first used in the field of immunology in the early 1970s. From these beginnings in the research laboratory the technology has expanded rapidly so that, 20 years on, flow cytometry has become a routine laboratory procedure in many clinical immunology and haematology laboratories. Perhaps the most significant factor contributing to this development was the introduction of hybridoma technology for the production of monoclonal antibodies. The availability of these standardized reagents allowed dissection of the cellular immune system on the basis of identification of distinctive surface membrane antigens which are present on functionally different but morphologically similar lymphoid cells. From this pioneering work developments came quickly as a result of (i) expansion in the range of monoclonal antibodies available for distinguishing haemopoietic cells and their progenitors; (ii) increasing awareness of the clinical relevance of lymphocyte subset and malignant haemopoietic cell identification and enumeration; and (iii) technical advances in instrumentation.

Flow cytometry has largely replaced conventional fluorescence microscopy for immunophenotypic analyses. With the latter technique, subjective assessments of membrane antigen expression and the delineation of individual cell populations are necessarily restricted to broad divisions, whereas using flow cytometry automated measurements are able reproducibly to discriminate minor differences in membrane fluorescent intensities. As a result, the relative fluorescence of all events analysed can be visualized in the form of a histogram. Consequently, although manual procedures may be able accurately to determine the proportion of cells with membrane fluorescence exceeding any given arbitrary limit (defined as positive), automated analyses are further able to measure the complete spectrum of positivity, the level of fluorescence of antigen-negative populations and the relative fluorescent staining levels of cells with intermediate staining.

The advantages of flow cytometry for the investigation of normal and malignant haemopoietic cells include: (i) a high degree of objectivity; (ii) multiparameter analysis; (iii) an ability to measure and analyse a large (and theoretically unlimited) number of events (cells) as list mode data; (iv) an ability to examine the phenotype characteristic of morphologically defined populations of leucocytes, without interference from contaminating cells which may express the same antigen(s), including the ability to combine and relate morphometric and fluorescence measurements; and (v) a capability to perform complex statistical analyses of acquired data (individual events) which not only provide an indication of the number of cells to which a fluorochrome-conjugated label (e.g., antibody) has been bound but also a semiquantitative measurement of the amount of bound label per cell. This ability to 'visualize' statistically all levels of membrane fluorescence clearly offers significant advantages over traditional 'positive' versus 'negative' assessments.

In this chapter we have concentrated on the application of flow cytometry in the clinical immunology and haematology laboratories. Three areas have been considered in detail:

1 immunofluorescence analyses for immunophenotypic investigations, including methods available, data acquisition and interpretation, quality assurance procedures;
2 immunophenotypic analyses of haemopoietic cells with particular reference to the leukaemias, and enumeration of lymphocyte subsets in acquired immunodeficiency syndrome (AIDS);
3 the use of flow cytometry in various functional and quantitative assays of immune function.

12.1 IMMUNOFLUORESCENT FLOW CYTOMETRIC ANALYSES

Immunophenotypic analyses of lymphoid and other haemopoietic cells comprise the vast majority of flow cytometric applications in the diagnostic immunology or immunohaematology laboratory. A number of elements which are important for successful immunophenotypic analysis have been identified. These include: (i) sample preparation; (ii) immunofluorescence labelling techniques; (iii) data acquisition and interpretation; and (iv) quality control procedures. Each of these is considered in detail below.

12.1.1 Sample preparation

Single cell suspensions are an absolute prerequisite for flow cytometric analyses. The presence of monodispersed cells in peripheral blood and its accessibility have made it the primary source for leucocyte immunophenotyping studies. Removal of excess erythrocytes prior to analysis may be achieved by the use of density gradient separation techniques. Gradients of Ficoll (polysucrose)–Hypaque (sodium metrizoate) are commonly used for this purpose as well as for isolating mononuclear cells (lymphocytes and monocytes). An alternative approach for removal of erythrocytes involves red-cell lysis by hypotonic shock (water, ammonium chloride), or with commercial detergent preparations supplied by the flow cytometer manufacturers. Provided care is exercised to prevent leucocyte damage, these methods offer advantages of simplicity and rapidity and, furthermore, can be performed following immunofluorescent labelling of whole-blood specimens.

Flow cytometric analyses of bone-marrow cells can present difficulties because of the complexity of the tissue. Isolation of low-density cells on Ficoll–Hypaque gradients may be used as a preliminary purification step. However, such is the heterogeneity in terms of cell lineage and maturation that cells isolated by this means must be identified by membrane marker analyses [1,2].

Lymphocytes may be obtained from lymphoid organs (spleen, thymus, lymph nodes) by mechanical disaggregation of the tissue. Further lymphocyte purification and removal of erythrocytes and dead cells may be accomplished with Ficoll–Hypaque gradients.

Practical guidelines for sample preparations from various sources have been published [3].

12.1.2 Immunofluorescent labelling of haemopoietic cells

In this section three aspects of immunofluorescent staining procedures will be discussed: (i) the range of monoclonal antibodies available for identification of leucocyte subpopulations; (ii) choice of fluorochromes; and (iii) labelling techniques.

12.1.3 Monoclonal antibodies

The increasing diversity of available monoclonal antibodies with specificity for leucocyte membrane determinants has necessitated their categorization into groups referred to as clusters of differentiation (CD). Each group of antibodies or cluster is essentially defined according to the nature of the antigen recognized, including its pattern of expression by different haemopoietic elements, and has been devised by a series of four international workshops on human leucocyte differentiation antigens [4–7]. To date, a total of 78 CD groups have been proposed. In this sense, the use of CD nomenclature can be viewed as providing a simplified form of communication, as monoclonal antibodies with different CD numbers show characteristic patterns of leucocyte specificity and generally precipitate a common or related antigen. Although this scheme of taxonomy has led to improvements in interpretation, it is still important to remember that individual monoclonal antibodies assigned to a single cluster do not always react with identical epitopes of the same parent antigen. This is of practical relevance as the expression of any given protein on a cell membrane may vary and some antigen sites can, as a result of differentiation or activation, be partially or completely inaccessible to monoclonal reagents. Consequently, this may occasionally lead to a situation where a cell may show distinct differences in reactivity with two monoclonal reagents of the same generic CD type.

In this chapter the general scheme of CD division proposed by the Fourth International Workshop is followed [7] which broadly subdivides currently defined clusters into: (i) B cell; (ii) T cell; (iii) activation; (iv) natural killer (NK) and non-lineage; (v) myeloid; and (vi) platelet antigens (see Table 12.1). The assignation of individual CD numbers to these groups does not necessarily imply that their reactivity is restricted entirely to leucocytes associated with that group. For example, many T-cell antigens are expressed by NK cells and some activation antigens may also be represented by various antibodies within the B-cell section. Nevertheless, although the relevance of some CD groups is as yet unclear, evidenced by a significant number of provisional (CD Workshop) clusters, there is considerable merit in the strategy of systematically documenting these monoclonal reagents and correlating, as far as possible, antigen expression with cellular function. Indeed, this approach may well prove to be fundamental in understanding the interrelationships between cells of different lineages as well as leading to insights into how cellular function is associated with differentiation. Although these processes are in continual flux, it is possible to delineate to a reasonable extent those antibody clusters which are of particular and current importance to the area of cell identification and characterization. In addition, a number of commercially available monoclonal antibodies remain 'unclustered', even though their reactivity and specificity may be well-understood. Examples of such antibodies include those against membrane determinants such as human leucocyte antigen (HLA)-DR [8]; glycophorin A [9,10]; FMC7 [11]; cytoplasmic enzymes, including myeloperoxidase [12] and elastase [13] and nuclear antigens such as TdT [14,15] and Ki-67 [16,17]. Details of appropriate applications for these reagents will be dealt with in the sections on normal haemopoietic cells and leukaemia classifications.

12.1.4 Fluorochromes

Fluorescein isothiocyanate (FITC) is the most widely used fluorescent probe. It is readily conjugated to proteins and its absorption maximum of 495 nm is close to the 488 nm output of the argon ion laser. Maximum emission occurs at 525 nm over a spectral region ranging from 500 to 600 nm.

The R form of phycoerythrin (PE) has an absorption peak at 490 nm, making it suitable for use with the argon laser. PE has been used most successfully for dual-colour labelling with FITC. Both dyes can be excited with a single laser (at 488 nm) but have sufficiently separate emission maxima (FITC, 525 nm; PE, 575 nm) to permit discrete signal analysis, provided that compensation for spectral overlap is allowed for.

The rhodamine derivative, Texas red (absorption maximum 596 nm) and the phycobiliprotein molecule, allophycocynin (absorption maximum 650 nm) are not efficiently excited at 488 nm. However, when used in a tandem conjugate system where PE is bound to Texas red and/or allophycocyanin, these dyes become readily excitable. Tandem reagents make use of the principle of fluorescence energy transfer whereby the PE component of the complex is excited at 488 nm and its emission at 575 nm is used to excite Texas red and/or allophycocyanin which subsequently emit at 618 and 660 nm, respectively. Thus, in combination with FITC these reagents make three or four colour analyses possible with a single laser source.

The use of the peridinin chlorophyll (PerCP) label (absorption maximum 470 nm; emission maximum 680 nm) in combination with FITC and PE also facilitates three-colour immunofluorescence analyses.

12.1.5 Labelling techniques

There are two basic techniques for immunofluorescence labelling of cells for flow cytometry: (i) direct labelling, which uses fluorochrome-conjugated antibodies; and (ii) indirect labelling, where

Table 12.1 Summary of currently defined monoclonal antibody-defined antigen clusters of differentiation (CD) of particular relevance to normal and leukaemic cell differentiation

Antigen cluster	Reactivity/specificity	Cellular distribution
B-cell antigens		
CD10	100 kDa neutral endopeptidase, CALLA	Early B, intranodal B; granulocytes
CD20	35/37 kDa protein ?involved in ion transport	Mature B
CD21	140 kDa CR2 receptor for C3d (EBV)	Mature B
CD22*	Immunoglobulin supergene family glycoprotein	Intermediate/late B
CD23	45/50 kDa low-affinity Fc-IgE receptor, ?BCGF receptor	Activated B
CD38	45 kDa type II integral glycoprotein	Late B (immunocytes); activated T
CD77	Burkitt's lymphoma-associated neutral glycosphingolipid	Follicle-centre B; activated B
T-cell antigens		
CD1(a–c)	Non-HLA 43–49 kDa membrane glycoproteins associated with β_2m	CD1a–c, immature T. CD1c, mature B
CD2	50 kDa transmembrane glycoprotein, LFA-3 receptor	Immature and mature T; NK cells
CD3*	Molecular complex associated with the T-cell receptor	Some immature and most mature T cells
CD4	59 kDa glycoprotein receptor for class II molecules, HIV receptor	Helper/inducer T cells; monocytes
CD5	67 kDa glycoprotein	Most immature and mature T cells; some B cells
CD7	40 kDa glycoprotein	Most immature and mature T cells
CD8	32 kDa disulphide-linked homo- (α/α) or heterodimer (α/β), receptor for class I molecules	Cytotoxic/suppressor T cells; some NK cells
CD27	110 kDa disulphide-linked homodimer	Major T-cell subset
CD28	44 kDa disulphide-linked homodimer	T-cell subsets
CDw29	Integrin β_1-chain, VLA β chain	Broad leucocyte reactivity
Activation antigens		
CD25	Interleukin-2 receptor	Early T-activation, intermediate/late B
CD26	Diaminopeptidase IV, ?involved in cellular proliferation	Activated T and B cells; macrophages
CD30	105 kDa glycoprotein, Ki-1 antigen	Activated T and B cells; Reed–Sternberg cells
CDw69	Activation inducer molecule	Activated T/B cells and macrophages; NK cells
CD70	Ki-24 antigen	Activated T/B cells; Reed–Sternberg cells
CD71	95 kDa membrane transferrin receptor, associated with cell activation/proliferation	Activated T/B cells and macrophages; proliferating cells
NK and non-lineage antigens		
CD11a	180 kDa α chain glycoprotein subunit of CD18, LFA-1	Most haemopoietic cells
CD11b	165 kDa α chain glycoprotein subunit of CD18, C3bi receptor (CR3)	Most myeloid/NK cells; some lymphoid cells
CD11c	150 kDa α chain glycoprotein subunit of CD18, ?C3bi receptor	Mature granulocytes; monocytes; intermediate/late B
CD16	50–65 kDa membrane receptor for IgG (FcR III)	Granulocytes and NK cells

Continued

Table 12.1 *Continued*

Antigen cluster	Reactivity/specificity	Cellular distribution
CDw32	40 kDa membrane receptor for IgG (FcR II)	Granulocytes; macrophages; B cells; eosinophils
CD45	Protein tyrosine phosphatase IB, leucocyte common antigen	Virtually all haemopoietic cells
CD45RA	220 kDa isoform of CD45 coded by exon A	Monocytes; B cells; unprimed ('virgin') T cells
CD45RO	180 kDa isoform of CD45 not encoded by exons A, B or C	B-cell subset; monocytes; primed ('memory') T cells
CDw52	Campath-1, *O*-linked carbohydrate	Most leucocytes; variable reactivity
CD54	90 kDa intracellular adhesion molecule-1, ligand for LFA-1 (CD11a)	Endothelial cells; many activated cell types
CD56	140 kDa N-CAM molecule	NK subpopulations; some plasma cells
CD57	110 kDa protein	NK subpopulations; some T cells
CD58	40–65 kDa glycoprotein ligand for membrane CD2	Many haemopoietic cell types
Myeloid antigens		
CD13	150 kDa glycoprotein; aminopeptidase N	Most myeloid cells
CD14	Phosphoinositol-linked membrane 55 kDa glycoprotein	Monocytes, macrophages
CD15	X-hapten	Mature granulocytes
CD33	67 kDa transmembrane protein	Most myeloid cells
CD34	105–120 kDa transmembrane glycoprotein	Haemopoietic precursor cells
CD35	Membrane receptor for C3b (CR1)	Granulocytes; monocytes; B cells; NK cells
CD64	75 kDa high-affinity membrane IgG receptor (FcR I)	Monocytes
Platelet antigens		
CD9	24 kDa protein	Early B; monocytes; platelets
CD41	Platelet glycoprotein IIb/IIIa complex (but not the vitronectin receptor)	Platelets
CD42a	GPIX, a 23 kDa glycoprotein non-covalently associated with GPIb	Platelets
CD42b	Platelet GPIb	Platelets
CD61	110 kDa integrin B3 chain (GPIIIa) of the vitronectin receptor and GPIIb/IIIa	Platelets

* Cytoplasmic expression of CD22 is detectable in immature B cells; cytoplasmic expression of CD3 is detectable in immature T cells.
BCGF, B cell growth factor; CALLA, common acute lymphoblastic leukaemia antigen; EBV, Epstein–Barr virus; GP, glycoprotein; HIV, human immunodeficiency virus; HLA, human leucocyte antigen; LFA, leucocyte functional antigen; N-CAM, neural cell adhesion molecule; NK, natural killer; VLA, very late antigen.

the non-fluorescent primary antibody is detected by the binding of secondary fluorochrome-conjugated reagents.

Direct labelling requires a single incubation step and thus is relatively quick and simple to perform. The procedure gives less intense staining than the indirect method but has the advantage of low non-specific staining. Automated processing of directly labelled blood samples is now possible with Coulter Cyto-Stat reagents and the Coulter Q-Prep workstation. Reduction in pre-analytical manipulation and significant time savings may be achieved with this technique.

Indirect labelling techniques are more time-consuming than direct staining by virtue of additional incubation and washing steps. However the resultant fluorescent intensity is generally higher with the method because two or more secondary antibodies may bind to each primary antibody. Non-specific background fluorescence due to inappropriate binding of the second step reagent may be problematic. To overcome this, biotinylated primary antibodies and avidin-fluorochrome conjugates may be used.

For dual-colour labelling it is simplest to use directly conjugated antibodies. Monoclonal antibody kits which incorporate FITC and PE conjugates are available, from several commercial sources, for simultaneous determination of lymphoid subpopulations and detection of activated cells. Indirect techniques must incorporate blocking steps to prevent binding secondary antibodies to the respective primary antibodies. Combination of direct and indirect (avidin/streptavidin–biotin system) methods can be used with success.

For all of the above techniques, appropriate control reagents (irrelevant antibodies of similar immunoglobulin class and isotype to the test reagents) must be incorporated in the labelling protocol. Practical details of the above procedures may be found elsewhere [3].

Increased sensitivity of detection of surface molecules may be achieved in an indirect labelling method by coupling the secondary antibodies to fluorescent liposomes [18]. Liposomes can carry up to 60 carboxyfluorescein molecules, whereas conventional conjugation results in two to four molecules bound to the secondary antibody. Thus these reagents have great potential for identifying molecules present at low densities on the cell surface, such as cytokine receptors which are normally detected using their fluoresceinated ligands.

Intracellular antigens may also be identified by flow cytometry. To enable labelling of intracellular antigens, cells must be fixed and the surface membrane permeabilized. This may be acheived in a single step by the use of 70% methanol [19] or by using a two-step (fixation/permeabilization) procedure. Formaldehyde/saponin [20] or paraformaldehyde/*n*-octyl-glucoside [21] combinations have been used for the simultaneous determination of surface and cytoplasmic antigens.

12.1.6 Data analysis and interpretation

In practical terms, the statistical measurements that are most often required involve the initial delineation of 'positive' and 'negative' components, together with analyses of fluorescent intensities. The first step in such procedures involves 'setting a gate' around the cell population being studied (based on forward-angle light scatter (FALS) and right-angle (90°LS) light scatter characteristics). The gates or windows are used by the computer to select for the accumulation of fluorescent events from the respective cell populations. Data can then be viewed as single histograms or dual-parameter plots. An example of the use of multiple gating is shown in Fig. 12.1, where immunofluorescence profiles for leucocyte functional antigen (LFA-1) (CD11a)-stained leucocytes have been derived from a single blood sample.

Threshold settings for positively and negatively labelled cells are made from information derived from a number of control procedures. These may be broadly subdivided into negative antibody controls and unstained cell controls, and are used to set the threshold on the histogram, above which cells are considered to be positive for the test antibody. The control antibody is usually an irrelevant antibody of the same immunoglobulin subclass (isotype) as the test antibody and conjugated with the same fluorochrome. In addition, if indirect (two-stage) staining procedures are used, then the test cells are also stained with the second-stage antibody alone to determine the contribution to background staining of this reagent. The marker point between 'positive' and 'negative' is therefore usually set at a position on the negative histogram so that less than 1% of the events are above the threshold. Examination of unstained cells is additionally used to give an indication of the autofluorescence of the test cells, and the background noise of the flow cytometer.

12.1.7 Single-colour immunophenotypic analysis

Histogram types of single-colour immunofluorescent staining patterns can broadly be subdivided into three main types.

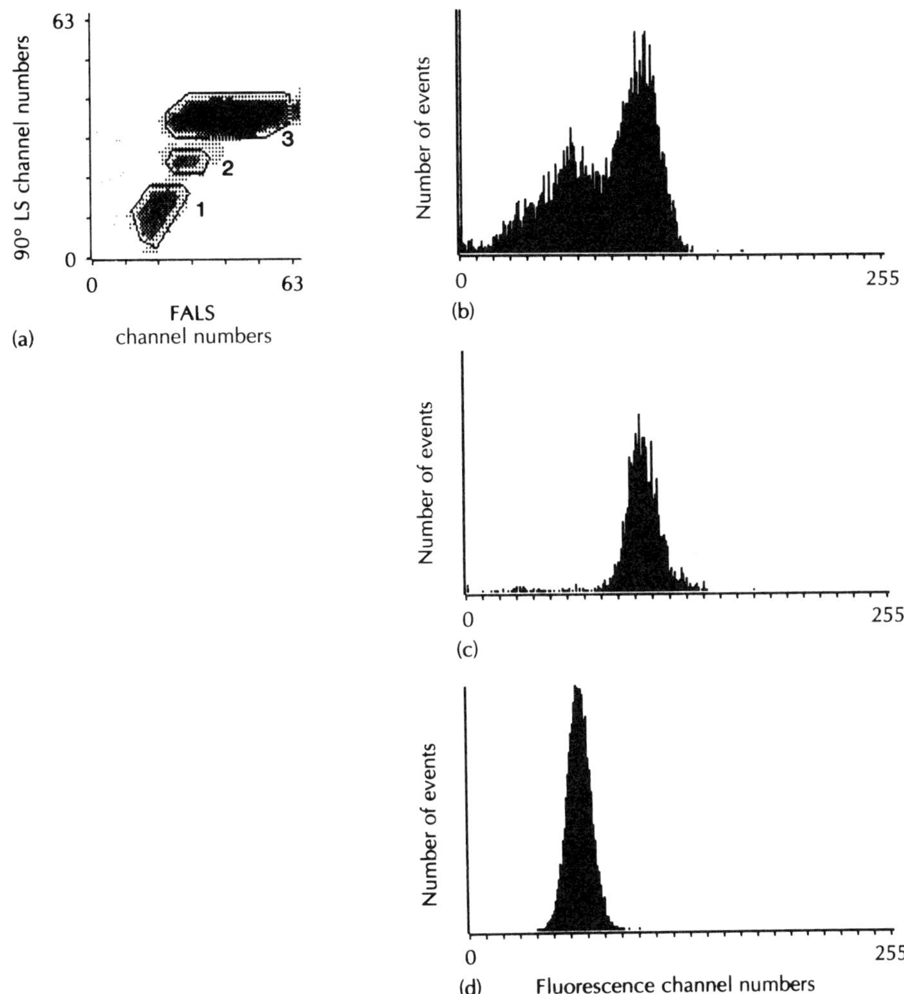

Fig. 12.1 Representative histograms from a peripheral blood leucocyte preparation indirectly labelled with anti-CD11a and goat antimouse fluorescein isothiocyanate (FITC) reagent, showing distinctive distribution of the leucocyte functional antigen (LFA)-1 on different leucocyte populations. (a) Two-parameter forward-angle light scatter (FALS) vs 90° light scatter (LS) plot showing (1) lymphocyte; (2) monocyte and (3) granulocyte populations. Fluorescence histograms obtained simultaneously from the gated populations: (b) lymphocyte, 92% positive median channel fluorescence (MCF) 88; (c) monocyte, 96% positive MCF 104; (d) granulocyte, 99% positive MCF 66.

1 The first of these histogram pattern types (S-type) is characterized by a homogeneous expression of antigen by the whole leukaemic cell fraction, or by homogeneous antigen expression by individual leukaemic subpopulations. In practice, this corresponds to situations where the antigen being investigated is absent (Fig. 12.2a) or consistently expressed with relatively high density (Fig. 12.2b).

2 The second staining pattern (SE-type) is characterized by a more heterogeneous distribution of antigen expression by the 'positive' component, in which a distinct antigen-negative fraction may or may not be apparent. In this latter situation, membrane staining is seen as a continuous spectrum of fluorescence in which there are no distinct subpopulations (Fig. 12.2c and d).

3 The third pattern type is characterized by the

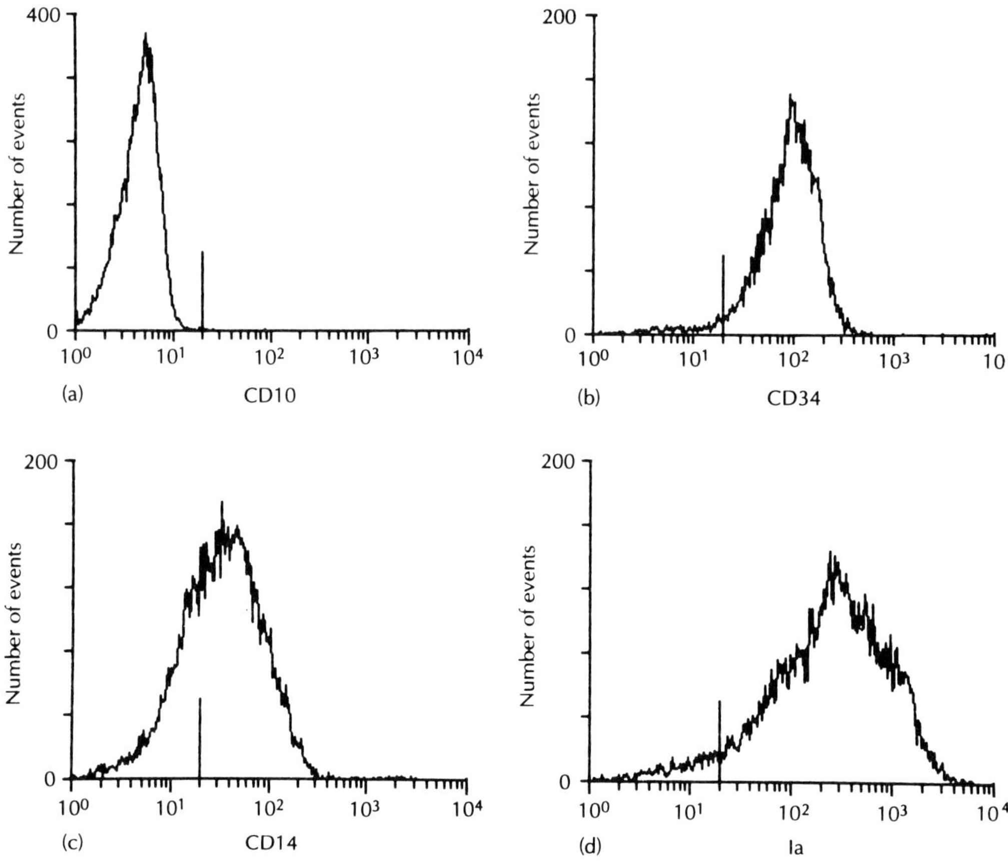

Fig. 12.2 Representative staining histograms of leukaemic cells illustrating: (a) a homogeneous distribution of CD10 antigen-negative cells; (b) a homogeneous distribution of CD34 antigen-positive cells; (c) a heterogeneous distribution of CD14 antigen-negative and antigen-positive cells with no evidence for the presence of distinct subpopulations; and (d) a heterogeneous distribution of Ia antigen-positive cells. Histograms (a) and (b) are defined as S-type, and histograms (c) and (d) as SE-type. Marker settings at 20 fluorescent units indicate the conventional level of discrimination between antigen-negative and antigen-positive components.

occurrence of two (B1-type; Fig. 12.3a and b) or three (TR1-type; Fig. 12.3c and d) subpopulations, each with a discrete level of membrane staining (usually including a negative fraction).

12.1.8 Two- and three-colour immunophenotypic analyses

For two-colour analysis, a dual-parameter data correlation gives more specific information than single histograms. This is best represented by a contour plot. A contour plot maps the events as contour lines representing a density distribution of cells. The result is similar to the height contour lines seen on geographical maps. Quadrant markers are set on the appropriate negative control sample stained with the appropriate FITC/PE isotype-matched irrelevant antibodies, dividing the graph into four areas. Statistical analysis of the quadrant settings gives the proportions (percentages) of cells which are single- or double-labelled or are unstained (Fig. 12.4).

Three-colour analyses may be carried out on instruments with software which permits the setting of multiple gates on histograms and dot plots. With simultaneous measurement of five parameters per

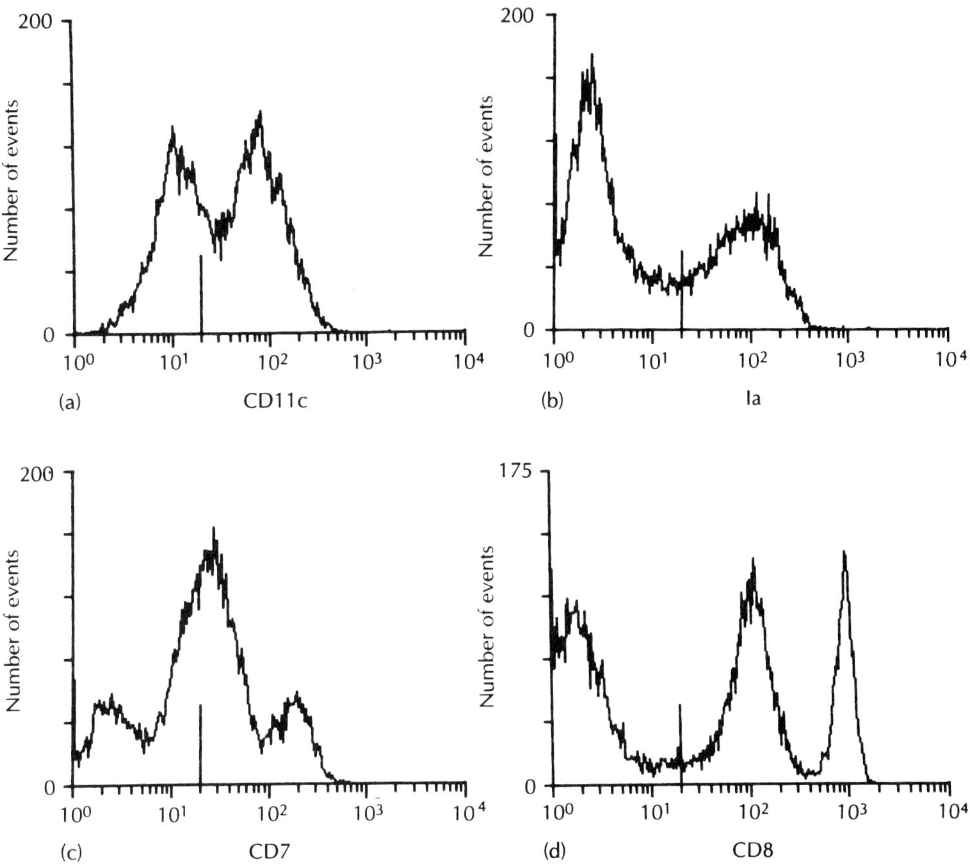

Fig. 12.3 Representative staining histograms of leukaemic cells illustrating the occurrence of subpopulations with distinct levels of antigen expression. Histograms (a) and (b) show bimodal distributions of CD11c and Ia expression, respectively; histograms (c) and (d) show trimodal distributions of CD7 and CD8 expression. Marker settings at 20 fluorescent units indicate the conventional level of discrimination between antigen-negative and antigen-positive components.

cell, the setting of multiple sequential gates is the easiest way to analyse data. For example, using FACSCAN (Becton Dickinson) research software, if a fluorescent histogram display for the expression of antigen X in the fluorochrome 3 (i.e., duochrome or dual-colour) mode indicates three levels of staining intensity, then a gate could be set around each population which could then be individually examined for the expression of the two other markers in the FL1 (FITC) and FL2 modes (PE). With this approach it is possible to obtain a numerical breakdown of $FL1^+FL2^-$, $FL1^+FL2^+$, $FL1^-FL2^+$ and $FL1^-FL2^-$ cell subpopulations of individual FL3 fractions (Fig. 12.5).

Fluorescence intensity may be acquired using either linear or logarithmic amplification of signals. Linear amplification allows direct estimation of fluorescence intensities, i.e., twice the mean channel number represents a doubling of fluorescence intensity. However, limitation of the measurement range results in uneven allocation in the histogram channel resolution of negative and positive cells and leads to a false emphasis on the negative population. This problem may be overcome using logarithmic amplification and this is the method of choice for leucocyte immunofluorescence studies. With this method, a more even emphasis of positive and negative cells is achieved

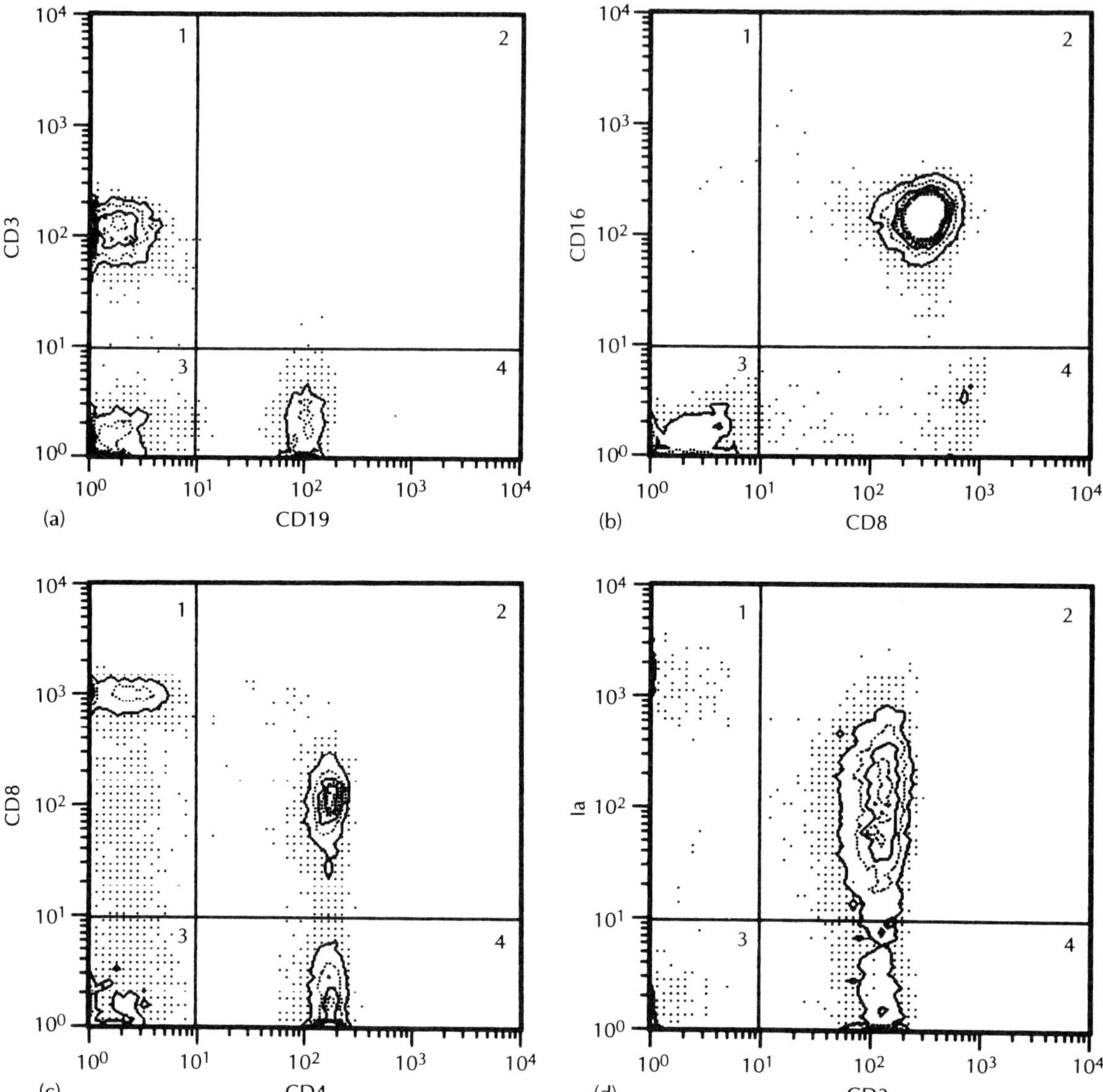

Fig. 12.4 Representative two-colour (fluorescein isothiocyanate, FITC; Fluorochrome 1; phycoerythrin, PE; Fluorochrome 2) immunocytometric contour plots: (a) CD8 (PE) versus CD19 (FITC) expression where distinct $CD3^+CD19^-$ (quadrant 1), $CD3^-$ $CD19^+$ (quadrant 4) and $CD3^-CD19^-$ (quadrant 3) components are seen; (b) CD8 (FITC) versus CD16 (PE) expression where a higher proportion of $CD8^+CD16^+$ (quadrant 2) cells are seen, together with smaller $CD8^-CD16^-$ (quadrant 3) and $CD8^+$ $CD16^-$ (quadrant 4) fractions; (c) CD4 (FITC) versus CD8 (PE) where four distinct populations are seen (note that the intensity of CD8 staining by $CD4^+CD8^+$ cells is less than that of the $CD4^-CD8^+$ component); (d) CD3 (FITC) versus Ia (PE), showing that virtually all cells analysed are $CD3^+$ and that the level of Ia expression is a continuous spectrum from negative to strong positive.

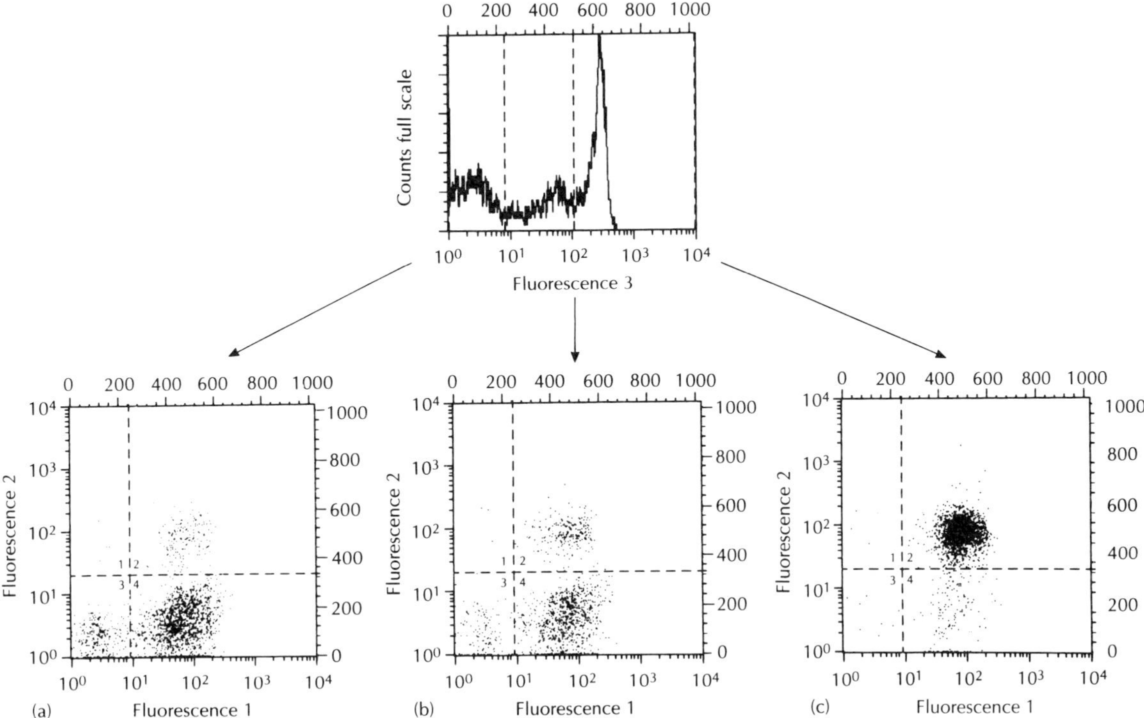

Fig. 12.5 Representative example of three-colour (fluorescein isothiocyanate, FITC; phycoerythrin, PE; and duochrome) analysis. In this case, membrane CD8 staining was achieved with duochrome (FL3) and visualized as a single histogram plot (upper diagram) in which are seen three apparently distinct levels of fluorescence (designated as negative, dim positive and positive, respectively). By setting a gate individually around each of these three CD8 subpopulations, it was possible to analyse each for the expression of CD2 (FL1, FITC) and CD3 (FL2, PE) determinants. Quadrant dot-plots (a) and (b) for the analyses of the $CD8^-$ and CD8 dim^+ fractions show that most of these cells have a $CD2^+CD3^-$ phenotype with minor proportions of $CD2^-CD3^-$ and $CD2^+CD3^+$ cells. In contrast, the $CD8^+$ component is predominantly (> 98%) of $CD2^+CD3^+$ phenotypic type (c), with only very occasional $CD2^+CD3^-$ cells.

and weak and intensely fluorescent cells may be displayed on the same scale. Comparison of fluorescent intensities is more difficult, however, with log amplified signals. Calibration of log amplifiers and linearization of fluorescence distribution for statistical analyses is required. A method which allows conversion of log channel numbers into relative fluorescence intensities has been described by Schmid *et al.* [22].

Fluorescence intensities may be quantified from standard calibration curves established from commercial preparations of microspheres of known fluorescence molecule concentrations. Microsphere preparations are also available; these can be used to measure antibody binding to cells (Simply Cellular microbeads; Flow Cytometry Standards). These beads, which have a predetermined number of mouse immunoglobulin G (IgG) antibody-binding sites on their surfaces, are stained by the same procedure as that used for the cells under study and the fluorescence intensity determined. From standard fluorescence calibration curves, the fluorescence intensity per antibody molecule (F/P ratio) can be determined. This F/P ratio may then be used to calculate the number of antibodies bound per cell and thus the number of available antibody-binding sites per cell.

12.1.9 Quality assurance procedures

In the clinical laboratory flow cytometric immunophenotyping analyses have become increasingly important procedures for identifying immunological abnormalities, diagnosing haemopoietic neoplasms and monitoring changes in immune status in relation to therapy. The precision and accuracy of results which are generated by the flow cytometry laboratory must, therefore, be guaranteed through the practice of adequate quality assurance schemes. Quality assurance procedures in flow cytometry should encompass all aspects of sample preparation, antibody labelling, instrument calibration, data analysis and interpretation. Comprehensive review of each of these is beyond the scope of this chapter, readers are referred to several overviews in the literature [23–26].

Two key areas of a flow cytometric quality assurance programme, instrument quality control and quality control of reagents and staining procedures, are considered below.

12.1.10 Instrument quality control

To ensure instrument reliability and precision, quality control schemes which incorporate the use of reference standards are employed. Examples of reference standards commonly used in flow cytometry are: (i) uniform monodisperse synthetic microspheres (beads) of known light scatter and fluorescence intensity; (ii) glutaraldehyde-fixed chicken erythrocytes; and (iii) fixed bovine thymocyte nuclei.

With all reference preparations it is important that the particles are uniform and remain stable over a period of time. In addition, the nature and intensity of the fluorochromes used in reference materials should be similar to those pertaining in the experimental situation. A routine instrument quality control programme should incorporate: (i) optical alignment with calibration beads or fixed erythrocytes; (ii) calibration of fluorescence intensity with particle mixtures of varying fluorescent intensities; and (iii) setting of compensation parameters for overlapping emission spectra of differing fluorochromes.

Monitoring and recording of these day-to-day performance indicators will ensure optimal instrument performance and allow initiation of trouble-shooting procedures when the limits of acceptability of the results are exceeded.

12.1.11 Quality control of staining procedures and reagents

Analyses of biological and reagent controls form the basis of quality control procedures for evaluating the quality of cell preparation methods, staining techniques and monitoring reagent performance.

Staining procedures

The establishment of optimal gating criteria for the selection of cell populations for analysis is critical for the accuracy of quantitative immunofluorescence analyses. By convention, leucocytes are identified on the basis of FALS and 90°LS characteristics and on these criteria immunofluorescent positivity is calculated for the populations of interest. In lymphocyte subset analyses, for example, it is essential to determine the proportion of cells within the lymphocyte gate which are, in fact, lymphocytes. The presence of non-lymphoid cells (e.g., erythrocytes) within the acquisition gate may give falsely depressed values. Alternatively, if the antibodies under study identify antigens which are not restricted to the lymphoid lineage, falsely elevated results will be obtained. As a means of improving lymphocyte gating efficiency, procedures which incorporate pan leucocyte (CD45) and monocytic (CD14) immunofluorescence labelling with light scatter parameters have been described [27].

For lymphocyte immunophenotypic analyses, peripheral blood lymphocytes obtained from normal subjects are commonly used as positive controls to demonstrate that reagent antibodies are binding to appropriate targets. As a means of minimizing variability it is preferable to use a small pool of donors. Alternatively, a pool of cryopreserved normal lymphocytes may be maintained which can be used over a period of time. Normal lymphocytes may also serve as negative controls for antibodies which are unreactive with lymphoid cells. Recently, commercial preparations of lyophilized human lymphocytes, such as CYTO-TROL control cells (Coulter Immunology), have become available. These cells exhibit surface antigens representative of those found on normal lymphocytes and can be used as standard preparations for indirect or direct staining procedures. Furthermore, as the light scatter and fluorescence properties are very similar to those observed with normal lymphocytes, these preparations appear to offer a useful source of standardized material for reagent/staining quality control procedures.

In situations where normal lymphocytes do not bind the antibodies under study, alternative controls must be sought. For example, positive controls for the common acute lymphoblastic leukaemia antigen (CALLA; CD10) may be a CALLA-positive cell line, such as Daudi, or cryopreserved aliquots of clinical specimens previously demonstrated as bearing the antigen

Reagents

The quality control programme for reagent antibodies should address both the storage of reagents and evaluation of specificity and sensitivity of staining.

Antibodies should be stored at 4 °C or in aliquots at −20 °C, with attention being paid to expiry dates. The specificity and staining intensity of new reagent lots should be compared with those of reagents in use before being adopted in ongoing protocols.

Appropriate reagent controls should always be employed to evaluate the specificity of all reagents. In direct immunofluorescence procedures, a fluorochrome-conjugated immunoglobulin which is unreactive with the cells under study, but is composed of the same immunoglobulin class and isotype as the test antibody, should be included in the reagent panel. For indirect staining, the primary antibody may be omitted or replaced with an irrelevant immunoglobulin of similar isotype and the fluorochrome-labelled second-step reagent added as usual. The fluorescence signals generated by the reagent controls are used to set the threshold on immunofluorescence histograms, above which cells are considered positive for antibody binding. It is usual to set the threshold at a position on the negative histogram such that less than 1% of events are above the threshold.

Finally, dead cells may represent a source of intense non-specific staining. Such cells may be labelled using vital dyes, such as propidium iodide, and by the use of selective gating, excluded from immunofluorescence analyses.

Standardization of flow cytometric analyses requires not only the application of intralaboratory quality control procedures as described above, but also the participation in interlaboratory quality control schemes. Such schemes are available in several countries both for lymphocyte subset enumerations and for leukaemia immunophenotyping. Because of the many variables associated with sample transportation, preparation and analysis, these programmes are still evolving. However, with careful study of each aspect of flow cytometric analysis, a consensus on these matters should eventually be reached.

12.2 IMMUNOPHENOTYPIC STUDIES OF LEUKAEMIA

12.2.1 Introduction

The diagnosis and classification of leukaemia are currently based on multiple characteristics defined by conventional morphology, cytochemistry, immunophenotyping, cytogenetics and, more recently, DNA analysis. Whilst the relative contribution of individual diagnostic elements to the consistency of any final scheme of classification varies in importance, it should be remembered that in examining these contributions there is no final arbiter or external reference with which such comparisons can be made. Nevertheless, there is little doubt that the characterization of malignant haemopoietic cells has been greatly advanced by monoclonal antibody immunophenotyping. Indeed, with a small number of notable exceptions, the diagnostic information provided by immunophenotypic analyses is rarely modified by the results of other investigations. Because of this consistency, and despite the limitations of membrane immunophenotyping discussed earlier, it is possible to state broadly the typical antigenic characteristics of most leukaemia subtypes. There are many comprehensive reviews on the application of monoclonal antibodies in the study of haemopoietic cells [28–31], but the following sections will summarize those areas in leukaemia diagnosis which are considered particularly relevant.

12.2.2 Acute lymphoblastic leukaemia (ALL)

There are currently five main immunological subgroups of ALL: (i) null-ALL; (ii) common-ALL (C-ALL); (iii) pre-B ALL; (iv) B-ALL; and (v) T-ALL. The typical immunophenotypic profiles for the non-T and T-ALL diagnostic groups, including analyses of cytoplasmic (μ chain) and nuclear (TdT) antigens, are shown in Tables 12.2 and 12.3, respectively. In this form, it can be seen that null-ALL is broadly differentiated from C-ALL and pre-B ALL on the basis of CD10 expression, and that pre-B ALL is phenotypically identical to C-ALL, with the exception that CTgμ is additionally present. The diagnosis of T-ALL, although relatively straightforward, is somewhat complicated by distinct maturation-associated differences in antigenic phenotypes. Thus, the developmental progression from pre-T-ALL is reflected by changes in the expression of membrane CD1, CD2, CD3, CD4 and CD8 in particular (Table 12.3). With reference to the expression of non-lymphoid-associated antigens by lymphoblastic leukaemia cells, this is currently a controversial area [34–36]. However, the general consensus is that most cases of ALL do not express myeloid-associated membrane determinants (CD13 and CD33), and the small proportion (approximately 5–10% [30,36,37]) of ALL cases that are labelled

Table 12.2 Immunophenotypic classification of acute lymphoblastic leukaemias (ALL) of non-T-cell type

	Null-ALL	C-ALL	Pre-B-ALL	B-ALL
Nuclear TdT	+	+	+	–
HLA-DR (Ia)	+	+	+	+
CD10	–	+	+	–
CD19	+	+	+	+
CD20	–	–	+	+
CD22	–	–	+	+
cCD22	+	+	na	na
CIgμ	–	–	+	na
SIgμ	–	–	–	+

Results for nuclear, membrane and cytoplasmic antigens are shown as: –, typically negative; +, typically positive; na, not applicable. Virtually all cases lack T-cell-associated membrane cluster of differentiation (CD2) and CD7, and cytoplasmic CD3 (cCD3). Approximately 5–10% of cases may show weak expression of membrane CD13 and/or CD33 myeloid-associated determinants. Membrane expression of CD20 by C-ALL (when present) and pre-B-ALL blasts is weak; cCD22 indicates cytoplasmic CD22 expression; CIgμ and SIgμ indicate cytoplasmic and surface expression of IgM heavy chains, respectively.
TdT, terminal deoxynucleotidyl transferase; HLA, human leucocyte antigen; Ig, immunoglobulin.

Table 12.3 Immunophenotypic classification of T-cell acute lymphoblastic leukaemias (T-ALL)

		T-ALL				
	Pre-T-ALL	Type A	Type B	Type C	Type D	Type E
Nuclear TdT	+	+	+	+	+	+
HLA-DR (Ia)	+	+	–	–	–	–
CD1a	–	–	+	+	–	–
CD2	–	+	+	+	+	+
CD3	–	–	–	–	–	+
cCD3	–	–	+	+	+	+
CD4/CD8	–	–	–	4 and 8	4 or 8	4 or 8
CD5	–	–	+	+	+	+
CD7	–	+	+	+	+	+

Results for membrane and cytoplasmic antigens are shown as; –, typically negative; +, typically positive. Phenotypic classification adapted from van Dongen *et al.* [31], and Drexler and Scott [32]. Virtually all cases are cluster of differentiation (CD)13- and CD33-negative, CD19-negative and cCD22-negative. cCD3 indicates cytoplasmic CD3 expression as assessed with monoclonal antibodies against the ε chain of the CD3 complex [33].
HLA, human leucocyte antigen.

with these pan-myeloid reagents may well correspond to what is becoming increasingly referred to as acute mixed-lineage leukaemia [38]). At present, the prognostic significance of myeloid antigen expression by ALL blasts is unclear [35,39]), although a relationship between the presence of myeloid antigens and membrane CD34 expression has been reported [40]. An analysis of correlations between morphological (French–American–British (FAB) subtypes L1, L2 and L3) and immunophenotypic classification schemes for over 1000 ALL cases [31] found wide morphological variability within the immunological groups (Table 12.4), although one fairly consistent observation was that most (78%) immunologically defined B-ALL cases were of L3 morphological type. Furthermore, with regards to the relative prognostic value of morphological and immunophenotypic classifications, there have been many conflicting reports [41–45]. Whilst many of these differences are attributable to case-group variables such as age, presenting leucocyte counts and treatment regimens, a number of consistent points have become apparent. For example, cases with L3 morphology [46] and/or immunologically defined B-ALL [47] have a particularly poor prognosis. Taking immunological classifications alone, the prognostic rank order for childhood ALL appears to be C-ALL > null-ALL > T-ALL > B-ALL [31,48], whereas for adults it appears to be T-ALL > C-ALL > null-ALL > B-ALL [31].

12.2.3 Acute myeloid leukaemia

The morphological classification of acute myeloid leukaemias currently consist of eight main subtypes [49–52]. These are: (i–iii) acute myeloblastic leukaemia (AML; M0, M1 and M2); (iv) acute promyelocytic leukaemia (APL; subtypes M3-hyper and M3-hypo); (v) acute myelomonocytic leukaemia (AMML; M4); (vi) acute monocytic leukaemia (AMoL; M5); (vii) erythroleukaemia (including acute erythroblastic leukaemia, AEL; M6); and (viii) acute megakaryoblastic leukaemia (AMegaL; M7). The three AML subtypes can effectively be viewed as reflecting early stages of the granulocytic maturational spectrum, where M0 is the most immature (morphologically agranular and cytochemically undifferentiated) and M2 the most mature (morphologically granular and cytochemically well-differentiated). Leukaemic promyelocytes of the M3 variants can be regarded as representing a further stage of this differentiation sequence and, similarly, the monocytic subtypes (M4 and M5) correspond to proliferations with characteristics of early and late monocytic differentiation respectively. Typical erythroleukaemia (M6) is often diagnosed without the need for immunological investigations, although such studies can be particularly informative when the erythroid cells are apparently undifferentiated (i.e., AEL [53]). AMegaL (M7) is a proliferation of immature cells which, because of the absence of distinct morphological or conventional cytochemical diagnostic indicators, is usually defined by immunological (or electron microscope, EM) studies [53–55].

Monoclonal antibody immunophenotyping of non-monocytic AML variants (M0–M3) should be regarded as a two-stage process which: (i) confirms with lineage-specific markers that the blast cells are expressing myeloid-associated determinants (e.g., CD13 and CD33), and lack those associated with lymphoid commitment (e.g., CD1, CD3 and CD19); and (ii) determines the expression of differentiation markers, that may not be lineage-specific, in order to assess the level of maturation corresponding to the various stages of granulocytic maturation designated by morphological criteria. The M4 and M5 AMoL are subject to the same diagnostic strategies, but these additionally require evaluation of monocyte lineage-specific CD14 expression. Similarly, AEL and AMegaL are defined by the expression of the lineage-specific antigens such as glycophorin A

Table 12.4 Correlations between morphological and immunological subtypes of acute lymphoblastic leukaemia (ALL)

	Morphological (FAB) subtype		
Immunological group*	L1 (%)	L2 (%)	L3 (%)
Null-ALL (n = 32)	34	65	1
C-ALL (n = 360)	52	26	2
B-ALL (n = 60)	7	15	78
T-ALL (n = 297)	65	34	1

* The C-ALL group includes pre-B-ALL cases.
FAB, French–American–British classification.

(unclustered) and CD41/CD42/CD61, respectively. In addition to basing leukaemic classifications on phenotypic characteristics, these studies are being increasingly used to evaluate potential prognostic features. For example, there is some evidence that CD34 expression by myeloid leukaemia blasts may have a lower complete remission (CR) induction rate than CD34 cases and that patterns of CD34 expression seen at initial clinical presentation are retained on relapse [56]. A simplified diagnostic scheme, based on immunophenotypic features, for the eight myeloid leukaemia variants is shown in Table 12.5.

12.2.4 Chronic lymphoid leukaemias (CLLs)

Chronic B-cell malignancies, in particular, are relatively common and have been the subject of extensive immunophenotypic analyses. As with the acute leukaemias, malignant cells in any given case of chronic B- or T-cell proliferation represent a maturational spectrum which, although showing a predominant phenotypic pattern of antigen expression, may show some maturational overlap. Thus, while typical phenotypic profiles for each diagnostic subgroup can be given, there are many individual exceptions and the final diagnostic categorization may be dependent on conclusions derived from all those investigations undertaken. For example, whilst an absence of membrane CD23 expression can reliably be interpreted as being inconsistent with typical B-CLL, its presence (without taking into account other phenotypic characteristics) is far less informative. For the most frequently encountered chronic lymphocytic malignancies, a number of phenotypic indicators can be provided. Although the number of potential clusters which can be applied to the analytical subdivision of such malignancies will no doubt increase, it also has to be accepted that this may not necessarily lead to more simplified and reproducible diagnostic schemes. In effect, this could only be achieved by the availability of monoclonal antibodies with specificity restricted to very narrow levels of lymphocytic differentiation and even then, this would not resolve the problems of maturational heterogeneity typical of many such disorders. The following sections briefly summarize the main diagnostic characteristics of chronic lymphocytic leukaemias, although it should perhaps be stressed that maturational overlap between related lymphoid proliferations may cause difficulties with regards to phenotypic interpretation.

12.2.5 Chronic B-cell disorders

The typically monomorphous lymphocytes which characterize B-CLL are at a relatively early stage of

Table 12.5 Phenotypic characteristics of blast cells in acute myeloid leukaemia (AML) subtypes defined by monoclonal antibodies against nuclear (TdT), membrane (human leucocyte antigen (HLA)-DR, cluster of differentiation (CD)13/CD33, CD14, CD15, CD41/CD42/CD61 and glycophorin A) and cytoplasmic (myeloperoxidase and elastase) antigens*

	AML-M0	AML-M1	AML-M2	APL-M3	AMML-M4	AMoL-M5	AEL-M6	AMegaL-M7
Nuclear TdT	41	31	16	11	16	13	?	?
HLA-DR (Ia)	+	+	+	−	+	+	−	+
CD13/CD33	+	+	+	+	+	+	+	−
CD14	−	−	−	−	V	+	−	−
CD15	−	−	+	+	+	+	+	?
CD41/CD42/CD61	−	−	−	−	−	−	−	+
Glycophorin A	−	−	−	−	−	−	+	−
Myeloperoxidase	−	V	+	+	+	+	−	−
Elastase	−	−	+	+	+	?	−	−

* Results for TdT are shown as the proportion of cases within each AML subtype with detectable nuclear TdT expression. Results for membrane and cytoplasmic antigens are shown as: −, typically negative; +, typically positive; V, variable expression; ?, not known.

APL, Acute promyelocytic leukaemia; AMML, acute myelomonocytic leukaemia; AMoL, acute monocytic leukaemia; AEL, acute erythroblastic leukaemia; AMegaL, acute megakaryoblastic leukaemia; TdT, terminal deoxynucleotidyl transferase.

differentiation. In phenotypic terms (Table 12.6), they appear to correspond to a subpopulation of normal B cells that are found in normal adult lymph nodes, the periphery of germinal centres and occasionally in normal blood and tonsil [57,58], and there is increasing evidence to suggest that B-CLL cells functionally resemble populations of normal activated B cells [59]. They are also phenotypically analogous to a major subset of fetal B cells and are sometimes seen in the peripheral blood of marrow transplant patients during the early stages of recovery [57,58,60]. For comparison, the prolymphocytoid variant (CLL-Pro) shares many of the phenotypic features of typical B-CLL (Table 12.6), despite the morphological presence of increased proportions of nucleolated cells, which in some cases is as low as 10% and in others may be the predominant morphological form [61]. The third type of chronic B-cell malignancy represents a later stage of B-differentiation and is termed prolymphocytic leukaemia (B-PLL) because of the presence of high proportions of nucleolated lymphoid cells. This particular malignancy has distinct clinical and immunophenotypic features (Table 12.6), as do the 'hairy cells' which characterize hairy-cell leukaemia (HCL). However, although the diagnosis of HCL is generally straightforward, the differential diagnosis also needs to consider the possibility of the morphologically similar but phenotypically different splenic lymphoma with circulating villous lymphocytes (SLVL) [62] and a proliferative HCL variant which shows morphological features intermediate between that of PLL and HCL [63,64].

12.2.6 Chronic T-cell disorders

Although malignancies of well-differentiated T cells are relatively rare, compared to those of B-cell origin, it is becoming increasingly apparent that chronic lymphocytic leukaemia of T-cell type (T-CLL) is perhaps far more common than previously thought. In particular, there is mounting evidence

Table 12.6 Immunophenotypic features of chronic B-cell malignancies*

	B-CLL	CLL-Pro	B-PLL	HCL	B-NHL
Nuclear antigens					
TdT	–	–	–	–	– or +†
Ki-67	–	–	–	–	– or +†
Membrane antigens					
FMC7	–	+	+	+	V
CD1c	–	+	+	+	+
CD2/CD3	–	–	–	–	–
CD5	+	+	–	–	V
CD10	–	–	–	–	–
CD11c‡	–	–	–	+	V
CD19	+	+	+	+	+
CD20	+	+	+	+	+
CD21	+	+	+	+	+
CD22§	+	+	+	+	+
CD23	+	+	–	–	V
CD24	+	+	+	–	+
CD25	–	–	–	+	–

* Results are shown as typical patterns of antigen expression in each diagnostic group: –, typically negative; +, typically positive; V, variable expression by diagnostic subtypes of B-NHL.
† Nuclear TdT and/or Ki-67 expression associated with B-NHL cases of high-grade type.
‡ Membrane CD11c expression strong in typical HCL cases and weak in B-NHL.
§ CD22 expressed weakly on the membrane of B-CLL and CLL-Pro cells, but strongly expressed in the cytoplasm.
B-CLL, B-cell chronic lymphoid leukaemia; CLL-Pro, prolymphocytoid chronic lymphoid leukaemia; B-PLL, B-cell prolymphocytic leukaemia; HCL, hairy-cell leukaemia; B-NHL, B-cell non-Hodgkin's lymphoma; TdT, terminal deoxynucleotidyl transferase.

that such disorders may well be associated with a significant proportion of autoimmune diseases and that the variable clinical, morphological and immunophenotypic features of T-CLL appear to reflect the diversity of disorders to which the generic term T-CLL has been ascribed. Although there is the difficulty in some cases of distinguishing between reactive and malignant T-cell proliferations [65,66], recent advances in the application of molecular biology (T-cell receptor gene probes) may be of particular help in equivocal $CD3^+$ cases. T-CLL broadly encompasses two main groups of lymphocytic proliferation, which can be differentiated by morphological and immunophenotypic features (Table 12.7). A minor proportion of cases are morphologically indistinguishable from B-CLL, although smear cells may be less evident. Some investigators have proposed that such $CD4^+CD8^-$ T-CLL cases, which morphologically show indented or convoluted nuclei and have a particularly poor prognosis [67], may well be variant forms of T-cell prolymphocytic leukaemia (T-PLL) [68]. Most cases of T-CLL are however morphologically characterized by the presence of cytoplasmic granulation and resemble large granular lymphocytes (LGL), and it has been suggested that LGL expansions (lymphoproliferative diseases of granular lymphocytes; LGDL) and non-LGL T-CLL cases should be considered separate clinicopathological entities [65,69]. The other two main malignant disorders of mature T cells are adult T-cell leukaemia-lymphoma (ATLL) and Sézary's syndrome (SS). Both of these have distinct morphological and clinical features, and their immunophenotypic characteristics are summarized in Table 12.7.

Table 12.7 Immunophenotypic features of chronic T-cell malignancies*

	T-CLL	LDGL†	T-PLL	ATLL	SS
Nuclear antigens					
TdT	–	–	–	–	–
Ki-67	–	–	–	–	–
Membrane antigens					
HLA-DR	–	V	–	–	–
CD1a	–	–	–	–	–
CD2	+	+	+	+	+
CD3	+	V	+	+	+
CD5	+	–	+	+	+
CD7	+	+	+	–	–
CD25	–	–	–	+	–
CD11b	–	+	V	–	–
CD16	–	V	–	–	–
CD56	–	V	–	–	–
CD57	–	V	–	–	–
CD4/CD8 composite phenotypes‡					
CD4+CD8–	Infrequent	Infrequent	Common	Common	Common
CD4–CD8+	Common	Common	Infrequent	None	Rare
CD4+CD8+	Rare	Some	Some	Infrequent	Infrequent
CD4–CD8–	Rare	Common	Infrequent	Some	Infrequent

* Results are shown as typical patterns of antigen expression in each diagnostic group: –, typically negative; +, typically positive; V, variable expression.
† Lymphoproliferative diseases of large granular lymphocytes (LDGL).
‡ Relative frequencies of CD4/CD8 phenotypes.
T-CLL, T-cell chronic lymphocytic leukaemia; T-PLL, T-cell prolymphocytic leukaemia; ATLL, adult T-cell leukaemia–lymphoma; SS, Sézary's syndrome; HLA, human leucocyte antigen; CD, cluster of differentiation; TdT, terminal deoxynucleotidyl transferase.

12.3 AIDS

Infection with the human immunodeficiency viruses (HIV) causes the profound immunosuppression responsible for most of the clinical features associated with AIDS. The immunopathogenic mechanisms associated with HIV infection have been reviewed extensively elsewhere [70–72]. However, as a means of introducing the role of flow cytometry in monitoring disease progression, the salient features of the immunopathogenic procedures are described briefly below.

HIV devastates the immune system because its main target, the CD4 lymphocyte, is the key component in generating and regulating an immune response. The initial event in the life cycle of HIV is the binding of the HIV envelope glycoprotein (gp 120) to the CD4 molecule which is present primarily, but not exclusively, on T-helper cells. Entry of the virus into the cell is accomplished by endocytosis or through direct fusion of the HIV envelope with the host cell membrane. Within the target cell the virus may remain latent until the cell becomes activated, following which, virus replication is initiated and the host cell destroyed.

Monocytes and macrophages in their role as phagocytes and by virtue of expression, to a variable extent, of the CD4 receptor are susceptible targets for HIV infection [73]. Unlike CD4 lymphocytes, cells of the macrophage lineage are not generally destroyed by HIV infection but act as reservoirs for virus dissemination to the lungs and brain.

The mechanisms of viral persistence, conversion to productive infection and consequent collapse of the immune system remain areas of intense investigation. However, host factors which may affect clinical outcome and immunological markers which may predict disease progression are currently being delineated. Important among these is the enumeration of circulating CD4 lymphocytes in patients with HIV infection, and this topic is discussed in the following section.

12.3.1 CD4 lymphocytes

The selective and progressive depletion of CD4 lymphocytes following HIV infection (Fig. 12.6) has been clearly linked to patient morbidity and mortality. Evidence for this has come from several cohort studies which have assessed various clinical and laboratory parameters in relation to disease progression and manifestations, and to therapeutic efficacy. Thus the levels of circulating CD4 lymphocytes have been reported as having prognostic value in (i) predicting progression to AIDS [74–82];

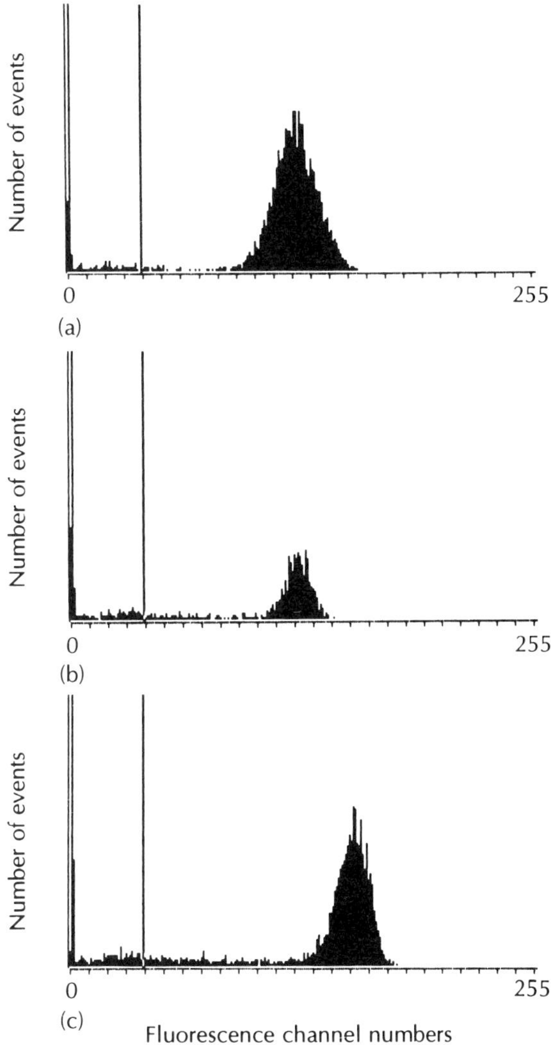

Fig. 12.6 Fluorescence histograms obtained following labelling of peripheral blood lymphocytes from a human immunodeficiency virus-1 (HIV-1) positive patient with (a) anti-CD3 (80%); (b) anti-CD4 (24%); and (c) anti-CD8 (60%) reagents. Note the characteristic depletion of $CD4^+$ cells with concomitant elevation in $CD8^+$ cells.

and (ii) identifying patients at risk of developing opportunistic infections [83] and monitoring therapeutic regimes [84]. The consequence of these reports has been to heighten interest in using CD4 counts in clinical decision-making and in placing demands on the flow cytometry laboratory to provide this information.

The question as to which form of CD4 lymphocyte count (a percentage, absolute count or CD4/CD8 ratio) provides the most useful information is debatable. Conventionally, absolute members of CD4 lymphocytes are reported by most investigators. These values, which are derived from percentage positivity with anti-CD4 reagents and total lymphocyte counts, are conceptually the preferred option. However, variations in white-cell counts due to normal physiological phenomena must be appreciated [85], and the procedures for obtaining total lymphocyte counts strictly controlled [86]. Because of these potential difficulties it has been suggested that the determination of CD4 percentages, which are less prone to variability, is more reliable for long-term studies [87].

Given these caveats, important advances in the understanding of the pathogenesis of HIV infection have been made through careful monitoring of CD4 lymphocyte levels. Data from a number of prospective studies [74–77,79,80] indicate that over a 3-year period of follow-up, few HIV-infected individuals with CD4 lymphocyte counts at presentation of $> 500/mm^3$ progress to AIDS, whereas the majority of patients with initial counts of $< 200/mm^3$ will do so. In an evaluation of eight immunological parameters as prognostic indicators in HIV infection, the CD4 lymphocyte count was found to be the best single predictor of progression to AIDS [88]. Combination of CD4 lymphocyte counts with either serum neopterin or β-microglobulin levels may provide additional predictive power [88].

Regular monitoring of CD4 lymphocyte levels may also be important in predicting the likelihood of the development of opportunistic infections. In a retrospective study [83] of 100 HIV-positive subjects with pulmonary dysfunction, it was shown that opportunistic pneumonias were commonest in patients whose CD4 lymphocyte counts were $< 200/mm^3$ in the 60-day period prior to pulmonary evaluation. Thus, the identification of such patients may warrant the commencement of antipneumocystis prophylaxis.

With the emergence of CD4 lymphocyte measurements as an important parameter in clinical management of HIV-infected individuals, the accuracy and precision of such measurements must be guaranteed and the results correctly interpreted. For the laboratory this entails following recommended procedural guidelines for measurement of lymphocyte subsets in HIV-positive blood samples [89,90], and the adoption of and adherence to stringent quality control programmes (see above). For the clinician, this involves an appreciation of the factors, both clinical and methodological, which influence lymphocyte subset measurements to avoid misinterpretation of results.

12.3.2 CD8 lymphocytes

The immune response to HIV is characterized by a 'reactive' increase in CD8 cells early in infection (see Fig. 12.6) which often precedes the decline in the CD4 population. These increased levels are maintained, irrespective of falling CD4 numbers, during opportunistic infections and through to end-stage disease [79]. Dual-colour immunofluorescence analyses have revealed a progressive increase in the numbers of CD8 cells bearing activation antigens (CD38 and HLA-DR) during the course of the disease. In asymptomatic patients high levels of $CD8^+$ $CD38^+$ cells appear to distinguish those individuals who will have more rapid and aggressive disease progression [91].

12.3.3 B cells

B-cell numbers have been variously reported as being normal [92], elevated [93] or decreased [94] in HIV-infected subjects. An intriguing observation, however, is the high incidence of B-cell lymphomas associated with HIV disease [95]. Whether this is due directly to virus infection or loss of T-cell regulation is unknown.

12.3.4 Detection of HIV-infected peripheral blood mononuclear cells

A flow cytometric assay has been described [96]

which can detect and quantify HIV-infected peripheral blood mononuclear cells from HIV-seropositive patients. The assay is based on the identification, by immunofluorescence, of p24 or nef antigens in affected cells. Using this technique of cell-associated antigen detection by flow cytometry, it has been possible to determine the proportion of circulating mononuclear cells infected by HIV. The assay shows a high degree of correlation with clinical status and is superior to conventional serological antigen capture assays which are prone to interference by immune complexes.

It is likely that assays such as this, which will more accurately determine the antigen status of HIV-infected individuals, will become of increasing importance.

12.4 ASSESSMENT OF POLYMORPHONUCLEAR (PMN) LEUCOCYTE FUNCTIONS BY FLOW CYTOMETRY

PMN leucocytes are primarily responsible for maintaining normal host defences against bacterial infections. The cellular response to microbial invasion can be divided into a number of stages (adherence, chemotaxis, phagocytosis and intracellular killing) on the basis of assays which have been devised to investigate aspects of PMN cell function. The availability of such functional assays has proved useful in the diagnosis of congenital and acquired defects of PMN cells and in the management of infectious and inflammatory diseases.

The application of flow cytometric technology to functional investigations of PMN cells has resulted in significant growth in the tests available and improvements in assay specificity. A description of several flow cytometric assays covering distinctive stages of PMN cell functions is given below. Comprehensive reviews of the subject may be found elsewhere [97,98].

12.4.1 Surface membrane receptors

A number of membrane receptors which mediate attachment of micro-organisms to PMN cells or are involved in regulation of PMN cell function may be identified by monoclonal antibody labelling and flow cytometry. Receptors for complement components and immunoglobulin have been the most thoroughly investigated because of their key role in the phagocytosis of opsonized particles.

Expression of receptors for C3 breakdown products, C3b and C3bi (designated CR1 and CR3, respectively) are increased following PMN cell activation. This has been demonstrated *in vitro* with various stimulants such as *N*-formyl-methionyl-leucyl-phenylalanine (FMLP) [99,100], C5a des Arg [99] and phorbol myristate acetate (PMA) [101,102]. Increased expression of CR1 and CR3 *in vivo* has been observed on PMN cells from inflammatory joints fluids [103] (see Fig. 12.7), bronchoalveolar fluids from cystic fibrosis patients [104] and in patients with thermal injuries [105,106].

CR3 is a member of a family of membrane glycoproteins, which includes LFA-1 and the p150,95 antigen, collectively known as leucocyte integrins or leucocyte adhesion molecules [107–109]. The receptors are heterodimeric structures consisting of variable α chains and a common β chain. The β subunit has been given the cluster differentiation number CD18 and the α subunits for LFA-1, CR3 and p150,95, the cluster differentiation numbers CD11a, CD11b and CD11c, respectively. Defective expression of the common β subunit (CD18) has been identified in patients with leucocyte adhesion deficiency [110,111]. Affected patients are prone to recurrent, life-threatening infections due to failure of leucocyte chemotaxis, infiltration of extravascular sites and adhesion of opsonized particles.

Three forms of Fc and receptor (FcR I, II and III) have been identified [112]. FcR II and III are present on resting PMN cells and, along with FcR I, are inducible by various inflammatory mediators [113]. Decreased FcR III expression on PMN cells from premature neonates has been described [114,115]. The reduction is most marked in preterm babies with severe respiratory distress syndrome or septicaemia. Thus, abnormalities in phagocytosis and bacterial killing in premature neonates may, in part, be a consequence of reduced FcR III expression.

12.4.2 Phagocytosis

Flow cytometric phagocytosis assays are based on the uptake of fluorescent particles such as latex

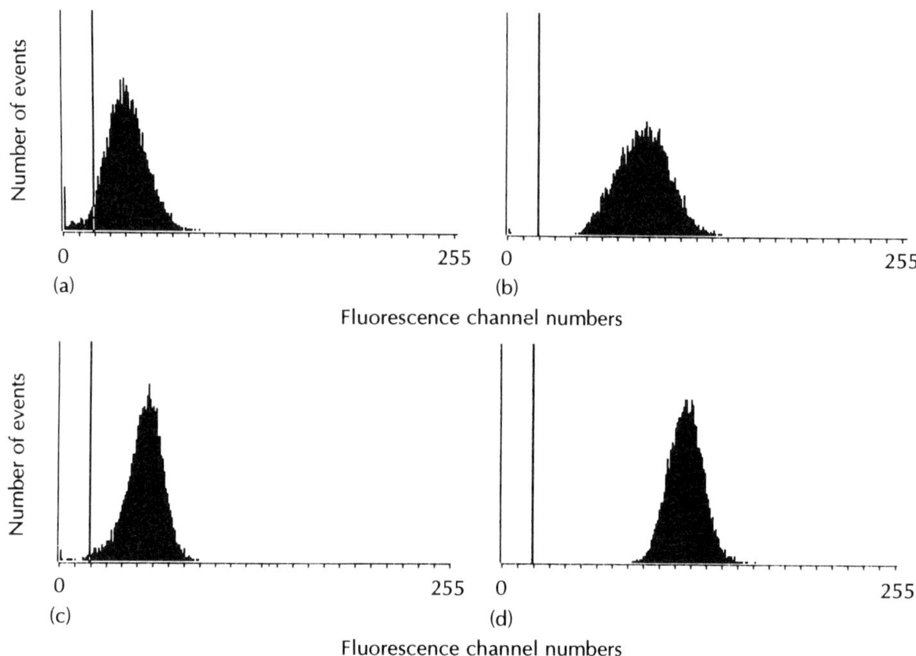

Fig. 12.7 Complement receptor expression, defined by anti-CR1 (CD35) and anti-CR3 (CD11b) reagents, on granulocytes from a patient with rheumatoid arthritis. Marked elevation in CR1 and CR3 expression is observed on granulocytes obtained from inflamed synovial fluid, compared with those from the corresponding peripheral blood sample. Peripheral blood: (a) CR1 (MCF 43); (b) CR3 (MCF 85). Synovial fluid: (c) CR1 (MCF 56); (d) CR3 (MCF 118). MCF, median-channel fluorescence.

microbeads, dye-labelled bacteria or yeast cells [116–119]. Phagocytic activity is determined from comparative measurement of intensities of cell populations containing ingested fluorescent particles with those of a control population. In circumstances where pH-sensitive fluorochromes are used and there is a reduction in fluorescence intensity because of phagolysosomal acidification, the number of particles ingested may be calculated from the loss of free extracellular particles [117,118].

In order to distinguish between particles attached to the cell surface and those actually internalized, flow cytometric quenching techniques have been developed [120,121]. In these procedures trypan blue or crystal violet dye added to the suspension of cells and fluorescein-labelled bacteria or yeasts before analysis on the flow cytometer quenches the fluorescence of all extracellular organisms but has no effect on the fluorescence of internalized particles. In another approach, receptor-mediated and non-specific phagocytosis may be determined by a dual-colour assay incorporating opsonized microspheres [122]. The method involves incubation of PMN cells with 'green' fluorescent microspheres in buffer alone or with cytochalasin D to inhibit phagocytosis, followed by labelling of externally bound beads with red fluorescent antibodies to the immobilized ligand. Discrimination of red and green fluorescence signals identifies adherence (red) and ingestion (green).

Intracellular killing of phagocytosed microorganisms may be assessed in an assay which combines phagocytic functions (fluorescein-conjugated yeast cells) with identification of killed organisms (propidium iodide labelling) [123].

12.4.3 Oxidative metabolism

The recognition and ingestion of opsonized microorganisms by PMN cells results in a burst of oxidative metabolic activity with the generation of a series of reactive oxygen species (hydrogen peroxide;

hydroxyl radical; hydroperoxyl radical; singlet oxygen) [124]. This oxidative respiratory burst is in large part responsible for the killing of ingested bacteria as well as a major portion of tissue damage that results from acute inflammation.

Measurement of respiratory burst activity in PMN cells by flow cytometry was first described by Bass *et al.* [125]. In the assay, PMN cells are incubated with 2-dichlorofluorescein diacetate (DCF-DA), a non-fluorescent analogue of fluorescein diacetate. Owing to its non-polar properties, DCF-DA readily traverses cell membranes. Cytoplasmic esterases act to deacetylate the DCF-DA to form the polar molecule 2,7-dichlorofluorescin, which becomes trapped intracellularly. The generation of hydrogen peroxide during the respiratory burst results in the conversion of the non-fluorescent DCF to highly fluorescent DCF. The flow cytometer measures the extent of respiratory burst activity by quantitating the green DCF fluorescence generated in stimulated DCF-DA loaded cells compared with unstimulated DCF-DA loaded cells. The assay is analogous to the nitroblue tetrazolium (NBT) dye reduction test used in the screening of patients for leucocyte oxidase deficiency, such as that found in chronic granulomatous disease.

Modifications to the assay have allowed simultaneous measurement of phagocytosis and respiratory burst activity to be performed by dual-colour fluorescence analysis [126,127]. Bacteria which have been labelled with Texas red or propidium iodide are incubated with DCF-DA-loaded PMN cells. Phagocytosis is measured by the generation of red fluorescence owing to the ingested organisms, which in turn trigger the oxidative burst and subsequent development of green DCF fluorescence.

A flow cytometric NBT reduction assay has also been described for the measurement of respiratory burst activity [128].

12.4.4 Phagocytic vacuole protein digestion

The assessment of protein digestion within phagocytic vacuoles by flow cytometry has recently been described [129]. In the assay, rhodamine-conjugated albumin, at a sufficiently high dye/protein concentration to cause fluorescence quenching, is bound to opsonized carrier microbeads. Following phagocytosis by PMN cells, digestion of the protein component results in liberation of free rhodamine whose fluorescence intensity may be determined. Information from such assays may provide an indication of the integrity of primary degranulation and the condition of the microenvironment within the phagocytic vacuole.

12.5 FLOW CYTOMETRIC CELL-MEDIATED CYTOTOXICITY ASSAYS

Various forms of cell-mediated cytotoxicity, including antibody-dependent cell-mediated cytotoxicity (ADCC), macrophage cytotoxicity and NK cell cytotoxicity have been documented. Description of these various activities was largely based on so-called chromium release assays [130,131]. In these assays, target cells loaded with radioactive chromium were subjected to lysis by effector cells and the released radioactivity measured. Improvements in the reliability and specificity of these original tests have been made by the introduction of flow cytometric detection methods.

Flow cytometric NK cytotoxicity assays have been described in which K562 target cells are labelled with fluorescein diacetate (FDA) [132,133]. Cytoplasmic esterase activity converts FDA to free fluorescein which remains trapped within the cells. Incubation of these intensely fluorescent cells with effector (NK) cells results in target cell lysis. This may be monitored by reduction in fluorescent signals due to leakage through damaged membranes. Dual-colour assays which incorporate selective plasma membrane dyes and propidium iodide have been described [134,135]. These assays permit the discrimination of live and dead target or effector cells and consequently offer a more accurate estimation of cytotoxic activity. NK cell activity has also been estimated on the basis of morphological changes, detected by 90°LS measurements, which occur as a result of target cell disruption [136].

The quantitation of conjugate formation between effector and target cells by a dual-colour fluorescence technique has been described [137]. The method has been applied to the study of lymphokine-activated killer cell functions.

12.6 DETERMINATION OF IMMUNE COMPLEXES BY FLOW CYTOMETRY

Immune complexes have been implicated in a wide range of diseases, including glomerulonephritis, vasculitis, systemic lupus erythematosus and rheumatoid arthritis [138–140]. Serial measurement of circulating immune complexes in these diseases can be useful in monitoring disease activity and response to therapy. Many methods exist for the detection of immune complexes and these vary greatly in sensitivity and predictive value in various diseases [141]. This reflects, to a large extent, the heterogeneity of the complexes with regard to size, immunoglobulin composition and different principles on which the assays are based.

A number of flow cytometric immune complex assays have been described which may offer improved sensitivity and specificity. Flow cytometric assays based on the binding of complement-activated immune complexes to Raji cells have been developed [143,143] (Fig. 12.8). An important advantage of these assays over the conventional immunoradiometric assays is the ability to 'gate out' dead cells thus minimizing false-positive results caused by binding of autoantibodies to accessible nuclear or cytoplasmic antigens in dead cells. In a further adaption of the flow cytometric Raji cell assay, the immunoglobulin isotype composition of the circulating immune complexes can be detected [144]. As the immunoglobulin class of the antibody component of circulating immune complexes may be an important determinant in their pathogenicity, this technique may be useful in identifying the immunoglobulin isotype composition of circulating immune complexes in various disease states. Furthermore, comparative analyses of the immunoglobulin composition of immune complexes from different sites may be undertaken. From such analyses in rheumatoid arthritis patients, it appears that circulating immune complexes may not always arise simply from spill-over from the inflamed articular sites [145].

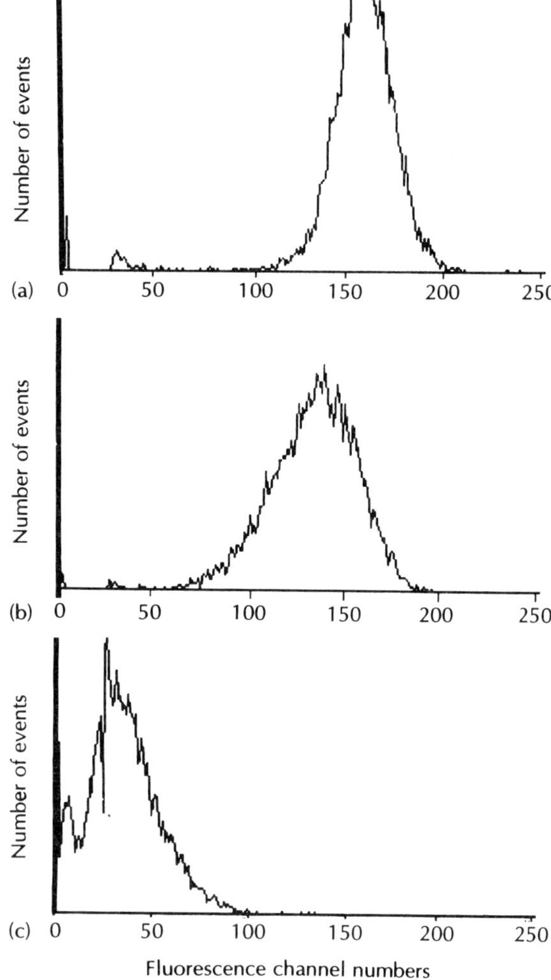

Fig. 12.8 Detection of immune complexes bound to Raji cells by fluorescein-conjugated antihuman immunoglobulin G (IgG) reagent. Fluorescence histograms were obtained following the flow cytometric analysis of Raji cells which had been incubated with serum samples from (a) systemic lupus erythematosus patient (MCF 158); (b) rheumatoid arthritis patient (MCF 134); (c) control subject (MCF 40). Application of MCF values to a standard aggregated γ-globulin curve allows quantification of immune complex levels [143]. MCF, median-channel fluorescence.

Flow cytometric detection of immune complexes using human C1q-coated microspheres has been reported [146]. Provided uniform coating of the beads can be attained, this technique would appear to offer a rapid and sensitive method of quantifying complement-binding immune complexes.

12.7 MICROSPHERE-BASED FLOW CYTOMETRIC ASSAYS

The application of flow cytometric analysis to quantitative and qualitative non-cellular immunoassays is an area of potential development in flow cytometry [147,148]. In microsphere-based assays, the microspheres (uniform latex particles) are used as a solid matrix to bind antibody, antigen or other biological compounds. A variety of immunoassays can thus be performed using the coated microspheres and fluorescence detection probes. The ability of the flow cytometer to discriminate and selectively analyse particles of varying sizes supports the potential for development of simultaneous detection systems using differing sizes of microsphere. It should be possible, therefore, to develop assays which can measure multiple antigens or antibodies simultaneously.

Essentially all assays which use a plastic support medium (e.g., antibody antigen capture; antibody competition; antibody/antibody sandwich assays) have the potential to be modified for microsphere/flow cytometric analysis. Requirements for successful development of such assays are the ability to absorb the appropriate protein or compound to the microsphere, and the availability of appropriate fluorescent probes.

Using this technology, a number of assays of potential interest to the clinical immunology laboratory have been reported: measurement of soluble IgG [149]; immune complexes [146]; Fc receptors [150]; and κ light-chain immunoglobulin [151].

Acknowledgements

We are grateful to Stephen Richards and Peter Master for their helpful comments and assistance in preparing this chapter, and to Phyllis McKenna for expert preparation of the manuscript.

References

1 Lorken MR, Shah VO, Dattilio KL, Civin CI. Flow cytometric analysis of human bone marrow. I. Normal erythroid development. *Blood* 1987; 69: 255–263.

2 Lorken MR, Shah VO, Dattilio KL, Civin CI. Flow cytometric analysis of human bone marrow. II Normal B lymphocyte development. *Blood* 1987; 70: 1316–1324.

3 Carter NP. Measurement of cellular subsets using antibodies. In: Ormerod MG (ed.) *Flow Cytometry: A Practical Approach.* IRL Press, Oxford, 1990: 45–67.

4 Bernard A, Boumsell L, Dausset J, Milstein C, Schlossman SF. (eds) *Leucocyte Typing.* Berlin: Springer, 1984.

5 Reinherz EL, Haynes BF, Nadler LM, Bernstein ID. (eds) *Leucocyte Typing II*, vol 1–3. Berlin: Springer, 1986.

6 McMichael AJ. (ed.) *Leucocyte Typing III. White Cell Differentiation Antigens.* Oxford: Oxford University Press, 1987.

7 Knapp W, Dorken B, Gilks WR, Rieber EP, Schmidt RE, Stein H, von dem Borne AEG. (eds) *Leucocyte Typing IV.* Oxford: Oxford University Press, 1989.

8 Winchester RJ, Ross GD, Jarowski CI, Wang CY, Halper J, Broxmeyer HE. Expression of Ia-like antigen molecules on human granulocytes during early phases of differentiation. *Proc Natl Acad Sci USA* 1977; 74: 4012–4016.

9 Edwards PAW. Monoclonal antibodies that bind to the human erthrocyte-membrane glycoproteins glycophorin A and band 3. *Biochem Soc Transact* 1980; 8: 198–199.

10 Greaves MF, Sieff C, Edwards PAW. Monoclonal anti-glycophorin as a probe for erythroleukaemias. *Blood* 1983; 61: 645–646.

11 Zola H, Neah SH, Potter A, Melo JV, De Oliveira SP, Catovsky D. Markers of differentiated B cell leukaemia: CD22 antibodies and FMC7 react with different molecules. *Dis Markers* 1987; 5: 227–235.

12 Morishta Y, Morishima Y, Ogura M, Yoshiyuki N, Ohno R. Biochemical characterization of human myeloperoxidase using three specific monoclonal antibodies. *Br J Haematol* 1986; 63: 435–444.

13 Erber WN. Applications of immunocytochemistry in leukaemia diagnosis. In: Scott CS (ed.) *Leukaemia Cytochemistry and Diagnosis: Principles and Practice.* Chichester: Ellis Harwood, 1989: 342–361.

14 Bollum FJ. Antibody to terminal deoxynucleotidyl transferase. *Proc Natl Acad Sci USA* 1975; 72: 4119–4122.

15 Bollum FJ. Terminal deoxynucleotidyl transferase as a haemopoietic cell marker. *Blood* 1979; 54: 1203–1215.

16 Gerdes J, Schwab U, Lemke H, Stein H. Production of a mouse monoclonal antibody reactive with a human nuclear antigen associated with cell proliferation. *Int J Cancer* 1983; 31: 13–20.

17 Scott CS, Ramsden W, Limbert HJ, Master PS, Roberts BE. Membrane transferrin receptor (TfR) and nuclear proliferation-associated Ki-67 expression in haemopoietic malignancies. *Leukemia* 1988; 2: 238–442.

18 Gray AG, Morgan J, Linch DC, Huehns ER. Enhanced fluorescence in indirect immunophenotyping by the

use of fluorescent liposomes. *J Immunol Methods* 1989; 121: 1–7.
19 Levitt D, King M. Methanol fixation permits flow cytometric analysis of immunofluorescent stained intracellular antigens. *J Immunol Methods* 1987; 96: 233–237.
20 Sander B, Andersson J, Andersson U. Assessment of cytokines by immunofluorescence and the paraformaldehyde-saporin procedure. *Immunol Rev* 1991; 119: 65–93.
21 Chikanza IC, Corrigal V, Kingsley G, Panayi GS. Enumeration of interleukin-1 alpha and beta producing cells by flow cytometry. *J Immunol Methods* 1992; 154: 173–178.
22 Schmid I, Schmid P, Giorgi JV. Conversion of logarithmic channel numbers into relative linear fluorescence intensity. *Cytometry* 1988; 9: 533–538.
23 Harvath L. Quality control in clinical flow cytometry. *Pathol Immunopathol Res* 1988; 7: 338–344.
24 McCarthy RC, Fetterhoff TJ. Issues for quality assurance in clinical flow cytometry. *Arch Pathol Lab Med* 1989; 113: 658–666.
25 McCoy JP, Carey JL, Krause JR. Quality control in flow cytometry for diagnostic pathology. I. Cell surface phenotyping and general laboratory procedures. *Am J Clin Pathol* 1990; 93: S27–S37.
26 Horan PK, Muirhead KA, Slezak SE. Standards and controls in flow cytometry. In: Melamed MR, Lindmo T, Mendelsohn ML (eds) *Flow Cytometry and Sorting*, 2nd edn. New York: Wiley–Liss, 1990: 392–414.
27 Lorken MR, Brosnan JM, Back BA, Ault KA. Establishing optimal lymphocyte gates for immunophenotyping by flow cytometry. *Cytometry* 1990; 11: 453–459.
28 Catovsky D, Melo JV, Matutes E. Biological markers in lymphoproliferative disorders. In: *Chronic and Acute Leukemias in Adults*. Boston: Martinus-Nijhoff, 1985: 69–112.
29 Foon KA, Tood RF. Immunologic classification of leukemia and lymphoma. *Blood* 1986; 68: 1–31.
30 Drexler HG. Classification of acute myeloid leukemias — a comparison of FAB and immunophenotyping. *Leukemia* 1987; 1: 697–705.
31 Van Dongen JJM, Quertermous T, Bartram CR *et al.* T cell receptor-CD3 complex during early T cell differentiation. Analysis of immature T cell acute lymphoblastic leukaemias (T-ALL) at DNA, RNA and cell membrane level. *J Immunol* 1987, 138: 1260–1269.
32 Drexler HG, Scott CS. Morphological and immunological aspects of leukaemia diagnosis. In: Scott CS (ed.) *Leukaemia and Diagnosis: Principles and Practice*. Chichester: Ellis Harwood, 1989: 13–67.
33 Campana D, Thompson JS, Amlot P, Brown S, Janossy G. The cytoplasmic expression of CD3 antigens in normal and malignant cells of the T lymphoid lineage. *J Immunol* 1987; 138: 648–655.
34 Stass SA, Mirro J. Lineage heterogeneity in acute leukaemia: acute mixed-lineage leukaemia and lineage switch. *Clin Haematol* 1986; 15: 811–827.
35 Sobol RE, Mick R, Royston I *et al.* Clinical importance of myeloid antigen expression in adult acute lymphoblastic leukaemia. *N Engl J Med* 1987; 316: 1111–1117.
36 Drexler HG. Myeloid-antigen expression in adult ALL. *N Engl J Med* 1987; 317: 1156.
37 Bradstock KF, Kirk J, Grimsley PG, Kabral A, Hughes WG. Unusual immunophenotypes in acute leukaemias: incidence and clinical correlations. *Br J Haematol* 1989; 72: 512–518.
38 Mirro J, Kitchingman GR. The morphology, cytochemistry, molecular characteristics and clinical significance of acute mixed-lineage leukaemia. In: Scott CS (ed.) *Leukaemia Cytochemistry and Diagnosis: Principles and Practice*. Chichester: Ellis Horwood, 1989: 155–179.
39 Pui CH, Behm FG, Singh B *et al.* Myeloid-associated antigen expression lacks prognostic value in childhood acute lymphoblastic leukemia. *Blood* 1990; 75: 198–202.
40 Guyotat D, Campos L, Shi ZH *et al.* Myeloid surface antigen expression in adult acute lymphoblastic leukemia. *Leukemia* 1990; 4: 664–666.
41 Keleti J, Revesz T, Schuler D. Morphological diagnosis in childhood leukaemia. *Br J Haematol* 1978; 40: 501–502.
42 Hann IM, Evans DIK, Palmer MK, Morris Jones PJ, Haworth C. The prognostic significance of morphological features in childhood acute lymphoblastic leukaemia. *Clin Lab Haematol* 1979; 1: 215–226.
43 Pullen DJ, Boyett JM, Crist WM *et al.* Pediatric Oncology Group utilisation of immunologic markers in the designation of acute lymphocytic leukemia (ALL) subgroups: influence on treatment response. *Ann NY Acad Sci* 1983; 428: 26–48.
44 Crist W, Boyett J, Roper M *et al.* Pre B-cell leukemia responds poorly to treatment: a Pediatric Oncology Group study. *Blood* 1984; 63: 407–414.
45 Van Eys J, Pullen J, Head D *et al.* The French–American–British (FAB) classification of leukemia. The Pediatric Oncology Group experience with lymphocytic leukemia. *Cancer* 1986; 57: 1046–1051.
46 Lister TA, Whitehouse JMA, Beard MEJ *et al.* Combination chemotherapy for acute lymphoblastic leukaemia in adults. *Br Med J* 1978; i: 199–203.
47 Flandrin G, Brouet JC, Daniel MT, Preud'homme JL. (1975) Acute leukemia with Burkitt's tumor cells: a study of six cases with special reference to lymphocyte surface markers. *Blood* 1975; 45: 183–188.
48 Greaves MF, Janossy G, Peto J, Kay H. Immunologically defined subclasses of acute lymphoblastic leukaemia in children: their relationship to presentation features and prognosis. *Br J Haematol* 1981; 48: 179–197.
49 Bennett JM, Catovsky D, Daniel MT *et al.* Proposals

for the classification of the acute leukaemias. *Br J Haematol* 1976; 33: 451–458.

50 Bennett JM, Catovsky D, Daniel MT *et al.* A variant form of hypergranular promyelocytic leukaemia (M3). *Br J Haematol* 1980; 44: 169–170.

51 Bennett JM, Catovsky D, Daniel MT *et al.* Criteria for the diagnosis of acute leukemia of megakaryocyte lineage (M7). *Ann Intern Med* 1985; 103: 460–462.

52 Bennett JM, Catovsky D, Daniel MT, Flandrin G, Galton DAG. Proposed revised criteria for the classification of acute myeloid leukaemia: a report of the French–American–British co-operative group. *Ann Intern Med* 1985; 103: 626–629.

53 de Oliveira MSP, Matutes E, Catovsky D. The cytochemistry, membrane markers and ultrastructure of megakaryoblastic (M7) and erythro (M6) leukaemias. In: Scott CS (ed.) *Leukaemia Cytochemistry and Diagnosis: Principles and Practice.* Chichester: Ellis Harwood, 1989: 137–154.

54 Vainchenker W, Villeval JL, Tabilio A *et al.* Immunophenotype of leukemic blasts with small peroxidase-positive granules detected by electron microscopy. *Leukemia* 1988; 2: 274–281.

55 Scott CS. Cytochemistry of acute myeloid leukemia with particular reference to myeloperoxidase (MPO). In: Scott CS (ed.) *Leukaemia Cytochemistry and Diagnosis: Principles and Practice.* Chichester: Ellis Harwood, 1989: 91–102.

56 Geller RB, Zahurak M, Hurwithz CA *et al.* Prognostic importance of immunophenotyping in adults with acute myelocytic leukaemia: the significance of the stem cell glycoprotein CD34 (My10). *Br J Haematol* 1990; 76: 340–347.

57 Galigaris-Cappio F, Gobbi M, Bofill M, Janossy G. Infrequent normal B lymphocytes express features of B chronic lymphocytic leukemia. *J Exp Med* 1982; 155: 623–627.

58 Ault KA, Antin JH, Ginsburg D *et al.* Phenotype of recovering lymphoid populations after marrow transplantation. *J Exp Med* 1985; 161: 1483–1502.

59 Freedman AS, Nadler LM. The relationship of chronic lymphocytic leukemia to normal activated B cells. *Leuk Lymph* 1990; 1: 293–300.

60 Bofill M, Janossy G, Janossa M *et al.* Human B cell development. II. Subpopulations in the human fetus. *J Immunol* 1985; 134: 1531–1538.

61 Scott CS, Limbert HJ, Roberts BE, Stark AN. Prolymphocytoid variants of chronic lymphocytic leukaemia: an immunological and morphological survey. *Leuk Res* 1987; 11: 135–140.

62 Melo JV, Robinson DSF, Gregory C, Catovsky D. Splenic B cell lymphoma with 'villous' lymphocytes in the peripheral blood. A disorder distinct from hairy cell leukemia. *Leukemia* 1987; 1: 294–299.

63 Catovsky D, O'Brien M, Melo M, Wardle J, Brosovic M. Hairy cell leukemia (HCL) variant: an intermediate disease between HCL and B-prolymphocytic leukemia. *Semin Oncol* 1984; 11: 362–369.

64 Scott CS, Hunt KM, Jones RA, Gignac SM, Matutes E, Drexler HG. Proliferative hairy cell leukaemia (HCL-v) resistant to alpha-interferon: clinical, diagnostic and *in-vitro* cellular characteristics. *Leuk Lymph* 1990; 1: 307–317.

65 Pandolfi F. T-CLL and allied disease: new insights into classification and pathogenesis. *Diagn Immunol* 1986; 4: 61–74.

66 Semenzato G, Pandolfi F, Chisesi T *et al.* The lymphoproliferative disease of granular lymphocytes. A heterogenous disorder ranging from indolent to aggressive conditions. *Cancer* 1987; 60: 2917–2928.

67 Witzig TE, Phyliky RL, Li C-Y, Hamburger HA, Dewald GW, Handwegar BS. T-cell chronic lymphocytic leukemia with a helper/inducer membrane phenotype: a distinct clinicopathologic subtype with a poor prognosis. *Am J Hematol* 1986; 21: 139–155.

68 Matutes E, Talavera JG, O'Brien M, Catovsky D. The morphological spectrum of T-prolymphocytic leukaemia. *Br J Haematol* 1986; 64: 111–124.

69 Reynolds CW, Foon KA. T-lymphoproliferative disease and related disorders in humans and experimental animals: a review of the clinical, cellular and functional characteristics. *Blood* 1984; 64: 1146–1158.

70 Sattentau QT. HIV infection and the immune system. *Biochim Biophys Acta* 1989; 989: 255–268.

71 Rosenberg ZF, Fauci AS. The immunopathogenesis of HIV infection. *Adv Immunol* 1989; 47: 377–431.

72 Seligmann M. Immunological features of human immunodeficiency virus disease. *Clin Haematol* 1990; 3: 37–63.

73 Meltzer MS, Skillman DR, Hoover DL *et al.* Macrophages and the human immunodeficiency virus. *Immunol Today* 1990; 11: 217–223.

74 Polk BF, Fox R, Brookmeyer R *et al.* Predictors of the acquired immunodeficiency syndrome developing in a cohort of seropositive homosexual men. *N Engl J Med* 1987; 316: 62–66.

75 Eyster ME, Gail MH, Ballard JO, Al-Mondhirg H, Goedert JJ. Natural history of human immunodeficiency virus infections in hemophiliacs: effects of T cell subsets, platelet counts and age. *Ann Intern Med* 1987; 107: 1–6.

76 Moss AR, Bacchetti P, Osmond D *et al.* Seropositivity for HIV and the development of AIDS or AIDS related condition: 3 years follow up of the San Francisco General Hospital cohort. *Br Med J* 1988; 296: 745–750.

77 Goedert JJ, Kessler CM, Aledort LM *et al.* A prospective study of human immunodeficiency virus type 1 infection and the development of AIDS in subjects with hemophilia. *N Engl J Med* 1989; 321: 1141–1148.

78 Lang W, Perkins H, Anderson RE, Royce R, Jewell N, Winhelstein W. Patterns of T lymphocyte changes with human immunodeficiency virus infection: from seroconversion to the development of AIDS. *J AIDS*

1989; 2: 63–69.
79 Giorgi JV, Detels R. T cell subset alterations in HIV infected homosexual men: NIAID multicentre AIDS cohort study. *Clin Immunol Immunopathol* 1989; 52: 10–18.
80 Fahey JL, Taylor JMG, Detels R *et al.* The prognostic value of cellular and serological markers in infection with human immunodeficiency virus type 1. *N Engl J Med* 1990; 322: 166–172.
81 Phillips AN, Lee CA, Elford J *et al.* Serial CD4 lymphocyte counts and development of AIDS. *Lancet* 1991; 337: 389–392.
82 Bird AG. Clinical and immunological assessment of HIV infection. *J Clin Pathol* 1992; 45: 850–854.
83 Masur H, Ognibene FP, Yarchoan R *et al.* CD4 counts as predictors of opportunistic pneumonias in human immunodeficiency virus (HIV) infection. *Ann Intern Med* 1989; 111: 223–231.
84 Volberding PA, Lagokos SW, Kock MA *et al.* Zidovudine in asymptomatic human immunodeficiency virus infection. *N Engl J Med* 1990; 322: 941–949.
85 Bird AG. Monitoring of lymphocyte subpopulation changes in the assessment of HIV infection. *Genitourin Med* 1990; 66: 133–137.
86 Koepke JA, Landay AL. Precision and accuracy of absolute lymphocyte counts. *Clin Immunol Immunopathol* 1989; 52: 19–27.
87 Taylor JMG, Fahey JL, Detels R, Giorgi JV. CD4 percentage, CD4 number and CD4:CD8 ratio in HIV infection; which to choose and how to use. *J AIDS* 1989; 2: 114–124.
88 Fahey JL, Taylor JMG, Detels R *et al.* The prognostic value of cellular and serological markers in infection with human immunodeficiency virus type 1. *N Engl J Med* 1990; 322: 166–172.
89 Giorgi JV, Cheng HL, Margolick JB *et al.* Quality control in the flow cytometric measurement of T lymphocyte subsets: the multicentre AIDS cohort study experience. *Clin Immunol Immunopathol* 1990; 55: 173–186.
90 CDC Guidelines for the performance of CD4+ T-cell determinations in persons with human immunodeficiency virus infection. *MMWR* 1992; 41: 1–17.
91 Hulstaert F, Strauss K, Levacher M, Vanham G, Kestens L, Bach BA. The staging and prognostic value of subset markers on CD8 cells in HIV disease. In: Janossy G, Autran B, Miedema F (eds) *Immunodeficiency in HIV Infection and AIDS.* Basel: S Karger, 1992; 185–194.
92 Stites DP, Casavant CH, McHugh TM *et al.* Flow cytometric analysis of lymphocyte phenotypes in AIDS using monoclonal antibodies and simultaneous dual immunofluorescence. *Clin Immunol Immunopathol* 1986; 38: 161–177.
93 Baron GC, Klimas NG, Fischi MA, Fletcher MA. Decreased natural cell-mediated cytotoxicity for effector cell in acquired immunodeficiency syndrome. *Diagn Immunol* 1985; 3: 197–204.
94 Wood GS, Burns BF, Dorfman RF, Warnke RA. The immunohistology of non-T cells in the acquired immunodeficiency syndrome. *Am J Pathol* 1985; 120: 371–378.
95 Levine AM, Meyer PR, Begandy MK *et al.* Development of B cell lymphoma in homosexual men: clinical and immunological findings. *Ann Intern Med* 1984; 100: 7–13.
96 McSharry JJ, Costantino R, Robbiano E, Echols R, Stevens R, Lehman JM. Detection and quantitation of human immunodeficiency virus-infected peripheral blood mononuclear cells by flow cytometry. *J Clin Microbiol* 1990; 28: 724–733.
97 Duque RE, Ward PA. Quantitative assessment of neutrophil function by flow cytometry. *Anal Quant Cytol Histol* 1987; 9: 42–48.
98 Bjerknes R, Bassoe CF, Sjursen H, Laerum OD, Solberg CO. Flow cytometry for the study of phagocyte functions. *Rev Infect Dis* 1989; 11: 16–33.
99 Fearon DT, Collins LA. Increased expression of C3b receptors on polymorphonuclear leukocytes induced by chemotactic factors and by purification procedures. *J Immunol* 1983; 130: 370–375.
100 Berger M, O'Shea J, Cross AS *et al.* Human neutrophils increase expression of C3bi as well as C3b receptors upon activation. *J Clin Invest* 1984; 74: 1566–1571.
101 O'Shea JJ, Brown EJ, Seligmann BE, Metcalf JA, Frank MM, Gallin JI. Evidence for distinct intracellular pools of receptors for C3b and C3bi in human neutrophils. *J Immunol* 1985; 134: 2580–2587.
102 Wright SD, Meyer BC. Phorbol esters cause sequential activation and deactivation of complement receptors on polymorphonuclear leukocytes. *J Immunol* 1986; 136: 1759–1764.
103 Crockard AD, Thompson JM, McBride SJ, Edgar JD, McNeill TA, Bell AL. Markers of inflammatory activation: upregulation of complement receptors CR1 and CR3 on synovial fluid neutrophils from patients with inflammatory joint disease. *Clin Immunol Immunopathol* 1992; 65: 135–142.
104 Berger M, Sorensen RU, Tosi MF, Dearborn G, Doring F. Complement receptor expression on neutrophils at an inflammatory site, the *Pseudomonas*-infected lung in cystic fibrosis. *J Clin Invest* 1989; 84: 1302–1313.
105 Moore FD, Davis C, Rodrick M, Mannick JA, Fearon DT. Neutrophil activation in thermal injury as assessed by expression of complement receptors. *N Engl J Med* 1986; 314: 948–953.
106 Babcock GF, Alexander JW, Warden GD. Flow cytometric analysis of neutrophil subsets in thermally injured patients developing infection. *Clin Immunol Immunopathol* 1990; 54: 117–125.
107 Kishimoto TK, Larson RS, Corbi AL, Dustin ML, Staunton DE, Springer TA. The leukocyte integrins. *Adv Immunol* 1989; 46: 149–182.
108 Arnaout MA. Structure and function of the leukocyte

adhesion molecules CD11/CD18. *Blood* 1990; 75: 1037–1050.
109 Springer TA. Adhesion receptors of the immune system. *Nature* 1990; 346: 425–434.
110 Springer TA, Thompson WS, Miller LJ, Schmalstieg FC, Anderson DC. Inherited deficiency of the Mac-1, LFA-1, p150-95 glycoprotein family and its molecular basis. *J Exp Med* 1984; 160: 1901–1918.
111 Anderson DC, Springer TA. Leukocyte adhesion deficiency and inherited defect in the Mac-1, LFA-1 and p150,95 glycoproteins. *Annu Rev Med* 1987; 38: 175–194.
112 Unkeless JC. Function and heterogeneity of human Fc receptors for immunoglobulin G. *J Clin Invest* 1989; 83: 355–361.
113 Huizinga TWJ, Ross D, von dem Borne AEG. Neutrophil Fc receptors: a two-way bridge in the immune system. *Blood* 1990; 75: 1211–1214.
114 Carr R, Davis JM. Abnormal FcR III expression by neutrophils from very preterm infants. *Blood* 1990; 76: 607–611.
115 Smith JB, Campbell DE, Ludomirsky A *et al.* Expression of the complement receptors CR1 and CR3 and the type III Fc gamma receptor on neutrophils from newborn infants and from fetuses with Rh disease. *Pediatr Res* 1990; 28: 120–126.
116 Dunn PA, Tyrer HW. Quantitation of neutrophil phagocytosis using fluorescent latex beads. Correlations of microscopy and flow cytometry. *J Lab Clin Med* 1981; 98: 374–381.
117 Bjerknnes R, Bassoe CF. Human leukocyte phagocytosis of zymosan particles measured by flow cytometry. *Acta Pathol Microbiol Immun Scand (C)* 1983; 91: 341–348.
118 Bassoe CF, Laerum OD, Solberg CO, Hanesberg B. Phagocytosis of bacteria by leucocytes measured by flow cytometry. *Proc Soc Exp Biol Med* 1983; 174: 182–186.
119 Steinkamp JA, Wilson JS, Saunders GC, Stewart CC. Phagocytosis: flow cytometric quantitation with fluorescent microspheres. *Science* 1982; 215: 64–66.
120 Bjerknes R. Flow cytometric assay for combined measurement of phagocytosis and intracellular killing of *Candida albicans. J Immunol Methods* 1984; 72: 229–241.
121 Hed J, Hallden G, Johansson SGO, Larsson P. The use of fluorescence quenching in flow cytofluorometry to measure the attachment and ingestion phases in phagocytosis in peripheral blood without prior cell separation. *J Immunol Methods* 1987; 101: 119–125.
122 Ogle JD, Noel JG, Sramkoski RM, Ogle CK, Alexander JW. Phagocytosis of opsonized fluorescent microspheres by human neutrophils. A two color flow cytometric method for the determination of attachment and ingestion *J Immunol Method* 1988; 115: 17–29.
123 Buschmann H, Winters M. Assessment of phagocytic activity of granulocytes using laser flow cytometry. *J Immunol Methods* 1989; 124: 231–234.
124 Babior BM. Oxygen-dependent microbial killing by phagocytes. *N Engl J Med* 1978; 298: 659–668.
125 Bass DA, Parce JW, De Chatelet LR, Szejda P, Seeds MC, Thomas M. Flow cytometric studies of oxidative product formation by neutrophils: a graded response to membrane stimulation. *J Immunol* 1983; 130: 1910–1917.
126 Trinkle LS, Wellhausen SR, McLeish KR. A simultaneous flow cytometric measurement of neutrophil phagocytosis and oxidative burst in whole blood. *Diagn Clin Immunol* 1987; 5: 62–68.
127 Hasui M, Hirabayashi Y, Kobayashi Y. Simultaneous measurement of flow cytometry of phagocytosis and hydrogen peroxide production of neutrophils in whole blood. *J Immunol Methods* 1989; 117: 53–58.
128 Blair OC, Carbone R, Sartorelli AC. Differentiation of ML-60 promyelocytic leukemia cells monitored by flow cytometric measurement of nitro blue tetrazolium (NBT) reduction. *Cytometry* 1985; 6: 54–61.
129 Haynes AP, Fletcher J, Garnett M, Robins A. A novel flow cytometric method for measuring protein digestion within the phagocytic vacuole of polymorphonuclear neutrophils. *J Immunol Methods* 1990; 135: 155–161.
130 Herberman RB. Natural killer cell activity and antibody-dependent cell-mediated cytotoxicity. In: Rose NR, Friedman H, Fahey JL (eds) *Manual of Clinical Laboratory Immunology*, 3rd edn. Washington: American Society for Microbiology, 1986: 308–314.
131 Rosenwasser LJ. Monocyte and macrophage function. In: Rose NR, Friedman H, Fahey JL (eds) *Manual of Clinical Laboratory Immunology*, 3rd edn. Washington: American Society for Microbiology, 1986: 321–325.
132 McGinnes K, Chapman G, Marks R, Penny R. A fluorescence NK assay using flow cytometry. *J Immunol Methods* 1986; 86: 7–15.
133 Shi TX, Tong MJ, Bohman R. The application of flow cytometry in the study of natural killer cell cytotoxicity. *Clin Immunol Immunopathol* 1987; 45: 356–365.
134 Slezak SE, Horan PK. Cell-mediated cytotoxicity. A highly sensitive and informative flow cytometric assay. *J Immunol Methods* 1989; 117: 205–214.
135 Radosevic K, Garritsen HSP, Van Graft M, De Grooth BG, Greve J. A simple and sensitive flow cytometric assay for the determination of the cytotoxic activity of human natural killer cells. *J Immunol Methods* 1990; 135: 81–89.
136 Vitale M, Neri LM, Comani S *et al.* Natural killer function in flow cytometry. II Evaluation of NK lytic activity by means of target cell morphological changes detected by right angle light scatter. *J Immunol Methods* 1989; 121: 115–120.
137 Cavarec L, Quillet MA, Fradelizi D, Conjeaud H. An improved double fluorescence flow cytometry method

for the quantification of killer cell/target cell conjugate formation. *J Immunol Methods* 1990; 130: 251–261.
138 McDougal JS, McDuffie FC. Immune complexes in man: detection and clinical significance. *Adv Clin Chem* 1985; 24: 1–60.
139 Barnett EV. Circulating immune complexes: their biological and clinical significance. *J Allergy Clin Immunol* 1986; 78: 1089–1096.
140 Phillips TM. Immune complex assays: diagnostic and clinical application. *Crit Rev Clin Lab Sci* 1989; 27: 237–264.
141 Lambert PH, Dixon FJ, Zubler RH *et al.* A WHO collaborative study for the evaluation of 18 methods for detecting immune complexes in serum. *J Clin Lab Immunol* 1978; 1: 1–15.
142 Lightfoot M, Folks TM, Redfield R *et al.* Flow cytometric detection of circulating immune complexes. *J Immunol Methods* 1986; 95: 107–112.
143 Kingsmore SF, Crockard AD, Fay AC, McNeill TA, Roberts SD, Thompson JM. Detection of circulating immune complexes by Raji cell assay: comparison of flow cytometric and radiometric techniques. *Diagn Clin Immunol* 1988; 5: 289–296.
144 Kingsmore SF, Thompson JM, Crockard AD *et al.* Measurement of circulating immune complexes containing IgE, IgM, IgA and IgE by flow cytometry: correlation with disease activity in patients with systemic lupus erythematosus. *J Clin Lab Immunol* 1989; 30: 45–52.
145 Crockard AD, Thompson JM, Finch MB, McNeill TA, Bell AL, Roberts SD. Immunoglobulin isotype composition of circulating and intra-articular immune complexes in patients with inflammatory joint disease. *Rheumatol Int* 1989; 11: 169–174.
146 McHugh TM, Stites DP, Casavant CH, Fulwyler MJ. Flow cytometric detection and quantitation of immune complexes using human C1q-coated microspheres. *J Immunol Methods* 1986; 95: 57–61.
147 Cook L, Irving D. Microsphere-based flow cytometric assays. *J Clin Immunoassay* 1989; 12; 36–39.
148 Lea T, O'Connell JP, Nustad K, Funderud S, Berge A, Rembaum A. In: Melamed MR, Lindmo T, Mendelsohn ML (eds) *Flow Cytometry and Sorting*, 2nd edn. New York: Wiley–Liss, 1990: 367–380.
149 Wilson MR, Witherspoon JS. A new microsphere-based immunofluorescence assay using flow cytometry. *J Immunol Methods* 1988; 107: 225–230.
150 Bonnefoy JY, Banchereau J, Aubry JP, Wijdenes J. A flow cytometric micromethod for the detection of Fc receptors and IgE binding factors using fluorescent microspheres. *J Immunol Methods* 1986; 88: 25–32.
151 Lisi PJ, Huang CW, Hoffman RA, Teipel JW. A fluorescence immunoassay for soluble antigens employing flow cytometric detection. *Clin Chim Acta* 1982; 120: 171–179.

PART 3
CURRENT DEVELOPMENTS

13

EXPERT SYSTEMS FOR HISTOPATHOLOGY

P. H. BARTELS, J. E. WEBER, D. THOMPSON, P. W. HAMILTON AND R. MONTIRONI

When we are faced with a situation made difficult because we find ourselves unable to make a decision, we consult experts. This difficulty in making a decision may be due to our lack of experience for a given unusual case or to ambiguities in the evidence presented. Probably it is also due to the lack of a clearly defined step-by-step procedure that will lead to an unequivocal decision, and so we turn to the expert.

Based on long-term experience, the expert may quickly arrive at a solution. The expert may, in fact, be quite capable of explaining the reasons for the decision which, on the whole, usually make sense. The way in which the expert is led from the evaluation of one piece of evidence to the selection of the next relevant piece of information may not follow any seemingly logical reasoning. The expert simply 'knows' from past experience that the process leads to success.

Consultation with the expert may take different forms. The expert may simply examine the situation, arrive at a decision, and then explain, as well as possible, why that decision was reached. The consultation may also take the form of an interchange, during which the expert is asked specific questions and, in turn, the expert requests additional information, until a final decision is reached. Human experts are often difficult to reach and, for a given domain, they may be rare. Also, their expertise usually is expensive, and eventually it is lost when they leave their profession. Expert systems are computer programs that are designed to replace a human expert. At their best, one should be able to communicate with an expert system as though one had a highly experienced human expert right there.

Expert systems are computer programs, but they are distinctly different in both structure and function from the usual algorithmic procedures. A conventional computer program is written and compiled. The algorithm processes data in a fixed deterministic manner, following a pre-established path to the solution. Each processing step follows the preceding step in a logical manner. The results of such algorithmic processing are predictable in all but their numerical values. The algorithm may be based on brute force and arrive at a solution by exhaustive number crunching or extensive iterations. Missing data cannot be tolerated; the entire procedure is predetermined and inexorable.

Expert system software has a basically different structure. There is a compiled, algorithmic program portion, the *expert system shell* with its inference engine, and there is the completely separated knowledge base. The program shell controls, in an algorithmic manner, the inference processing. The knowledge base holds facts and procedural information. This information is interpreted at run time, thus there really is no fixed processing sequence since the next step depends on the interpretation of the preceding step. The rules may be based on heuristic insight (and they often are), therefore the selection of the next step may be well-justified on heuristic grounds, but may not follow logically at all. If data are missing, the expert system will utilize other information to continue. The knowledge base may contain prior information specifying heuristic short-cuts under certain conditions. Expert systems do not go into brute force iterations or exhaustive searches, but rather rely on insight and prior knowledge, much like the human expert would. The reasoning process conducted by an expert system may involve judgement calls, as contained in its knowledge base, so the final results are not logically predictable. The system may find a number of different solutions to a problem. Some expert systems offer an explanation for the reasoning sequence which they followed. This illustrates, better than anything else, the difference in functioning between a heuristic search for a solution and an algorithmic procedure.

The development of expert systems followed from research in artificial intelligence and has come a long way. In diagnostic pathology, most published developments were understandably aimed at diagnostic decision-making. It has been said that diagnostic expert systems may consistently perform at the level of an average specialist. In those cases where performance was found to be better than that of a human specialist, it was because the expert system used the available knowledge exhaustively and did not neglect consideration of any possibly relevant diagnostic clue or possible outcome. Even though the emphasis in ongoing developments of expert systems for histopathology has been on diagnostic decision support, one should really view the methodology in a broader context.

The overwhelming majority of knowledge in histopathology is based on image information, descriptive terms, words, concepts and the understanding of processes. Only a small proportion of knowledge in pathology is presented in numerical form. Data in histopathology thus are predominantly non-numerical. We have extensive methodology for analysis of numerical data, for example, descriptive statistics, analysis of variance, statistical classification techniques, trend analysis methods, and measures of distance and typicality, to name a few. There also exists some methodology to analyse and accommodate categorical data.

For the vast bulk of knowledge in histopathology though, its representation in symbolic form, as linguistic descriptive terms, has precluded systematic manipulation and evaluation. Expert systems methodology, with its symbolic processing, offers this capability, and the potential exceeds by far the mere role of diagnostic decision support. In fact, it offers the potential for systematic representation and manipulation of histopathological knowledge. This includes, of course, the capability for diagnostic decision-making and for descriptive classification, with their advantages of specificity and ability to accommodate a large number of alternative outcomes and to tolerate missing information.

Expert systems methodology also is the key to the management of options offered by advances in information technology. Quantitative image analysis has been shown to provide valuable diagnostic and possibly prognostic clues. However, the evaluation of diagnostically representative areas of a section, at high resolution, may involve the digitizing and recording of hundreds of video frames. The information can indeed be recorded and digitized within a few minutes. However, algorithmic image processing has been found unable to cope with the multitudinous problems of scene segmentation, which is the prerequisite for the extraction of diagnostic histometric or karyometric data. While segmentation problems can be corrected interactively on a few frames, this is no longer a practical option when hundreds of frames are involved. Expert-system-guided, intelligent and adaptive scene segmentation software has been shown to provide machine vision capabilities to diagnostic and prognostic expert systems [1]. With the general introduction of shared computer databases, we can also expect that very extensive databases on patient anamnestic data, diagnostic information, treatment regimen and, eventually, clinical outcome will accumulate worldwide. It is now technically feasible to store very large amounts of digitized imagery of histological sections or cytological preparations using such records. However, the search through databases on such a scale, the retrieval of relevant information and appropriate analysis are all tasks requiring highly specialized knowledge. Here, expert systems may well serve as consultants to medical researchers, advising on proper study design, researching availability of data and providing guidance in the choice of analytical procedures as well as in the interpretation of results.

There exists a rich literature on expert system principles, design, mode of operation and applications [2–7]. For the histopathologist, there are three major aspects of the methodology that require careful examination before the implementation or even use of an expert system is considered. These are the manner in which the inference process is conducted in a system, how uncertainty is managed by the system and the way in which knowledge is represented.

13.1 INFERENCE

Inference is the process by which observations and knowledge about the problem domain are related in such a way that each inference step brings an advance toward a solution. It seems necessary here to elaborate on what is meant by a solution to a problem. Reaching a solution could involve procedures of vastly differing complexity. In the simplest case, the solution to a problem might be the determination of whether an assertion is true or false. In a much more difficult case, obtaining a solution might involve making a long sequence of intermediate decisions, taking into account not only the order in which these intermediate decisions should be made but, even more importantly, which intermediate decisions should be chosen. When combined, the accumulated evidence would suggest a solution to the problem.

Thus, a solution to a problem may involve no more than determining whether or not a clinical cytological preparation contains cells with large nuclei; or it may involve the suggestion of a diagnostic outcome, based on numerous observed diagnostic clues and patient anamnestic data.

In much of the early work in artificial intelligence, finding the solution to a problem is approached as a 'search through a state space' [8]. Every fact or chunk of knowledge about a problem is seen as an island in a space; by traversing the space and evaluating the situation at hand and then comparing it with the information offered in the knowledge base of the system, evidence is combined and accumulated until the system arrives at a state where all the evidence needed to make a decision has been obtained.

There are two important aspects here which need to be considered. The first is the efficiency of the search for a solution; the second is the management of uncertainty.

The search for a problem's solution may take either of two extreme routes, given that the correct answer is indeed represented among the many possible combinations of facts and assertions in the state space. The first extreme approach would be an exhaustive, brute-force search. Every piece of evidence would be evaluated and combined with every other piece of evidence. This is an approach that is guaranteed to find the best solution assuming, of course, that a criterion for what is best can be defined. However, it is an approach that, for all but the most trivial problems, is not feasible. For example, for only 32 facts, and assuming the only possible outcomes for each fact to be true or false, the number of combinations that must be evaluated to obtain a solution is astronomically large – in excess of 4 billion. Yet, exhaustive search is the process used in many algorithmic problem-solving tasks.

Another approach might be taken by a decision-maker with considerable understanding of the problem area. It utilizes prior knowledge about which facts and which combinations of evidence are relevant for a decision, and then a highly directed search for only those pieces of evidence is pursued. It is a heuristic search and can be highly efficient. Heuristic search is the procedure followed by human experts. They frequently may not be able to state precisely why they proceed from one piece of evidence to another particular piece of evidence, other than the fact that their long-term experience has taught them that this will lead to the desired answer. It is this heuristic reasoning and heuristic knowledge that one tries to imitate in an expert system.

Heuristic does not imply a search that is totally non-systematic. On the contrary, human experts usually pursue the search for useful evidence using a well-suited strategy. They may consider a multitude of observations and facts that support a particular conclusion rather than any of a number of other possible conclusions. Then, they may proceed in an analogous manner until only a very limited number of alternative solutions remain, from which the final solution is chosen. It may be a bottom-up, data-driven process, also known in expert system design as a forward-chaining strategy. This is a good strategy when there are a large number of pieces of evidence and a limited number of alternative outcomes.

On the other hand, bottom-up is not a good strategy when the number of alternative outcomes is large. One would then have to evaluate all of the numerous pieces of evidence for all of the many possible outcomes. In this case, it is more efficient to start with each possible outcome and ask whether there is any evidence to suggest that this outcome is likely. One can then concentrate on those outcomes for which there is some high level of evidence, and go down in a decision sequence to the more detailed evidence supporting each alternative. This is a top-down goal-driven strategy, also known as backward chaining in expert systems methodology.

Clearly, human experts alternate in their search strategies between bottom-up and top-down reasoning, as different aspects of a complex problem are examined. Mixed strategies can also be pursued in many expert systems. They are initiated and controlled by so-called metarules which direct the inferencing strategy.

One important determinant in the development of an inference and decision sequence is the criterion for measuring how far one has come towards the goal of an unequivocal final decision. This criterion is based on a measure of uncertainty.

13.2 THE MANAGEMENT OF UNCERTAINTY

It is time to return in the discussion to a crucial aspect of inferencing – the management of uncertainty [9]. One may look at the process of finding a solution to a problem from another point of view and see it as a process of reducing uncertainty. For a given problem, there may be some initial knowledge of the relative likelihood of different outcomes. This knowledge exists before any observations are made for a particular case. For example, for any particular clinical pathology laboratory, the proportions of colon biopsies which turn out to be normal, to show an adenomatous lesion or to indicate an adenocarcinoma are well-known. This initial knowledge can be expressed as *prior probabilities* for the alternative diagnostic outcomes. This prior knowledge can also be used as a measure of uncertainty for each diagnostic outcome for a newly received biopsy. The process of making a diagnostic decision, by considering different diagnostic clues, thus may be seen as an attempt to reduce uncertainty to the point where one diagnostic outcome has almost no remaining uncertainty, and can be chosen as the diagnostic decision.

One of the most useful capabilities of an expert system is the ability to derive decisions in the face of uncertainty. Uncertainties affect nearly all aspects of knowledge in histopathology and arise from many different causes. There is uncertainty due to randomness which can be managed by probability theory. Uncertainty due to vagueness of linguistic and descriptive terms can be managed by fuzzy set and possibility theory.

For an expert system, each chunk of knowledge in a knowledge base is afflicted with some uncertainty. As the expert system derives a decision, it evaluates various pieces of evidence in view of these uncertainties and, of course, even the final decision has uncertainty associated with it. The management of uncertainty in an expert system thus is a crucial aspect of the methodology.

Two major points must be considered here. The first is the definition of a numerical measure of uncertainty; the second is the choice of methodology for combining evidence so that the final conclusion has a minimum of uncertainty.

For uncertainty due to randomness, probability theory offers a scientifically rigorous measure. Many eminent researchers in probability theory suggest that probability measures are the only acceptable assessments of uncertainty [10]. Probabilities are based on observations of how often, in a large number of trials, a given event occurred, i.e., probabilities are based on frequency counts. Frequency-count-based probabilities are well-defined and scientifically well-respected measures of uncertainty – where they are practical and applicable. Unfortunately, the use of frequency-count-based probabilities in expert systems often is not feasible, not appropriate, and very often not applicable, as discussed below.

In probability theory, it is assumed that the observed sample is homogeneous. Yet, however well-matched for covariables the patients may be in a given cohort for which a probability is estimated, the assumption that they are as homogeneous as 'fair coins' may not be valid at all. It is possible to model the presence of subpopulations having, for example, different immune competence, by using Weibull statistics [11], but thus far no one has even suggested such an approach in an expert system.

A more serious problem though is posed by the need to consider the conditional dependence of probabilities, as evidence is combined. When different diagnostic clues entering a decision sequence are conditionally independent, one may indeed obtain a reliable estimate for the probability of the correctness of a final decision. However, if such conditional independence cannot be assumed, as is practically always the case, it becomes computationally infeasible to compute a reliable estimate of the posterior probability of a final decision.

Many commercial expert systems offer an inadequate Bayesian updating of the posterior probability, as each piece of evidence is considered, in which the full conditional dependence structure is neglected. This can have unpredictable consequences. For example, if a certain diagnostic outcome is indicated but the observation of a given diagnostic clue and subsequent clues suggest the same diagnosis, the cumulative, confirming information may preclude the consideration of alternative diagnostic outcomes. However, if all of the subsequent clues are highly correlated, both with the first clue suggesting a particular diagnostic outcome and with each other, they really do not offer additional independent information, and should not substantially increase the probability that this diagnostic outcome is best supported by the evidence. This is a serious problem.

Moreover, probabilities entered into the knowledge base of an expert system often are not based on frequency counts. Instead, they may be merely subjective estimates made by an expert – so-called personal probabilities. Although these estimates are by no means arbitrary, it is difficult to assess their error and, if they are entered into a decision sequence, the cumulative error is even more difficult to predict.

These problems also affect certainty assessments which are based on measures of belief and measures of disbelief and are defined so that they may resemble a probabilistic measure of uncertainty. Certainty factors defined in this manner are available in many expert systems and generally provide satisfactory performance, even though they are, at best, only heuristic approximations to probabilities [12].

There is a basic discrepancy, though, between the requirement of complete independence of rules in a rule-based expert system and the use of a probability-based measure of uncertainty, for which conditional independence should not simply be postulated.

Furthermore, in probability theory, evidence which supports an assertion is always complemented by the remainder, which brings the total probability to unity. This remainder evidence is then counted as not supporting the assertion, because the event did not occur. However, there is a difference between a statement saying 'not so' and a statement saying 'no information', i.e., simple ignorance without judgement. Probability theory cannot model ignorance very well. This deficiency has been felt to be unsatisfactory in the use of probability for the measurement of uncertainty.

The desire to model ignorance in the combining of evidence was one of the motives in the development of the Dempster–Shafer theory of evidence. In this theory, exact probabilities are replaced by probability intervals and provisions are made to hold remainder evidence in reserve, without suggesting that it countermands the assertion. In the Dempster–Shafer theory [13,14], emphasis is placed on confirming evidence that is obtained from a different source.

The Dempster–Shafer methodology for combining evidence may be seen as bridging probability theory and possibility theory. It offers a theoretically rather encompassing approach to the management of uncertainty. Yet, it has not found widespread implementation in expert systems. This may be to do with an extraordinary sensitivity to the choice of numerical values for representing the uncertainty of given assertions. It has been shown, in admittedly unusual cases, that the Dempster–Shafer methodology can lead to intuitively grossly erroneous assessments of the uncertainty of a final diagnosis [15].

Uncertainty due to vagueness of linguistic expressions cannot really be measured by probabilities. Here, fuzzy set and possibility theory [16,17] offer an effective means of assigning numerical values to uncertainty and combining evidence. The underlying basic idea is best illustrated by drawing the distinction between a *crisp set* and a *fuzzy set*. Members of crisp set are unequivocally members of that set and cannot possibly be considered to belong to another set as well. For example, erythrocytes may be seen as forming a crisp set in distinguishing them from epithelial cells, and vice versa. Unequivocal membership is no longer clear for an ectocervical 'slightly dysplastic cell'. It may be considered by some cytopathologists to be an immature metaplastic cell. On the other hand, there certainly are immature metaplastic cells which some cytopathologists might see as slightly dysplastic. Thus, immature metaplastic and slightly dysplastic cells form two fuzzy sets with an intersection. For cells falling in the intersection, it is not 100% true that they are immature metaplastic cells or that they are slightly dysplastic cells.

The same logic applies to assertions in a knowledge base. If a rule is absolutely true, it is a member of a crisp set and involves no uncertainty. However, if the facts or the linguistic terms used in the rule are inherently ambiguous, then the rule is not 100% true and is afflicted with uncertainty: it is a fuzzy rule.

One can express such uncertainty using certainty factors; however, then the rules for combining evidence are very different from those used with certainty measures based on probabilistic assumptions. In fuzzy-set theory, the uncertainty of pieces of evidence combined by the 'AND' clause is defined as the minimum of the certainty factors associated with each piece of evidence; this reflects the intersection of the two assertions. For two pieces of evidence combined by the 'OR' operator, the maximum of the certainty factors is the measure of uncertainty. This is the case because the union of the two sets is involved [18].

Thus, in an expert system, certainty measures may have similar-appearing values, but their definition and updating may follow drastically different rationales, depending on whether a probabilistic or a possibilistic model is used. There is no consideration of full conditional dependence of evidence in either methodology.

The need to consider the conditional dependence of evidence in a computationally feasible manner led to the development of inference networks [19]. Peare [20], in particular, provides an extensive study of Bayesian belief networks. In a Bayesian belief network, the prior knowledge of the expert is used to identify those dependencies which are relevant. This is a task which human experts perform very well, and it results in a drastic reduction in the number of combinations of evidence that need to be evaluated as new pieces of evidence accumulate in the decision sequence.

The assertions in the knowledge base are ordered as a network – actually as a directed acyclic graph. A node is established for each assertion. Stored at the node are all possible outcomes for the assertion, with their assessed probabilities. A node 'cytological diagnosis' for example, may have as outcomes 'normal cytology', 'atypical cytology' and 'CIN III' (cervical intraepithelial neoplasia III) with respective probabilities 0.95, 0.045 and 0.005.

The conditional dependencies with respect to the next node are stored as a conditional probability matrix, which relates the probability of each outcome at the first node to the probability of each outcome at the next dependent node. In addition, a likelihood vector is stored at each node: it accepts the new evidence as it is observed for a particular case and entered into the network.

The dynamic behaviour of a Bayesian belief network then involves the following stages. New evidence is observed and is expressed as a relative likelihood vector for the different possible outcomes at a given node. This new evidence is used to update the belief in the alternative outcomes at that node. However, since the belief in the assertion has now changed, the belief in the different assertions at the parent node must be updated. Thus, the effect of an input, at a node anywhere in the network, percolates up to the root node, updating all beliefs. Furthermore, since the beliefs have changed, the prior probabilities of all descendent nodes must be changed throughout the tree, with the exception of the branch from which the updating started, as that would initiate an endless loop. In this fashion, the conditional dependencies are considered for all relevant assertions in the knowledge base, without creating a non-feasible computational burden.

Bayesian belief networks are performing well in practice. They have, in their graph structure, a

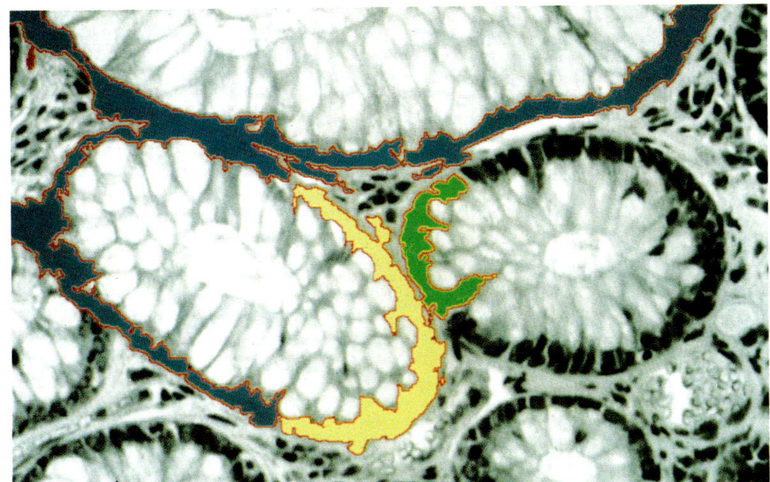

Plate 13.1 Automated segmentation of cross-sectioned glands in colorectal tissue. Associating gland-wall segments with the correct lumen.

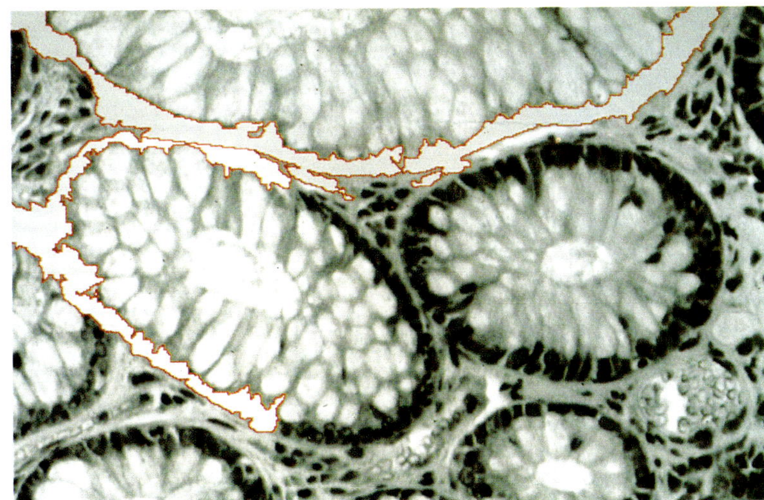

Plate 13.2 Automated segmentation of cross-sectioned glands in colorectal tissue. Separation of two joined gland-wall segments allowing the correct association of segments with respective lumen and assembly of complete gland objects.

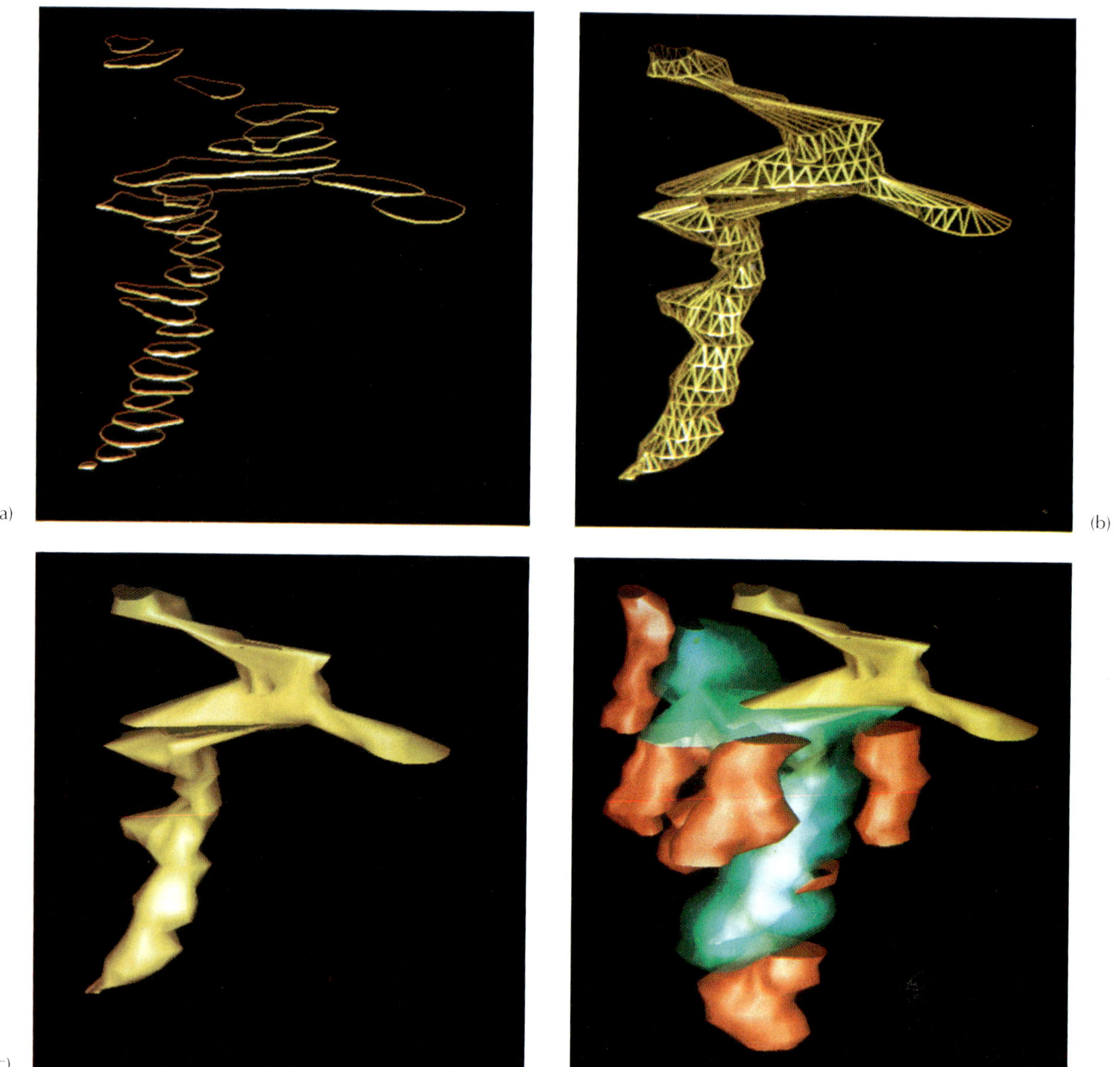

Plate 14.1 Bronchial gland reconstruction. (a) Lumen: wire frame mode. (b) Lumen: triangulation mode. (c) Lumen: surface rendering. (d) Serous cells (red) and mucus cells (blue) in transparent mode to visualize lumen.

serendipitous compatibility with some knowledge representation schemes, and thus lend themselves to integration into the reasoning sequence of an expert system.

To illustrate their role in decision support, a simple inference network for combining evidence in the assessment of tissue sections of prostate shall be considered [21]. The alternative diagnostic outcomes at the decision node of the inference network are benign prostatic hyperplasia (BPH), low-grade prostatic intraepithelial neoplasia (PIN low), high-grade PIN (PIN high), large acinar-gland adenocarcinoma (lgac AC) and adenocarcinoma exhibiting cribriform glands (crib AC). The network has a shallow topology, with only a single layer of descendent nodes, representing seven diagnostic clues, as shown in Fig. 13.1. These clues, with their alternative outcomes, are listed in Table 13.1.

Figure 13.2 shows the cumulative development of belief at the decision node for a section from a cribriform gland adenocarcinoma for the two diagnostic outcomes of PIN high and crib AC. In Fig. 13.3 an example is shown of a case of low-grade PIN and the development of belief after observation of the seven diagnostic clues for two alternative diagnostic outcomes, low-grade and high-grade PIN.

Table 13.1 Diagnostic clues and their outcomes for the diagnosis of prostate neoplasia

Gland pattern changes	None/moderate/severe
Cribriformity of glands	Absent/present
Basal-cell nuclei recognition	Recognizable/difficult to recognize/unrecognizable
Prominence of basal-cell nuclei	Mild/moderate/marked/none
Enlargement of secretory-cell nuclei	None/moderate
Substantial secretory-cell nuclei stratification	None/mild/moderate/heavy
Secretory-cell cytoplasm	Clear/moderately clear/granular

13.3 KNOWLEDGE REPRESENTATION [22]

The manner in which the knowledge about a system's domain is represented has a very significant impact on the human expert's ability to formulate his/her knowledge base. The objective of a knowledge representation scheme is to make the information in the knowledge base available to the inference module. Thus it is understood that the

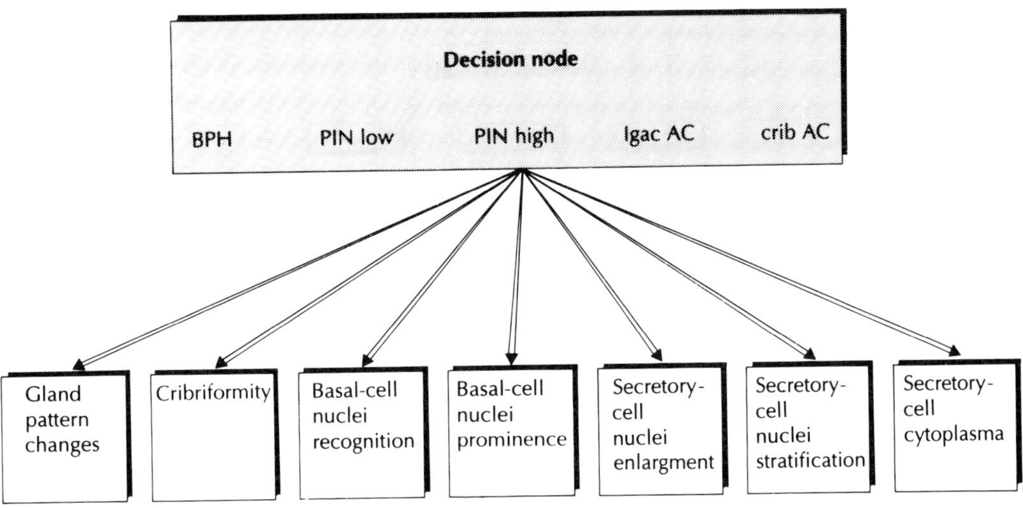

Fig. 13.1 Bayesian belief network topology for diagnostic decision-making in prostate neoplasia. BPH, benign prostatic hyperplasia; PIN, prostatic intraephithelial neoplasia; lgac AC, large acinar-gland adenocarcinoma; crib AC, cribriform-gland adenocarcinoma.

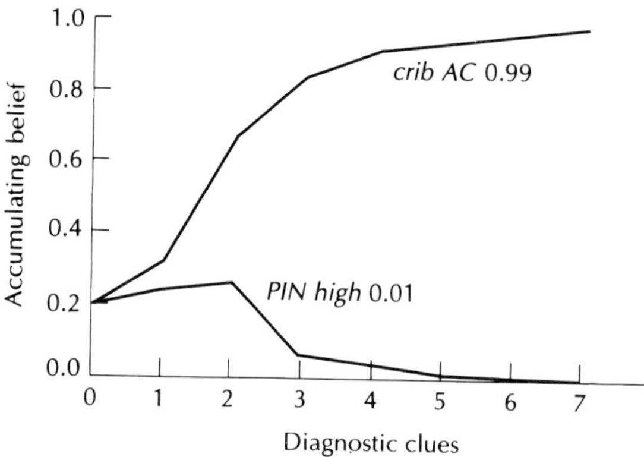

Fig. 13.2 Cumulative belief curve for a prostate lesion showing cribriform-gland adenocarcinoma. crib AC, cribriform-gland adenocarcinoma; PIN, prostatic intraepithelial neoplasia.

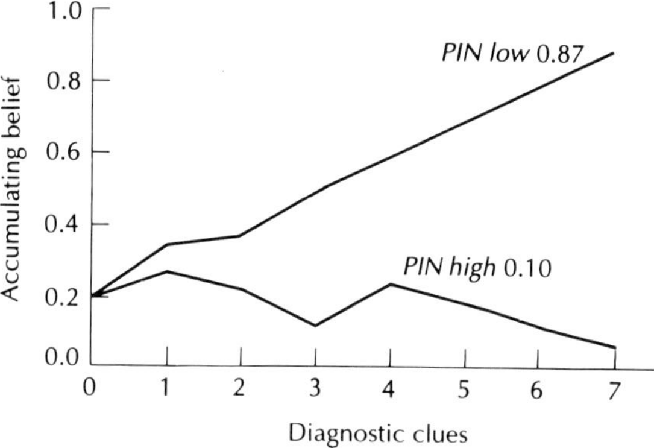

Fig. 13.3 Cumulative belief curve for a prostate sample with low-grade prostatic intraepithelial neoplasia (PIN).

knowledge must be represented obeying certain conventions, i.e., a certain grammar. The inference engine, after all, has very little latitude in handling input and carries out a strictly algorithmic procedure. The inference engine in a simple expert system may merely match some input about a situation to a corresponding symbolic representation in a knowledge base by string comparison. It may then look up a pointer to additional strings to check whether a match is possible, and establish whether or not the assertion is true for the situation at hand. If the assertion is true, the expert system follows another pointer and finds the appropriate symbol string that now determines the next cycle in the inferencing process. There are numerous variations on this theme, but the basic mode of operation is the same. Before a decision is made concerning which step to take next in the inference process, the inference engine may make a numerical evaluation to determine which step would most reduce the uncertainty for the alternative outcomes.

In more complex inference modules, the determination of the 'truth' of an assertion may involve examination of extensive sequences of assertions, satisfaction of numeric constraints, and the ability to handle a complex grammar of knowledge representation, as well as interpretive capabilities to determine which pointers to follow.

We see a trade-off here, in the design of expert system shells, between simplicity of grammar and ability of human experts to express their knowledge so that it can be integrated into a knowledge base. If the human expert is permitted a rich and complex set of expressions, the inference module must have extensive interpretive capabilities to process the assertions made. The advantage is that the human expert has much more control and understanding of how his/her knowledge is to be used.

If the inference module is restricted to a very sparse grammar, either only very simple expert systems can be built, or a knowledge engineer may be needed to express the wealth and complexity of human diagnostic knowledge using this very restrictive grammar. This can lead to misinterpretations and implied assumptions, with subsequent problems during validation of the completed system's performance.

Researchers in a given field go through a number of stages in the development of their expertise [23]. When confronted with a totally new domain, they first acquire knowledge about typical situations – 'textbook' examples of alternatives, i.e., they develop a rather insular knowledge. As a more representative collection of instances is encountered, their knowledge increases to allow assessment of less typical situations falling in between typical situations. Also, as insight is gained into the mutual dependence structure of assertions supporting the various alternative outcomes, understanding of the domain begins to develop. Real understanding is reached when the dependence structure is fully appreciated, so that even missing information would not seriously impede the appropriate assessment of accumulating evidence.

Understanding the domain thus constitutes a significant aspect of the human expert's competence. Incorporating a model of human competence into an expert system requires that knowledge about the dependence structure of facts, procedures and assertions concerning the domain can be incorporated at the design stage [24]. This, in turn, requires a rich representational scheme, structure and grammar. Reasoning about a domain is often aided by incorporating a model of the domain into the knowledge base.

The relationship between the ability to express understanding of a domain and the simplicity of representation is best illustrated by some practical examples of expert system knowledge representations.

In the simplest case, knowledge representation may be in the form of a table. The system offers a spreadsheet, and the user may enter the alternative outcomes, or diagnoses, e.g., as column headings. The user enters diagnostic clues as row headings, with a separate row for each diagnostic clue value or attribute. Also entered are a set of numerical values which represent the designer's belief concerning the way in which the observation of a given attribute for a particular diagnostic clue would relate to each diagnostic outcome. Each user can choose his/her own linguistic terms. The inference module will simply accept each linguistic term as a string – a symbolic representation.

In a system like this, the clue that promises the greatest reduction in uncertainty is always chosen next. As a clue attribute is observed, the measures of belief for all alternative diagnostic outcomes are updated; this suggests which clue would now bring the greatest reduction in uncertainty. Eventually, one of the diagnostic alternatives will exceed a preset threshold in the accumulating measure of certainty for a given alternative outcome, and the alternative will be chosen as the system's diagnostic decision.

Systems of this kind are suitable for short decision sequences, and their value may be primarily in making a diagnostic pathologist aware of which clues are being considered and how much each clue contributes to the diagnostic process. Systems having this very simple architecture may be most useful in controlling an automated assessment by a machine vision system.

Most commercially available expert system shells offer a rule-based knowledge representation. For many domains, rules allow a human expert to express knowledge adequately. The grammar is simple. An assertion is stated in the form:

if object logical operator attribute *then* action.

The inference engine interprets such a string by knowing that the *if* symbol is followed by the object, and it can match the object string to an entry in the working memory. Next follows a logical operator, such as larger than, or equal to, and this is followed by the attribute. An example is:

if nucleus = large *then*. . .

The part preceding the *then* symbol is tested for its truth: the user may be asked whether the nucleus should be called large or not, and the truth is considered to be established if the user input verifies the assertion as true. In an automatic system, the nuclear area may be computed and compared to a membership function to determine the truth value of its being large, and the truth value will enter the decision sequence as a measure of uncertainty. In a rule-based system, objects usually are nouns accompanied by a verb, such as 'patient has' or 'nucleus is'. Logical operators are, for example, equal to, larger than, smaller than, and so on. Attributes may be numerical, they may be adjectives, they may be categorical, they could be membership in a Boolean expression, and so forth.

Uncertainty in a rule-based system is frequently managed by certainty factors. These are assigned to each assertion, since an assertion is not expected to be unequivocally true or absolutely certain. Certainty factors are also assigned to each rule as a whole, because rules can have widely varying truth values. For example, the rule '*if* frank tumour cells = present, *then* patient has malignant lesion' would have a high certainty factor. However, the same facts when presented in a rule such as '*if* patient has malignant lesion *then* frank tumour cells are present' is a far from certain assertion.

Rule-based knowledge representation thus allows a fairly rich expression of knowledge. The decision process creates a sequence of rules, 'chained together', which state conditions that must be true or for which other assertions could be substituted. A given situation is finally represented by an *and/or* graph (CF = certainty factor):

if assertion I is true (CF 0.3)
  and assertion II is true (CF 0.5)
  and assertion III is true (CF 0.2)
  or assertion IV is true (CF 0.6)
  and assertion V is true (CF 0.4)
then conclusion (CF 0.6)

Rules are presumed to express independent information, to allow incremental building of a knowledge base and to allow some basis for estimating a final certainty assessment. In practice, rule independence is rarely even approximated. The very domain to which the *if–then* form of knowledge representation lends itself, evaluation of a sequence of diagnostic pieces of evidence, is usually characterized by a high degree of mutual dependence of facts and procedures.

The rule format is not well-suited to representing image information, such as the topography and topology of a histopathological section. Domains in which facts and procedures are not related either by a cause-and-effect relationship or by condition and consequence expressions are better represented by a set of declarative statements. These statements in turn may then be related to each other, in a manner corresponding to their spatial arrangement or functional relationship.

Such knowledge representations are known as associative networks, with facts and procedures forming the nodes of a network and relationships (represented by the arcs) connecting the nodes. In histopathology, a simple associative network is usually not adequate to represent image information. In that case, each node in an associative network may be replaced by a frame, so that one has, *de facto*, an associative network of frames. A frame is a data structure offering a set of slots – a large variety of records can be kept in an organized scheme in each frame. Frames were originally introduced to allow all information characterizing a complex situation to be stored in a single structure. An associative network with frames at every node thus allows a very rich representation of knowledge, including the causal or topographical relationship between frames.

In practice, the implementation of such a knowledge representation scheme must allow for an even more detailed structure. The challenge of effective and exhaustive knowledge representation is faced most directly in the design of machine vision systems, for the following reasons.

In an interactive expert system the program, with its inferencing module, provides very efficient and possibly complex string-matching capabilities and assessments of uncertainties. The expert system *per se*, however, has no need for and no understanding of the histopathological meaning of the symbol strings it manipulates: all such knowledge is supplied by the designer and the user of the system. However, when one wishes the expert system to embody at least a partial model of the histopathological reasoning of a human expert, all concepts used by a human expert must be available in the knowledge base of the expert system, with their definitions and dependencies. This includes knowledge of facts and procedures that may have little to do with the histopathological domain, but are required for the appropriate use of facts and procedures relevant to the domain.

In a machine vision system, reasoning must proceed without any interaction with a human expert; all of the information needed must be in the knowledge base. A term such as 'differentiated' is meaningful to the system and useful to its reasoning capability only if it is defined in terms of other entities that the system can compute from imagery or can be directed to retrieve from the knowledge file.

Thus, knowledge representations in competent expert systems or machine vision systems typically are not merely a network of nodes where each node is expanded into a frame. In practice, each of the nodes of this conceptual organization is implemented as a cluster of nodes, with each node remaining a frame. For example, a declarative statement concerning a thyroid follicle will begin with an entity declaration node. Immediately, though, there is a need to have pointers to an associated definition node where the terms used in the declarative statement are defined. This, in turn, may require further definition nodes, including those identifying algorithmic procedures needed to compute the histometric entities involved. In addition, some definition nodes may point to constraint nodes, where restricting conditions are declared and imposed. Figure 13.4 shows such a hierarchic structure [25]. It organizes the knowledge about the facts of the domain and the procedures required to relate different aspects of these facts to each other. Every concept or entity is declared, defined and, if necessary, constrained. The structure as seen in Fig. 13.4 is automatically set up by the expert system interpreter when it reads in the knowledge file.

The user need not be concerned with any of this, although an insight into the constraints are necessary. The designer, though, must very carefully research each and every concept, term, relationship, constraint, exception and procedure that is necessary to enable the system's independent reasoning.

The knowledge file is entered into the knowledge base as a sequence of declarative statements. The expert system then interprets these statements. This must follow a well-defined grammar, but may allow a great diversity of expressions. As the knowledge file is read in and interpreted, the system sets up

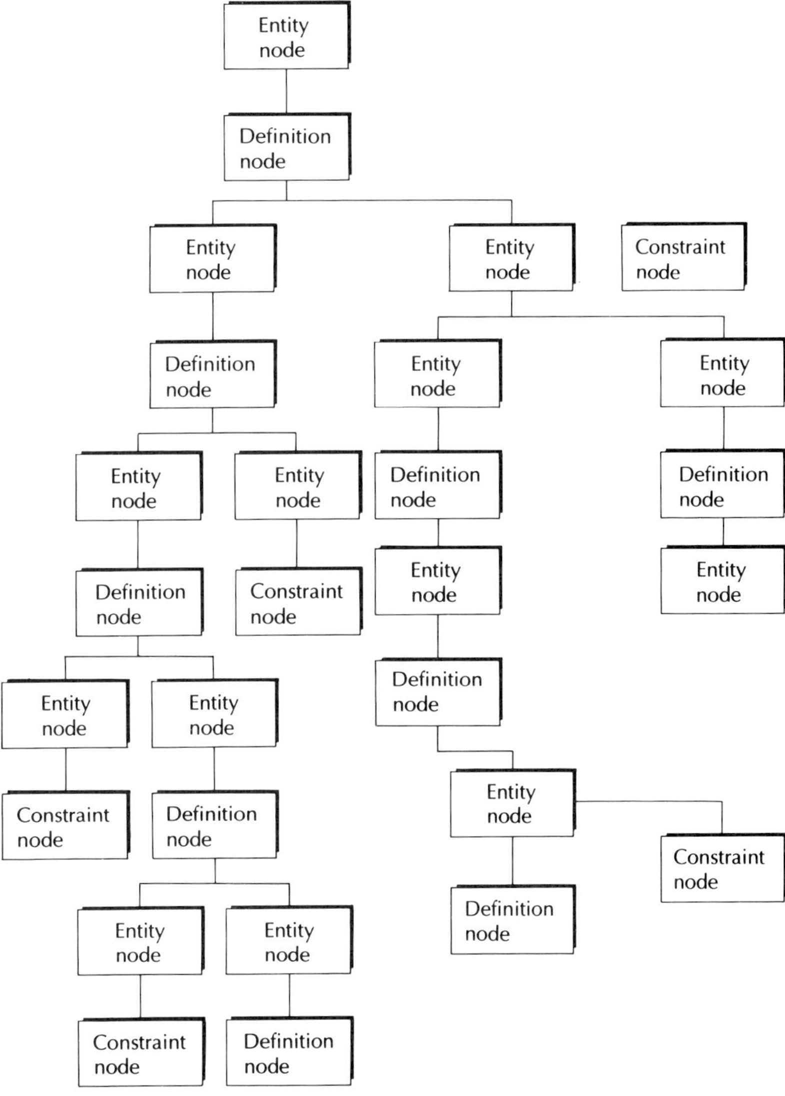

Fig. 13.4 Hierarchical structure for the organization of knowledge.

the pointers and stores them in certain slots of each node's frame. This occurs automatically, as a result of the interpretation of the grammar of each declarative statement. After the structure of the network is set up, the system is ready to process data. It traverses the model of the histological situation described by the declarative statements in the knowledge file from the root node down, examining and satisfying the assertions at each node in comparison with the observed data, in a forward-chaining manner, until a conclusion is reached. The uncertainty management, either as certainty factors based on fuzzy-set theory or as a Bayesian belief network, is associated with and part of the information in a given slot at each frame.

To give a practical example, the knowledge file for an automated segmentation of images of adenomatous colonic lesions is presented [26]. It lists 33 object types, e.g., the entities gland, glandular epithelial layer, cytoplasm, lumen and stroma. Other object types are necessary to relate to scene segmentation procedures, e.g., object group, or gland wall segment, denoting a segment of glandular epithelium detected during segmentation. Another entity is a 'set of wall segments', a collection of segments of glandular epithelium tentatively assembled to form a gland, provided an associated lumen fulfills certain conditions. If so, the reasoning process will declare the set as a gland.

Then, there are image-related concepts among the declared object types, e.g., original image and thresholded image. There are also entities relating to intermediate representations of image components during segmentation, such as segments of glandular epithelium associated with two or more lumina. There are several types of such entities which the knowledge base distinguishes, since they require different segmentation procedures and they are related to one or more lumina in different ways. There could be several lumina, i.e., the segmentation so far has failed to separate glandular epithelium from at least two different glands. They may also belong to glands cut by the edge of the field of view, and these require different segmentation procedures.

The knowledge base defines 18 functions, such as the FIND OBJECT, the FIND LUMEN, the VERIFY and the CLOSE HOLE functions, to name a few. For example, the SPLIT SEGMENT function is based on mathematical morphology. It applies skeletonization, followed by erosion operations to separate object groups associated with two or more different lumina.

The knowledge file defines six features and provides 44 object definitions, further defined by 28 constraints. An example is the object definition 'a multi-2 gland wall segment IS A single SPLIT SEGMENT.FCT remnant WITH FIND ASSOCIATED LUMEN >1'. This statement, written in the grammar based on declarative IS A statements used in the scene segmentation expert system SES (1), says that the function which finds the lumina associated with a segment of glandular epithelium, as it resulted from a particular processing step, must find more than one, i.e., two or more different lumina, to confirm and verify that the segmentation procedure has correctly analysed the local segmentation problem before the SES should proceed. A 'multi-2 gland wall segment' is an example of such a specific kind of intermediate histological component's fragment as is generated during processing.

The knowledge file must provide directives for any eventuality that the reasoning process might encounter. Its design requires considerable analysis of the kind of scenes found in a given domain of application. It must allow the system to sort out, on a logical basis, which object groups resulting from the image processing belong together and form histological components, and where the segmentation has produced object groups which are logically not allowed and need to be corrected, such as segments of glandular epithelium containing glandular nuclei from different glands.

Two graphic examples may illustrate different stages of these processes. In Plate 13.1 (opposite p. 278), the glandular epithelium for the cut gland on the right bottom has been correctly identified and excluded from the analysis. For the gland in the right centre, two epithelium segments have not yet been cleared for assembly into a gland. The gland on centre left has a large epithelial segment still not separated from the glandular epithelial layer lining the large cut gland at the top of the scene. Only the right half of the left centre gland's epithelium is recognized as associated exclusively with its lumen.

Plate 13.2 (opposite p. 278) shows the next stage. All of the glandular epithelium for the gland at right centre has now been confirmed as being associated with the same lumen, and a gland has been assembled (not shown). The joined glandular epithelium segments from the gland at centre left and top of the scene have been separated and are ready to be verified in their association with their respective lumina.

Figure 13.5 demonstrates how complete lining of a tentative lumen by an epithelial layer is checked before a set of image components is accepted for assembly into a gland. Here, the local threshold for area of a piece of glandular epithelium is being lowered. The small set of glandular nuclei can now be accepted. The next step is checking whether the tentative lumen is completely lined by glandular epithelium.

The table-driven, rule-based and associative network knowledge representation schemes show the wide range of complexity of the conceptual structures on which autonomous reasoning and, considering uncertainty management, 'approximate reasoning' are carried out in expert systems.

In addition to these basic knowledge representation schemes, systems employing hierarchic architectures have been developed. Multiple context expert systems [27] first determine the context in which an expert assessment is sought, and then select an appropriate module from the knowledge base. Machine vision systems may employ multiple knowledge representations, from table-driven modules to rule-based modules to frame based modules, in order to enable different components to accomplish their missions. So-called blackboard systems [28] were designed to allow integration of information from diverse, multiple data sources, all of which can, in such a system, present relevant information to a common blackboard, from which all other components of the system can select useful information to advance the inference process.

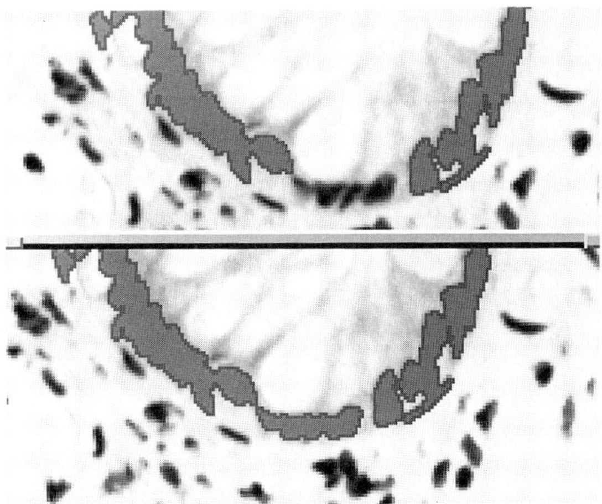

Fig. 13.5 The knowledge file checks for missing pieces in the gland wall and attempts to 'fill in' these areas by adjusting the segmentation threshold.

13.4 VALIDATION

Expert systems are applied to problems where the path to a solution is not obvious, is not always the same and is hard to predict. To write algorithmic procedures for poorly defined problems is an almost non-feasible task. It was, therefore, an ingenious software engineering solution to separate the knowledge, or data, completely from the expert system itself, thus making the development of expert systems practical. The developer or the user can alter the knowledge base at any time to improve the performance of the system, without the need to recompile and debug a program. This separation of the knowledge base and the expert system shell itself represents a significant difference between conventional computer programs and expert system software.

While it is true that the essential flexibility and ease of modification of the knowledge base allow a gradual iteration of performance to the level of a human expert, this ease of access and entering of additional knowledge can also create problems. Assertions may be entered which affect the validity of assertions already in the knowledge base, or declarative statements may be added which even directly contradict knowledge entered earlier, possibly by another expert consulted for the development of the system.

In some of their methodology, expert systems grew out of the so-called 'productions' employed by early researchers in artificial intelligence work. In efforts to develop descriptive classification schemes and to use categorical rather than numerical data, so-called productions were formulated as simple declarative statements, such as: 'If a patient had more than two positive Pap smears in the past, she is a member of a high-risk group'. Productions were based on and validated by frequency count data, i.e., actual experimental evidence. They were implemented only after the validity of each statement had been established for the general case, on a training set and cross-validation test data.

Later, the frequency count validation was replaced by an expert's personal probability estimate for the truth of a production. Early expert systems were formulated with uncertainty assessments based merely on subjective personal judgement. Expert systems provide extremely powerful classification capabilities. Nevertheless, an expert system's performance as a classifier must be validated just like the performance of any other classifier [29]. Datasets or knowledge used in training an expert system in the development phase are kept separate. Then facts, procedures, constraints and/or measures of uncertainty are altered or tuned until the system performs at a level comparable to that of a human expert. Then, the system is tested on cases not included in the training data and its performance is observed.

A question that comes up frequently is the sample size/outcome/dimensionality ratio that is required in a descriptive classifier of this nature. In statistical classification, the multivariate feature vectors representing the members of each training set are used to estimate a multivariate probability density distribution. One may allow for the covariance structure of the dataset and consider only the intrinsic dimensionality of the problem. However, there still should be at least five to 10 observations for each pattern class for each feature used in the classification rule, in order to obtain a somewhat realistic estimate of the true error rate of the classifier.

A descriptive classifier is not based on the values observed for a given feature set common to all classes. Rather, each category is characterized by the features it exhibits, e.g., which path is taken through an and/or tree. If, in fact, each assertion were absolutely certain, then a very modest number of instances could define a category, enough to represent every path through the and/or tree that is a member of the category.

However, since facts, assertions and features used in a descriptive classifier are fuzzy objects, distribution theory again applies. Training samples of a size sufficient to provide a reasonable representation of the overlap of membership functions are required.

For larger systems involving hundreds of rules or nodes, it is no longer feasible to check exhaustively the impact of newly added knowledge on the already existing knowledge base. Some training can be done by means of examining decision sequences in a 'what if' mode, when test situations directly involving the newly added information are set up. However, this is of limited efficacy. In very large systems, the issue of validation assumes a new complexity. So-called truth maintenance systems are then incorporated; these are software modules which trace automatically and exhaustively the logical compatibility of newly added knowledge. While necessary and effective, this clearly will slow the development effort.

13.5 CONCLUSION

Expert systems surely will be applied to diagnostic and quantitative histopathology, but it is difficult to assess where the impact of the methodology will be most significant. It may turn out that the capability for systematic manipulation of symbolic information will open the way for an encompassing management of histopathological knowledge. As far as interactive diagnostic expert systems are concerned, the information loss from two-dimensional imagery to one-dimensional descriptive linguistic terms is hard to bridge, and there is no technological reason why quantitatively assessed imagery, computer graphics and expert system displays could not be integrated. Thus one would expect that diagnostic expert systems will be integrated with large, intelligently managed image databases. While it is academically interesting to have an interactive discourse with an expert system, one would imagine that a clinical diagnostic histopathologist would prefer and would feel safer using his/her superb ability to assess diagnostic imagery in interaction with the expert system. One can expect to see expert-system-guided grading systems designed on that basis.

In diagnostic expert systems, the crucial issue is management of uncertainty, with proper consideration of the conditional dependence of evidence. Bayesian belief networks may offer a practical and scientifically rigorous approach to this problem, but their implementation is still in the research stage.

The use of expert system guidance in machine vision systems and as process control in automated image processing, information extraction, evaluation and interpretation is another area of substantial potential for expert system methodology. As information technologies will permit storage of very large image databases, the processing of diagnostically representative areas of sections may become feasible and more common. Expert systems providing guidance in the search through and analysis of large-scale patient databases may make a valuable contribution to research in pathology. It is simply not practical for most researchers in pathology to assemble a team of consultants in image photometry, image analysis, statistical analysis, multivariate analysis, classification theory and uncertainty management, and computer science in general. Yet, advice from specialists in most, if not all, of these disciplines is required to take full advantage of the information that is available. It is quite possible that expert system methodology will be able to provide such interdisciplinary insight to researchers in quantitative pathology.

Acknowledgements

This work has been supported by two grants from the National Institutes of Health, National Cancer Institute, Bethesda, MD, 1PO 1 CA 38548 and R 35 CA 53877.

References

1 Bartels PH, Bibbo M, Graham A, Paplanus S, Shoemaker RL, Thompson D. Image understanding system for histopathology. *Anal Cell Pathol* 1989; 1: 195–214.

2 Buchanan BG, Shortliffe EH. *Rule-based Expert Systems.* Reading: Addison Wesley, 1984.

3 Forsyth R. *Expert Systems.* London: Chapman and Hall, 1984.

4 Harmon P, King D. *Expert Systems.* New York: John Wiley, 1985.

5 Hayes-Roth F, Waterman DA, Lenat DB. *Building Expert Systems.* London: Addison-Wesley, 1983.

6 Jackson P. *Introduction to Expert Systems.* Reading: Addison Wesley, 1986.

7 Walters JR, Nielson NR. *Crafting Knowledge Based Systems.* New York: John Wiley, 1988.

8 Rich E. *Artificial Intelligence.* New York: McGraw Hill, 1983.

9 Kanal LN, Lemmer JF. *Uncertainty in Artificial Intelligence.* Amsterdam: North Holland, 1986.

10 Lindley D. The probability approach to the treatment of uncertainty in artificial intelligence and expert systems. *Stat Sci* 1987; 2: 17–24.

11 Byar DP. Analysis of survival data: Cox and Weibull models with covariance. In: Mike V, Stanley KE (eds) *Statistics in Medical Research.* New York: John Wiley, 1982: 365–401.

12 Lopez de Mantaras R. *Approximate Reasoning Models.* Chichester: Ellis Horwood, 1990.

13 Giarratano J, Riley G. *Expert Systems.* Boston: PWS Kent, 1989.

14 Shafer G. *A Mathematical Theory of Evidence.* Princeton, NJ: Princeton Press, 1976.

15 Zadeh LA. Is probability theory sufficient for dealing with uncertainty in AI: a negative view. In: Kanal LN, Lemmer JF (eds) *Uncertainty in Artificial Intelligence.* Amsterdam: North Holland, 1986: 103–112.

16 Dubois D, Prade H. *Possibility Theory.* New York: Plenum Press, 1986.

17 Zadeh LA. *Fuzzy Sets. Information and Control.* 1965; 8: 338–353.

18 Levine RI, Drang DE, Edelson B. *AI and Expert Systems.* New York: McGraw Hill, 1990.

19 Duda RO, Hart PE, Nilsson NJ. Subjective Bayesian methods for rule-based inference systems. *Proc Natl Comp Conf AFIPS* 1976; 45: 1075–1082.

20 Pearl J. *Probabilistic Reasoning in Intelligent Systems.* San Mateo, CA: Morgan Kaufman, 1988.

21 Montironi R, Bartels PH, Thompson D, Scarpelli M, Hamilton PW. Prostate intraepithelial neoplasia, development of Bayesian network for diagnosis and grading. *Anal Quant Cytol Histol* 1994; 16: 101–112.

22 Brachman RJ, Levesque HJ. *Readings in Knowledge Representation.* Los Altos: Morgan Kaufman, 1985.

23 Feltovich PL, Johnson PF, Moller LH, Swanson DB. LCS: the role and development of medical knowledge in diagnostic expertise. In: Clancey WJ, Shortliffe EH, (eds) *Readings in Medical AI: The First Decade.* Reading: Addison Wesley, 1984: 275–319.

24 Keravnou ET, Johnson L. *Competent Expert Systems.* New York: McGraw Hill, 1986.

25 Bartels PH, Thompson D, Weber JE. Construction of the knowledge file for an image understanding system. *Pathol Res Pract* 1992; 188: 396–404.

26 Thompson D, Bartels PH, Bartels HG, Hamilton PW, Sloan JM. Knowledge guided segmentation of colorectal histopathologic imagery. *Anal Quant Cytol Histol* 1993; 15: 236–246.

27 Waterman DA. *A Guide to Expert Systems*. Reading: Addison Wesley, 1986.

28 Nii HP. Blackboard systems. The blackboard model of problem solving and the evolution of blackboard architectures. *AI Magazine* 1986; Summer: 39–53.

29 Weiss SM, Kulikowski CA. *Computer Systems that Learn*. San Mateo: Morgan Kaufman, 1991.

14

THREE-DIMENSIONAL RECONSTRUCTION

W. F. WHIMSTER AND M. J. COOKSON

14.1 INTRODUCTION

The aim of this chapter is to outline what has been done with computer assistance in the field of three-dimensional reconstruction (3DR), visualization and image analysis of biological structures, to indicate the problems and potential for applications in pathology.

Serial sectioning combined with 3DR is used to help anatomists and others understand the structure of individual organs, tissues and cells, the structure of the components hidden within them and the relationships and connections between these structures. His [1] in the late 19th century may have been the first to use two-dimensional (2D) serial sections to produce precise 3D models (of embryos) to gain anatomical insights. Since then many workers have laboriously reconstructed tissues and organs from stacks of 2D photographs or drawings of macroscopic or microscopic slices or sections. Such models are usually fragile and difficult to examine or measure. Nevertheless, they have helped in the comprehension of individual structures and the relationships and connections between structures.

Gaunt in 1971 [2], Ware and LoPresti in 1975 [3] and Gaunt and Gaunt [4] give comprehensive accounts of the methods tried and the results obtained during the postwar era before the widespread use of computers.

The advent of newer microscopical and imaging techniques, including computed tomography (CT scanning), positron emission tomography (PET), magnetic resonance imaging (MRI), confocal laser scanning microscopy (CLSM) and tandem scanning confocal optical microscopy (TSOM), has led to an explosion in the numbers of 3D datasets available. The data may be microscopic structures visualized using conventional light sources (as in TSOM) or lasers (CLSM) or electron micrographs of serial sections, photographs or drawings, or data in digital form derived from scanning systems or tomography. The existence of these datasets has encouraged a vast volume of work concerned with 3D visualization and 3D measurements. The technology will soon become readily available to allow these techniques to be applied as routine tools for the pathologist.

The problems of visualizing these data are formidable. It is difficult to recreate a mental 3D picture of an organ after it has been sliced, or of a tubular structure that has been opened or of a solid structure that has been serially sectioned. Such mental reconstructions that can be produced suffer from serious limitations. Their accuracy is not accessible to independent verification or measurement and the results of these studies are impossible to communicate accurately to others. It is furthermore infeasible, with even a fairly simple object, to visualize the spatial relationships between components and subunits embedded within it. The common observation that 'experts' are almost always surprised by some unthought-of aspect of a 3DR suggests that people tend to exaggerate their understanding of 3D structures. Some people in addition have very limited 3D visualization abilities, and many never acquire any significant skill in visualization.

The central problem of 3D visualization methods

is to provide visual cues in a 2D image of a 3D structure. The nature of these cues determines the degree of 'realism' of the reconstruction. There are two major problems: (i) creation of the 3D illusion; and (ii) ensuring the accuracy of the impression of the structure it creates. It is easy to produce images that give 3D monocular cues which are basically misleading about aspects of the structure such as concavity/convexity, surface texture and detail.

14.2 STAGES IN THE RECONSTRUCTION PROCESS

The production of 3DRs follows a sequence of stages. These are:

1 sample acquisition and preparation;
2 serial section production;
3 data entry;
4 model construction;
5 image generation and display.

For stage 1 little benefit has as yet been derived from the application of computer technology. In the other areas, computer technology has proved to be effective.

14.2.1 Sample acquisition and preparation

Computer technology has made no significant contribution to the problem of acquisition of biological data. The production of the appropriately sectioned biological material to be reconstructed, except from scanning systems, generally remains a slow, laborious process. The reconstruction process requires identification, from the specimen, of the plane in which sectioning is to be performed. The first problem is to understand the alignment of the specimen. This may be difficult. An important decision is whether coronal, transverse or sagittal sections are to be produced. If physical sectioning is to be the basis for the reconstruction, the plane is generally chosen which is likely to give the most sections. This choice may, however, be inappropriate if the orientation chosen increases the difficulties of constructing the 3D model. This can occur where reconstruction of the image in one plane is a more complex task than in another. With techniques such as CT scanning, where sectioning is non-destructive, individual sections in different orientations can be produced to assess the best orientation for serial section production. A further factor which may affect the choice of orientation for the serial sections is the sampling resolution achievable. In all the sectioning methodologies discussed, the overall sampling frequency is generally limited by the section thickness, i.e., the sampling frequency along the z-axis. Ideally the sampling frequency should be the same in all directions. In reality, the sampling frequency attainable in the $x-y$-plane is usually greater than in the z-plane. In this case consideration of the resolution achievable may affect the choice of orientation of the specimen prior to sectioning.

In a dissected piece of soft tissue such as a whole organ, serial slicing may readily reveal the structure and allow production of suitable slices. An example is the reconstruction by Yaegashi *et al.* [5] of cirrhotic liver nodules. Difficulties arise, however, if the structure has to be found and removed from within an organ to be serially sliced or sectioned. The locating cut may not be well-oriented. The two parts containing the structure may then have to be serially sliced independently and may be difficult to realign.

14.2.2 Serial section production

Data from physical slices

The process of physically sectioning objects creates several potential sources of error that non-destructive sectioning (using scanning or tomographic systems) avoids. These errors include loss of slices, distortion introduced by staining, fixation or sectioning processes, faulty alignment of adjacent sections and incorrect estimation of slice thickness. Producing serial sections without losses or ordering errors in the section sequence requires considerable technical skill.

Sectioning

For reconstruction of macroscopic structures, it may be sufficient to slice and photograph the organ without fixation. Fixation of whole organs or large pieces of tissue may be ineffective and fixation of individual slices can cause unacceptable distortion.

Nevertheless, fixation is usually necessary for macroscopic studies and is essential for light and electron microscopic studies. For these, the tissue must be processed and embedded in paraffin wax or resin and serially sectioned. Success here is reported to be dependent on close quality control, for example, ensuring that a straight leading edge is presented to the microtome knife and the floating-out time and temperature are standardized [6].

Section alignment

Orienting successive sections in relation to each other, so that their components have exactly the same relationships that they had before slicing took place, is a potential source of inaccuracy. For orientation to be achieved, at least two standard markers have to be present in each section so that successive sections can be aligned with each other. *Translational* misalignment, in the x- or y-axes, and/or *rotational* misalignment, around the z-axis, may occur between two slices, and may, by occurring between further slices, cause cumulative errors. On the other hand, intuitive corrections of translational and/or rotational misalignment (using the eye of the reconstructor) may also lead to errors. For example, a reconstructed tubular structure may appear straight and cylindrical by injudicious 'corrections' when it is really oblique and irregular. The alignment problem for soft tissues is often solved by incorporating markers into the blocks to be sectioned. To overcome these alignment difficulties, registration points of various kinds have been proposed. Holes have been drilled in the wax or resin [7], but these are generally too large. Burston and Thurley [8] drilled holes and inserted nerve fibres, but this is a difficult technique. Others [9] recommended using endogenous structures such as blood vessels, but these are also seldom conveniently oriented. Clarke *et al.* [10] have shown that laser-generated holes are a very appropriate alignment tool for tissue sections (Fig. 14.1a). With the increasing use of electronic image capture in electron microscopy, an integrated approach to the generation of 3D datasets is possible. Bron *et al.* [11] have demonstrated the digital processing of electron microscopic images from serial sections containing laser-induced topographical references. This permits 3DR at a depth resolution of 30–40 nm of entire cells by the use of image analysis methods for both transmission electron microscopy [12] and scanning transmission electron microscopy (STEM) [11]. They used computer algorithms to correct artefacts arising from the use of STEM and the serial sectioning process to reconstruct automatically the third dimension of the cells. They used a minimum of three fiducial markers as references per section created using an Excimer laser in tissues largely devoid of usable internal correlation points. The results of Bron *et al.* show that digital processing of electron microscopic images combined with the laser technique is a powerful tool which will eventually be usable for the routine generation of 3D electron microscopic reconstructions. The results of Clarke *et al.* [10] and Bron *et al.* [11] suggest that laser-based techniques will in future play an important role in the generation of accurate alignment of serial section data. Deverell and Whimster [13] have confirmed the advantages of introducing artificial registration points into the tissue block before embedding, and have successfully used cactus spines of the genus *Mammillaria* to make artificial registration points (Fig. 14.1b and c). These are particularly suitable by virtue of their straightness, narrow cross-section, cutting texture and birefringence. The technique is applicable to a wide range of tissues but the technique using cactus spines does not work well in brain tissue because the tissue is damaged by the spine during sectioning.

For hard tissues, such as teeth or bone, which can be sawn or ground, alignment may be ensured by milling parallel v-shaped grooves into one external face of the block within which the subject of the investigation is embedded [14–16]. On sectioning, the two parallel fiducial markers can be used to align adjacent sections.

For specimens which do not have external markers, internal structures which show little variation in position in adjacent sections may be used. This can be successful if the slices are thin enough that there is a high degree of coherence between adjacent sections. For electron microscopy-based reconstruction using thin slices, this may be useful. Equally, where a structure of known shape or little variation is present (e.g., the femur in a leg

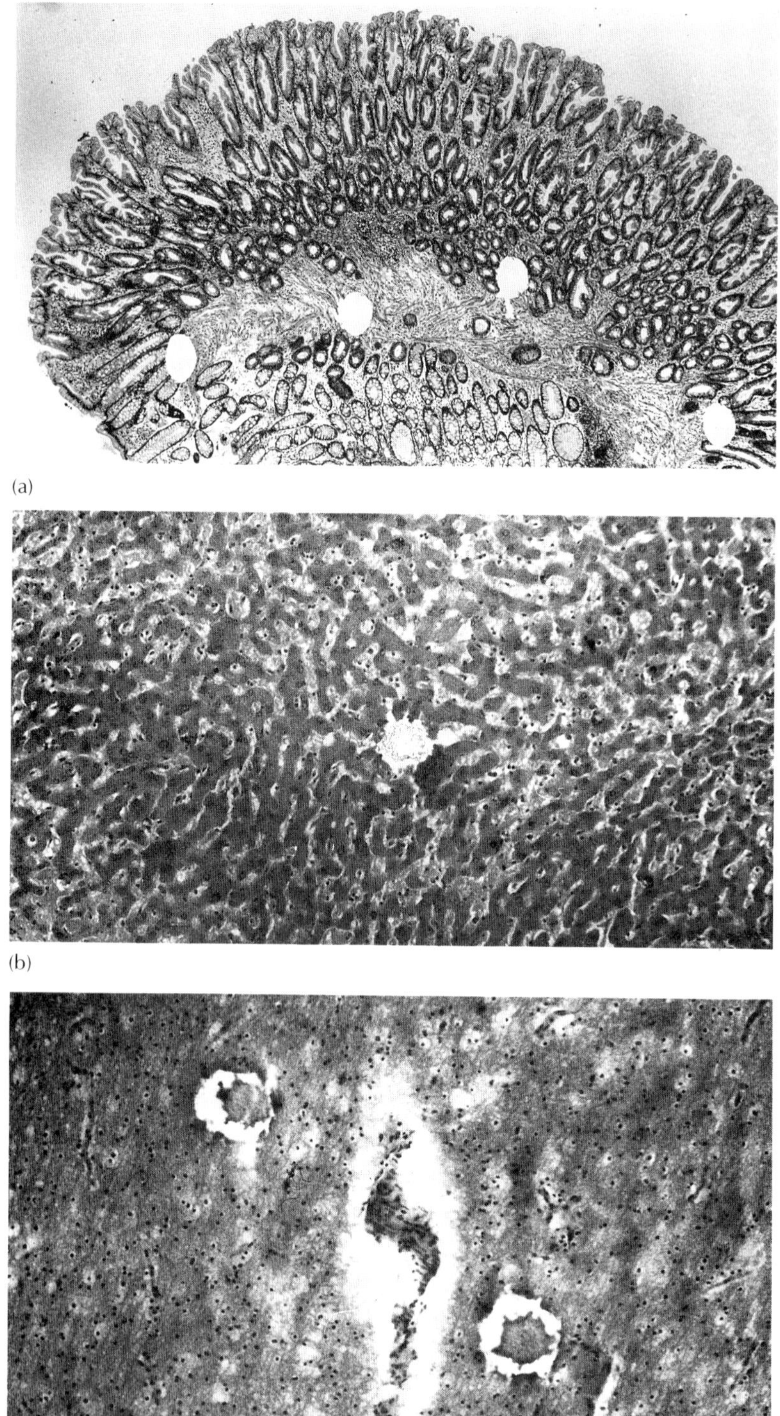

(a)

(b)

(c)

Fig. 14.1 Markers for tissue section alignment. (a) Micrograph of laser-generated holes in colorectal tissue. Courtesy of Mr G. Clarke. (b) Fiducial marker *Mamillaria* spine inserted into liver tissue and (c) central nervous system tissue. Cutting and staining produce minimal tissue distortion and, being birefringent, the spines are easily found on light microscopy. Courtesy of Dr M.H. Deverell.

reconstruction), this can be used as an alignment guide.

If the sections to be aligned are stored in digital form on the computer it may be possible to align them by using correlation methods or boundary matching, by moving adjacent sections relative to each other until some acceptable criterion is satisfied.

Hibbard and Hawkins [17] have evaluated two image-processing techniques for objective image alignment for 3DR of digital autoradiograms. The techniques used were principal axis transformation and cross-correlation, of which the latter proved the more effective. Where no form of fiducial markers is available, these techniques probably have the best chance of producing good alignment.

The least accurate method of alignment is to photograph each section, transfer the details to tracing paper and superimpose sections by eye for the best fit. On the tracing paper a minimum of two reference points corresponding to equivalent points in adjacent sections can be used to align the stack of slices. This was the method routinely employed during the late 19th century, although its limitations were recognized very quickly.

The methods described above all assume that distortions are due to misalignment. In reality, for soft tissue there may be in addition distortion created by the staining or fixation techniques or by the sectioning process due to compression and shearing. Some attempts have been made to deal with these problems but they present formidable difficulties. The effects of artefacts due to staining procedures can be compensated for by recording the section digitally before sectioning and staining and after all the histochemical procedures have been applied [18]. The use of multiple reference points is one approach, calculating for each point a vector representing the correction to be applied at that point. Using these vectors and treating the image mathematically as an elastic plate undergoing deformation, it is possible to calculate corrections to be applied over the whole image [19].

Estimating section separation

Estimating the distance between sections may also be a source of difficulty. Cutting techniques usually cause losses of material and so specific markers need to be incorporated to indicate depth. For softer materials, if the section thickness is known and no sections have been lost, the z parameter can be obtained by summation, i.e., adding the thicknesses of all the slices. If the dimensions of the unprocessed tissue sample are known, allowances can be made for distortion, compression and tissue loss. For hard tissues where alignment is assured by parallel milled grooves as described above, a third groove can be provided running diagonally between the two parallel grooves. Simple trigonometry allows the calculation of the position of the section in the block [20]. The same principle has been applied to allow the alignment of MRI, CT and digital subtraction angiography scans of the human head [21].

In some circumstances, for example with sawn or ground sectioning, precise measurement of the z value is often more difficult. For hard materials which are ground to produce sections, the accuracy of the z parameter depends on how accurately the grinding machine can be set. Typically, micrometer settings are used to ensure sufficient accuracy. As a last resort for section material which does not have fiducial markers, estimates or measurements of the thickness of saw cut may be used to estimate the approximate size of the missing materials.

Isolation and orientation of the structure to be reconstructed

Having prepared the slices, the structures of interest have to be distinguished from the rest of the material. This procedure varies according to the nature of the slices and the complexity of the structures. For example, in reconstructing a small tumour, tooth or fetal heart, all the material in the slices may be used. Microscopic structures, such as glands in gastric dysplasia and carcinoma, however, may have to be magnified and recorded [22,23]. The recording can be done photographically and the structures of interest separated from the rest later, or, with the help of projection or a drawing arm, the structures of interest can be selectively drawn out, although this can be tedious and prone to error. Ultramicroscopic structures such as neurons and intracellular organelles have to be viewed at high magnification and photographed. The photographs or drawings have to be aligned within the stack. Elaborate systems have been devised to ensure that the sections are properly aligned for photography [24], although this can be very laborious and time-consuming.

14.3 DATA ENTRY

14.3.1 The process of digitization

In order to produce 3DR by computer from the 2D sections of the object under examination, a 3D representation can be produced by recording the positions of parts of the object, volumes or surfaces of interest as numerical values or co-ordinates in 3D space. Various devices are commonly used to collect digitized data for computer processing.

14.3.2 The graphics tablet

(see also Section 2.1)

A digitizing tablet is the most frequently used tool for manual data entry and typically consists of a mesh of criss-cross wires and a separate cursor. The principle of the digitizing tablet is that the electromagnetic field produced by a coil in the cursor is detected at the nearest intersection of the wires in the digitizing tablet. Since individual wires in the mesh can be identified, the 2D co-ordinates can be found. An outline is digitized by moving the cursor around the outline and recording x, y co-ordinates (usually by pressing a button on the cursor). A great advantage of using a digitizing tablet is that sampling frequency can be adjusted locally to take into account regions of highly variable local curvature embedded in less complex regions. The output from the tablet is a set of x, y co-ordinates. The third co-ordinate, the z co-ordinate, is a position of the slices within the object.

14.3.3 The digitizing microscope

A digitizing microscope is an optical microscope with a specimen stage which is movable in two directions at right angles to each other (the x and the y directions). Movement of the stage is accomplished by means of stage micrometers which, when rotated, translate the stage in the appropriate direction. If an optical encoder, which translates rotational movement into a series of pulses, is attached to each of the x- and y-stage micrometers, pulses can be added or subtracted depending on the direction of movement of the micrometer. At any position of the stage the number of pulses stored in the computer gives the x and y positions of the stage relative to the fixed cross-wires in the eyepiece of the microscope.

To digitize an outline when viewed down the microscope, the stage is moved by rotating the micrometers so that the cross-wires in the eyepiece of the microscope are coincident with part of the outline. This x, y co-ordinate is then stored. The stage is then moved so that the next position which is to be recorded along the outline is coincident with the cross-wires. This point is again stored. In this way the outline is converted into a series of x, y co-ordinates which define the outline traced.

14.3.4 Image data from point digitization systems

For 2D images of physical sections, especially cut section surfaces, for example those produced by sectioning by grinding away and polishing, structures are represented as contours and edges. In cases where the section thickness is very small in relation to the separation between sections along the z-axis (i.e., the sampling frequency in the z direction), the 2D images can be considered as 'true' 2D representations. From the physical slices, the images of the 2D slices may be visible through the microscope or in micrographs. With a drawing arm, microscope images can be traced and digitized using a digitizing table on which the image is projected. The cursor is used to 'draw' (i.e., transmit the successive x, y co-ordinates of the cursor on the tablet to the computer) the structures of interest. An effective way of using a digitizing tablet is to trace around the images on a photomicrograph or projection arm-drawing system and then digitize these drawings. Separation of the identification of the contour from its digitization makes the digitizing process less subject to error. The use of projection drawing systems is prone to error since the outlines are often faint and may be difficult to follow. With micrographs and projection drawing systems there may be distortion at the edges of the field due to barrel or pincushion distortion in the optical system. These errors can be avoided by using a digitizing microscope [25] which records x, y co-ordinates using cross-hairs in the centre of the field of view, thereby avoiding problems due to optical distortion. Micrographs may be captured into a computer system using a video camera with a frame-grabber card which records and stores the image the camera acquires, typically with a 256×256 or 512×512 pixel resolution. Each image in a 3D dataset has to be accurately aligned prior to capture. For quantitative work the characteristics of the camera and imaging system should be determined so that allowance can be made for instrumental errors.

Contour data can be extracted from scanning systems such as CLSM; however, the extraction of contours presents problems. Edges may be extracted from these data by 2D or 3D edge-detection algorithms, or by manual delineation. The automatic detection of edges in images with a low signal/noise ratio can be difficult. Using thresholding to produce bilevel images allows the effects of different threshold values on the accuracy of edge determination to be examined. Edge enhancement can be performed using Laplacian, Sobel or Roberts filters in two or three dimensions [26]. Median smoothing allows subjective improvement in the image quality but with loss of edge clarity. Automatic methods for generating contours may be computationally tractable but often fail, particularly when dealing with laminar or complex structures. For these reasons, manual methods such as using digitizing tablets are often preferred for data entry. The tracing of the contours from the scanned image by graphics tablet allows the user to apply his/her judgement to the location of the boundaries of the objects. Since these boundaries may be inadequately represented by changes in adjacent voxel values, this allows the experimenter to use this higher-level knowledge of the structures to make meaningful representations of the individual objects.

14.3.5 Images as data arrays from scanning systems

Slice data from scanning systems (CT, MRI or CLSM) are usually acquired in the form of arrays of numbers, each of which represents the value of a volume element or voxel. The voxels of each slice form a 2D array of numbers representing the values of some parameter such as absorbance throughout the thickness of a slice. For a single slice with a reasonable resolution of 512×512 voxels, for example, over 250 000 numbers have to be stored. For the number of slices needed to form a 3DR the computer storage requirements may be considerable. Since the processing of large volumes of data is computationally intensive, systems that process these data must have large memories, disk sizes and processing power. Manipulating these data requires expensive computer systems if results are to be obtained within reasonable time scales.

Although the output from scanning systems resembles superficially that of the 2D images referred to above, it differs in significant ways. The scanned image does not represent a surface because each building block of the image represents the average or integrated intensity or some other parameter over a small finite volume of space, the voxel or volume element. Thus the image seen is the 2D projection of a 3D volume. In addition, the sampling frequency in the x–y plane is commonly higher than in the z plane, which means that these voxels are not cubic in shape. To avoid the distortion caused by the anisotropy in sampling, interpolation of extra slices may be used to provide displays based on cubic elements. Linear interpolation is commonly used to compute these but this may be inaccurate and may not be scientifically justified. Interpolating extra slices into the dataset increases the storage requirements markedly and is, of course, creating 'ficticious' data. Not interpolating usually results in images of poor visual quality.

For systems which base their imaging on the display of collections of voxels, methods for the isolation of the collections of voxels of interest are needed. The process of identifying separate regions is termed segmentation (see Section 7.3). Numerous algorithms for image segmentation are available, but the problems are formidable and in general far from solved. Segmenting data simply on the values of voxels (thresholding) is not usually sufficient since differences in data values in the image may not reflect the boundaries of structures as identified anatomically.

It should be noted that the collections of voxels which form one slice from a scanning system represent a digitized image. Taking the scan, and digitizing it using a digitizing tablet for example, is a redigitizing process. As such it may be expected to introduce error. The size of error is dependent upon the sampling density and the accuracy of estimating the true contour of the object of interest. Redigitizing scanner data is only acceptable if quantitative assessment of the errors induced is performed, by using test objects of accurately known dimensions, using standardized sampling procedures on objects of very similar size to the objects whose scans have been redigitized.

14.4 MODEL CONSTRUCTION

14.4.1 Contour-based models

Digitizing tablets and similar devices output a set of points which in 3D space represents the boundary of an object. In their most primitive form contour-based systems represent the boundary as a set of piecewise-connected lines.

14.4.2 Models constructed of surface elements

To create 3D images which have a solid appearance from digitized boundary data, adjacent sections must be joined by surfaces. A simple method of doing this is to extrude the serial section as a solid slice. This gives only a very limited visualization of the surface, and can reveal no surface detail

The most common method of constructing a model of the surface is by triangulating the surface between the contours. For simple contours the generation of the strip of triangles joining the contours can be completely automated. Difficulties arise where branches and joins between multiple objects are to be created. Manual intervention in the triangulation process is usually necessary. Reliable automated triangulation procedures are under development, but have so far not been applied widely enough for potential users to be assured that they will work satisfactorily in practice [27].

14.4.3 Voxel models

The geometric basis for the voxel model is the collection of cuboids forming the voxels. No additional structure is added to the voxels and these form the basis for the display techniques used.

14.5 IMAGE GENERATION AND DISPLAY

14.5.1 Contour display techniques

Simple display programs show contours drawn on the computer screen or graph plotter as piecewise-connected lines as they would appear from different 3D viewpoints (Plate 14.1a, opposite p. 278). The more sophisticated of these programs perform hidden line removal, that is, lines which would be obscured by opaque slices from the viewing position are not drawn. This improves the 3D illusion by providing better depth cues. Many such programs have been developed for large computers [28–30]. More recently such systems have also become available on microcomputers [31,32].

When an object is represented by a line drawing of its contours, reconstruction of the surface connecting the contours is dependent on the imagination and experience of the viewer. If the contours overlap from the chosen viewpoint and the object is fairly simple, the illusion of three-dimensionality can be sustained and the image is usually relatively easy to interpret. Difficulties arise when the scene is more complex or contours do not overlap significantly. When several objects are present confusion can arise over which contours belong to which object. These difficulties are due to the lack of adequate depth and shape cues.

An improvement is to draw the sections as flat-shaded filled contours [33]. This provides significantly better cues than hidden line techniques since colour can be more effectively used to shade different structures in the drawn sections.

This is also technically very simple and easy to

achieve but suffers the same fundamental limitations as line-drawing techniques.

14.5.2 Surface display techniques

Displaying 3D surfaces made up of triangular patches can be done with classical computer graphics techniques (Plate 14.1b). Each triangle is oriented in 3D space and its orientation can be represented by estimating the direction in which the face of the triangle is pointing (the surface normal). The angle between the estimated surface normal and light source can be used to shade the triangle. The normals at the vertices of the triangles are estimated using the calculated normals of the surrounding triangles to give an averaged value at each vertex. A smooth appearance is achieved (Plate 14.1c) either by calculating the shade at each vertex of a triangle and interpolating the shades necessary to fill the whole triangle (Gouraud shading) [34] or by interpolating between the vertex normals and calculating the correct shade at each point on the triangle (Phong shading) [35]. The latter technique provides better-quality images (Plate 14.1d) but is more computationally expensive. Highlighting is very important in providing depth cues. If such highlighting is not provided, the images can give a misleading impression, for example that a surface is concave when it is convex [36].

Software to model and display 3D structures based on surface tiles with hidden surface removal is complex and difficult to produce and was initially available only on expensive mini- and mainframe computers. The fall in price and the increase in power of microcomputers has meant that high-quality 3DRs are possible on standard IBM PC-compatible systems [37,38].

14.5.3 Voxel-based display techniques

With the advent of many tomographic and other scanning systems the development of display methods for voxel data has been rapid and a number of methods have been produced. Since the geometric basis for display is the box-like voxel in the more primitive display systems, the images often have a 'boxy' appearance or serrated edges. One simple division of voxel methods is into two types – surface and volume methods. In the surface methods only those voxels which form the surface of the object are stored for display. This reduces the volume of data which needs to be stored, but does mean that an extra step, of identifying the surface voxels, is necessary before display. For speed, voxel-based images are often shaded solely in terms of the distance of the voxel from the observer's viewpoint – depth-shaded images. These can give an impression of structure but, since surfaces at the same distance from the observer have the same shade, vital information may be lost. The orientation of edges is also not readily appreciated from these images. The grey-level values associated with each voxel are not stored, so that voxels can be stored as values in a 3D binary array, reducing the storage requirements considerably. Because the volumes of data are reduced, fast processing is possible even on modest computer systems. These techniques have the merit of speed but the images are crude in comparison with surface-shaded images from models based on triangular tiles, or other surface elements. Better-quality images can be derived from the voxel data by approximating as accurately as possible the shape of the surface in the neighbourhood of a surface voxel, using a similar approach to the shading of the triangular tiling models to shade the surface. Many studies have been performed on the comparison of surface-shading algorithms for voxel data [39,40].

A second class of methods of volume rendering retains grey-level information about each voxel and generates the image directly from this array without explicitly extracting the object surfaces. This allows more flexibility in the images that can be produced – for example, in the use of transparency and slicing through internal structures – but at a cost of greater memory requirements and processor speed. Some of these methods are particularly well-suited to data in which the surfaces are ill-defined, and take care to avoid artefacts due to sampling errors [41,42]. Typical voxel-rendering packages offer many options for data display. It is not correct to assert that one particular method is best, because different types of data and different features of the same data can be illuminated by different display techniques. It is, for example, unlikely that the shading method most suited to displaying the surface of the human skull would be as suitable for displaying filamentous structures derived from CLSM of single cells.

14.6 3DR USING OPTICAL SECTIONING

It will have become clear from the previous discussion that physical sectioning of biological materials causes a variety of problems which make successful 3DR difficult. Non-destructive techniques for sectioning would have enormous value. Tomographical techniques have revolutionized medicine and it is possible that optical serial sectioning, if properly realized, could do the same for biomedical research based on light microscopy.

14.6.1 Confocal optical microscopy

3DR is possible by stacking 2D planes acquired by through-focusing serially in light microscopy. Results of such procedures have been disappointing due to out-of-focus contributions from image planes above and below the plane of focus. Such blurring is an unavoidable consequence of the microscope optical system. Minsky [43] proposed to reduce these problems using the principle of confocal microscopy. Confocal microscopy improves image resolution by passing the light through one (CLSM) or many (TSOM) small apertures, which has the effect of reducing the out-of-focus contribution. This leaves a thin, highly focused plane. Since the image is built up from many small samples, the light from CLSM images is digitized and stored on a computer. As the distance between the specimen and microscope changes, a new focal plane is produced. In this way a series of images can be collected, digitized and stored. The specimen can then be reconstructed in the computer as a 3D volume and displayed using voxel display techniques. Since this method involves no physical sectioning and consequent physical distortion and the adjacent slices are automatically aligned, good serial section datasets can be easily generated. However, the confocal microscope is a complex instrument and the effects of errors in alignment of the components, uncertainties over the true depth of the optical sections, mechanical errors in scanning systems, optical aberrations, etc., need to be assessed, especially before quantitative measurements are applied.

14.6.2 Deconvolution of light microscope images

Because of the cost and complexity of confocal microscopes, attempts have been made to remove out-of-focus blur computationally. Agard [44] showed that it is computationally possible to remove blurring from the digitized images without using confocal scanning systems. Using computational techniques has a number of advantages: lower light intensities can be used, high rates of data acquisition can be achieved, many different methods of illumination and light sources can be used and less photo bleaching occurs in fluorescence microscopy. All the 3D information is not recoverable computationally; some is lost. One major problem with this technique is that deconvolution is computationally intensive. However, the ready availability of more powerful computer systems means that the computation is now more feasible. In addition, the simple nearest-neighbour algorithm [45] has simplified this computational task, giving acceptable results at the risk of generating some artefacts. Both confocal microscopy and optical sectioning have major significance for studies in pathology. To be able to perform 3DR very readily means that 3D morphological studies and measurements could be made on populations of cells and their components in health and disease. At lower magnifications the organization of tissues and their components would become accessible.

14.7 QUANTITATIVE MEASUREMENT

Since in voxel systems counting voxels can give accurate volume estimations, this is available on many systems. Assessing surface areas is more difficult [46]. The construction of a model of the surface of a structure as triangular elements can, in addition to accurate volumes, give good estimates of surface areas of the structure. However, even on simple convex bodies it can also lead to significant errors [46,47]. Calculating volumes and surfaces of objects using tiling algorithms is subject to errors dependent on the local concavity/convexity of the surface. On a convex surface a tiled covering underestimates the volume; on a concave surface a tiled covering locally overestimates the volume. Corrections for these errors are possible where the surface normals of the adjacent triangles are known, which is the case, for example, where the model is to be displayed using surface-shading techniques. Alternatively, representations based on other types of surface patches may prove more suitable.

14.8 CONCLUSION

3DR techniques are under continuous development, as is the technology which supports them. Systems developed for engineering and other applications are coming within the price range of many users. Recently publications have started to appear using standard high-quality graphics workstations [48]. As these are coming down in price, more applications will be possible. The advent of new computer technology, notably highly parallel systems and chips such as the Intel i860, offer the prospect of very fast reconstructions and the software to make 3DR a routine technique. Most significant however is the continuing increase in type and numbers of scanning systems, both macroscopic and microscopic. Prior to these systems becoming available, the critical limiting factor inhibiting the wide application of 3DR was generating adequately registered, undistorted, complete sets of serial section data for the reconstruction process. The fact that scanning optical microscopes can produce such datasets easily means that the everyday use of 3DR for studies of pathology is now feasible.

Concerning the benefits from 3DR, Los in 1973 [49] quoted His as follows:

> Even now having occupied myself for so many years with embryonic sections and their reconstruction, I dare not form myself a complete image of the real form from studying those sections only. And again and again, with each reconstruction, I stumble upon some completely unexpected surprise or other.

References

1 His W. *Anatomie Menschlicher Embryonen*. Leipzig: Vogel, 1880.

2 Gaunt WA. *Microreconstruction*. London: Pitman Medical, 1971.

3 Ware RW, LoPresti V. Three-dimensional reconstruction from serial sections. *Int Rev Cytol* 1975; 40: 323–440.

4 Gaunt PM, Gaunt WA. *Three-dimensional Reconstruction in Biology*. Baltimore: University Park Press, 1978.

5 Yaegashi HJ, Takahashi T, Kawasaki M. Microcomputer-aided reconstruction — a system designed for the study of 3-D microstructure in histology and histopathology. *J Microsc* 1987; 146: 55–65.

6 Deverell MH, Bailey N, Whimster WF. Tissue distortion in three-dimensional reconstruction of wax or plastic embedded microscopic structures. *Pathol Res Pract* 1989; 185: 598.

7 Gough NG. A method for the accurate localisation and orientation of structures studied by the use of serial microscopic structures. *J R Microsc Soc* 1967; 88: 291–300.

8 Burston WR, Thurley K. A technique for the orientation of serial histological sections. *J Anat* 1957; 91: 409–412.

9 Street H, Mize RR. A simple microcomputer based three-dimensional reconstruction system (MICROS). *J Neurosci Methods* 1983; 7: 359–375.

10 Clarke GE, Hamilton PW, Montgomery WA. Aligning histological serial sections for three-dimensional reconstruction using an Excimer laser beam. *Pathol Res Pract* 1993; 189: 563–566.

11 Bron C, Gremillet P, Launay D *et al*. Scanning transmission and computer aided volumic electron microscopy: 3D modelling of entire cells by electronic imaging. *SPIE Proc Biomed Image Proc* 1990; 1245: 61–67.

12 Bron C, Gremillet P, Launay D *et al*. Three dimensional electron microscopy of entire cells. *J Microsc* 1990; 157: 21–35.

13 Deverell MH, Whimster WF. A method of image registration for three-dimensional reconstruction of microscopic structures using an IBAS 2000 image analysis system. *Pathol Res Pract* 1989; 185: 602–605.

14 Kimura O, Dykes E, Fearnhead RW. The relationship between the surface area of the enamel crowns of human teeth and that of the dentine-enamel junction. *Arch Oral Biol* 1977; 22: 677–683.

15 Sullivan PG. Growth of the canine mandible. PhD Thesis. University of London, 1976.

16 Dykes E, Afshar F. Computer generated three-dimensional reconstruction from serial sections. *Acta Stereol* 1982; 82: 289–296.

17 Hibbard LS, Hawkins RA. Objective image alignment

for three-dimensional reconstruction of digital autoradiograms. *J Neurosci Methods* 1988; 26: 55–74.

18 Laan AC, Lamers WH, Huijsmans DP *et al.* Deformation-corrected computer-aided three-dimensional reconstruction of immunohistochemically stained organs: application to the rat heart during early organogenesis. *Anat Rec* 1989; 224: 443–457.

19 Durr R, Peterhans E, Von der Heydt R. Correction of distorted image pairs with elastic models. *Eur J Cell Biol* 1988; 48(suppl 25): 85–88.

20 Gillings B, Buonocore M. An investigation of enamel thickness in human lower incisor teeth. *J Dent Res* 1961; 40: 105–118.

21 Peters TM, Clerk JA, Olivier A *et al.* Integrated stereotaxic imaging with CT, MR imaging and digital subtraction angiography. *Radiology* 1986; 161: 821–826.

22 Takahashi T, Iwama N. Atypical glands in gastric adenoma: three-dimensional architecture compared with carcinomatous and metaplastic glands. *Virchows Arch [A]* 1984; 403: 135–148.

23 Takahashi T, Iwama N. Architectural pattern of gastric adenocarcinoma: a three-dimensional reconstruction study. *Virchows Arch [A]* 1984; 403: 127–134.

24 Prothero JS, Prothero JW. Three-dimensional reconstruction from serial sections. IV. The reassembly problem. *Comput Biomed Res* 1986; 19: 361–373.

25 Dykes E, Clement JG. The construction and applications of an *x-y* coordinate plotting microscope. *J Dent Res* 1980; 59: 1800.

26 Gonzalez RC, Wintz P. *Digital Image Processing.* Reading: Addison-Wesley, 1987.

27 Boissonat J-D. Shape reconstruction from planar cross sections. *Comput Vision, Graphics Image Proc* 1988; 44: 1–29.

28 Afshar F, Dykes ED. A three-dimensional reconstruction of the human brain stem. *J Neurosurg* 1982; 57: 491–495.

29 Cahan LD, Trombka BT. Computer graphics — three-dimensional reconstruction of thalamic anatomy from serial sections. *Comp Prog Biomed* 1975; 5: 91–98.

30 Johnson EM, Capowski JJ. A system for the three-dimensional reconstruction of biological structures. *Comp Biomed Res* 1983; 16: 79–87.

31 Vanden Berghe W, Aerts P, Claeys H, Verraes W. A microcomputer-based graphical reconstruction technique for serial sectioned objects. *Anat Rec* 1986; 215: 84–91.

32 Gras H. A 'hidden line' algorithm for 3d-reconstruction from serial sections — an extension of the Neurec program package for a microcomputer. *Comp Prog Biomed* 1984; 18: 217–226.

33 Runham NW, Davies DA, Roberts D. Computer-aided three dimensional reconstructions from serial sections *Microsc Anal* 1990; 16: 15–18.

34 Gouraud H. Continuous shading of curved surfaces. *IEEE Trans Comput* 1971; 20: 623–628.

35 Bui-Tuong P. Illumination for computer-generated pictures. *Comm ACM* 1975; 18(6): 311–317.

36 Gregory RL, Gombrich EH (eds) *Illusion in Nature and Art.* London: Duckworth, 1973.

37 Cookson MJ, Dykes E, Holman JG. A microcomputer based system for generating realistic shaded images reconstructed from serial sections. *Eur J Cell Biol* 1988; 48(suppl 25): 69–72.

38 Holman JG, Cookson MJ, Dykes E. Applications of a microcomputer-based reconstruction system to produce realistic three-dimensional shaded images from serial sections. *Med Inform* 1989; 14: 173–184.

39 Chen LS, Herman GT, Reynolds RA, Udupa JK. Surface shading in the cuberille environment. *IEEE Comput Graphics Appl* 1985; 5(12): 33–43.

40 Pommert A, Tiede U, Wiebecke G, Hohne KH. Surface shading in tomographic volume visualisation: a comparative study. In: Ezquerra N, Garcia E, Arkin ER (eds) *Proceedings of the First Conference on Visualisation in Biomedical Computing, Atlanta, Georgia.* May 22–25, 1990. IEEE Computer Society Press: 1990: 19–26.

41 Levoy M. Display of surfaces from volume data. *IEEE Comput Graphics Appl* 1988; 3: 29–37.

42 Drebin RA, Carpenter L, Hanrahan P. Volume rendering. *Comput Graphics* 1988; 22(4): 65–74.

43 Minsky M. US Patent 3013467, 1961.

44 Agard DA. Optical sectioning microscopy: cellular architecture in three dimensions. *Ann Rev Biophys Bieong* 1984; 13: 191–219.

45 Agard DA, Hiraoka Y, Sedat JW. Three dimensional Microscopy: image processing for high resolution subcellular imaging. Proceedings SPIE, The International Society for Photo-Optical Engineers, Bellingham, WA, Vol. 1161, In: Wampler JE (ed.) *New Methods in Microscopy and Low Light Imaging.* 24–30.

46 Fahle M, Palm G. Calculation of surface areas from serial sections. *J Neurosci Methods* 1983; 9: 75–85.

47 Funnell WRJ. On the calculation of surface areas of objects reconstructed from serial sections. *J Neurosci Methods* 1984; 11: 205–210.

48 Winslow JL, Bjerknes M, Cheng H. Three-dimensional reconstruction of biological objects using a graphics engine. *Comput Biomed Res* 1987; 20: 583–602.

49 Los JA. Reconstructive morphology — possibilities and limitations. *Acta Morphol Neerl Scand* 1973; 11: 263–268.

15

FRACTAL GEOMETRIC ANALYSIS IN PATHOLOGY

S. S. CROSS

There are many objects in clinical pathology which it would be desirable to quantitate but which have irregular and complex boundaries or surfaces. Integer-dimensional geometry, such as the Euclidean system, is not an effective method of measuring the dimensions of such objects because their irregular boundaries have to be approximated to smooth regular shapes, such as circles or spheres, before measurement can be made [1]. Fractal geometric analysis is a non-integer-dimensional system which can describe the irregularity of such objects more appropriately [1,2].

15.1 FRACTAL GEOMETRY

Before the fractal properties of objects in clinical pathology are discussed it is best to illustrate the general properties of fractal objects using mathematical fractal sets. The mathematical images can be regarded as visual images without recourse to the theory of their formation or mathematical significance. Figure 15.1 shows an image of a mathematical fractal structure, in this example a Julia set, with the whole set shown in Fig. 15.1a and successive magnifications of the area enclosed in the boxes in (b–d). It can be seen that, even with a total magnification of 15 625× from (a) to (d), the boundary between the black and white areas is still of the same complexity, it is not becoming a smoother line. It is also apparent that similar shapes, such as curved units like seahorse tails, appear at all levels of magnifications – a property known as scaling self-similarity [1]. The complexity of the boundary presents a problem if its length is to be measured; it is easy to see that if the perimeter of the dark area measured at the resolution in Fig. 15.1a was compared with a measurement made at the resolution in 1d, then the latter value would be larger because more of the complexity of the boundary would be available to the measuring device. A mathematical fractal object has the same level of complexity at all levels of magnification [1,3], so the boundary length of the Julia set illustrated in Fig. 15.1 will be infinite but its space-filling properties can be described by a fractal dimension. A fractal dimension differs from Euclidean dimensions in that it may not be an integer: the topological dimension of the line boundary of the black area in Fig. 15.1 would be 1 and the topological dimension of the plane in which it is drawn is 2 but the fractal dimension lies between 1 and 2. The fractal dimension has specialized significance for mathematicians [1] but for the quantitative clinical pathologist it can be seen as an index of the space-filling properties [2,4] of an object which has fractal properties. Thus the boundary in Fig. 15.1 is more complex than a smooth line (which would have a fractal dimension of 1) but does not completely fill the plane in which it is embedded (when it would have a fractal dimension of 2). The closer the fractal dimension is to the dimension of the space in which it is embedded then the greater its space-filling properties (which is synonymous with its boundary or surface complexity). The fractal dimension also gives the formal mathematical definition of a fractal object as being one in which the fractal (or Hausdorff–Besicovitch) dimension exceeds the topological dimension [1]. The important

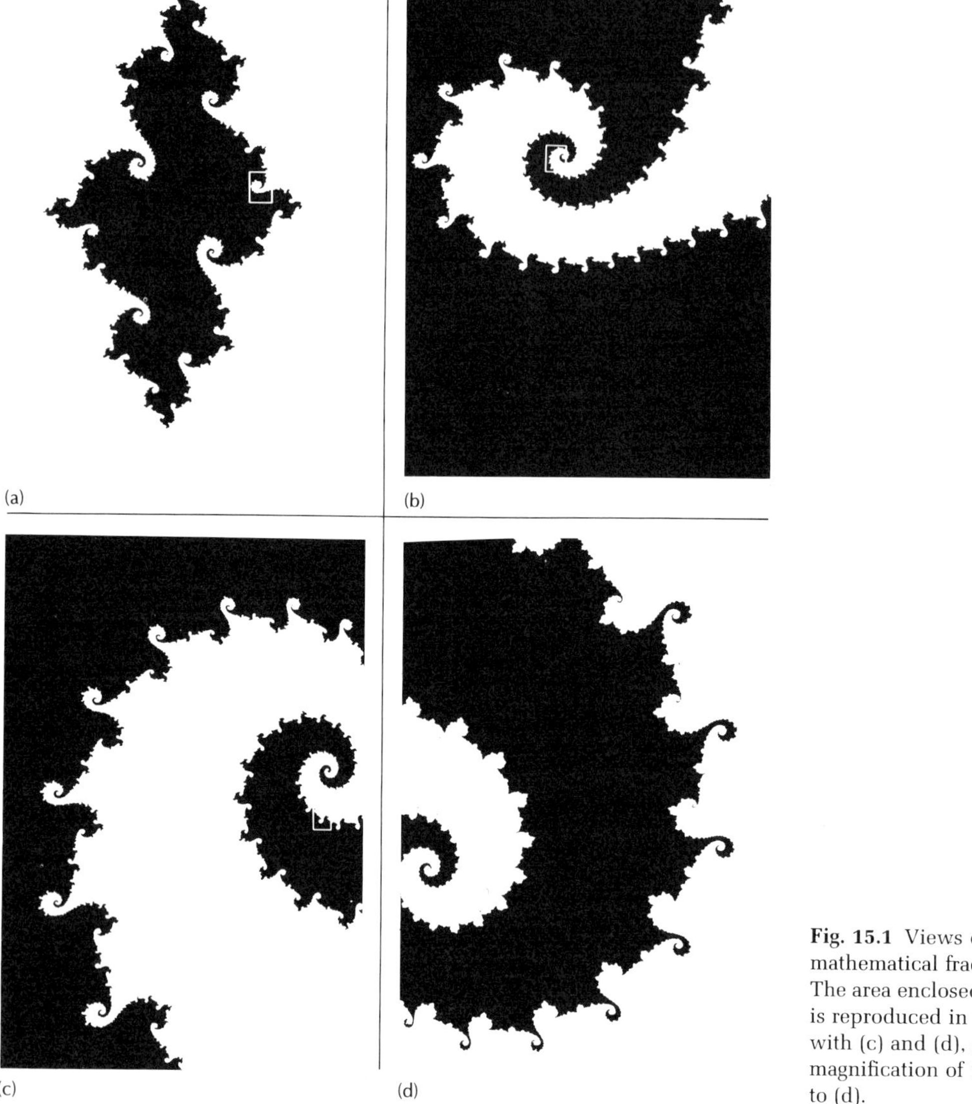

Fig. 15.1 Views of a Julia set, a mathematical fractal structure. The area enclosed in the box in (a) is reproduced in (b) and similarly with (c) and (d), giving a total magnification of 15 625× from (a) to (d).

difference between mathematical fractal objects and natural objects with fractal properties is that mathematical fractal objects retain the same level of boundary complexity at all levels of magnification, but with natural objects there is some point where magnification reveals the basic unit of construction and there is loss of boundary complexity [5]. In clinical pathological objects examined by light microscopy this limit occurs when single cells are filling the field of view but until this point is reached, fractal analysis may be appropriate.

15.2 MEASURING THE FRACTAL DIMENSION

The most widely used method of measuring the fractal dimension in the biological sciences is the box-counting method [2,4,6,7] given by:

$$D_B = \lim_{\varepsilon \to 0} \frac{\log N(\varepsilon)}{\log(1/\varepsilon)}$$

where D_B is the box-counting fractal dimension of the object, ε is the side length of the box and $N(\varepsilon)$ is the smallest number of boxes of side length ε required completely to cover the outline of the object being measured. The limit 0 cannot be applied to natural objects, so the dimension is calculated by:

$$D_B = d$$

where d is the slope of the graph of log $[N(\varepsilon)]$ against log $1/\varepsilon$. This method is illustrated in Fig. 15.2. An object is imaged (a) and its outline defined (b). Grids of differing sizes (c and d) are placed over the image and the number of outline-containing squares is counted. The gradient of the linear segment on an appropriate log–log graph gives D_B.

Figure 15.3 is a log–log graph for the three different types of colorectal polyps. It can be seen that the gradient of the lines for the adenomatous and metaplastic polyps is steeper than that for the inflammatory polyp, indicating that these have greater fractal dimensions. This method can be performed manually with prints of images and grids printed on transparent sheets but is easily implemented on microcomputer-based image analysis systems. An implementation of the box-counting method has been described in a non-microscopic context [8] which was accurate when tested with objects of known fractal dimension (errors: circle +0.5%, square +0.1%, quadric Koch island −1.2%) and reproducible with a reliability coefficient of 0.968 (95% confidence limits 0.911–0.984). An alternative method is the divider or perimeter-stepping algorithm [9].

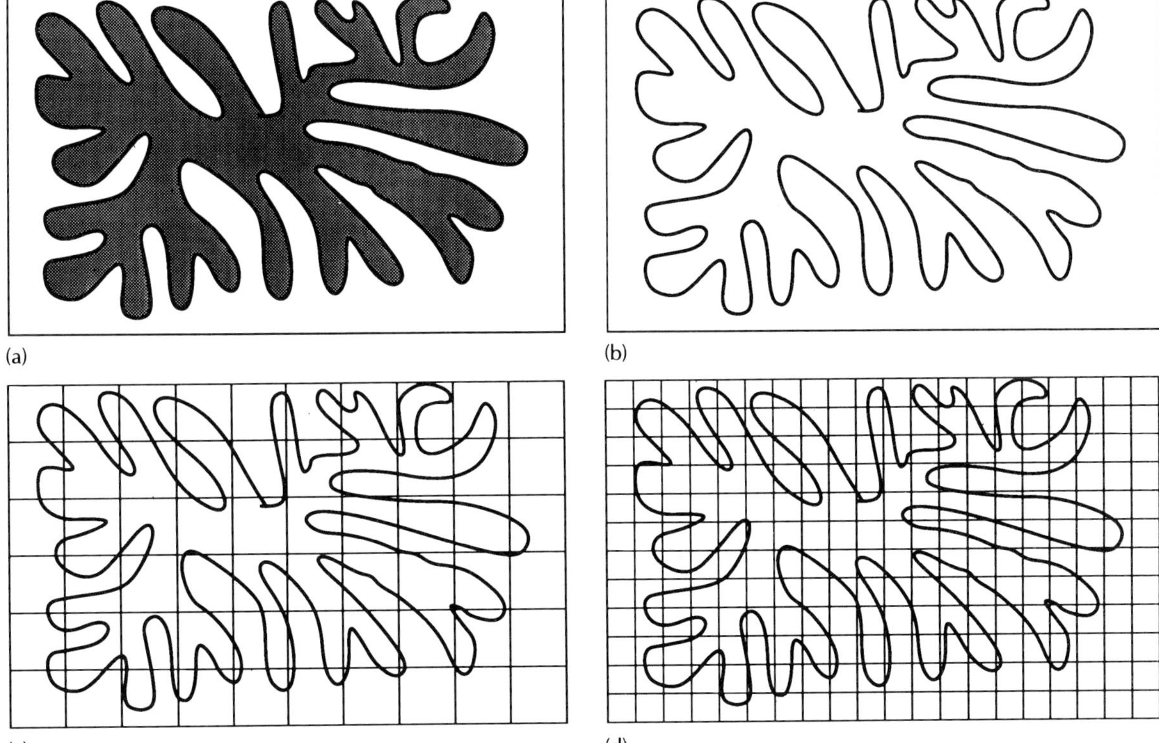

Fig. 15.2 Diagrammatic representation of the box-counting method. The image of a convoluted object (a) is reduced to its outline (b), grids of differing sizes (c and d) are applied and the number of outline-containing squares is counted.

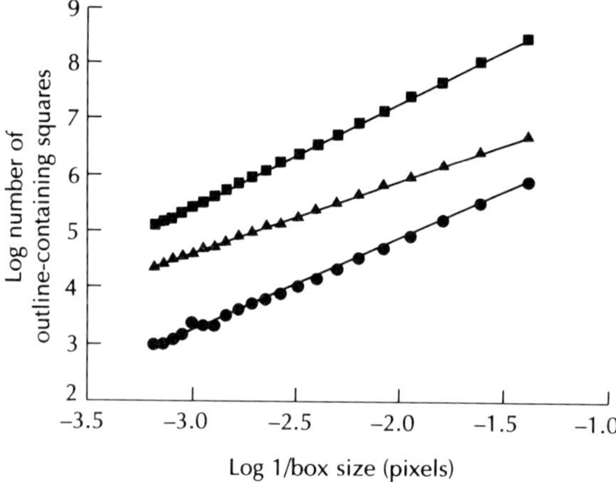

Fig. 15.3 Log–log graph of 1/box size (pixels) plotted against the number of outline-containing squares showing single examples of three different colorectal polyps. Each plot produces a set of points which lie very close to a straight line and the gradient of these lines (which is taken to be D_B) varies for different polyp types. In these examples the gradient of the line for the inflammatory polyp (▲) is less than the other two polyps.

The box-counting method is the method of choice for line boundaries but for whole-image grey-scale values, the fractal texture or area is more appropriate [10] and is given by:

$$A(\varepsilon) = \lambda\varepsilon^{2-D_a}$$

where $A(\varepsilon)$ is the area of the surface measured with a square of side length ε, λ is a scaling factor and D_a is the fractal dimension, or texture, of the surface. In microcomputer implementations [11] an algorithm for calculating this takes each point of a digitized image and imagines a pillar with a height corresponding to its grey-scale value. The differences between the height of adjacent pixels is measured and the overall area or fractal texture is calculated, as expressed by:

$$A(\varepsilon) = \sum_{x,y}\varepsilon^2 + \sum_{x,y}\varepsilon\{abs[I(x,y) - I(x+1,y)] + abs[I(x,y) - I(x,y+1)]\}$$

where $I(x,y)$ is the height of a column found for a particular value of ε by averaging the values stored in adjacent pixels to produce blocks with a side length of ε. The fractal dimension of the surface is determined by plotting a graph of log $[A(\varepsilon)]$ versus log $1/\varepsilon$ and measuring the gradient.

15.3 APPLICATIONS IN CLINICAL PATHOLOGY

15.3.1 Trabecular bone

The first step in the application of fractal geometry to microscopic images must be to establish whether the examined object has a fractal structure over the range of magnifications under consideration. Subjective examination can suggest fractal properties by the identification of self-similarity and retention of boundary complexity at higher magnifications but this must be proved empirically by measurement of the fractal dimension to show that it is greater than the topological dimension. The interconnected struts of trabecular bone might give a subjective impression of fractal properties but the trabeculae have a smooth surface on light microscopic examination and the measured fractal dimension is 1 [12], so equaling the topological dimension. Such negative findings are important since they show that integer-dimensional geometric measurements can continue to be made on such structures, as they are in the assessment of metabolic bone disease (see Chapter 4).

15.3.2 Exfoliative cervical cytology

The subjective assessment of the pattern of nuclear chromatin is an integral part of the assessment of clinical pathological specimens and the fractal texture dimension may provide an objective measure of this. MacAulay and Palcic [13] have used a fractal texture method to analyse the nuclear chromatin pattern of Feulgen-stained normal and dysplastic cervical epithelial cells. Their results on 31 subjects showed that the values for fractal texture were less discriminating than nuclear area or the integrated optical density of the nucleus. This suggests that the amount of nuclear DNA is more important than its distribution, but the numbers in this study are relatively small and further investigations are needed.

15.3.3 Ophthalmic pathology

The retinal arterial system is finely branching with self-similar units and is well-characterized by fractal analysis [14]. Whilst this area is the province of ophthalmologists, similar methodologies could be used when quantitating blood vessels in studies of tumour angiogenesis. The irregular shape of corneal ulcers in herpes simplex keratitis has also been analysed by fractal methods [15].

15.3.4 Neuropathology

The fractal dimension has found extensive use in the quantitation of neurite branching and outgrowth, but most of this work has been in experimental situations [16,17]. Such studies are illustrated by that of Wingate *et al.* [18] who have characterized the dendritic morphology of retinal ganglion cells in the ferret. Retinal ganglion cells were identified by the retrograde transport of microspheres and then injected with lucifer yellow to visualize the dendrites. The images were digitized on to a 256 × 256 pixel array and the fractal dimension was calculated by a pixel dilation protocol. The investigators found that α cells had a mean fractal dimension of 1.455 and this dimension was significantly different from the values for β and γ cells. Tomas *et al.* [19] have examined many different morphometric parameters, including a fractal dimension, in attempts to quantitate the pattern of arborization of the motor nerve terminals in fast and slow mammalian muscles. The soleus and extensor digitorum longus muscles of rats were stained using the Bielschowsky–Gros silver method to visualize intramuscular axons and endings. Camera lucida drawings were made of the nerve terminal arborizations and the fractal dimension was measured after digitization in an automatic image analysis system. This process of tracing does pose the risk of losing some image detail with artefactual reduction in the fractal dimension. Tomas *et al.* [19] found that the fractal dimension was 1.54 (range 1.40–1.65) for slow-twitch muscle (soleus) and 1.55 (range 1.41–1.77) for fast-twitch muscle (extensor digitorum longus). Despite the very similar figures for the two types of muscle they did calculate a statistically significant difference ($P = 0.008$) but there were large numbers of samples in each group (489 and 492).

15.3.5 Renal arterial tree

The finely branching structure of the arterial vasculature is difficult to describe using measurements such as area or length of vessels but can be quantitated by fractal geometry. Cross *et al.* [8] measured the fractal dimension of postmortem renal angiograms using a box-counting method. In 36 satisfactory angiograms the mean fractal dimension was 1.61, which was significantly greater than the topological dimension (1), indicating that the renal arterial tree does have a fractal structure over the examined range of magnification. There was no significant relationship between age, sex, systolic or diastolic blood pressure but two congenitally abnormal kidneys (hypoplastic dysplasia and renal artery stenosis) had fractal dimensions on the third centile of the normal range. These results suggest that the overall structure of the renal arterial tree is little changed by disease after its initial development. The mean fractal dimension (1.61) was similar to that obtained for the retinal arterial tree [14] and is close to that of model trees produced by the process of diffusion-limited aggregation [20], a process which can be translated into a biological frame of reference with gradients of growth factors and migration of embryonic cells. The images in this study were projections of a three-dimensional structure on to the two-dimensional plane of the radiograph film but fractal objects retain the fractal component of their dimensions when undergoing such projections [21] – another advantage of fractal geometric analysis.

15.3.6 Colorectal polyps

The fractal dimension has been examined as a morphometric discriminant between different diagnostic groups [22]. The fractal dimension of 368 colorectal polyps was measured using a box-counting method. In all polyps, the measured fractal dimension exceeded the topological dimension, indicating that they had a fractal structure over the examined range of magnification. There were significant differences in the fractal dimensions between adenomatous, metaplastic and inflammatory polyps and if fractal dimension and polyp size were used to assign polyps to the diagnostic group then there was an acceptable degree of accuracy (κ statistic = 0.60). This is one of the first studies that confirms the practical use of the fractal dimension in quantitative clinical pathology.

15.4 CONCLUSION

Fractal geometry has yet to be widely applied in quantitative clinical pathology but there are strong theoretical reasons for using fractal dimensionality as an integral part of many morphometric studies [23]. There are many areas where this should prove fruitful, including the characterization of tumour boundaries [24–28], tumour angiogenesis, dispersal of cells in fine-needle aspirates [29] and the grey-scale texture of pathological images.

References

1 Mandelbrot BB. *The Fractal Geometry of Nature*. New York: WH Freeman, 1981.

2 Gulick G. Fractals. In: Gulick D (ed.) *Encounters with Chaos*. New York: McGraw-Hill, 1992: 188–239.

3 Peitgen H, Richter PH. *The Beauty of Fractals: Images of Complex Dynamical Systems*. Berlin: Springer-Verlag, 1986.

4 Froyland J. Fractals. In: Froyland J (ed.) *Introduction to Chaos and Coherence*. Bristol: Institute of Physics Publishing, 1992: 3–8.

5 Avnir D, Farin D. Molecular fractal surfaces. *Nature* 1984; 308: 261–263.

6 Peitgen H, Jurgens H, Saupe D. Length, area and dimension: measuring complexity and scaling properties. In: Peitgen H, Jurgens H, Saupe D (eds) *Chaos and Fractals: New Frontiers of Science*. New York: Springer-Verlag, 1992: 183–228.

7 Peitgen H, Jurgens H, Saupe D. Length, area and dimension: measuring complexity and scaling properties. In: Peitgen H, Jurgens H, Saupe D (eds) *Fractals for the Classroom: Part 1 – Introduction to Fractals and Chaos*. New York: Springer-Verlag, 1992: 209–254.

8 Cross SS, Start RD, Silcocks PB, Bull AD, Cotton DWK, Underwood JCE. Quantitation of the renal arterial tree by fractal analysis. *J Pathol* 1993; 170: 479–484.

9 Sanders H, Crocker J. A simple technique for the measurement of fractal dimensions in histopathological specimens. *J Pathol* 1993; 169: 383–385.

10 Bartlett ML. Comparison of methods for measuring fractal dimension. *Australas Phys Eng Sci Med* 1991; 14: 146–152.

11 Ruttimann UE, Webber RL, Hazelrig JB. Fractal dimension from radiographs of peridontal alveolar bone. A possible diagnostic indicator of osteoporosis. *Oral Surg Oral Med Oral Pathol* 1992; 74: 98–110.

12 Cross SS, Rogers S, Silcocks PB, Cotton DWK. Trabecular bone does not have a fractal structure on light microscopic examination. *J Pathol* 1993; 170: 311–313.

13 MacAulay C, Palcic B. Fractal texture features based on optical density surface area. Use in image analysis of cervical cells. *Anal Quant Cytol Histol* 1990; 12: 394–398.

14 Landini G, Misson GP, Murray PI. Fractal analysis of the normal human retinal fluorescein angiogram. *Curr Eye Res* 1993; 12: 23–27.

15 Landini G, Mission GP, Murray PI. Fractal properties of herpes simplex dendritic keratitis. *Cornea* 1992; 11: 510–514.

16 Caserta F, Hausman RE, Eldred WD, Kimmel C, Stanley HE. Effect of viscosity on neurite outgrowth and fractal dimension. *Neurosci Lett* 1992; 136: 198–202.

17 Neale EA, Bowers LM, Smith TG Jr. Early dendrite development in spinal cord cell cultures: a quantitative study. *J Neurosci Res* 1993; 34: 54–66.

18 Wingate RJ, Fitzgibbon T, Thompson ID. Lucifer yellow, retrograde tracers, and fractal analysis characterise adult ferret retinal ganglion cells. *J Comp Neurol* 1992; 323: 449–474.

19 Tomas J, Santafe M, Fenoll R *et al.* Pattern of arborization of the motor nerve terminals in the fast and slow mammalian muscles. *Biol Cell* 1992; 74: 299–305.

20 Meakin P. A new model for biological pattern formation. *J Theor Biol* 1986; 118: 101–113.

21 Falconer K. *Fractal Geometry: Mathematical Foundations and Applications*. Chicester: John Wiley, Chicester: 1990.

22 Cross SS, Bury JP, Silcocks PB, Stephenson TJ, Cotton DWK, Underwood JCE. Fractal and Euclidean geometric analysis of colorectal polyps. *J Pathol* 1993; 170: 359A.

23 Cross SS, Cotton DW. The fractal dimension may be a useful morphometric discriminant in histopathology. *J Pathol* 1992; 166: 409–411.

24 Claridge E, Hall PN, Keefe M, Allen JP. Shape analysis for classification of malignant melanoma. *J Biomed Eng* 1992; 14: 229–234.

25 Cross SS, McDonagh AJ, Cotton DWK. The fractal dimension of the boundary of pigmented skin lesions. *J Pathol* 1992; 168: 116A.

26 Cross SS, Scholfield JH, Kennedy A, Cotton DWK. Measuring the fractal dimension of tumour borders. *J Pathol* 1992; 168: 117A.

27 Cross SS, Scholfield JH, Kennedy A, Stephenson TJ, Cotton DWK, Underwood JCE. Measuring the fractal dimension of tumour boundaries: implementation on an image analysis system using colour separation techniques. *J Pathol* 1993; 170: 379A.
28 Lumb PD, Cross SS, Stephenson TJ. Comparison of the Euclidean and fractal geometric properties of breast carcinomas in histological sections. *J Pathol* 1993; 169: 170A.
29 Lumb PD, Stephenson TJ, Cross SS. Fractal texture analysis of breast cytology. *J Pathol* 1993; 170: 383A.

PART 4
STUDY DESIGN AND STATISTICAL CONSIDERATIONS

16

DESIGNING A MORPHOMETRIC STUDY

P. W. HAMILTON

It is important at the outset of a morphometric study to give consideration to its design and pay particular attention to those factors which may introduce bias, variation or inaccuracies in the data. These factors need to be removed or, if that cannot be done, their effect on the data should be recorded and taken into account in any conclusions that are made. The major factors that need to be investigated are: (i) tissue processing; (ii) sample selection; and (iii) sample size.

In order properly to examine these factors, a *pilot study* on the tissue in question is vital and this is discussed in Section 16.4.4.

16.1 TISSUE PROCESSING

If morphometry is to be accepted as a common diagnostic tool in different centres, standardization of technique is vital [1–3]. In prospective morphometric studies, all the tissue under examination should be processed in an identical manner, thus excluding any variation which may be introduced by tissue handling, fixation, embedding and storage. Many morphometric studies in pathology, however, are based on archival, stored tissue. Here, control over standardized processing techniques is lost. This represents a potential source of variation, the effects of which are unknown, and under these conditions one must rely on the consistency of laboratory practice for uniformity in tissue processing. Before pursuing retrospective studies, therefore, it is worthwhile discovering the history of tissue-processing techniques within the laboratory. This will determine if any major changes have occurred which may affect the set of cases under examination.

16.1.1 Fixation and embedding

Formaldehyde fixation has been shown to cause swelling of tissues while dehydration and paraffin embedding causes the tissue to shrink [4,5]. In cervical tissue, shrinkage can reduce the original dimensions by as much as 15% [6]. Morphometric examination of nuclear area, however, has shown little variation between tissue treated using different fixatives [3], although the pH of the fixative is vital [7]: a pH of 7 should be maintained with a lower pH resulting in reduced nuclear area. While delay in fixation is not likely to affect nuclear measurements in large specimens, it may result in reduced nuclear area in small tissue samples, e.g., biopsies, due to rapid dehydration [7]. Prompt fixation of tissue should be maintained and this can be critical in studies quantifying cell proliferation markers, e.g., mitoses. The effects of fixation shrinkage on larger tissue components (e.g., stromal or epithelial area) have yet to be studied in detail. In cytology, air drying and wet fixation have very different effects on nuclear size [8].

16.1.2 Section thickness

Many histopathological investigations have examined nuclear morphometry in tissue sections. This introduces a problem in that by sectioning, some nuclei will be sliced above or below their point of maximum girth (i.e., 'capped'), so that only a

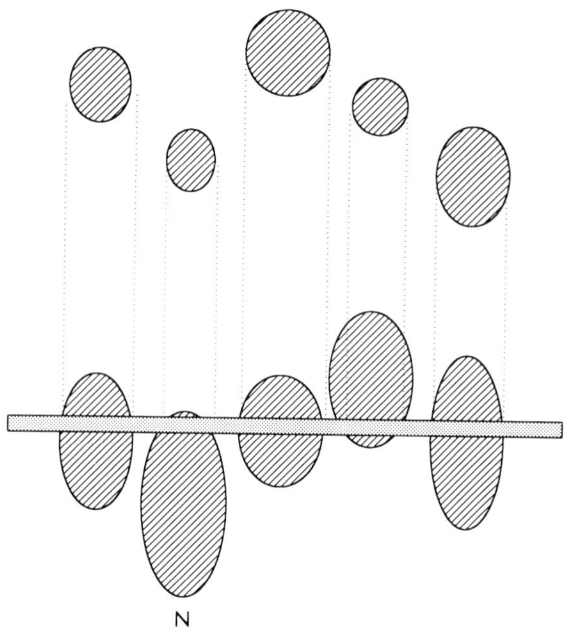

Fig. 16.1 'Capped' nuclei as a result of sectioning. It can be seen that the nucleus (N) has not been sectioned at the point of maximum girth, providing a smaller profile on tissue section.

reduced profile will be evident in the section (Fig. 16.1). This is called the Holmes effect [9]. Therefore, measurements of mean nuclear size (area, perimeter, maximum diameter, etc.) will be smaller than the actual mean value. This problem tends to increase as the section thickness decreases. Increasing the section thickness may reduce the proportion of capped nuclei but increased nuclear overlap will diminish the ability accurately to define nuclear boundaries. Various correction factors can be applied to overcome the Holmes effect [9,10]. Generally, however, it is accepted as a consistent bias which is present in all work and does not negate the relevance of nuclear morphometry, provided section thickness is kept as constant as possible. Standard 5–7 μm sections have been found acceptable for many studies.

Problems of sectioning are not encountered in cytological preparations of whole cells/nuclei. However, tissue morphology is lost and the nuclear shape and size of free nuclei in cytology will vary from those seen *in situ* on tissue section.

16.2 SAMPLE SELECTION

Samples may constitute patients, biopsies, tissue sections, microscopic fields, cells, points (in stereology), etc. In order to exclude bias from results, it is important that samples are randomly selected at each sampling level of the study. This can be easily carried out at the higher levels of sampling but becomes more difficult in the selection of microscopic fields or objects for examination and measurement.

If the aim of the study is to measure features from specific focal pathognomonic areas of the sample (e.g., foci of dysplasia) then these fields must be selected by the observer. Unfortunately, such selection is often based on subjective criteria. In studies which it is necessary to select specific areas for measurement and, if this must be done, strict criteria should be defined as to how these areas are to be chosen, or better, a quantitative definition should be used.

When the tissue to be sampled is relatively homogeneous, a random method of field selection is necessary. The basis of random sampling is that each field has an equal probability of being selected for measurement. This may be attempted by randomly moving the microscopic stage and measuring the features within the field of view. This method has two limitations: (i) it may result in the unconscious yet biased selection of specific fields, e.g., those containing larger nuclei [11]; and (ii) by totally random movement, the same field may be measured twice, therefore reducing the number of original samples (Fig. 16.2). A more appropriate method is found by *stratified random sampling* (Fig. 16.2). By superimposing a series of parallel lines over the specimen and chosing a specified number of random fields along each of the lines, bias can be removed [11], duplicate fields can be avoided and the whole specimen can be adequately sampled.

A similar random approach is required in selecting objects (e.g., nuclei) within a field. If the numbers are small then all objects within the field can be measured (see Chapter 1 for the appropriate method). Alternatively, methods such as measuring the first 10 encountered nuclei moving from the top of the field down can be used. Use of graticule lines

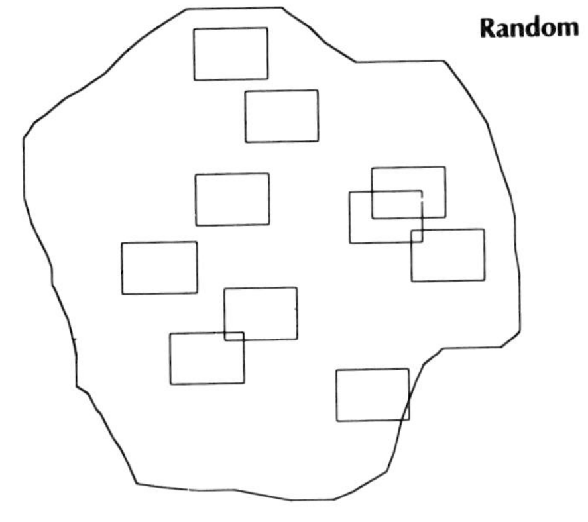

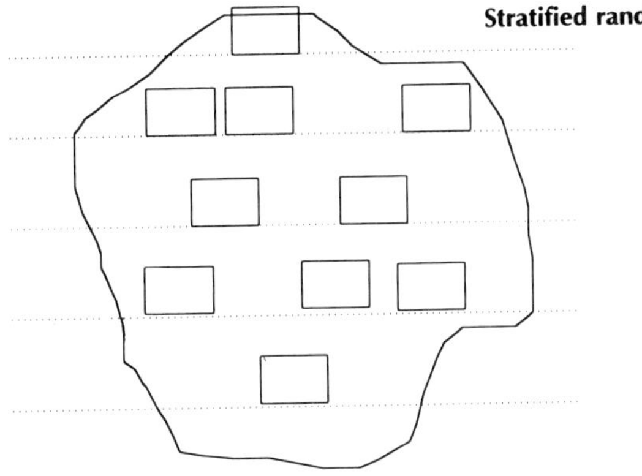

Fig. 16.2 Random and stratified random sampling methods.

for the selection of nuclei has been employed but may give slightly biased results as larger nuclei have a greater chance of touching the lines. All things considered, it is important to ensure that the same sampling procedure is applied to all specimens in the study.

16.3 SAMPLE SIZE

The variation seen in object shape, size and number dictates the size of sample required to obtain a defined level of precision (see Chapter 17). If too few samples are taken for measurement then results may be imprecise. At the other extreme, examining too many samples will be expensive in terms of time and resources and may not improve the precision of results. It is generally found that increasing the number of samples at the higher levels of sampling (e.g., patients) is better than increasing numbers at the lower levels (e.g., nuclei). It is important to determine how many samples are required for a particular study and various methods for determining this are given in Chapter 17.

A useful method for determining the efficiency of sample selection procedures and sample size is by assessing the reproducibility of results. As with any quantitative statement, it is important to show that the results obtained by morphometric measurement can be reproduced by the same person, by different persons and ultimately by different laboratories with different equipment. While one of the proposed advantages of morphometry over conventional visual assessment is that it gives repeatable results, many workers fail to test this assumption. Reproducibility tests should be carried out as part of the pilot study.

16.4 PLANNING A MORPHOMETRIC STUDY

16.4.1 Defining the problem

The first step in a morphometric study is to define the problem. Generally, projects can be divided into those examining: (i) diagnosis; (ii) prognosis; and (iii) biological function or a combination of these, and how morphometry may be used to investigate these factors. Aims should be well-defined prior to analysis and, as with any scientific study, a hypothesis should be devised. The morphometric features to be measured should be defined at an early stage.

16.4.2 Prospective or retrospective?

The next question is whether the study is going to be carried out on retrospective stored histological tissue or on prospectively collected material. Retrospective studies usually provide a wealth of material for analysis but tissue processing has not been standardized. If cases of a specific diagnosis are being examined it is best to have them reviewed by a single pathologist rather than rely on the original diagnoses from a myriad of individuals.

In prospective studies, collection, handling, fixation, embedding, sectioning and staining of tissue samples should be standardized. If possible, a single laboratory technician should be recruited who is familiar with your requirements and will process the tissue with a degree of consistency.

16.4.3 Method of measurement

It must be decided how the measurements are to be made. If stereology is to be used then appropriate grids should be chosen. These may be purchased as eyepiece graticules for direct microscopic assessment, or can be drawn or photocopied on to acetate sheets for overlaying on photographs. In some prospective stereological applications the organ volume needs to be determined before sectioning. This requires consideration at an early stage! Computerized morphometry generally gives higher accuracy measurements at the lower levels of sampling (e.g., nuclei). This may be of little benefit to your study, in which case stereological methods might provide faster and cheaper results. If interactive computerized image analysis is used, check the accuracy of the equipment with profiles and lengths of known dimensions. The use of automated image analysis in the analysis of complex histological images is often investigated as a more rapid means of measurement for previously established morphometric findings (often using interactive systems). Automation, particularly in histopathology, can be problematic and generally requires more sophisticated software.

Regardless of the measuring technique it is important to become fully familiar and well-practised with the methods prior to any study. Several weeks of experience may be required to reach the plateau of the learning curve. It is sometimes useful for specific microscopic fields to be selected by the pathologist and the images digitally stored. These images form a consistent record of the areas of pathognomic interest which can be measured later either by the pathologist or by a trained technician. Once the images are stored, they can be measured using interactive methods or alternatively segmentation algorithms can be designed for automated measurement.

16.4.4 The pilot study

It is essential in the design of any morphometric study to include a pilot investigative study prior to the main study. The pilot study should be carried out on a subset of the available cases and is primarily designed to provide information on the factors discussed in Sections 16.1–16.3, i.e., tissue processing, sampling, sample numbers. As part of the pilot study it is important that the reproducibility of results is determined. A set of cases should be remeasured by the same individual to assess intraobserver variation and by a different person to assess interobserver variation in results. This will also help determine the efficiency of your sampling regime.

16.4.5 The main study

In the main study it is important that all measurements are made by one individual to avoid the effects of interobserver variation. Care should be made in the collection and cataloguing of results. At an early stage, advice should be sought on the study design and statistical analysis of the data. If a specific statistical software package is to be used (see Section 17.7), one must ensure that data can be easily converted from the format used by the image analysis system to the file format used by the statistical package.

16.5 CONCLUSION

Study design is essential to any scientific experiment. It studies carried out on histopathological tissues attention needs to be paid to tissue fixation, embedding and section thickness. These problems are less important in cytological preparations but histological context is often lost. The sampling protocol is important and should be random. However, in some applications, measurements need to be made from selected areas. A pilot study is often a useful approach to determining sampling methods, sample size and reproducibility and statistical advice should be sought at an early stage. These considerations should not discourage individuals from pursuing morphometric studies but should advocate the collection of reliable and meaningful quantitative data.

References

1 Loud AV, Anversa P. Morphometric analysis of biological processes. *Lab Invest* 1984; 50: 250–261.

2 Smeulders AWM, Dorst L. Measurement issues in morphometry. *Anal Quant Cytol Histol* 1985; 7: 242–249.

3 Collan Y, Torkkeli T, Pesonen E, Jantunen E, Kosma V-M. Application of morphometry in tumour pathology. *Anal Quant Cytol Histol* 1987; 9: 79–88.

4 Bahr GF, Bloom G, Friberg U. Volume changes of tissues in physiological fluids during fixation in osmium tetroxide or formaldehyde and during subsequent treatment. *Exp Cell Res* 1957; 12: 342–335.

5 Pentilla A, McDowell EM, Trump BF. Effects of fixation and postfixation treatments on the volume of injured cells. *J Histochem Cytochem* 1975; 23: 251–270.

6 Boonstra H, Ossterhuis JW, Oosterhuis AM, Fleuren GJ. Cervical tissue shrinkage by formaldehyde fixation, paraffin wax embedding, section cutting and mounting. *Virchows Arch [A]* 1983; 402: 195–201.

7 Baak JPA, Noteboom E. Koevoets JJM. The influence of fixatives and other variations in tissue processing on nuclear morphometric features. *Anal Quant Cytol Histol* 1989; 11: 219–224.

8 Beyer-Boon ME, van der Voorn-Den Hollander MJA, Arentz PW, Cornellisse CJ, Schaberg A, Fox CH. Effect of various routine cytopreparatory techniques on normal urothelial cells and their nuclei. *Acta Pathol Microbiol Scand [A]* 1979; 87: 63–69.

9 Beck JS, Anderson JM. Quantitative methods as an aid to diagnosis in histopathology. In: Anthony PP, MacSween RNM (eds) *Recent Advances in Histopathology*, vol. 13. Edinburgh: Churchill Livingstone, 1987: 255–269.

10 Stephenson TJ. Quantitation of the nucleus. In: Underwood JC (ed) *Current Topics in Pathology: Pathology of the Nucleus*. Berlin: Springer-Verlag, 1990: 151–213.

11 van Diest PJ, Smeulders AWM, Thunnissen FBJM, Baak JPA. Cytomorphometry: a methodological study on preparation techniques, selection methods and sample size. *Anal Quant Cytol Histol* 1989; 11: 225–231.

17

STATISTICAL ANALYSIS OF MORPHOMETRIC AND CLINICAL DATA

C. C. PATTERSON

17.1 INTRODUCTION

17.1.1 The need for statistical analysis of morphometric data

The role that quantitative methods have to play in maximizing the objectivity and reproducibility of pathologists' assessments of morphology has already been advanced throughout in this book. If this role is accepted, the argument for the need to submit data obtained in quantitative morphometric studies to statistical scrutiny hardly needs elaboration. Appropriate statistical methodology contributes both objectivity and reproducibility to the interpretation of results.

17.1.2 Aims of the chapter

Experience indicates that the use of statistics in the medical literature has not been without problem. The selection of inappropriate statistical techniques and the incorrect interpretation of statistical analyses are commonplace [1]. The primary aim of this chapter is, therefore, to help those involved in quantitative pathology to employ statistical methodology in an appropriate way.

Space does not permit a detailed description of the numerous statistical methods available. Fortunately, most of these methods have already been described in a non-theoretical fashion either in articles published in medical journals or in widely available textbooks on statistics. This chapter includes many such references.

17.1.3 Outline of the chapter

Section 17.2 provides some background and introduces statistical terminology used later in the chapter. Section 17.3 discusses some important statistical issues that must be considered at the planning stage of an investigation, addressing among other things how large a study should be. Section 17.4 deals with some of the simpler, more commonly used statistical methods, the majority of which are described in any introductory statistical textbook.

The remaining sections deal with some of the more specialized statistical methods that are of particular relevance to clinical morphometric studies. Section 17.5 considers *principal components analysis* which is used in an attempt to reduce the number of variables under consideration in a morphometric study. Also considered are methods for classification, concentrating particularly on the techniques of *discriminant analysis* (where classes are decided in advance) and *cluster analysis* (in which there is no imposition of preconceived classes). Section 17.6 discusses some methods for *survival analysis* which may be used to identify morphometric variables that are indicative of patient prognosis.

Finally, Section 17.7 discusses the use of statistical software packages which are capable of performing the various analyses considered in the chapter.

17.2 BACKGROUND AND TERMINOLOGY

17.2.1 Scales of measurement

Any qualitative or quantitative assessment in pathology belongs to one of four scales of measurement: nominal, ordinal, interval or ratio.

The lowest scale of measurement is *nominal* scale. This is the scale of measurement for categorical variables. Any assignment of numbers to the categories of such a variable is arbitrary. Examples are the cell type of a tumour of the bronchus (squamous cell, oat cell, adenocarcinoma, etc.) or the site of a carcinoma of the large bowel (ascending colon, transverse colon, descending colon).

In the *ordinal* scale of measurement, the assignment of numbers to categories is again arbitrary, but does impose an ordering on the categories. Examples are the degree of differentiation in a specimen (well, moderate, poor) or the level of experience of the surgeon performing a biopsy (novice, intermediate, expert).

For statistical purposes it is seldom necessary to distinguish between the remaining two scales of measurement. Both *interval* and *ratio* scales require an underlying metric of measurement, so that differences and averages may be validly calculated. Many variables in quantitative pathology (e.g., cell area, maximum cell diameter) belong to one of these two scales of measurement. A ratio scale measurement must also have a true zero as its origin, so permitting the calculation of ratios.

A fuller explanation of these scales of measurement, their formal properties and the operations that are admissible on each scale is given by Siegel and Castellan [2]. Smeulders and Dorst [3] discuss scales of measurement, together with some other measurement issues in a morphometric context.

As will be explained in Section 17.3, the scale of measurement is an important consideration in selecting appropriate techniques for statistical analysis.

17.2.2 Statistical inference

Statistical techniques generally require the assumption that groups under study may be considered to be *random samples* from the populations about which inferences are to be made. The potential for biased conclusions resulting from not using random samples (as is often the case in practice) must be carefully assessed by the investigator. Statistical methods only take account of *sampling error* (i.e., variation arising from the process of random sampling); they cannot quantify the extent of biases attributable to non-random sampling. The investigator must be cautious about extrapolating findings beyond the population from which the sample was drawn.

A proper understanding of *significance tests* is vital for the successful application of statistical methods in clinical research. Any significance test is a decision-making process. Formally a test begins with the supposition that a *null hypothesis* is true. Typically, this might state that two samples are drawn from populations with the same mean, or alternatively that any difference between two sample means may reasonably be ascribed to sampling error. An *alternative hypothesis* is also necessary, although it is often simply a negation of the null hypothesis. The test of significance is a method for deciding between the following two courses of action: (i) reject the null hypothesis in favour of the alternative; or (ii) continue to accept the null hypothesis in the absence of sufficient evidence to reject it.

Under the assumption that the null hypothesis is true, the probability, P, of encountering (in repetitions of the study) as large a difference in sample means as that observed is obtained. Modern computer software will usually supply the value of P directly. If P is small, then a difference between sample means of the magnitude observed will only occur very rarely by chance. Sampling error is therefore an unlikely explanation for the observed difference, and the null hypothesis is rejected (action i). However, if P is large, then the observed difference may very reasonably be ascribed to chance, and there is no evidence to reject the null hypothesis (action ii). Values of P which are considered small depend on the *significance level* (α) chosen for the test. A test at the conventional 5% significance level will therefore result in rejection of the null hypothesis if $P < 0.05$.

Unfortunately errors do occur in this decision-making process. A *type I error* occurs if the null hypothesis is rejected when it is true. By choosing the 5% level of significance, the investigator accepts a one in 20 chance of rejecting the null hypothesis when it is true. On the other hand, a *type II error* occurs if the null hypothesis is accepted when it should have been rejected. The risk of a type II error (β) depends on the choice of the alternative hypothesis. The probability of *not* committing a type II error is called the *power* of the test and is $(1-\beta)$. This concept of power is important in ensuring that a study is of adequate size (see Section 17.3.4).

Although much emphasis has been placed in the medical literature on significance tests, the additional knowledge to be gained from the calculation of *confidence intervals* has been stressed [4–6], and many journals now request contributors to use them when appropriate. In comparison with significance tests, such intervals provide more useful information about the likely magnitude of the true differences between groups. Additionally confidence intervals usually allow a test of significance to be conducted implicitly.

17.2.3 Methods of sampling

Suppose that a sample of patients has provided specimens for study. It is usually not possible to examine the entire specimen from any given patient. Rather than taking a random sample of the specimen, a *hierarchical sampling design* (taking samples within samples) is usually adopted. Sections or blocks selected from the specimen might constitute the first level of the hierarchy. The second level could be zones or areas selected from a given section, and the third level cells selected from a given zone.

Suppose the aim of such a sampling design is to provide an estimate of the mean cell area of a specimen. At each level of the hierarchy it is desirable from the statistical perspective that a *random selection* is made. In choosing sections, such a selection might be made using either tables of random sampling digits or the random number function provided in many calculators. A modification which helps to ensure that all parts of the specimen are represented is a *systematic random selection* in which a random start is taken but samples are then selected at regular intervals throughout the specimen. The random selection of areas from a given section poses a more difficult problem since sampling must take place in two dimensions. Randomly selected x and y co-ordinates may be generated as indicated previously, and these may be used in conjunction with the graduations of the microscope stage to select the centre of an area for further study. The random selection of cells from a given area may be achieved using a similar approach, but this time with the assistance of a graticule (see Section 16.2).

Inevitably the surgeon and pathologist exert some influence on the selection of material for examination. Some researchers advocate that, rather than using random selection, the pathologist should select those portions of the specimen that are most interesting or which show the greatest changes. It is argued that such a *purposive selection* procedure provides more relevant measurements, and avoids the dilution of findings by measurements taken from less interesting portions of the specimen. However, from the statistical viewpoint, such selection introduces subjectivity and can compromise the interpretation of the statistical analysis. In either case it is recommended that a detailed description of the selection process is supplied in the final report.

17.3 CONSIDERATIONS AT THE PLANNING STAGE

17.3.1 Study design

The design should be summarized in a study *protocol* which, among other things, should address the following statistical issues: (i) statement of aims; (ii) specific hypotheses to be tested; (iii) entry and exclusion criteria; (iv) necessary study size; (v) method of sampling; and (vi) approach to the statistical analysis.

When the aims have been clarified, possible ways of acquiring the necessary study material must be considered. There are advantages and disadvantages in using material that is already available. In terms of cost and convenience, such *retrospective* assembly of study material may seem attractive.

However, the *prospective* approach permits a greater degree of control over the selection of patients for study, the collection of associated patient information and the methods of specimen selection, preparation and storage. Irrespective of the approach used for its collection, it is imperative that the study material is adequately characterized in terms of demographic and clinical characteristics.

Often it will be necessary to collect information from a *control* group consisting of patients without the disease under investigation. It may be desirable for this control group to be *matched* to the diseased group on characteristics that are relevant to the morphometric results but which are of no intrinsic interest to the study (e.g., age and sex of the patient). If possible, *pairwise* matching should be attempted in preference to group matching, and it should be noted that this has important implications in the selection of the method for statistical analysis (see Section 17.4).

17.3.2 Assessing measurement error

Measurement error in the interval scale variables encountered in morphometric studies may be considered as consisting of two components: (i) the systematic component (*inaccuracy* or *bias*); and (ii) the random component (*imprecision* or *unreliability*).

Bias typically arises through faulty measurement technique or from the use of incorrectly calibrated instruments. Increasing the number of measurements does nothing to reduce the magnitude of the bias. In certain comparative studies the presence of bias may be tolerable since all measurements will be equally affected, and any comparisons made within the study should therefore be valid. However, measurements will not be comparable with those from other centres; if such comparability is important then techniques and instruments must be validated by conducting calibration studies [7]. There is also the possibility that an operator may introduce systematic error into the measurement process through knowledge of the origin of the specimen. Such bias is best avoided by *blinding* the operator, perhaps by presenting coded specimens in a random order.

In contrast to the systematic component, there is potential to reduce the magnitude of the random component of error by increasing the number of measurements. An important preliminary step for any study in quantitative pathology is therefore to assess the reliability or precision of the measurement process.

Several different statistical methods for assessing precision are in widespread use, and terminology is not standardized. If a series of measurements is repeated then a simple method is available for obtaining the standard deviation, s, and the coefficient of variation for measurement error [8]. The value $2\sqrt{2s^2} = 2.83s$ has the advantage of a more direct interpretation than does s. Assuming measurement error is normally distributed, the difference between a pair of measurements will exceed this value in only 5% of occasions. It has been proposed [9] that this value be called the *repeatability*. The use of the correlation coefficient in these circumstances is not recommended; its value reflects not only the magnitude of s, but also the degree of scatter in the true values of the measurements.

If measurements are taken three or more times, the necessary calculations are more complex and are best handled using analysis of variance [10]. *Components of variance* may be derived; the measurement-to-measurement component assumes the role of s in the previous paragraph. Alternatively an *intraclass correlation coefficient* may be calculated, representing the proportion of the total variation in the results not attributable to measurement error; coefficients close to unity therefore indicate high measurement reliability.

Note that if the measurements are repeated by a different observer or using a different method, then *interobserver error* (bias between the observers) or *method comparison* may be of primary interest. A rather different approach to statistical analysis is then appropriate [11].

Subjective clinical grading, the type of measurement more traditionally used by pathologists, typically gives rise to nominal or ordinal-scale data. Such measurements can be assessed for reliability and interobserver error using a κ *statistic* [12] or a *weighted* κ *statistic* [13]. Such statistics provide measures of agreement on a scale from 0 to 1 which have been corrected for the amount of agreement expected to occur simply by chance.

Although some authors have suggested ranges of κ representing fair, moderate and almost perfect agreement [14,15], the values obtained are probably best judged in the context of previous work in the same field.

17.3.3 Assessing variability in the study material

It is important to appreciate that there are many potential sources of variability in the material assembled for morphometric analysis. Foremost among these will usually be patient-to-patient variability, but there may also be considerable variation between specimens from a given patient, and even between portions of the same specimen. Any changes attributable to the disease process will generally have to be assessed against this masking *biological variation.*

It is useful to quantify the contributions to variability from these different sources in a pilot investigation. A typical example might involve the measurement of cell area in specimens from patients with colonic carcinoma. Such an investigation can provide answers to questions such as the following.

1 How many blocks of a specimen should be examined?

2 How many zones should be studied from each block?

3 How many cells should be measured in each zone?

Specimens of tissue from a number of representative patients are obtained, and n blocks taken at random from each specimen for microscopic examination. From each block a fixed number, m, of zones is selected, and in each zone the areas of k cells measured. The resulting data permit an analysis of variance to be performed, and the following *components of variance* estimates to be derived:

1 s_p^2 = patient-to-patient variation;

2 s_b^2 = block-to-block variation within a patient;

3 s_z^2 = zone-to-zone variation within a block;

4 s_c^2 = cell-to-cell variation within a zone.

An estimate of the standard error of the mean area, $SE(\bar{x})$, calculated for any given patient may then be obtained as:

$$SE(\bar{x}) = \sqrt{\frac{s_b^2}{n} + \frac{s_z^2}{nm} + \frac{s_c^2}{nmk}}$$

If costs can be assigned (for example, in min) to counting an extra cell (C_c), to considering another zone (C_z) and to examining a further block (C_b), then the total cost, C, per patient may be expressed as:

$$C = nC_b + nmC_z + nmkC_c$$

The values of k, m and n which minimize the standard error for a given overall cost per patient may be found. Assuming resources are constrained to C_{max} min per patient, a simple spreadsheet program could be used to establish quickly by trial and error which protocol provides most precision (i.e., minimizes the standard error) for any given cost constraint. For example, the protocol might specify the examination of three zones from each of two blocks and allow time for the examination of 15 cells per zone. Further details of the computations involved are given by Shay [16].

It is often found that concentration of effort in the lowest level of the hierarchy (e.g., counting a large number of cells per zone) is not cost-effective, and that the time available would be better spent studying specimens from a larger number of patients or examining a greater number of sections per specimen. Dunnill discusses these and other aspects of sampling in morphometry [17].

17.3.4 Size of the investigation

The importance of ensuring a proposed study is of adequate size cannot be overemphasized. If a study is too small its findings may be inconclusive (or, worse still, misleading), while too large a study is wasteful of resources. Although useful information about the adequacy of study size may be obtained at the analysis stage through consideration of the width of confidence intervals, this does not obviate the need for a proper assessment of study size at the planning stage.

The unit for the final statistical analysis in most studies will be the patient, so this section addresses the issue of the number of patients required in an investigation. The primary aim of most studies is the comparison of two groups, although the methods to be described can be extended to the comparison of three or more groups [18,19].

Techniques are available both for outcome variables that are interval scale, and so typically summarized for a group of patients using the mean, and for outcomes that are binary, nominal scale (yes or no, present or absent) and so typically summarized using a proportion. In the former case information is required about the magnitude of patient-to-patient variability (e.g., SE($\bar{x}$) in Section 17.3.3), while in the latter a crude estimate of the magnitude of the proportion is necessary. Such information may be obtained either from a pilot study or from previous work in the same field. The numbers required for a study to have a high power (e.g., 80 or 90%) to detect a clinically worthwhile difference as statistically significant may be estimated by formula [20,21], by tables [22,23] or by nomogram [24].

17.4 SIMPLE STATISTICAL METHODS

17.4.1 Preliminary analysis

The first step in the statistical analysis of quantitative data is pictorial presentation and the calculation of summary statistics. A histogram will indicate whether or not a variable has a frequency distribution that is skewed. If this is the case, the median and interquartile range are more appropriate summary statistics than are the mean and standard deviation. At this stage associations between variables can also be investigated using scatter diagrams and correlation analyses (see Section 17.4.3).

17.4.2 Comparisons between groups

As indicated in Section 17.2.2, the use of confidence intervals in the statistical comparison of groups has much to commend it. A comprehensive account of the calculation and interpretation of confidence intervals for between group comparisons is available [25]. The selection of an appropriate statistical technique for comparing groups depends on the study design, on the scale of measurement of the variable in question, and on whether or not certain assumptions are satisfied. Table 17.1 provides a guide to selection of tests of hypothesis. Descriptions of the methods can be found in standard statistical texts. Lentner provides a very concise presentation [26].

The techniques shown in the first line of Table 17.1 are called *parametric methods*. These methods typically require certain parametric assumptions.

Table 17.1 A guide to selecting the appropriate statistical test for comparisons between groups

Scale of measurement	Two samples		*R* samples ($R > 2$)	
	Independent	Paired	Independent	Matched
Interval scale (parametric assumptions satisfied)	Independent samples *t*-test*	Paired samples *t*-test*	One-way analysis of variance	Randomized block analysis of variance
Ordinal scale *Interval scale* (parametric assumptions not satisfied)	Mann–Whitney U-test *or* Wilcoxon rank-sum test	Wilcoxon signed-rank test	Kruskal–Wallis analysis of variance	Friedman two-way analysis of variance
Nominal scale Two categories	χ^2 test for 2×2 table *or* Fisher's exact probability test	McNemar's test	χ^2 test for $R \times 2$ table	Cochran's *Q* test
C categories ($C > 2$)	χ^2 test for $2 \times C$ table	—	χ^2 test for $R \times C$ table	—

* Or equivalent large-samples z-test.

For example, in addition to the need for the variable to be interval scale, the independent samples *t*-test and one-way analysis of variance require that: (i) the samples should be drawn from populations with a normal (Gaussian) distribution; and (ii) the samples should be drawn from populations with the same variance.

Although statistical methods can help in the assessment of whether or not a variable follows the normal distribution, the techniques are not as useful as they might appear. Tests of hypothesis [27,28] are insensitive unless sample sizes are large, and in this situation the normality requirement is often less critical. Normal and half-normal plots provide graphical methods for assessing normality [29,30], but require subjective interpretation. In the two-sample situation the equality of variance assumption is less important since alternative tests are available [20].

A more useful approach may be to find a *transformation* which gives results which more closely satisfy the necessary assumptions. Often the *logarithmic* transformation is used to rectify positive skew, and it also permits a convenient interpretation in terms of multiplicative effects [31]. The *square root* and *arcsin* transformations are also relevant for morphometric data since they will tend to equalize the variance of counts and proportions, respectively [30,31].

If no suitable transformation can be found, then the *non-parametric methods* shown in the second line of Table 17.1 may still be employed [32,33]. These methods are also suitable for the analysis of ordinal-scale variables. When used for interval-scale data, the methods are slightly less efficient (i.e., there is a small sacrifice in power in using a non-parametric method on occasions when a parametric method could have been employed). Also methods for calculating confidence intervals for means are much simpler and more widely known than are the corresponding methods for medians [25]. Parametric methods are therefore recommended when the necessary assumptions can be justified.

For nominal-scale variables, the tests shown in the final line of Table 17.1 may be used. Most of these tests are *contingency table methods*. The calculation of confidence intervals for proportions is also relevant in such instances [25].

The interpretation of analyses involving more than two groups is sometimes complicated by the *multiple comparison* problem. If the aim of the analysis is to test only a small number of hypotheses that were specified in advance and stated in the protocol, then the multiple comparisons are less of an issue. However, for the investigator who is testing hypotheses other than these (e.g., hypotheses formulated after looking at the data), a conservative approach is necessary to limit the risk of occurrence of type I errors. Typically a significant F statistic in a one-way or randomized block analysis of variance leads to the desire to state which groups differ from which other groups. The *Bonferroni criterion* provides a particularly simple technique which is applicable in a wide range of circumstances. It requires that the significance level should be reduced from α to α/k, where k is the number of comparisons which are performed. Other more specialized procedures have been devised to address this problem [18,23,34]. Each procedure permits certain types of comparison to be performed whilst offering different safeguards against type I errors. Corresponding methods are also available for non-parametric techniques [32,33].

17.4.3 Studies of association

A prerequisite for the interpretation of results obtained using multivariate statistical methods is a clear understanding of associations that are present between the variables in the dataset. This section deals with the examination of association between quantitative (interval-scale) variables.

Correlation analysis is appropriate if the relationship is linear, so a vital preliminary step is to plot a scatter diagram. The *correlation coefficient*, r, provides a measure, on a scale from -1 (perfect negative relationship) through 0 (no association) to $+1$ (perfect positive relationship), of the degree of linear relationship. Most computer packages provide a test of whether or not the correlation coefficient differs significantly from zero, and methods are also available for calculating 95% confidence limits [35,36]. The square of r is referred to as the *coefficient of determination*, and may be interpreted as the proportion of variation in either variable which may be explained by the other. *Partial correlation coefficients* are sometimes used to assess the degree of relationship between two variables adjusting for a third variable [29,37].

Often *regression analysis* is more informative than correlation analysis, allowing the estimation of effects and the making of predictions. The *simple regression* model specifies that the following linear relationship exists between a *dependent* (response or outcome) variable, y, and an *independent* (explanatory or predictor) variable, x:

$$y = a + bx$$

where a is the intercept (on the y-axis) and b is the slope, the increase in the y variable associated with unit increase in the x variable.

This basic model may be extended in a number of ways. If the relationship between y and x is non-linear, then *polynomial regression* [38] involves the addition of extra terms to the model representing higher powers of the variable x. Alternatively, new x variables may be added to the basic model to give a *multiple regression* analysis with the following associated model.

$$y = a + b_1x_1 + b_2x_2 + \ldots + b_nx_n$$

Note that x variables may be correlated, even though they are referred to as independent variables. Multiple regression is helpful in distinguishing between two types of x variable, those that are predictive of y independently of other x variables, and those that are associated with y only through relationship with other x variables. Usually an x variable of the first type is of more interest.

Computer algorithms have been developed to assist the user with *variable selection*, the process by which x variables are chosen for inclusion in the final regression model. *Forward selection* options build up the model by successively adding the most significant x variable until none of the remaining variables can make any further significant contribution. In contrast, *backward elimination* begins with all x variables in the model and successively eliminates those variables making least contribution until any further elimination would result in a variable that contributes significantly to the model being removed. *Stepwise* options provide a combination of these two approaches, so that a variable which is initially selected may sometimes be rejected at a later stage. *Best subsets* options offer the user the best-fitting regression equation for any specified number of variables in the model. However, there are many occasions when a fuller understanding will be obtained by taking control of the variable selection process and using combinations of x variables not considered by these automatic approaches.

Certain assumptions are required for the hypothesis tests and confidence limits obtained in correlation and regression analyses to be valid. In regression analysis these are best checked through the graphical examination of *residuals* [29,36]. Such examination may suggest the need for transformations. Although non-parametric measures of association are available [32,33], they are generally rather limited and less informative than their parametric counterparts.

Tests for association between qualitative (nominal-scale) variables may be obtained using the contingency table method already mentioned in Table 17.1, or any one of a number of measures of association may be calculated [32,33].

17.5 MULTIVARIATE METHODS

17.5.1 Principal components analysis

A common problem faced by investigators engaged in quantitative pathological studies is the large number of variables available for analysis, some of which may be highly correlated. A consequence of this is that type I errors are likely to occur if the tests of hypothesis described in the previous section are simply applied to each variable in turn.

One way round this multiple testing problem is to reduce the significance level of each test. The *Bonferroni criterion* can once more be used and dictates that, in the analyses of p variables, each test should be conducted at the α/p level to ensure that the chance of any type I error occurring is kept below the α level. However, this approach can be very conservative.

An alternative is to use multivariate tests of significance, although the results from these techniques are often difficult to interpret. *Hotelling's* T^2 provides a multivariate generalization of the independent samples t-test and *multivariate analysis of variance* is also possible. Bartels [39,40] provides details of the calculations in a morphometric context, although the availability of computer packages makes these details of limited relevance. Applications of these techniques in the clinical literature are rare.

A more practical multivariate solution to this problem of high dimensionality is to attempt to summarize the data using a technique such as *principal components analysis*. The aim is to define a small number of composite variables called *principal components* which may be analysed in place of the original variables. The first component is a weighted combination of the original variables with weights chosen to capture the largest possible percentage of the variation in the data. The second component is constructed so that, subject to being uncorrelated with the first component, it captures the largest possible percentage of the remaining variation in the data. This process continues with the aim of defining a small number of components that describe the majority of the variation in the data. The concept is illustrated in Fig. 17.1 for the simple case of two variables.

For three variables, the principal components have been likened to the axes of an airship whose shape is that of the cloud formed by plotting the observations in three-dimensional space [38]. The principal components define the axes of the airship, the first representing the major axis (the airship's length), the second and third representing the minor axes (the airship's width and height). Should the first two components account for most of the variation (as would be the case if the observations formed a flat saucer-shaped cloud), the position of any observation may be approximated by its values on these two components. Further analysis may then be conducted, without serious loss of information, using only these two components.

Since a change in the scale of measurement of a variable will alter the principal components, it is usually desirable to *standardize* each variable to have zero mean and unit variance before conducting the analysis. This is achieved by subtracting the mean from each observation and dividing by the standard deviation. In this case the weights for any given component indicate the relative contribution of the variables to that component. By examining the magnitudes and signs of the weights, it may be possible to attach an interpretation to each component. For example, in one study of 28 morphometric variables it was found that 75% of the variation was accounted for by just four principal components, each of which could be assigned an interpretation [41].

A point to note is that the results of any principal components analysis inevitably reflect the selection of variables for inclusion in the analysis. For instance, if the variables chosen for analysis are predominantly measures of cell size, then it would not

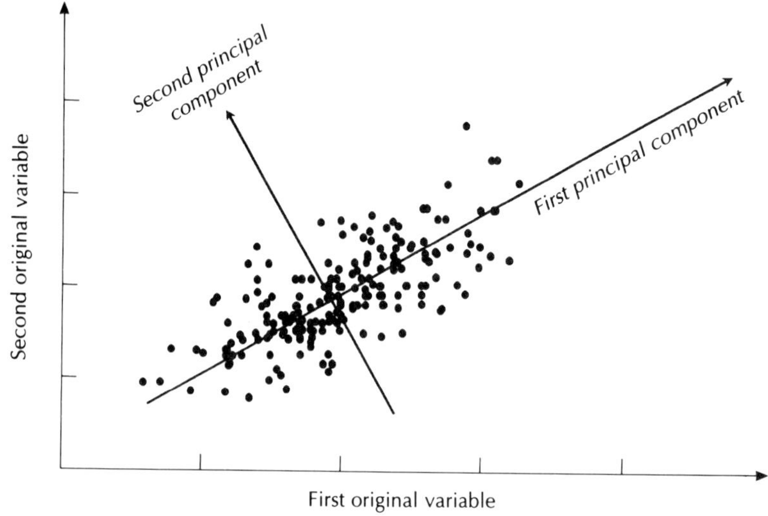

Fig. 17.1 Definition of principal components in a two-dimensional space.

be surprising to find that the interpretation of the first component is as a measure of cell size.

Principal components analysis may be regarded simply as a tool for extracting and summarizing the major components of variation from a set of data. However, any such summary inevitably runs a risk of discarding useful information [42]. Sometimes the principal components may be *rotated* in the hope that the resulting new components will be more easily interpreted. However, the principal components technique should not be confused with the apparently similar method of *factor analysis* which requires a complex model structure with potentially unwarranted assumptions [38,43].

17.5.2 Discriminant function analysis

By far the most commonly used multivariate statistical technique in quantitative clinical pathology is *discriminant function analysis*, which has the potential to provide objective differential diagnoses which mimic those of an expert pathologist. Typically morphometric data are obtained from representative samples of cases which are known to belong to one of two diagnostic groups. Discriminant function analysis then provides an allocation rule which will assign any new case to one or other group.

Suppose that p morphometric variables (x_1, $x_2 \ldots x_p$) are available for each case. One method of derivation specifies that the *linear discriminant function* is that combination of the variables, $z = a_1x_1 + a_2x_1 \ldots a_px_p$ which best discriminates between the groups in the sense that the *coefficients* ($a_1, a_2 \ldots a_p$) are chosen to maximize the ratio of between-group variation in z to within-group variation in z. In addition to providing values for the coefficients, some software packages also provide *standardized coefficients* which help to identify which variables contribute most to the discriminant function.

In general only those variables whose contribution to the discrimination attains statistical significance should be retained in the final discriminant function. The addition of non-significant variables may actually lead to a deterioration in performance when the derived allocation rule is applied to a fresh dataset [44]. Some computer packages provide stepwise selection procedures similar in nature to those for multiple regression. Although very convenient, as noted in Section 17.4.3, these procedures tend to be rather inflexible.

The results of discriminant function analyses are usually summarized using an *allocation* (or *confusion*) *matrix*, a table showing the association between actual and predicted group membership. Sometimes only the overall percentage of successful allocations is quoted, but examination of the success rates within each group is more informative. In simple situations, pictorial presentation of results may be helpful. Figure 17.2 illustrates an

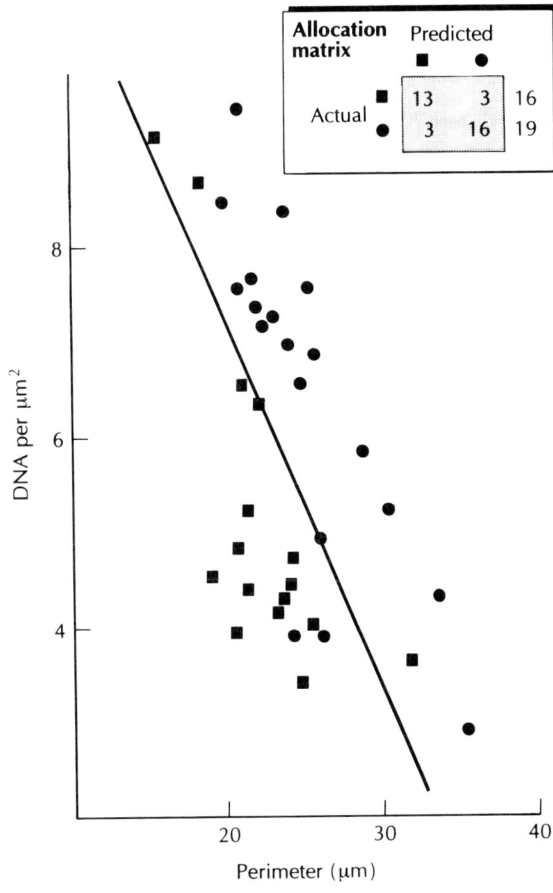

Fig. 17.2 Discriminant function derived from DNA per μm^2 and nuclear perimeter to distinguish between 16 well-differentiated intraductal carcinomas (■) and 19 intraductal carcinomas with atypia (●). From Norris *et al.* [45].

allocation rule based on two variables (nuclear perimeter and DNA content per μm^2) for discriminating between well-differentiated intraductal carcinoma of the breast and intraductal carcinoma with cytological atypia [45].

Unfortunately, the straightforward application of an allocation rule to the dataset from which it was derived (the *training* set) will tend to provide a falsely optimistic impression of the rule's performance. For a fairer assessment, the derived procedure must either be applied to a fresh set of cases (a *test set*) or reapplied to the training set using a cross-validation technique such as the *leaving-one-out* or *jack-knife* method [44]. The method allocates each case in turn by a modified rule derived using only the remaining cases.

Sometimes the relative frequency of a group in the dataset may not reflect its true relative frequency (i.e., the relative frequency likely to be encountered in practical application of the allocation rule). For example, cases in rarer diagnostic groups may have been preferentially selected to ensure that the numbers in each group were sufficiently large. This must be taken into account during the allocation phase of the analysis by specifying *prior probabilities* equal to the true relative frequencies. Most software packages permit the user to set these probabilities.

An alternative theoretical derivation of the discriminant function requires assumptions of multivariate normality and equality of variance–covariance matrices. Unfortunately these assumptions are not easily verified. Dropping the latter assumption leads to a *quadratic discriminant function* [46] which provides a non-linear boundary, in contrast to the linear boundary arising from the usual approach. The method has been illustrated in the two-group, two-variable situation [47], and what has been termed a *Bayesian decision boundary* derived.

In the event of failure of the assumptions, although allocations made by the linear discriminant function may often be reasonable, any allocation probabilities assigned to individual cases should not be relied upon. Transformations should first be considered, but if reliable allocation probabilities are required, a non-parametric approach may be desirable [44]. When categorical variables are to be included in the discrimination, *logistic regression analysis* [48,49] provides a more appropriate methodology.

Discriminant analysis may easily be extended to the problem of distinguishing among three or more groups, although implementation of the allocation rule and visual presentation of the results become more difficult. In such situations the technique is sometimes referred to as *canonical variates analysis*. Comprehensive accounts of the discriminant analysis method are available [44,46].

17.5.3 Cluster analysis

Even if no predefined diagnosis is available to permit a discriminant function analysis, it may still be possible to classify cases into groups with similar pathological characteristics using *cluster analysis*. In contrast to the well-defined techniques in the previous two sections, cluster analysis has a wide range of variations and options. This means that analyses are best regard as exploratory, and any clusters that are identified should be carefully scrutinized in the light of existing knowledge about the condition under study.

Fundamental to the technique is the choice of a measure of *similarity* or *distance* between any pair of cases. If all variables are continuous, then this measure could be based on Euclidean distance calculated using the standardized variables. However, there are numerous possible measures both for continuous and categorical variables [44,50,51]. Also required is some measure of intercluster similarity, such as the Euclidean distance between two cluster centroids or between nearest neighbours in the two clusters.

Most applications employ a hierarchical approach to cluster formation, although non-hierarchical approaches are also available. *Agglomerative* methods begin with each case forming a separate cluster, nearby clusters then being fused to form larger clusters. At each stage the two clusters with the smallest intercluster distance are fused. *Divisive* methods start with all cases in a single cluster which is then subdivided into smaller clusters. Results of the analysis may be conveniently summarized by a *tree diagram* or *dendrogram* which shows the intergroup distance at which each fusion or division occurs. Examination of the dendrogram may suggest a suitable breakpoint in the process, so defining the number of clusters that should be considered. For example, Fig. 17.3 shows a dendro-

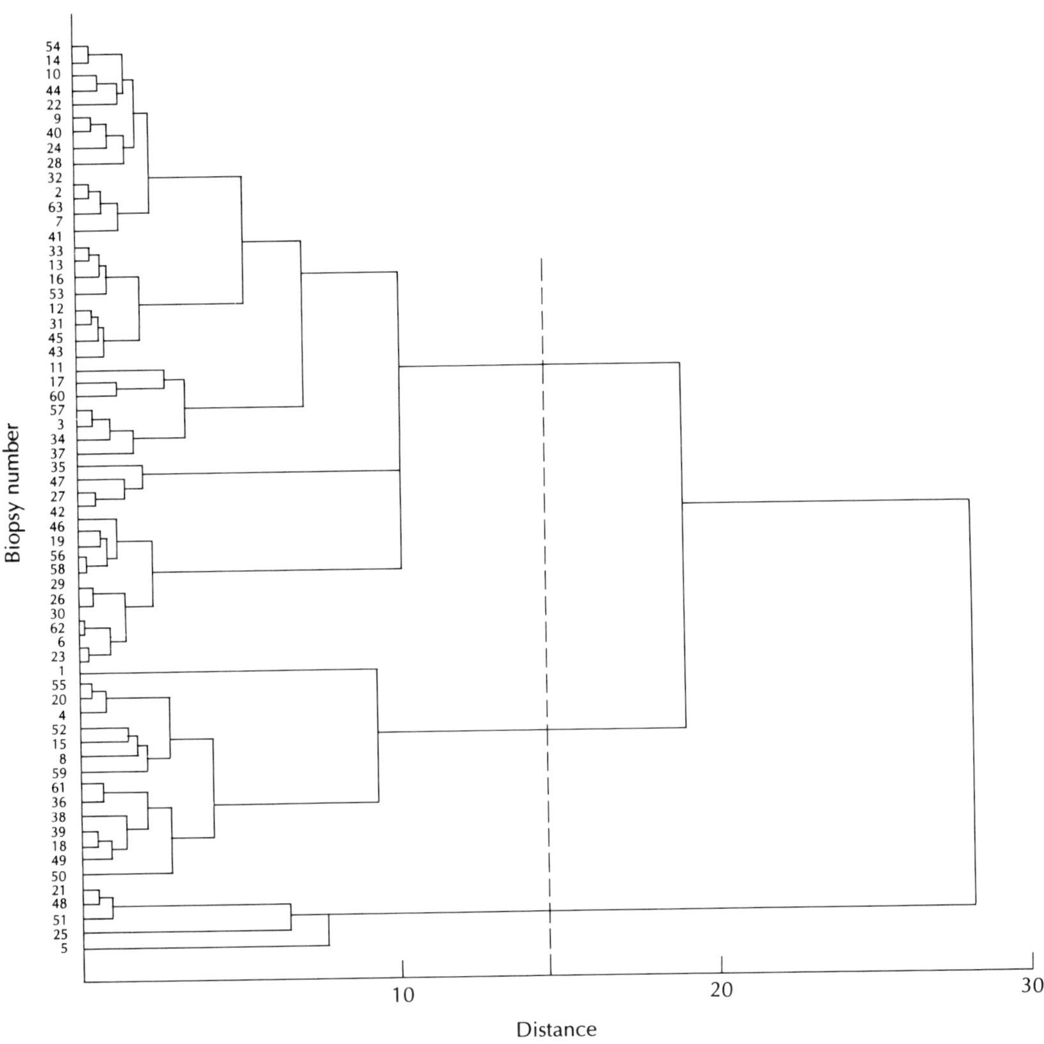

Fig. 17.3 Dendrogram showing hierarchical cluster formation by distance measure among 63 duodenal biopsies, resulting in three clusters of 43, 15 and five biopsies. From Jenkins *et al.* [52].

gram from a quantitative histological study of 63 duodenal biopsies [52]. The distance measure increases markedly between the three-cluster fusion and the two-cluster fusion, and the authors therefore chose to study three clusters of patients.

Cluster analysis may also be applied to identify groups of similar variables, so providing some insight into relationships between variables.

Everitt [51] provides a good introductory text on cluster analysis, while Sneath and Sokal [50] give a more comprehensive account with a review of applications in biology.

17.6 SURVIVAL ANALYSIS

17.6.1 Life tables and survival curves

Studies that seek to establish pathological factors indicative of prognosis often require patients to be followed for lengthy periods until some end-point or event, such as death or disease recurrence, is observed. A characteristic of these studies is that typically many patients will not have experienced the event by the time of data analysis, and all that can be said is that the patient's *survival time* (defined as the interval from diagnosis or entry to the study until occurrence of the event) exceeds some value. Such patients are said to have survival times which are *censored* and special methods of statistical analysis must be employed. In the remainder of this section it is assumed that the event in question is the death of the patient.

Often estimates of the 5-year survival rate will be required. Such estimates can be obtained using only data from patients who were followed (or had the potential to be followed) for 5 years. However, this approach does not make best use of the available data, and an alternative approach based on the *life-table* method is more appropriate. The *actuarial method* for constructing a life table requires the period of follow-up to be arbitrarily divided into a number of intervals. Within each interval, an estimate of the probability of surviving to the end of the interval (conditional on having survived to the start of the interval) is obtained from the numbers surviving at the start of the interval, the numbers censored during the interval and the numbers dying during the interval. The probability of surviving to any given time after entry is then obtained as the product of the probabilities for all preceding intervals. Details of the calculations are available in standard texts [53,54].

When the survival times are recorded with sufficient accuracy, the *Kaplan–Meier method* [54,55] provides an alternative estimate which does not require arbitrary division of the follow-up period. Figure 17.4 illustrates Kaplan–Meier survival plots for 104 patients with breast cancer in three subgroups defined by mean nuclear area [56]. Another advantage of the Kaplan–Meier approach is that individual deaths and censorings can be incorporated in the pictorial presentation.

With either method the numbers of patients still under follow-up (or 'at risk') in each subgroup at various times can be inserted beneath the horizontal axis. Confidence limits may be calculated to provide a measure of the precision of the survival estimate at any specified time. Precision usually declines as the number of patients remaining at risk reduces, so little emphasis should be placed on estimates from the tail of a survival plot where the numbers at risk are often small.

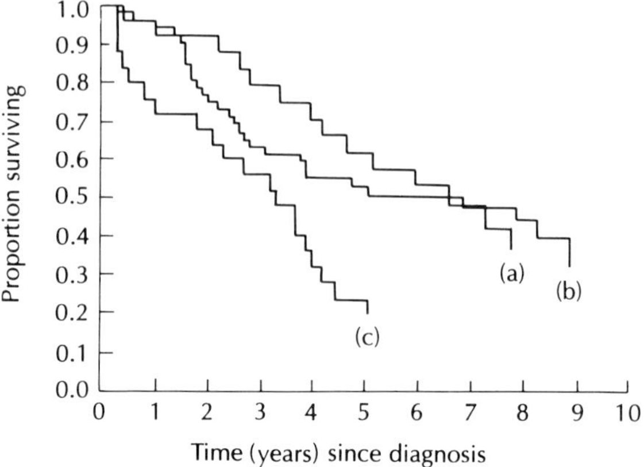

Fig. 17.4 Kaplan–Meier survival plots for 104 breast cancer patients in subgroups defined by quartiles of mean nuclear area. (a) Less than first quartile (25%); (b) between first and third quartiles (50%); (c) greater than third quartile (25%). From Böcking *et al.* [56].

17.6.2 Log-rank test

The standard errors referred to in the previous section permit a significance test for the comparison of survival estimates in two samples to be conducted at any specified follow-up time [53]. However, a better approach is to use methods that compare survival over the entire period of follow-up. One such method, the *log-rank test*, requires the calculation of *extents of exposure* in each sample, which may be loosely interpreted as the numbers of deaths expected in the samples on the assumption that they are exposed to the same mortality rates. The test is obtained by comparing the numbers of observed and expected deaths [54,55,57]. Alternative tests are available but, because of its simplicity and intuitive appeal, the log-rank test is the most popular.

17.6.3 Cox's proportional hazards model

Although the log-rank test may be refined by stratifying the analysis to take account of the effects of a potentially confounding variable, a more sophisticated approach is to use regression-based methodology. The method in most widespread use is *Cox's proportional hazards model*, which requires minimal parametric assumptions. It specifies that variables (or *covariates*) $x_1, x_2 \ldots x_n$ should have a multiplicative effect on the *hazard function*, $\lambda(t)$, the risk of death at time t. Covariates may be either continuous variables or indicator binary (0/1) variables contrasting the levels of a categorical covariate [29,38]. The model may be written as:

$$\lambda(t) = \lambda_0(t) \exp(b_1x_1 + b_2x_2 + \ldots b_nx_n)$$

where $b_1, b_2 \ldots b_n$ are coefficients estimated from the data and $\lambda_0(t)$ is the baseline hazard which is the risk of death in an individual whose covariate values are all zero.

Programs that fit the model provide estimates of $b_1, b_2 \ldots b_n$ and their standard errors. The value $\exp(b_i)$ provides an estimate of the multiplicative increase in the risk of death (or *relative hazard*) associated with unit increase in x_i. Such estimates are adjusted for the confounding influence of other covariates in the model. The standard errors may be used to derive 95% confidence limits for the relative hazard according to the formula $\exp[b_i + 1.96\,\mathrm{SE}(b_i)]$. Significance tests of the contribution made by each covariate to any given model are also possible, and may be used to construct a parsimonious final model. Estimates of baseline hazard, $\lambda_0(t)$, may also be obtained, permitting the risk of death (and consequently the pattern of survival) for individuals with given covariate values to be predicted.

Both introductory [54,57,58] and comprehensive [59,60] accounts of the proportional hazards model are available.

17.7 REVIEW OF STATISTICAL SOFTWARE PACKAGES

17.7.1 Scope of the review

The process of conducting statistical analyses has been greatly simplified by the availability of powerful, well-documented and easy-to-use software packages. Initially these packages were only available on mainframe computers, and their use therefore necessitated some familiarity with the mainframe operating system. Today many powerful microcomputer packages are available which can be used even by those with very limited computer experience.

However, this increased accessibility has associated risks, since there is potential for selection of the wrong statistical procedure and for misinterpretation of the output supplied by the package. Although careful reading of the manual may help, anyone who is in doubt would be well-advised to seek the advice of a statistician.

17.7.2 Practical advice about data analysis

Before analysis can begin, data must be input to the package. Many packages are supplied with facilities for direct data entry. However, most will also accept (or *import*) data in the format of popular database and spreadsheet programs, and many users will prefer to enter their data in this way.

An indispensable first step in advance of conducting any data analysis is to check that the data have been correctly entered. For small datasets this may be done by visual inspection, but if the data are extensive it is advisable to use the computer to conduct *validity checks*. These take the form of *range checks*, which ensure that all results take values in a sensible range, and *consistency checks*, which ensure that the data for two variables are not contradictory (e.g., minimum cell diameter exceeding maximum cell diameter).

17.7.3 Software packages

This section primarily considers non-specialist microcomputer packages which provide a broad range of analyses (including most of the techniques listed in Table 17.1), which permit graphical examination of the data (e.g., histograms and scatter diagrams) and which incorporate comprehensive facilities for data management (e.g., editing, selecting, recoding, transforming). Many (BMDP, CSS, MINITAB, SAS, SOLO, SPSS, STATGRAPHICS, SYSTAT) are available for the IBM PC and compatibles, and some (CSS, MINITAB, SPSS, STATVIEW, SYSTAT) for the Apple Macintosh. In a few cases optional modules may need to be purchased in addition to the basic package. Some were originally developed for mainframe computers, and as a result the microcomputer user interface of early versions was sometimes cumbersome. However, with more and more packages being released to run under Microsoft

Windows, easy access to powerful software is now a reality. A few (e.g., CSS, SAS, STATGRAPHICS, SYSTAT) can execute programming language instructions which permit the sophisticated user to implement new statistical procedures.

Comprehensive analysis of variance facilities are provided by the majority of the packages, although a good background knowledge of the topic is a prerequisite. BMDP, CSS, SOLO, SPSS and STATGRAPHICS provide good facilities for multiple-range tests. SAS and STATGRAPHICS provide options for the calculations of components of variance for hierarchical designs.

All the packages perform principal components analysis, although in many (BMDP, CSS, SOLO, SPSS, STATVIEW, SYSTAT) the technique is found as an option in factor analysis.

BMDP, SAS, SOLO and SPSS provide excellent facilities for discriminant function analysis, including stepwise variable selection, while MINITAB, STATGRAPHICS and SYSTAT provide good, but rather less comprehensive facilities. In CSS, the discriminant function analysis is provided within the multivariate analysis of variance section, and is weak. BMDP, MINITAB and SAS implement the jack-knife or cross-validation procedure (see Section 17.5.2). Quadratic discriminant analysis is available in MINITAB, and logistic discriminant analysis is provided in BMDP, SAS, SOLO, SPSS and SYSTAT.

With the exception of MINITAB and STATVIEW, all the packages perform cluster analysis, many offering numerous variations of the technique. CLUSTAN, a specialist package which is widely available on larger computers, provides perhaps the most comprehensive range of cluster analysis options and produces high-quality dendrograms.

For survival analysis, BMDP, SAS and SPSS are probably the most comprehensive packages, and are capable of constructing actuarial and Kaplan–Meier life tables, performing log-rank tests and fitting proportional hazards models. CSS and optional modules in SOLO and SYSTAT also provide good facilities. A specialist epidemiological package called EGRET performs survival analysis and logistic discriminant analysis, but few of its other facilities are likely to be of much interest.

17.8 CONCLUSION

Those who observe the statistical advice given in this chapter should avoid many of the pitfalls and mistakes which have been described in past reviews of statistical methodology in the medical literature. In the future, the widespread availability of sophisticated statistical software may result in an even greater risk of performing an inappropriate analysis or misinterpreting a correctly performed analysis. However, statistical help should not be sought only at the analysis stage of a study; at the planning stage the statistician can provide worthwhile advice which may considerably enhance the validity of the work.

References

1 Altman DG. Statistics in medical journals. *Stat Med* 1982; 1: 59–71.

2 Siegel S, Castellan NJ. *Nonparametric Statistics for the Behavioral Sciences*, 2nd edn. New York: McGraw-Hill, 1988: 19–36.

3 Smeulders AWM, Dorst L. Measurement issues in morphometry. *Anal Quant Cytol Histol* 1985; 7: 242–249.

4 Rothman KJ. A show of confidence. *N Engl J Med* 1978; 299: 1362–1363.

5 Gardner MJ, Altman DG. Confidence intervals rather than *P* values: estimation rather than hypothesis testing. *Br Med J* 1986; 292: 746–750.

6 Bulpitt CJ. Confidence intervals. *Lancet* 1987; i: 494–497.

7 Bland JM, Altman DG. Statistical methods for assessing agreement between two methods of clinical measurement. *Lancet* 1986; i: 307–310.

8 Bland JM. *An Introduction to Medical Statistics*. Oxford: Oxford University Press, 1987: 276–278.

9 British Standards Institution. *Precision of Test Methods I: Guide for the Determination and Reproducibility for a Standard Test Method (BS 5497, part 1)*. London: British Standards Institution, 1979.

10 Snedecor GW, Cochran WG. *Statistical Methods*, 6th edn. Iowa: Iowa State University Press, 1967: 258–298.

11 Bland JM, Altman DG. Statistical methods for assessing agreement between two methods of clinical measurement. *Lancet* 1986; i: 307–310.

12 Fleiss JL. *Statistical Methods for Rates and Proportions*, 2nd edn. New York: Wiley, 1981.

13 Dunn G. *Design and Analysis of Reliability Studies*. New York: Oxford University Press, 1989.

14 Landis JR, Koch GG. The measurement of observer

agreement for categorical data. *Biometrics* 1977; 33: 159–174.

15 Selkainaho K. Statistics in stereology and morphometry. *Acta Stereol* 1983; 2: 239–249.

16 Shay J. Economy of effort in electron microscope morphometry. *Am J Pathol* 1975; 81: 503–511.

17 Dunnill MS. Some statistical aspects of sampling in morphometry. *Anal Quant Cytol Histol* 1985; 7: 250–255.

18 Winer BJ. *Statistical Principles in Experimental Design*, 2nd edn. New York: McGraw-Hill, 1971: 149–260.

19 Day SJ, Graham DF. Sample size and power for comparing two or more treatment groups in clinical trials. *Br Med J* 1989; 299: 663–665.

20 Snedecor GW, Cochran WG. *Statistical Methods*, 6th edn. Iowa: Iowa State University Press, 1967: 91–119.

21 Armitage P, Berry G. *Statistical Methods in Medical Research*, 2nd edn. Oxford: Blackwell Scientific Publications, 1987: 160–185.

22 Cochran WG, Cox GM. *Experimental Designs*, 2nd edn. New York: Wiley, 1957: 15–44.

23 Fleiss JL. *The Design and Analysis of Clinical Experiments*. New York: Wiley, 1986.

24 Altman DG. How large a sample? In: Gore SM, Altman DG (eds) *Statistics in Practice*. London: British Medical Journal, 1982.

25 Gardner MJ, Altman DG. (eds) *Statistics with Confidence*. London: British Medical Journal, 1989.

26 Lentner C. *Geigy Scientific Tables* vol. 2. *Introduction to Statistics, Statistical Tables and Mathematical Formulae*, 8th edn. Basle: Ciba-Geigy, 1982.

27 Snedecor FW, Cochran WG. *Statistical Methods*, 6th edn. Iowa: Iowa State University Press, 1967: 66–90.

28 Conover WJ. *Practical Nonparametric Statistics*, 2nd edn. New York: Wiley, 1980: 363–367.

29 Draper NR, Smith H. *Applied Regression Analysis*, 2nd edn. New York: Wiley, 1981.

30 Armitage P, Berry G. Data editing. In: *Statistical Methods in Medical Research*, 2nd edn. Oxford: Blackwell Scientific Publications, 1987: 358–370.

31 Fleiss JL. *The Design and Analysis of Clinical Experiments*. New York: Wiley, 1986: 59–68.

32 Conover WJ. *Practical Nonparametric Statistics*, 2nd edn. New York: Wiley, 1980.

33 Siegel S, Castellan NJ. *Nonparametric Statistics for the Behavioral Sciences*, 2nd edn. New York: McGraw-Hill, 1988.

34 Armitage P, Berry G. *Statistical Methods in Medical Research*, 2nd edn. Oxford: Blackwell Scientific Publications, 1987: 186–213.

35 Snedecor GW, Cochran WG. *Statistical Methods*, 6th edn. Iowa: Iowa State University Press, 1967: 172–198.

36 Armitage P, Berry G. *Statistical Methods in Medical Research*, 2nd edn. Oxford: Blackwell Scientific Publications, 1987: 141–159.

37 Snedecor GW, Cochran WG. *Statistical Methods*, 6th edn. Iowa: Iowa State University Press, 1967: 381–418.

38 Armitage P, Berry G. *Statistical Methods in Medical Research*, 2nd edn. Oxford: Blackwell Scientific Publications, 1987: 296–357.

39 Bartels PH. Numerical evaluation of cytologic data. VII. Multivariate significance tests. *Anal Quant Cytol* 1981; 3: 1–7.

40 Bartels PH. Numerical evaluation of cytologic data. X. Introduction to multivariate analysis of variance. *Anal Quant Cytol* 1981; 3: 251–260.

41 Hamilton PW, Allen DC, Watt PCH, Patterson CC, Biggart JD. Classification of normal colorectal mucosa and adenocarcinoma by morphometry. *Histopathology* 1987; 11: 901–911.

42 Bartels PH. Numerical evaluation of cytologic data. IX. Search for data structure by principal components transformation. *Anal Quant Cytol* 1981; 3: 167–177.

43 Reyment RA, Blackith RE, Campbell NA. *Multivariate Morphometrics*, 2nd edn. London: Academic Press, 1984.

44 Hand DJ. *Discrimination and Classification*. Chichester: Wiley, 1981.

45 Norris HJ, Bahr GF, Mikel UV. A comparative morphometric and cytophotometric study of intraductual hyperplasia and intraductual carcinoma of the breast. *Anal Quant Cytol Histol* 1988; 10: 1–9.

46 Lachenbruch PA. *Discriminant Analysis*. New York: Hafner, 1975.

47 Bartels PH. Numerical evaluation of cytologic data. V. Bivariate distributions and the Bayesian decision boundary. *Anal Quant Cytol* 1980; 2: 77–83.

48 Brown BW. Prediction analysis for binary data. In: Miller RG, Efron B, Brown BW, Moses LE (eds) *Biostatistics Casebook*. New York: Wiley, 1980: 3–18.

49 Armitage P, Berry G. Generalized linear models. In: *Statistical Methods in Medical Research*, 2nd edn. Oxford: Blackwell Scientific Publications, 1987: 386–399.

50 Sneath PHA, Sokal RR. *Numerical Taxonomy. The Principles and Practice of Numerical Classification*. San Francisco: WH Freeman, 1973.

51 Everitt BS. *Cluster Analysis*, 2nd edn. London: Heinemann Educational Books, 1980.

52 Jenkins D, Goodall A, Gillet FR, Scott BB. Defining duodenitis: quantitative histological study of mucosal responses and their correlations. *J Clin Pathol* 1985; 38: 1119–1126.

53 Colton T. *Statistics in Medicine*. Boston: Little, Brown, 1974: 237–250.

54 Armitage P, Berry G. *Statistical Methods in Medical Research*, 2nd edn. Oxford: Blackwell Scientific Publications, 1987: 421–439.

55 Peto R, Pike MC, Armitage P *et al*. Design and analysis of randomised clinical trials requiring prolonged observation of the patient. II. Analysis and examples. *Br J Cancer* 1977; 35: 1–39.

56 Böcking A, Chatelain R, Biesterfeld S *et al.* DNA grading of malignancy in breast cancer. Prognostic validity, reproducibility and comparison with other classifications. *Anal Quant Cytol Histol* 1989; 11: 73–80.
57 Anderson S, Auquier A, Hauck WW, Oakes D, Vandaele W, Weisberg HI. *Statistical Methods for Comparative Studies*. New York: Wiley, 1980.
58 Harris EK, Albert K. *Survivorship Analysis for Clinical Studies*. New York: Marcel Dekker, 1991.
59 Kalbfleisch JD, Prentice RL. *The Statistical Analysis of Failure Time Data*. New York: John Wiley, 1980.
60 Lawless JF. *Statistical Models and Methods for Lifetime Data*. New York: John Wiley, 1982.

INDEX

Page numbers in *italics* refer to figures or tables